The Newborn Lung: Neonatology Questions and Controversies

The Newborn Lung

Neonatology Questions and Controversies

Series Editor

Richard A. Polin, MD
Professor of Pediatrics
College of Physicians and Surgeons
Columbia University
Director, Division of Neonatology
Morgan Stanley Children's Hospital of New York-Presbyterian
Columbia University Medical Center
New York, New York

Other Volumes in the Neonatology Questions and Controversies Series

Cardiology
Gastroenterology and Nutrition
Hematology, Immunology and Infectious Disease
Nephrology and Fluid/Electrolyte Physiology
Neurology

The Newborn Lung
Neonatology Questions and Controversies

Eduardo Bancalari, MD
Professor of Pediatrics
Director, Division of Neonatology
University of Miami Miller School of Medicine
Miami, Florida

Consulting Editor

Richard A. Polin, MD
Professor of Pediatrics
College of Physicians and Surgeons
Columbia University
Director Division of Neonatology
Morgan Stanley Children's Hospital of New York-Presbyterian
Columbia University Medical Center
New York, New York

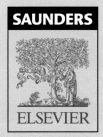

SAUNDERS

ELSEVIER

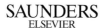

1600 John F. Kennedy Blvd.
Suite 1800
Philadelphia, PA 19103-2899

THE NEWBORN LUNG: Neonatology Questions and Controversies   ISBN: 978-1-4160-3166-6
Copyright © 2008 by Saunders, an imprint of Elsevier Inc.

Notice

Library of Congress Cataloging-in-Publication Data

The Newborn Lung : neonatology questions and controversies / [edited by] Eduardo Bancalari ; consulting editor, Richard A. Polin.—1st ed.
   p. ; cm.
  Includes bibliographical references.
  ISBN 978-1-4160-3166-6
  1. Pediatric respiratory diseases. 2. Newborn infants—Diseases. I. Bancalari, Eduardo. II. Polin, Richard A. (Richard Alan), 1945-
  [DNLM: 1. Infant, Newborn, Diseases. 2. Lung Diseases. 3. Infant, Newborn. 4. Lung—growth & development. 5. Respiration Disorders. WS 421 P982 2008]
  RJ312.P85 2008
  618.92'2—dc22

                                            2007043790

Acquisitions Editor: Judith Fletcher
Developmental Editor: Lisa Barnes
Associate Developmental Editor: Bernard Buckholtz
Senior Project Manager: David Saltzberg
Design Direction: Karen O'Keefe-Owens

Printed in China

Last digit is the print number: 9 8 7 6 5 4 3 2

Contents

Section I
LUNG DEVELOPMENT, 1

Chapter 1   **Molecular Basis for Normal and Abnormal Lung Development, 3**
Martin Rutter, BSc • Martin Post, PhD

Chapter 2   **Hereditary Disorders of Alveolar Homeostasis in the Newborn, 42**
Jeffrey A. Whitsett, MD • Timothy E. Weaver, PhD

Chapter 3   **Growth and Development of the Lung Circulation: Mechanisms and Clinical Implications, 50**
Steven H. Abman, MD • Christopher Baker, MD • Vivek Balasubramaniam, MD

Chapter 4   **Surfactant: The Basis for Clinical Treatment Strategies, 73**
Alan H. Jobe, MD PhD

Section II
INJURY IN THE DEVELOPING LUNG, 99

Chapter 5   **Susceptibility of the Immature Lung to Oxidative and Mechanical Injury, 101**
Jaques Belik, MD FRCPC

Chapter 6   **Inflammation/Infection: Effects on the Fetal/Newborn Lung, 119**
Alan H. Jobe, MD PhD • Suhas Kallapur, MD • Timothy J.M. Moss, PhD

Chapter 7   **Lung Fluid Balance During Development and in Neonatal Lung Disease, 141**
Richard D. Bland, MD • David P. Carlton, MD • Lucky Jain, MD MBA

Chapter 8   **Role of Inflammation in the Pathogenesis of Acute and Chronic Neonatal Lung Disease, 166**
Christian P. Speer, MD FRCPE

Chapter 9   **New Developments in the Presentation, Pathogenesis, Epidemiology and Prevention of Bronchopulmonary Dysplasia, 187**
Ilene R.S. Sosenko, MD • Eduardo Bancalari, MD

Chapter 10   **What is the Evidence for Drug Therapy in the Prevention and Management of Bronchopulmonary Dysplasia?, 208**
Henry L. Halliday, MD FRCPE FRCP FRCPCH • Conor O'Neill, MB BCh BAO MRCPCH

Chapter 11   **Definitions and Predictors of Bronchopulmonary Dysplasia, 233**
Michele C. Walsh, MD MS

Chapter 12   **New Developments in the Pathogenesis and Management of Neonatal Pulmonary Hypertension, 241**
Judy L. Aschner, MD • Candice D. Fike, MD

Chapter 13   **Impact of Perinatal Lung Injury in Later Life, 300**
Lex W. Doyle, MD FRACP • Peter J. Anderson, PhD

Section III
MANAGEMENT OF RESPIRATORY FAILURE, 315

Oxygen

Chapter 14   **The Oxygen Versus Room Air Controversy for Neonatal Resuscitation, 317**
Peter W. Fowlie, MB ChB MSc DRCOG MRCGP FRCPCH • Hannah Shore, MB ChB MRCPCH

Chapter 15   **Optimal Levels of Oxygenation in Preterm Infants: Impact on Short- and Long-Term Outcomes, 333**
Win Tin, MB BS FRCP FRCPCH • Samir Gupta, MB BS MD MRCP(Ire) FRCPCH

Mechanical Respiratory Support

Chapter 16   **Non-invasive Respiratory Support: An Alternative to Mechanical Ventilation in Preterm Infants, 361**
Peter G. Davis, MD FRACP • Colin J. Morley, MD FRACP FRCPCH

Chapter 17   **High-Frequency Ventilation in Neonatal Respiratory Failure, 377**
Ulrich H. Thome, MD • Waldemar A. Carlo, MD

Chapter 18   **New Modalities of Mechanical Ventilation in the Newborn, 392**
Nelson Claure, MSc PhD • Eduardo Bancalari, MD

Chapter 19   **Role of Pulmonary Function Testing in the Management of Neonates on Mechanical Ventilation, 419**
Tilo Gerhardt, MD • Nelson Claure, MSc PhD • Eduardo Bancalari, MD

Section IV
RESPIRATORY CONTROL AND APNEA OF PREMATURITY, 447

Chapter 20 **Neonatal Respiratory Control and Apnea of Prematurity, 449**
Oded Mesner, MD • Juliann M. Di Fiore, BSEE • Richard J. Martin, MBBS FRACP

Chapter 21 **Strategies for Prevention of Apneic Episodes in Preterm Infants: Are Respiratory Stimulants Worth the Risk?, 461**
Dirk Bassler, MD MSc • Barbara Schmidt, MD MSc

Index, 477

Contributors

Steven H. Abman, MD

Professor, Department of Pediatrics
Director, Pediatric Heart Lung Center
University of Colorado School of Medicine
The Children's Hospital
Denver, Colorado

Growth and Development of the Lung Circulation: Mechanisms and Clinical Implications

Peter J. Anderson, PhD

CR Roper Fellow
School of Behavioural Science
The University of Melbourne
Senior Research Fellow
The Murdoch Children's Research Institute
Melbourne, Australia

Impact of Perinatal Lung Injury in Later Life

Judy L. Aschner, MD

Professor of Pediatrics
Vanderbilt University Medical Center
Chief of Neonatology
The Monroe Carell Jr. Children's Hospital at Vanderbilt
Nashville, Tennessee

New Developments in the Pathogenesis and Management of Neonatal Pulmonary Hypertension

Christopher Baker, MD

Fellow, Pediatric Pulmonology
Department of Pediatric Pulmonology
University of Colorado Health Sciences Center
The Children's Hospital
Denver, Colorado

Growth and Development of the Lung Circulation: Mechanisms and Clinical Implications

Vivek Balasubramaniam, MD

Assistant Professor of Pediatrics
Director, Pediatric Heart Lung Center Laboratory
Department of Pediatric Pulmonology
University of Colorado Health Sciences Center
The Children's Hospital
Denver, Colorado

Growth and Development of the Lung Circulation: Mechanisms and Clinical Implications

Eduardo Bancalari, MD

Professor of Pediatrics
Director, Division of Neonatology
University of Miami
Miller School of Medicine
Miami, Florida

New Developments in the Presentation, Pathogenesis, Epidemiology and Prevention of Bronchopulmonary Dysplasia; New Modalities of Mechanical Ventilation in the Newborn; Role of Pulmonary Function Testing in the Management of Neonates on Mechanical Ventilation

Dirk Bassler, MD MSc

Neonatal Consultant and Clinical Epidemiologist
Department of Neonatology
University Children's Hospital
Tübingen, Germany

Strategies for Prevention of Apneic Episodes in Preterm Infants: Are Respiratory Stimulants Worth the Risk?

Jaques Belik, MD FRCPC

Professor of Pediatrics
Division of Neonatology
The Hospital for Sick Children
University of Toronto
Toronto, Canada

Susceptibility of the Immature Lung to Oxidative and Mechanical Injury

Richard D. Bland, MD

Professor of Pediatrics
Stanford University School of Medicine
Stanford, California

Lung Fluid Balance During Development and in Neonatal Lung Disease

Waldemar A. Carlo, MD

Edwin M. Dixon Professor of Pediatrics
Director, Division of Neonatology
Director, Newborn Nurseries
University of Alabama at Birmingham
Birmingham, Alabama

High-Frequency Ventilation in Neonatal Respiratory Failure

David P. Carlton, MD

Marcus Professor of Pediatrics
Division of Neonatal–Perinatal Medicine
Department of Pediatrics
Emory University School of Medicine
Atlanta, Georgia

Lung Fluid Balance During Development and in Neonatal Lung Disease

Nelson Claure, MSc PhD

Research Assistant Professor
Division of Neonatology
Department of Pediatrics
University of Miami
Miller School of Medicine
Miami, Florida

New Modalities of Mechanical Ventilation in the Newborn; Role of Pulmonary Function Testing in the Management of Neonates on Mechanical Ventilation

Peter G. Davis, MD FRACP

Consultant Neonatologist
Division of Newborn Services
Department of Obstetrics and Gynaecology
Royal Women's Hospital
Associate Professor
University of Melbourne
Melbourne, Australia

Non-invasive Respiratory Support: An Alternative to Mechanical Ventilation in Preterm Infants

Juliann M. Di Fiore, BSEE

Research Engineer
Department of Medicine
Case School of Medicine
Department of Pediatrics
Division of Neonatology
Rainbow Babies & Children's Hospital
Cleveland, Ohio

Neonatal Respiratory Control and Apnea of Prematurity

Lex W. Doyle, MD FRACP

Professor of Neonatal Pediatrics
Departments of Obstetrics and Gynaecology and Pediatrics
The University of Melbourne
Head, Clinical Research Development
Division of Newborn Services
The Royal Women's Hospital
Murdoch Children's Research Institute
Melbourne, Australia

> *Impact of Perinatal Lung Injury in Later Life*

Candice D. Fike, MD

Professor of Pediatrics
Division of Neonatology
Vanderbilt University Medical Center
Nashville, Tennessee

> *New Developments in the Pathogenesis and Management of Neonatal Pulmonary Hypertension*

Peter W. Fowlie, MB ChB MSc DRCOG MRCGP FRCPCH

Consultant Pediatrician
Neonatal Unit
Ninewells Hospital and Medical School
Dundee, United Kingdom

> *The Oxygen Versus Room Air Controversy for Neonatal Resuscitation*

Tilo Gerhardt, MD

Professor of Pediatrics
Division of Neonatology
University of Miami
Miller School of Medicine
Miami, Florida

> *Role of Pulmonary Function Testing in the Management of Neonates on Mechanical Ventilation*

Samir Gupta, MB BS MD MRCP(Ire) FRCPCH

Senior Research Fellow
Directorate of Neonatal Medicine
The James Cook University Hospital
Middlesborough, United Kingdom

> *Optimal Levels of Oxygenation in Preterm Infants: Impact on Short- and Long-Term Outcomes*

Henry L. Halliday, MD FRCPE FRCP FRCPCH

Honorary Professor of Child Health
Queen's University Belfast
Retired Consultant Neonatologist
Regional Neonatal Unit
Royal Maternity Hospital
Belfast, Northern Ireland
> *What is the Evidence for Drug Therapy in the Prevention and Management of Bronchopulmonary Dysplasia?*

Lucky Jain, MD MBA

Professor of Pediatrics
Executive Vice Chairman
Emory University School of Medicine
Atlanta, Georgia
> *Lung Fluid Balance During Development and in Neonatal Lung Disease*

Alan H. Jobe, MD PhD

Professor of Pediatrics/Neonatology
Cincinnati Children's Hospital
Cincinnati, Ohio
> *Surfactant: The Basis for Clinical Treatment Strategies; Inflammation/Infection: Effects on the Fetal/Newborn Lung*

Suhas Kallapur, MD

Associate Professor of Pediatrics
Cincinnati Children's Hospital Medical Center
Cincinnati, Ohio
> *Inflammation/Infection: Effects on the Fetal/Newborn Lung*

Richard J. Martin, MBBS FRACP

Professor, Pediatrics, Reproductive Biology, and
  Physiology & Biophysics
Case Western Reserve University School of Medicine
Director, Division of Neonatology
Drusinsky/Fanaroff Professor in Neonatology
Rainbow Babies and Children's Hospital
Cleveland, Ohio
> *Neonatal Respiratory Control and Apnea of Prematurity*

Oded Mesner, MD

Attending Neonatologist
Division of Neonatology
Soroka Medical Center
Ben-Gurion University
Beer Sheva, Israel
> *Neonatal Respiratory Control and Apnea of Prematurity*

Colin J. Morley, MD FRACP FRCPCH
Professor/Director of Neonatal Medicine
Neonatal Services
Royal Women's Hospital
Melbourne, Australia

Non-invasive Respiratory Support: An Alternative to Mechanical Ventilation in Preterm Infants

Timothy J.M. Moss, PhD
NHMRC RD Wright Fellow
Department of Physiology
Monash University
Melbourne, Australia

Inflammation/Infection: Effects on the Fetal/Newborn Lung

Conor P. O'Neill, MB BCh BAO MRCPCH
Specialist Registrar
Royal Jubilee Maternity Hospital
Belfast, Northern Ireland

What is the Evidence for Drug Therapy in the Prevention and Management of Bronchopulmonary Dysplasia?

Martin Post, PhD
Head, Physiology and Experimental Medicine Program
Lung Biology Research Group
Hospital for Sick Children Research Institute
Professor of Pediatrics
Physiology and Laboratory Medicine and Pathobiology
Department of Pediatrics
Faculty of Medicine
University of Toronto
Toronto, Canada

Molecular Basis for Normal and Abnormal Lung Development

Martin Rutter, BSc
Physiology and Experimental Medicine Program
Lung Biology Research Group
Hospital for Sick Children Research Institute
PhD Candidate
Institute of Medical Sciences
Faculty of Medicine
University of Toronto
Toronto, Canada

Molecular Basis for Normal and Abnormal Lung Development

Barbara Schmidt, MD MSc

Director of Clinical Research
Division of Neonatology
The Children's Hospital of Philadelphia
Professor of Pediatrics
University of Pennsylvania School of Medicine
Philadelphia, Pennsylvania
Professor of Clinical Epidemiology & Biostatistics
McMaster University
Hamilton, Ontario

> *Strategies for Prevention of Apneic Episodes in Preterm Infants: Are Respiratory Stimulants Worth the Risk?*

Hannah Shore, MB ChB MRCPCH

Jennifer Brown Research Fellow
Queens Medical Research Institute
Edinburgh Royal Infirmary
Edinburgh, United Kingdom

> *The Oxygen Versus Room Air Controversy for Neonatal Resuscitation*

Ilene R.S. Sosenko, MD

Professor of Pediatrics, Division of Neonatology
Department of Pediatrics
University of Miami
Miller School of Medicine
Miami, Florida

> *New Developments in the Presentation, Pathogenesis, Epidemiology and Prevention of Bronchopulmonary Dysplasia*

Christian P. Speer, MD FRCPE

Professor of Pediatrics
Director and Chairman
University Children's Hospital
Würzburg, Germany

> *Role of Inflammation in the Pathogenesis of Acute and Chronic Neonatal Lung Disease*

Ulrich H. Thome, MD

Privatdozent
Division of Neonatology and Pediatric Critical Care
University Hospital for Children and Adolescents
University of Ulm
Ulm, Germany

> *High-Frequency Ventilation in Neonatal Respiratory Failure*

Win Tin, MB BS FRCP FRCPCH

Consultant Pediatrician and Neonatologist
Directorate of Neonatal Medicine
The James Cook University Hospital
Middlesborough, United Kingdom

> *Optimal Levels of Oxygenation in Preterm Infants: Impact on Short- and Long-Term Outcomes*

Michele C. Walsh, MD MS

Medical Director, Neonatal Intensive Care Unit
Rainbow Babies & Children's Hospital
Case Medical Center
Professor, Department of Pediatrics
Case Western Reserve University
Cleveland, Ohio

> *Definitions and Predictors of Bronchopulmonary Dysplasia*

Timothy E. Weaver, PhD

Professor of Pediatrics
Cincinnati Children's Hospital Medical Center
Division of Pulmonary Biology
Cincinnati, Ohio

> *Hereditary Disorders of Alveolar Homeostasis in the Newborn*

Jeffrey A. Whitsett, MD

Chief, Section of Neonatology
Perinatal and Pulmonary Biology
Cincinnati Children's Hospital Medical Center
Cincinnati, Ohio

> *Hereditary Disorders of Alveolar Homeostasis in the Newborn*

Series Foreword

"Learn from yesterday, live for today, hope for tomorrow. The important thing is not to stop questioning."

ALBERT EINSTEIN

The art and science of asking questions is the source of all knowledge.

THOMAS BERGER

In the mid-1960s W.B. Saunders began publishing a series of books focused on the care of newborn infants. The series was entitled *Major Problems in Clinical Pediatrics*. The original series (1964–1979) consisted of ten titles dealing with problems of the newborn infant (*The Lung and its Disorders in the Newborn infant* edited by Mary Ellen Avery, *Disorders of Carbohydrate Metabolism in Infancy* edited by Marvin Cornblath and Robert Schwartz, *Hematologic Problems in the Newborn* edited by Frank A. Oski and J. Lawrence Naiman, *The Neonate with Congenital Heart Disease* edited by Richard D. Rowe and Ali Mehrizi, *Recognizable Patterns of Human Malformation* edited by David W. Smith, *Neonatal Dermatology* edited by Lawrence M. Solomon and Nancy B. Esterly, *Amino Acid Metabolism and its Disorders* edited by Charles L. Scriver and Leon E. Rosenberg, *The High Risk Infant* edited by Lula O. Lubchenco, *Gastrointestinal Problems in the Infant* edited by Joyce Gryboski and *Viral Diseases of the Fetus and Newborn* edited by James B. Hanshaw and John A. Dudgeon). Dr. Alexander J. Schaffer was asked to be the consulting editor for the entire series. Dr. Schaffer coined the term "neonatology" and edited the first clinical textbook of neonatology entitled *Diseases of the Newborn*. For those of us training in the 1970s, this series and Dr. Schaffer's textbook of neonatology provided exciting, up-to-date information that attracted many of us into the subspecialty. Dr. Schaffer's role as "consulting editor" allowed him to select leading scientists and practitioners to serve as editors for each individual volume. As the "consulting editor" for *Neonatology Questions and Controversies*, I had the challenge of identifying the topics and editors for each volume in this series. The six volumes encompass the major issues encountered in the neonatal intensive care unit (newborn lung, fluid and electrolytes, neonatal cardiology and hemodynamics, hematology, immunology and infectious disease, gastroenterology, and neurology). The editors for each volume were challenged to combine discussions of fetal and neonatal physiology with disease pathophysiology and selected controversial topics in clinical care. It is my hope that this series (like *Major Problems in Clinical Pediatrics*) will excite a new generation of trainees to question existing dogma (from my own generation) and seek new information through scientific investigation. I wish to congratulate and thank each of the volume editors (Drs. Bancalari, Oh, Guignard, Baumgart, Kleinman, Seri, Ohls, Yoder, Neu and Perlman) for their extraordinary effort and finished products. I also wish to acknowledge Judy Fletcher at Elsevier who conceived the idea for the series and who has been my "editor and friend" throughout my academic career.

Richard A. Polin, MD

Preface

Few areas in medicine have undergone such remarkable progress over the last two decades as the care of the neonate. Most of the improvement in outcome has been related to the advances in the respiratory care of the preterm infant. These advances have only been possible because of the dramatic progress in knowledge regarding the mechanisms that determine the normal development of the respiratory system as well as the alterations that can lead to respiratory failure and its multiple consequences. Because the improved care has resulted in better survival of the more immature infants, this population has become a major challenge to the clinician because of the immaturity of multiple organs and their susceptibility to long-term sequelae.

In this first edition of *The Newborn Lung* volume in the *Neonatology: Questions and Controversies Series* we have been fortunate to attract many of the leading scientists and clinicians who have been responsible for the dramatic progress in the care of the newborn infant. The aim of this book is not to address all aspects related to the newborn lung but to discuss those areas that are more novel or controversial or have been of greater relevance in the progress of neonatal respiratory care. While the early chapters deal primarily with developmental issues, the subsequent chapters address some of the most important clinical problems facing the neonatologist today. Therefore, this book should be useful to developmental biologists as well as clinicians caring for sick newborns.

I have greatly enjoyed working with each of the authors who contributed to this book and reading their state-of-the-art, comprehensive contributions. I hope the reader will share my appreciation for the outstanding quality of each of the chapters.

I acknowledge with great gratitude each of the authors for their outstanding contributions, Judith Fletcher and Lisa Barnes from Elsevier and Maureen Allen from Keyword Publishing Services for their great help. I am also extremely grateful to Maria Valles and Yami Douglas for their invaluable assistance with the editing of the book.

Finally I would like to dedicate this book to my wife Teresa and my children Eduardo, Claudia, Alejandro, and Pilar for being a constant inspiration.

Eduardo Bancalari, MD

Section I

Lung Development

Chapter 1

Molecular Basis for Normal and Abnormal Lung Development

Martin Rutter, BSc • Martin Post, PhD

Developmental Stages

Growth Factors

Morphogens

Receptors

Transcription Factors

Physical Determinants of Lung Development

Vascular Development

Final Remarks

Like water, molecular oxygen is one of the most essential components of our environment as it is crucial to the molecular reactions that provide us with the energy not only to move about, but to run the basic cellular machinery that allows us to survive. While other lesser animals have managed to subsist using simple gas-exchange organs or even their skin to absorb oxygen, the metabolic requirements of higher mammals demand a much more sophisticated system. To meet this requirement through simple epidermal diffusion is just not practical, even if our skin was capable of this feat. The adult human lung exchanges nearly 12 000 liters of air per day, transferring oxygen between two drastically different mediums. There is a remarkable amount of physics that go into making this gas-exchange process functional, and a unique laminated tripartite architecture has evolved throughout vertebrate evolution to create the mammalian lung. In fact it has been suggested that no other molecular factor has had a larger impact on our evolutionary development than oxygen has (1). To facilitate the diffusion of oxygen from the atmosphere to our blood, a vast network of branched airways is formed in a process termed branching morphogenesis. At the same time dual vascular networks develop, of which one will provide the non-respiratory parts of the lung with oxygenated blood and the other will absorb oxygen from the respiratory epithelium. The latter of the two systems is called the pulmonary vasculature and will undergo a complex process of formation and then remodeling to adapt to the growing airways and form in close proximity to them. The development of the airways and vasculature is carefully controlled through a multitude of molecular and physical factors. These factors include transcriptional regulators, growth factors, morphogens and extracellular matrix molecules (ECM), all of which must be carefully controlled in both time and space to form a properly functioning lung that will perform the critical task of gas exchange upon the transition from fetal to newborn life. If some of these developmental factors do not function at the right time and/or place then lung defects can occur, and can lead to reduced lung function or mortality due to respiratory failure at birth.

DEVELOPMENTAL STAGES

Typically lung development has been divided into five stages: embryonic, pseudoglandular, canalicular, saccular, and finally the alveolar period. However, more recently the alveolar period has been split in two and a sixth stage has been defined as the period of microvascular maturation (2, 3). Each of these stages is defined by a specific developmental milestone and each also requires a unique set of developmental factors to accomplish its specific end goal (Table 1-1). Much of what we know about lung development has arisen from studies in rodents; however, there is a great deal in common between mouse and human lung development, with only two major exceptions. During human fetal development, our lung is divided into five separate lobes, with two lobes deriving from the left primary bronchus and three from the right. This asymmetric layout is believed to exist to accommodate space for the heart. Mice on the other hand have a different pattern of lung lobation. While they still have five secondary bronchi (each secondary bronchi is the primary stem for a lung lobe), they have only one lobe off the left primary bronchi and four derived off of the right (Fig. 1-1). The second major difference between mouse and human pulmonary development involves the time frame for the different developmental stages. Human lung development is almost complete at birth, with only part of alveolarization and microvascular maturation occurring postnatally. Conversely, mice are born with a saccular lung: thus their lungs have to function in an air-breathing environment at a more primitive stage of maturation than humans. For the purposes of this chapter, the six stages of lung development will be grouped into early (embryonic and pseudoglandular), mid (canalicular and saccular) and late (alveolar and microvascular maturation) phases of lung development.

Early Lung Development

The human lung originates as a ventral endodermal pouch from the primitive foregut during the fourth week of embryonic life. The endodermal bud will then elongate, growing caudally, where it will bifurcate into the primary left and right lung buds. At the same time the position of the original diverticulum will then move in a rostral direction, separating the foregut into two tubes, the dorsal esophagus and the ventrally positioned trachea. The two lung buds (primary bronchi) will then grow out in a posterior-ventral direction into the splanchnic mesenchyme, where they will branch again, with the left bronchi forming two secondary bronchi and the right bronchi forming three secondary bronchi. Each of these secondary bronchi represents a future lobe of the mature lung, and will undergo further branching, thus expanding the major airways within each lobe of the lung.

In the mouse a slightly different process occurs. The mouse lung starts at 9.5 days post coitum (dpc) from two endodermal buds which will sprout from the ventral foregut just anterior to the stomach. At this same location, the single foregut tube will then invaginate and pinch into two separate tubes creating the trachea containing the two primary lung buds and the dorsally located esophagus. The two primary mouse lung bronchi will then grow out further into the splanchnic mesenchyme just as in humans; however, the right primary bronchi will create four secondary bronchi whereas the left will not branch at this point and will create only one lung lobe. All five secondary bronchi will then continue to undergo further branching to create the mature airway tree (Fig. 1-2). This process of directed endodermal outgrowth and reiterated airway branching is termed

Table 1-1   Stages of Lung Formation and Major Structural Developments and their Molecular Mediators

| Developmental stage | GESTATIONAL AGE | | Formation/induction of: | Molecular mediators |
	Human (weeks)	Mouse (days)		
Embryonic	3.5–7	9.5–14.2	Initial bud outgrowth Trachea Primary bronchi Major airways	SHH, PTC, GLI's, RA, RARs FGF10, FGF9, FGF7, FGFR2 LEFTY1, LEFTY2, PITX2, NODAL SPRY2, SPRY4, BMP4, HOXA5 TBX4/5, TITF1, FOX's, CRISPLD2
Pseudoglandular	5–17	14.2–16.6	Preacinar bronchial tree	SHH, PTC, TGFB, BMP4, RA, RARs FGF7, FGF9, CRISPLD2, TBX4/5 GATA6, SMADs, TITF1, FOX's
Canalicular	16–26	16.6–17.4	Completion of conducting airways Pulmonary acinus and gas exchange area Increase in capillary bed Start of epithelial differentiation	VEGF, FLT1, FLK1 HIF1A, ARNT, HIF2A GATA6, TITF1, ASCL1, HES1 FGF7, FOX's, MDK ANGPT1, ANGPT2, TIE1, TEK
Saccular	24–38	17.5 d–5 dpn	Saccules Alveolar ducts and air sacs Surfactant	VEGF, FLT1, FLK1 HIF1A, ARNT, HIF2A FOX's, HOXA5, MDK ANGPT1, ANGPT2, TIE1, TEK
Alveolar	36–2 ypn	4–14 dpn	Secondary crests and alveoli	FGFR3, FGFR4, RA, RARs, MDK ANGPT1, ANGPT2, TIE1, TEK
Microvascular maturation	Birth–3 ypn	14–21 dpn	Thinning of alveolar septa Remodeling of pulmonary vasculature Fusion of capillary bilayer	VEGF, FLT1, FLK1 ANGPT1, ANGPT2, TIE1, TEK FOX's

dpn, days postnatal; ypn, years postnatal.

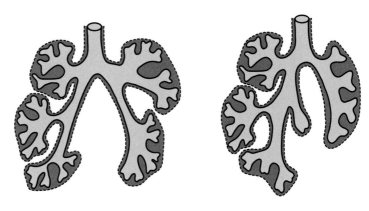

Human lung
(Late pseudoglandular stage)

Mouse lung
(Late pseudoglandular stage)

Figure 1-1 Anterior view model diagram illustrating the differences between human and murine lobar formation. The human lung has two left lobes and three right lobes. The mouse has one left lung lobe and four right side lung lobes.

branching morphogenesis. The lung will undergo 23 generations of branching during this process, of which the first 16 are reproducible and the latter half appear to have a more random distribution. It has been suggested and seems likely that the reproducible nature of these first 16 generations is genetically pre-programmed in humans and the term "hard-wiring" is used to refer to this developmentally predetermined construction of airway tree development (4). What separates early lung development into embryonic and pseudoglandular stages is the onset of cellular differentiation in the expanding network of airway branches. The embryonic stage is characterized by the formation of the lung bud(s), trachea, primary bronchi and major airways, which are lined with undifferentiated columnar epithelium. The pseudoglandular stage of lung development starts during the fifth week of human gestation (14.2 days in mice) and continues with the formation

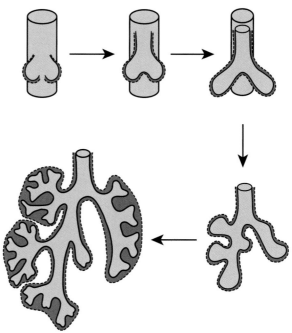

Figure 1-2 Anterior view model of early murine lung branching morphogenesis. Starting with initial bud outgrowth from the primitive foregut at 9.5 dpc into the surrounding mesenchyme.

of all conductive airways establishing the bronchial tree down to the terminal bronchi. However, a key developmental process also distinguishes this period of lung growth from the embryonic phase and that is the process of cellular differentiation. Pulmonary differentiation can be broken down into four major categories: proximal airway epithelium, distal airway epithelium, proximal mesenchyme and distal mesenchyme. Each of these groups of cells will undergo differentiation into specific cell types and/or are responsible for signaling other groups to undergo differentiation or morphological changes. The primary purpose of differentiation is to set up the functional characteristics of both the conducting airways (bronchial system) and the respiratory airways (pulmonary acinus). The proximal epithelium of the conducting airways is initially undifferentiated columnar epithelium and will differentiate into nonciliated columnar (Clara) cells, pulmonary neuroendocrine cells (PNECs), and ciliated cells. The distal respiratory epithelium is low columnar/cuboidal in nature and will differentiate into type II epithelial cells that will later give rise to type I epithelial cells (5, 6). Mesenchymal cells will differentiate into chondrocytes, fibroblasts and myoblasts. Specification of mesenchymal cell types starts around the trachea and primary bronchi laying out the cartilaginous rings to support the larger airways, then moving distally creating the complex vascular network and visceral pleura in the peripheral mesenchyme. One of the fundamental guiding principles of lung development is epithelial-mesenchymal cell interactions. Often referred to as "cross-talk," interactions between these two tissue layers are crucial to normal lung development, and both branching morphogenesis and cellular differentiation depend heavily on this process. Early experiments using tissue grafts demonstrated the unique ability of distal mesenchyme to induce epithelial budding from the trachea when denuded of its own mesenchyme (7, 8). Tracheal mesenchyme on the other hand could not induce budding when grafted onto distal lung epithelium. Further experimentation revealed that not only could branching morphogenesis be stimulated by the distal mesenchyme but also cytodifferentiation (9). These simple experiments demonstrate the physiological differences in the ability of proximal versus distal mesenchyme to induce growth and differentiation of the developing pulmonary epithelium. The theme of epithelial-mesenchymal cross-talk and its importance will be discussed later in areas of lung development such as sonic hedgehog (SHH) and fibroblast growth factor (FGF) signaling.

Mid Lung Development

During the 16th week of life for a human embryo (16.6 dpc in the mouse), lung development is well on its way and the fetal pulmonary system enters the canalicular period. The major defining characteristic of this phase in lung development is the growth of the respiratory epithelium and the formation of the respiratory bronchioles and the prospective pulmonary acinus. A second major development during this period is a large increase in the capillary bed of the distal lung. By the end of the canalicular period the human fetus is capable of surviving premature birth because it has the necessary respiratory epithelium and the associated vascular bed to support a minimal, yet life-permitting, level of gas exchange with the outside world. The major conducting airway branching pattern is now completed and development of the lung starts to focus on creating the necessary functional elements to facilitate gas exchange. Foremost is the rapid expansion of the lung vasculature through capillary formation in the primitive lung interstitium. Secondly, differentiation from cuboidal type II to squamous type I cells in the distal epithelium occurs (6). Differentiation of these cell types is an important step as the type II cells will be required to produce and secrete surfactant and the type I cells will form the thin cell layer to support future gas exchange. By the 24th week of gestation, the lung starts to gain its alveolar appearance under the microscope as the peripheral airspaces expand with a coordinate reduction in the surrounding mesenchyme, thus denoting the start of the saccular or terminal sac phase of lung development. Further cell differentiation occurs in both the conductive and respiratory epithelium, as well as the proximal and distal mesenchyme. This is evident through the increased appearance of ciliated, non-ciliated Clara, basal and neuroendocrine cells in the proximal epithelium and maturation of type I and type II cells in the distal epithelium. Structural support for the lung starts to form during this period as elastic fibers are laid down in the thinning interstitium and the larger vessels of the pulmonary vasculature start to muscularize (2).

Late Lung Development

While the initial part of alveolarization in human development occurs in utero, late lung development consisting of alveolarization and microvascular maturation occurs predominantly after parturition in an air-breathing environment. Formation of secondary crests in the terminal saccules is primarily responsible for dividing up the terminal air spaces into smaller units and is paramount for proper formation of mature alveoli. The secondary crests still contain a capillary bilayer and will need to undergo further modification to achieve an efficient diffusion distance between air and blood. Since complete alveolarization of the whole lung is a long process lasting for several years in humans, it heavily overlaps with the stage of microvascular maturation. When the process of alveolar formation is complete within a specific region of the lung, it will move onto the next phase of microvascular maturation while other areas of the lung may continue on in the process of alveolar formation. Microvascular maturation is the final step in lung formation which is necessary to create an efficient gas-exchange surface. The intraalveolar septa containing the capillary bilayer will now thin and in the process fuse the capillary bilayer into a single layered network with the mature blood vessels sitting 0.1 μm from the internal airspace of the lung.

GROWTH FACTORS

Growth factors are crucial signaling molecules for development and have been conserved across many diverse species throughout evolution. The mammalian lung is no exception, with effects ranging from mild to severe when their native expression is altered. FGFs are a class of secreted polypeptide ligands that when combined with their tyrosine kinase receptors (FGFR) regulate many cellular processes during embryonic, fetal and postnatal vertebrate development (10). FGFs have also been implicated in many areas of lung formation ranging across the developmental timeframe of pulmonary morphogenesis. Unless specifically mentioned, all discussion regarding expression patterns and developmental effects of morphogens, transcription and growth factors or any other developmental factors affecting lung development is specifically relevant to the murine lung; however, the functional relevance of these factors is theorized to exist in the human lung as well, although not proven.

Early Growth Factors

One of the most striking effects of how a single growth factor can shape lung development can be seen in the deletion of *Fgf10*. The *Fgf10* null mouse develops a trachea but has complete absence of the lung (lung agenesis), with the trachea ending in a mass of disorganized mesenchymal cells in which no primary lung buds are visible (11, 12). These mice die at birth due to respiratory failure, with other severe developmental defects such as complete truncation of the fore- and hind-limbs. When the distal endoderm of the trachea was examined, no expression of *Shh* or *bone morphogenetic protein 4 (Bmp4)* was found. Also, *wingless-type MMTV integration site family member 2 (Wnt2)* transcripts were absent from the surrounding mutant lung mesoderm. The lack of these other factors implicated in early lung development suggests that FGF10 is one of the most upstream regulators of lung development found to date (12). To comprehend the importance of FGF10 signaling during lung development we must also understand its expression pattern to complete the picture. High levels of *Fgf10* expression were initially discovered in 14 dpc rat lung mesenchymal cells (13). Bellusci and colleagues (14) further investigated *Fgf10* expression in mouse lungs using in situ hybridization. They demonstrated that *Fgf10* is expressed at the onset of lung development in the mouse at 9.75 dpc, in the splanchnic mesenchyme surrounding the small lung buds growing out from the ventral foregut. They also noted that the expression seemed to be higher around the larger right lung bud, possibly due to the fact that it will soon be creating four secondary bronchi whereas the left will create one. About a day later, around 10.5 dpc, *Fgf10* was found to be restricted to the distal mesenchyme of the two main bronchi. Twenty-four hours after that the expression pattern was restricted to the developing tips of the new secondary bronchi. As time progressed and the developing buds grew out into the mesenchyme, the level of *Fgf10* expression increased in the surrounding area of the bud. This was accompanied by an increase of expression in regions of the mesenchyme where the next bud will form. This spatial-temporal expression pattern suggests that FGF10 is directing the outgrowth of the branching airways, and then moving to new positions of future branch sites as morphogenesis progresses. This also indicates that the developing endoderm is signaling back to the mesenchyme to regulate *Fgf10* expression, possibly through interaction with the SHH pathway, which will be discussed later.

A splice variant for the FGFR2 receptor FGFR2b (FGFR2-IIIb) has been found in the developing lung (15). Since FGF10 has been shown to bind FGFR2b, it represented an ideal target for deletion to check for effects on lung development (14, 16). Early experiments using an overexpression of a dominant negative variant of *Fgfr2* using the human surfactant protein C (SFTPC) promoter created a mouse with a complete absence of normal lungs, resulting in perinatal death (17). The promoter for SFTPC has been demonstrated to drive expression of a downstream gene construct in the epithelial cells of primordial lung buds as early as day 10 dpc. Expression is then restricted to the distal epithelial elements of the branching bronchial tubules from days 13 to 16 post coitum, and finally is constrained to the type II cells in the terminal alveolar saccules in the late gestational lung (18, 19). These mice that were expressing the dominant negative *Fgfr2* construct had two undifferentiated epithelial tubes. Unfortunately a knockout of the *Fgfr2* receptor results in early embryonic lethality due to trophectoderm defects well before the start of lung development; therefore any effect on the lung could not be elucidated (20). This problem was overcome by Arman and colleagues (21), who created a mouse embryo via a fusion chimera to allow these mice to survive until term. Their discovery was quite interesting in that the phenotype that resulted was almost identical to the *Fgf10* null mouse. A normal trachea appeared to develop but then abruptly ended with no lung, thus restricting the airway defect to the bronchial tree. This discovery was further clarified when an *Fgfr2b* isoform-specific null mouse was generated, leaving the *Fgfr2c* splice variant to function normally (22). Unlike the mice generated with a loss of both *Fgfr2* isoforms, the *Fgfr2b* null mice survived to birth, but still suffered from a variety of developmental defects and died at parturition due to respiratory failure. The authors noticed that like the previously reported *Fgf10* null and the chimeric *Fgfr2*$^{-/-}$ mice, there was no lung formation, but just a tracheal bud without the establishment of primary bronchi.

This strongly suggests that FGFR2b is the receptor that transmits the signals from FGF10 during pulmonary morphogenesis to drive the initial primary branching events. However, new evidence suggests that this may not be the case, as both $Fgf10^{-/-}$ and $Fgfr2b^{-/-}$ mice have been found to initiate primary branching by 11.5 dpc (23). While the $Fgfr2b$ null mice appear to show continued growth of the right primary bud with a visible cleft between the left and right primary bronchi by 13.5 dpc, the $Fgf10$ null mice do not. By 13.5 dpc the $Fgf10$ knockout mice show only the right bronchus, with no visible cleft denoting a separate left bronchus.

Another FGF family member shown to have affects on early lung development is FGF9. $Fgf9$ expression is detected within the airway epithelium and visceral pleura at 10.5 dpc, and appears to be restricted to the pleura by 12.5 dpc (24). Colvin et al. (25) created an $Fgf9$ null mouse which had severe lung hypoplasia and consequently died shortly after parturition. Upon closer examination it was revealed that these lungs had reduced airway branching and a reduction in mesenchyme. Interestingly, there was still a significant amount of distal airspace formation and pneumocyte differentiation. The authors propose that FGF9 and FGF10 are involved in controlling lung growth through epithelial-mesenchymal signaling mechanisms, where FGF9's primary function is the regulation of mesenchymal proliferation (25). Recent developments have shed new light on the function of FGF9 in lung development, indicating that FGF9 may have a more significant role than originally thought. While previous reports indicated that $Fgf9$ expression was absent from the lung epithelium by 12.5 dpc, new evidence shows it is expressed at significant levels in 14.5 dpc lung epithelium (23). When recombinant FGF9 was added to 12.5 dpc lung explant cultures to mimic overexpression, it resulted in increased mesenchymal proliferation, inhibition of mesenchymal differentiation, epithelial dilatation and decreased epithelial branching. These effects were also shown in separate epithelial and mesenchymal lung tissue cultures when the two layers were separated from one another. This indicates that neither tissue layer is dependent on the other for responding to FGF9 signaling. Further experimentation revealed that FGF9 signaling in the lung epithelium is dependent on the FGFR2b receptor, independent of FGF10 signaling. Using a $Fgf10$ enhancer-trap $nlacZ$ transgene reporter in $Fgf9^{-/-}$ mice it was noticed that there was an increase in FGF10 expression, a result contrary to previous findings by Colvin and colleagues using in situ hybridization for $Fgf10$ (25). Del Moral et al. (23) also noticed an increase in $Fgf10$ expression in lungs treated with recombinant FGF9 and suggest that this FGF9-induced up-regulation of $Fgf10$ expression is likely to be mediated via T-box 4 (TBX4) and TBX5. Similar to the effects of recombinant FGF9 on cultured lungs, overexpression of $Fgf9$ using an inducible system spatially regulated by the SFTPC promoter induced a large mesenchymal expansion and a reduction in epithelial branching during early lung development (26). Interestingly, Shh and $patched$ (Ptc) expression was significantly up-regulated in these lungs. Since the opposite effect on Shh and Ptc expression was seen in the $Fgf9^{-/-}$ lung, it suggests that FGF9 is both necessary and sufficient to induce Shh expression and SHH signaling. $Fgf7$ and $Fgf10$ expression was also up-regulated in the $Fgf9$ overexpression mice with a loss of spatial restriction to $Fgf10$ transcripts, in agreement with the recombinant FGF9 culture experiments mentioned earlier. These results suggest that the lung phenotype resulting from increased levels of FGF9 may be mediated through changes in FGF7 and FGF10 signaling. Increased levels of $sprouty$ 2 ($Spry2$) and $Bmp4$ transcripts were also seen in the $Fgf9$ overexpression mouse, providing further evidence that epithelial-mesenchymal FGF signaling through FGF7 and FGF10 is mediating the effects of FGF9 (26).

It is clear that FGFs play an important role during branching morphogenesis through epithelial-mesenchymal signaling interactions. In $Drosophila$, a mutation in the $sprouty$ ($Spry$) gene results in enhanced branching of its respiratory system, and it was discovered that the *Spry* gene encodes a protein that antagonizes FGF signaling (27). Multiple homologues to *Spry* have been found in both humans and rodents and have been demonstrated to have effects on lung development. Antisense oligonucleotides of the murine *Spry* homologue *Spry2* used on cultured embryonic lung explants demonstrated a dramatic effect on branching morphogenesis, showing a 72% increase in epithelial branching as well as increased expression of epithelial differentiation markers (28). This relationship was further clarified through the use of two separate overexpression models which showed that an increase of *Spry2* expression results in decreased pulmonary branching morphogenesis (29). But the most potent effects of a *Spry* gene on lung development were observed in a transgenic mouse expressing an inducible lung epithelial specific *Spry4* construct. In these animals exogenous *Spry4* resulted in hypoplasia and defects in lobar formation when expressed throughout lung development. Furthermore, the aberrant effects of exogenous *Spry4* are variable depending on the specific phase of lung development it is expressed in. While *Spry4* expression during the pseudoglandular phase showed severe developmental defects resulting in perinatal lethality, expression of *Spry4* during the saccular and alveolar stages resulted in survival with mild non-inflammatory emphysema (30).

BMPs are a family of secreted growth and differentiation factors related to the transforming growth factor B (TGFB) superfamily. Expression of several BMPs has been found throughout the developing lung in both endodermal and mesodermal derived tissues. A *Bmp7* null mouse has been generated and suffers from a great deal of developmental defects, dying within one month after birth. Although *Bmp7* transcripts are detected throughout the lung epithelium with slightly higher expression seen at the developing bud tips, no lung aberrations are noted in the null mouse (31). *Bmp5* expression has been detected in the mesenchyme of the embryonic mouse lung around 10.5 dpc to 16.5 dpc. However, $Bmp5^{-/-}$ mice are viable and show no apparent lung phenotype (32). By far the most interesting member of the BMP family as far as lung development is concerned is BMP4. High levels of *Bmp4* transcripts can be seen in the distal tips of the developing epithelial buds early on (11.5 dpc) in lung development. Expression continues to at least 15.5 dpc with lower levels of expression also occurring in the mesenchyme adjacent to the developing epithelial bud tips; however, expression slowly declines thereafter towards 18.5 dpc (33). A *Bmp4* null mouse has been successfully generated, but these mice die early in gestation between 6.5 and 9.5 dpc (34). This experiment clearly demonstrates the importance of BMP4 during early mouse development; however, to investigate the effects on lung formation another approach will have to be used, as these mice die well before the initiation of lung development. Further insight into the influence of BMP4 signaling on lung development has resulted from expressing *Bmp4* in the distal lung epithelium using the SFTPC promoter (33). Analysis at 15.5 dpc revealed smaller lungs, apparently as the result of both reduced cellular proliferation and increased cell death as evident from BrdU and TUNEL labeling respectively. Morphologically these lungs showed fewer and grossly distended epithelial terminal buds separated by an abundance of mesenchyme. Further study revealed large epithelial sacs that were continuous with the bronchi and trachea, ultimately resulting in a lung incapable of supporting normal lung function at birth (33). The authors also noted that while differentiation was unaffected in the proximal airway epithelium, the distal pulmonary epithelial cells showed reduced differentiation to a type II cell fate. Finally, when the transgenic lungs were tested to see whether other regulatory molecules known to be involved in lung development were affected no changes were seen in the mRNA transcript levels of *forkhead box A2* (*Foxa2*), *Shh*, *Wnt2* or *Bmp7*.

When the potent effects of BMP4 on lung development were discovered, it led to other research to investigate the control mechanisms playing a role in

BMP4 signaling. In a study by Weaver and colleagues (35), they examined two mechanisms of inhibiting BMP signaling using the BMP agonist Xnoggin as well as a dominant negative type I BMP receptor called dnAlk6. Using the SFTPC promoter, each of these constructs were individually examined and found to have powerful effects on BMP signaling. Overexpression of *Xnoggin* was found to cause not only pre-natal lethality in almost all transgenic mice, but also a dramatic reduction in lung size, irregularities of lobar shape and abnormalities of proximal-distal differentiation, specifically with the adoption of a proximal airway phenotype in the distal lung epithelium. There was also the appearance of alpha smooth muscle actin (ACTA2) positive cells in the distal mesenchyme surrounding the proximalized distal tubules; however, no gross abnormalities in vasculogenesis were found. When *dnAlk6* was ectopically expressed with the SFTPC promoter it also resulted in no live-born pups and a disruption of normal proximal-distal patterning, which, however, was not quite as severe as in the SFTPC-*Xnoggin* transgenic mouse as the proximal mesenchyme appeared normal (35).

Another important regulator of BMP4 signaling has emerged over the past few years and is shedding new light on the role of BMP4 in lung branching morphogenesis. An important group of regulatory molecules known as the "can" family, named for a domain of homology initially identified in the *Xenopus cerberus* gene (*Cer1*), contains several important developmental regulators and is closely related to other influential factors such as the TGFB superfamily (for review see Pearce et al. (36)). Many of these "can" proteins have been demonstrated to inhibit BMP signaling, specifically by binding to and blocking BMP2/4 activity (37). It has been shown that the "can" family members *gremlin* (*Grem1*), *Grem2* (formerly *Prdc*), *Cer1*, and *Nbl1* (formerly *Dan*) are all expressed in the lung during fetal development (38). Further insight into "can" family regulation on BMP signaling was provided by two groups using different approaches to examine the effects of GREM1 on BMP4 signaling in the developing lung. In one approach, Lu and colleagues (38) used the SFTPC promoter to overexpress *Grem1* in the distal lung based on observations that *Grem1* was natively expressed in the proximal airways during pulmonary development. These transgenic lungs developed a proximalization of the distal lung as evident by the appearance of smooth muscle surrounding the distal airways and proximal airway markers *Ccsp* and *Foxj1* in the distal epithelium (38). Evidence from a second group (37) using antisense oligonucleotides to knockdown *Grem1* expression in lung explant cultures showed that potent growth and enhanced branching resulted from decreased *Grem1* expression. Since GREM1 is a powerful antagonist of BMP4 they examined the other half of the same principle using exogenous BMP4 on wild-type lung explant cultures and observed increased branching as well as an increase in the epithelial sac count, a phenotype not unlike that of the *Grem1* knockdown lung explant. Finally, using recombinant adenovirus to exogenously express *Grem1* the authors demonstrated a reduction in the BMP4-induced branching observed in the lung cultures (37). The combined results of these two groups clearly demonstrate the importance of BMP4 regulation via GREM1 during lung development. These findings also denote the need for more investigation into this area of pulmonary development, as there are several "can" family members expressed in the lung which have not been as intimately examined and may also be crucial regulators of lung development via BMP regulation.

Mid Growth Factors

FGF1, also called acidic fibroblast growth factor (aFGF), has definite effects on lung development. Early experiments by Nogawa and Ito (39) showed that mouse lung epithelium cultured under mesenchyme-free conditions underwent branching morphogenesis in medium containing FGF1. Further investigation demonstrated that FGF1 will induce not only branching, but also cell proliferation and differentiation in epithelial lung bud culture experiments (40). The appearance of differential cell proliferation in the lung epithelium does not appear to be the trigger for bud induction, as FGF1 induces budding prior to observable differences in regional BrdU incorporation (41). Another theory has been proposed in which FGF signaling could induce changes in cell motility and adhesion, thus allowing for cell rearrangements initiating budding (42).

FGF7, also called keratinocyte growth factor (KGF), is a member of the FGF family of signaling peptides whose expression has been studied across many diverse developmental systems. *Fgf7* transcripts were initially found in the mouse lung starting at 14.5 dpc. The transcripts were found to be localized to the lung mesenchyme and expression persisted into adulthood, although at lower levels (43). Experiments using mesenchyme-free epithelial lung cell cultures have shown that there are several interesting effects that FGF7 has on lung development. The mesenchyme surrounding the epithelial buds of 11 dpc mouse lungs was removed and the exposed lung buds were grown in culture containing exogenous FGF7 protein (40). It was found that exogenous FGF7 induced growth and lumen expansion in the explants, but resulted in dilated cyst-like structures, not characteristic of normal lung growth. It was noted that at higher concentrations FGF7 was also able to induce differentiation, evident via the appearance of type II-like cells with features of lamellar bodies, and induce expression of surfactant proteins A and B (SFTPA and SFTPB). However, when interpreting the effects of FGF7 early on in lung development, it must be noted that the FGF7 was administered at a time when native *Fgf7* expression in the lung is not detected. Therefore, the cyst-like growth pattern could have developed as a result of lack of a native control element in the FGF7 signaling pathway. This is in contrast to the rat, in which *Fgf7* can be detected in the mesenchyme via RT-PCR at the onset of lung development (44). Experiments using the SFTPC promoter to drive expression of FGF7 in the developing lung resulted in an abnormal growth pattern during the pseudoglandular stage of development, showing marked enlargement of the bronchial airspaces and a reduction in small airway branches (45). What was also noticed was a lack of mesenchyme and incomplete epithelial differentiation when compared to normal embryos during the same developmental time-frame. Similarly to the explants receiving exogenous FGF7, these lungs demonstrated increased SFTPB expression; however, protein levels did not coordinate with this observation as no detectable levels of SFTPB protein were evident. These mice die prior to 17.5 dpc, most likely due to the large cystadenoma-like lung morphology, in which the developing lung occupies almost the whole thoracic cavity and therefore is likely to impede cardiac function, leading to pre-natal lethality. But again, one must consider the fact that FGF7 was expressed in the type II epithelial cells, quite the opposite of its normal mesenchymal expression pattern. It appears more likely that FGF7 is responsible for growth and differentiation during later stages of lung development (40). But if this is true, then there must be other compensating or redundant factors, as an *Fgf7* null mouse has been generated and it shows no lung phenotype (46). Many FGFs signal through the same receptors, therefore it is possible that another related family member is compensating for the loss of FGF7. It has been demonstrated that FGF7 is expressed in rat lung mesenchyme and signals across to its receptor (FGFR2b) in the developing epithelium. It was shown that antisense oligonucleotides targeted towards the FGFR2b receptor resulted in a reduction of airway branching (44).

The TGFB superfamily is another classification of growth factors with important contributions to lung formation. Mediating a wide variety of effects in the developing lung, including, proliferation, differentiation, cell migration and ECM formation, they are intimately linked to glucocorticoid (GC) signaling (47).

Expressed during lung development, TGFB1, TGFB2 and TGFB3 have all been demonstrated to have unique contributions to lung development (48). While there is a vast amount of information about the effects that each of these isoforms and their receptors have, we will only highlight a few of the more prominent examples. TGFB1 has been demonstrated to be a negative regulator of lung development, as evident through lung culture experiments showing that exogenous TGFB1 can block the early stages of branching morphogenesis, most likely through inhibition of *Nmyc* (49). Further studies using the SFTPC promoter to test for the in vivo effects of exogenous *Tgfb1* expression demonstrated arrest of lung growth just prior to the mid-phase of lung development, with a mild reduction in branching morphogenesis (50). The variation seen between these two models with regard to the potency of the branching defect most likely results from differences in the absolute levels of exogenous TGFB1 supplied to the developing lung. Interestingly, inhibition of *Tgfb1* using antisense oligonucleotides on lung explants had no significant effect on branching morphogenesis (51). This also holds true for the *Tgfb1* null mouse, which displays no disruption in branching morphogenesis (52, 53). In the antisense *Tgfb1* knockdown study it was noted that TGFB3 also had no effect on branching when down-regulated in culture. However, the authors observed that loss of *Tgfb2* signaling using the antisense knockdown method resulted in a significant reduction in branching morphogenesis (51). This contrasts to the *Tgfb2* null mouse, which shows no branching defect during lung formation although it suffers from perinatal mortality due to a multitude of other defects, including collapsed conducting airways at birth (54). The lack of branching defect in the *Tgfb2* null mouse is theorized to result from a rescue effect due to maternal transmission of TGFB2 to the fetus during development (55). On the other hand, the *Tgfb3* null mouse unlike its related isoforms does suffer from defects in lung development, showing delayed pulmonary maturation and defective palatogenesis at birth (56). The phenotypic characteristics of this delay in lung development included mesenchymal thickening, alveolar hypoplasia, decreased septal formation and an overall reduction in the number of type II epithelial cells. Typically GC treatment via maternal administration of dexamethazone is used to speed up maturation of the lungs in human infants at risk of premature birth to prevent respiratory distress syndrome. Since the *Tgfb3* null lung appears immature at birth, GC treatment was used to see whether the immature lung phenotype could be rescued, based on earlier studies showing a link between GC treatment and *Tgfb3* expression levels (57). It has been previously shown that GC signaling exerts its stimulatory effects through a TGFB3-dependent mechanism (58). However, in the in vivo model GC treatment was able to induce expression of ECM molecules in the *Tgfb3* null lung, thus providing evidence that GC signaling does not exert its effects solely through TGFB3 (59).

SMAD (mothers against DPP (Smad)) proteins are intracellular signaling molecules that are intimately linked to signal transduction from TGFB isoforms. Therefore, they became excellent targets to examine for effects on lung development due to the emerging studies denoting the importance of TGFB signaling during lung formation. Indeed, attenuation of *Smad2* and *Smad3* transcripts concurrently resulted in an increase in lung branching morphogenesis in culture, as did the same experiment using *Smad4* alone. Exogenous TGFB1, which should show the opposite effect, was unable to reduce the increased branching, clearly demonstrating that SMAD2 and SMAD3, as well as SMAD4, are downstream and intricately linked to TGFB1 inhibition of branching morphogenesis during lung formation (60). Interestingly, another Smad family member, SMAD7, was shown to interrupt TGFB-induced inhibition of branching morphogenesis and cytodifferentiation in culture, through modulation of downstream SMAD2 activity in the TGFB signaling pathway (61).

Late Growth Factors

As mentioned earlier, all four FGFR receptors are expressed in the developing lung. However, effects from disruption of both *Fgfr1* and *Fgfr2* lead to early lethality in the developing mouse, prior to the events of lung development. A null mutant for *Fgfr3* has been created and produces a viable embryo but shows no lung phenotype, with only some skeletal overgrowth and inner ear anomalies (62). *Fgfr4* has been knocked out as well but shows no gross developmental defects, representing the mildest null phenotype of the four FGFR receptors (63). But when the *Fgfr3* and *Fgfr4* null mice are bred together creating a double knockout, the result is a unique mouse different from either single knockout condition. The double null mice suffered from severe growth defects and appeared dehydrated. When the authors investigated for a cause of this condition they discovered that the lungs, which looked outwardly normal, upon histological examination showed an emphysematous appearance with enlarged air spaces and a lack of alveoli (63). Further investigation revealed that these double mutant lungs, which looked normal up until postnatal day 2 of life, failed to undergo secondary septation during the alveolar period. These mice retained their simplified pre-alveolar saccules into adulthood, thus halting lung development resulting in an abnormal and immature lung.

MORPHOGENS

Morphogens are an interesting group of molecules that use concentration gradients to give different developmental cues to a growing organism. In 1952 a mathematician named Allan Turing described a type of signaling molecule released by organizing centers such as the notochord in developing animals, and posited that these molecules must meet two conditions. First, they must be released in such a way that they form a concentration gradient in their zone of influence. Second, they must be able to elicit distinct responses in surrounding cells at different concentrations (64). These molecules are the key to normal development in almost every complex organism, from fruit flies to humans, and impairment of their function can lead to dire consequences for a developing embryo.

SHH is a mammalian member of the hedgehog (HH) family of morphogens, which also includes Indian hedgehog (IHH) and desert hedgehog (DHH). HH itself was initially described in *Drosophila melanogaster* as a morphogen crucial to normal development. In mammals SHH, IHH and DHH are the functional evolution of their single *Drosophila* ancestor. SHH has shown itself to be the most potent of the three mammalian HH homologues, and an absolute requirement for normal mammalian development (65–69).

Perhaps ceding only to FGF10, SHH has been acknowledged to be one of the most crucial factors to early lung development. SHH is part of a larger group of proteins called the SHH signaling pathway/network, and is made up of many factors all working as one to accomplish the overall goal of transducing SHH signaling from one cell or tissue type to another. While there are many factors involved in this signaling mechanism, we will briefly outline the SHH pathway in its most basic form to help make further more detailed discussion clearer. SHH signaling originates from a source cell, from which it will travel to a receiving cell which has the membrane-bound receptor PTC. Binding of SHH to PTC will de-repress another membrane-bound protein called smoothened (SMO), which is natively inhibited by PTC. This release of SMO will ultimately result in the increased activity of the downstream SHH transcription factors (through a secondary mechanism), resulting in SHH signaling becoming active in the receiving cell.

Shh expression is detected as early as 9.5 dpc in the tracheal diverticulum, and continues to be expressed throughout pulmonary development (33, 70–72).

Expression of *Shh* transcripts expands from the tracheal diverticulum to the developing mouse lung epithelium by 10.5 dpc, with higher levels of expression seen at the tips of the developing buds. From 13.5 dpc to 15.5 dpc *Shh* expression appears to be restricted to the distal airway epithelium, where it will then start to appear in the bronchial epithelium at 16.5 dpc. *Shh* transcripts continue to increase in the proximal conducting airways towards birth, with expression in the distal respiratory epithelium remaining high until parturition. At birth *Shh* expression appreciably decreases in the distal epithelium; however, it is still maintained in the conducting airways. A few weeks later at postnatal day 24 *Shh* was undetectable in both the alveolar and bronchial epithelium (73). A homozygous targeted deletion of *Shh* results in severe defects in the developing mouse. While no defects are seen in their heterozygous siblings, $Shh^{-/-}$ mice die at or just prior to parturition with severe cranial, skeletal, neural and internal organ defects (74). Specifically relevant to this discussion are the severe pulmonary aberrations that result from the loss of SHH signaling. *Shh* null mice suffer from a variety of pulmonary malformations, including closure or narrowing of the esophagus (atresia and stenosis respectively), failure of the trachea and the esophagus to separate (tracheo-esophageal fistula), hypoplastic lung buds, and a loss of lung asymmetry which manifests as a left pulmonary isomerism (one lung lobe on each side). There is also no sign of epithelial airway branching or mesenchymal differentiation; however, proximal-distal differentiation of the lung epithelium appears normal (71, 75, 76). The mesenchyme of these lungs also shows a reduction in cellular proliferation and an increase in cell death, as evident with BrdU and TUNEL experiments (71). When expression levels of other SHH-related genes transcripts were analyzed it was found that *Ptc1*, *Wnt2*, *glioma-associated oncogene homolog 1* (*Gli1*) and *GLI-Kruppel family member GLI3* (*Gli3*) were all down-regulated. On the other hand, expression patterns for *Pct2*, *Gli2*, *Fgfr2*, *Wnt7b*, *thyroid transcription factor 1* (*Titf1*) and *Foxa2* appear unchanged. Also it was noted that while expression levels of *Fgf10* were unaltered, the pattern of expression was no longer spatially restricted, but rather expressed broadly throughout the mesenchyme bordering the epithelium (71, 75). One puzzling development in the investigation of the *Shh* null lung has arisen from conflicting reports on the analysis of *Bmp4* expression. While the pattern of expression appears to remain consistent, one group reports that the mesenchymal levels decrease while the epithelial levels are maintained in the *Shh* null lung and another reports an increase in the normal sites of *Bmp4* expression (71, 75).

To further shed light on the requirement for SHH signaling in lung development, Miller and colleagues (77) created a lung-specific *Shh* null mouse, in which the removal of *Shh* from the lung can also be temporally controlled. When *Shh* is removed prior to 13.5 dpc, severe lung defects are present, similar to those seen in the complete *Shh* knockout mouse, with defects found in the trachea, bronchi and peripheral lung. The authors were also able to demonstrate the requirement for proper spatial expression for SHH in cartilage formation of the conducting airways. On the other hand the requirement for SHH during later stages of lung development does not appear to be critical, with only mild defects in the peripheral lung structure occurring (77). However, this could also be due to the fact that a complete removal of SHH function from the lung is unlikely due to the spatial restrictions of the SFTPC promoter and efficiency of the reaction in excising the second exon of *Shh*.

Ectopic overexpression of *Shh* in the mouse lung endoderm has also been investigated using the SFTPC promoter. The lungs of these mice showed no obvious differences upon visual inspection when examined at several different gestational ages, ranging from 15.5 to 18.5 dpc. However, a day later at birth the lungs were noticeably smaller in size, only weighing half of the wet weight of their wild-type counterparts (78). Upon closer inspection it was found that at 16.5 dpc the mutant lungs had an increase in the ratio of interstitial mesenchyme to epithelial tubules, but epithelial organization still looked normal at higher levels of magnification. Normally, the lung starts to undergo major structural changes entering into the saccular period, with the expansion of the epithelial tubules into sac-like structures. This still holds true for lungs ectopically overexpressing *Shh* with the SFTPC promoter; however, at this stage the interstitial mesenchyme is much thicker than normal. At birth these mice die, succumbing to respiratory failure due to lack of functional alveoli, most likely the result of compaction from hyper-cellularity of the lung mesenchyme (78). In situ hybridization revealed that *Ptc* expression was relatively the same as in control animals up until 16.5 dpc; however, *Ptc* showed a dramatic increase in expression at 17.5 and 18.5 dpc in the mesenchyme of the transgenic lungs (78). The increase in *Ptc* expression in the transgenic mice suggests that the ectopic SHH is functionally active, as it is known that SHH increases *Ptc* expression natively (79). Another factor known to have elevated expression levels due to SHH signaling is its own downstream transcription factor *Gli1*. This was also observed in the SFTPC-Shh overexpressor mice, with an increase of *Gli1* expression of approximately 2.5-fold, but no changes in *Gli2* or *Gli3* expression (80).

An important regulator of SHH signal transduction is hedgehog-interacting protein 1 (HHIP1). Levels of HHIP1 increase due to SHH signaling and function as a negative feedback loop by binding and sequestering SHH, thus attenuating the signal (79). *Hhip1* expression overlaps with *Ptc* and is expressed in the lung mesenchyme near the epithelial border as well as in the epithelium itself (81). Expression levels of *Hhip1* directly coordinate with levels of SHH as they increase in the *Shh* overexpressor mouse and decrease in the *Shh* null mouse. In fact HHIP1 was found to attenuate IHH signaling when ectopically expressed in the developing endochondral skeletal system, and phenotypically resembled the *Ihh* null mouse (81). Further analysis using a *Hhip1* null mouse revealed that HHIP1 is crucial to normal lung development, as these mutant mice die shortly after birth due to respiratory failure. When the lungs were examined they displayed a phenotype quite similar to the *Shh* null lung, including defective branching morphogenesis, an increase in the number of mesenchymal cells, normal proximal-distal differentiation, and a left lobar isomerism (82). Molecular analysis revealed that many developmental factors affecting lung development were unchanged in the *Hhip1* null lung, except that of *Fgf10*, which showed a dramatic shift from its normal expression pattern. There was almost complete loss of normal *Fgf10* expression, resulting in the breakdown of branching morphogenesis due to failure of FGF10-mediated bud induction. This theory was confirmed using FGF10 soaked beads in *Hhip1*$^{-/-}$ lung cultures, where it induced significant epithelial budding towards the exogenous source of FGF10, indicating that the failure of branching morphogenesis in the *Hhip1* null lung in all probability results from defective FGF10 signaling as a result of excessive SHH activity (82).

Continuing with the topic of epithelial-mesenchymal signaling factors, a new player in lung development has emerged through studies looking for novel GC-inducible factors during lung development. Cysteine-rich secretory protein LCCL domain containing 2 (CRISPLD2), also known as late gestation lung 1 (LGL1), is a member of the CRISP family of cysteine-rich extra-cellular proteins that is expressed in the pulmonary fibroblasts in both humans and rodents (83). In situ hybridization demonstrated expression of *Crispld2* transcripts as early as 13 dpc throughout the mesenchyme of fetal rat lungs. Expression was maintained throughout gestation in the mesenchyme of these animals, with levels slightly elevated in *Acta2*-expressing cells. CRISPLD2 protein was first detected at 16 dpc and its levels showed a steady increase towards birth. Using 13 dpc fetal rat lung explant cultures, the authors demonstrated a dose-dependent reduction in airway branching using antisense oligonucleotides targeted towards *Crispld2*, as evident by the number of terminal airway buds after a 2-day incubation (84). The effect was more pronounced when 12 dpc rat lung rudiments were cultured in the presence of antisense *Crispld2*, which showed a complete cessation of branching morphogenesis. Considering the marked effect observed on epithelial airway branching, further studies were performed to examine CRISPLD2 as a secreted signaling factor. Indeed CRISPLD2 was found to co-localize with the Golgi apparatus and the endoplasmic reticulum, consistent with proteins that function as secreted signaling molecules. The functional relevance of CRISPLD2 being secreted by mesenchymal cells was further supported by cell culture experiments demonstrating that late-gestation lung epithelial cells will take up CRISPLD2 from their surrounding medium (85). These experiments clearly denote CRISPLD2 as an important epithelial-mesenchymal regulator of lung development.

RECEPTORS

The mouse PTC receptor is a cell surface receptor that is an integral part of the SHH pathway. Also called PTC1 after a second homologue PTC2 was discovered, PTC is a 12 pass transmembrane receptor protein that is responsible for signaling the arrival of SHH to a receiving cell (86). *Ptc* is expressed at high levels in the mesenchyme near the epithelial border of the developing lung, juxtaposed to *Shh* expression in the epithelial bud tips (78). This pattern of expression between morphogen and receptor illustrates the importance of SHH signaling across the epithelial-mesenchymal border during lung development. Lower levels of *Ptc* expression can also be detected in the epithelium, possibly denoting paracrine signaling mechanisms in the SHH signaling network. As seen with other factors crucial to development, a *Ptc* null mouse dies early in gestation, in this case at the start of lung formation 9.0–10.5 dpc (87). Experiments using a viral-introduced DNA construct expressing *Ptc* in skin cells demonstrated that increased levels of PTC could modulate SHH signaling, specifically causing a down-regulation of SHH signaling and thus a reduction in the expression of native *Ptc* and *Gli1* levels (88). Since further experiments investigating the role of PTC in the lung have not yet been performed we can only theorize what effects might result if PTC was manipulated during lung development. If a lung-specific knockout of *Ptc* was generated, it would most likely resemble the *Shh* null lung as this is the only receptor known to transduce SHH signaling during lung development. One of the other important functions of PTC is to sequester SHH signaling, thus limiting the range of expression (89, 90). Therefore, a secondary effect that might occur in a *Ptc* null lung could be a more widely spread area of SHH levels. Alternatively, an overexpression of *Ptc* in the lung at the onset of development might also resemble the *Shh* null lung. Since PTC can attenuate SHH signaling if expressed at high enough levels it could negate effective SHH signaling and, thus, result in a phenotype potentially similar to the *Shh* null lung (91).

Retinoic acid (RA), although not a receptor itself, will be discussed in this section, for much of what we know of this signaling pathway has been determined from experimentation with its receptors. RA and its two families of receptors, RARs and RXRs, have been shown to be crucial to developmental processes throughout formation of many different organs, including the lung (92). RA, a derivative of vitamin A, has been clearly demonstrated to have dramatic effects on lung development, including severe hypoplasia and left lung agenesis. This was shown through double knockout mice for RARA and RARB receptors, which established early on the critical role of RA signal transduction through RARA and RARB during lung development (93). Interestingly, RA signaling has both beneficial and detrimental effects on lung development and must be temporally and spatially regulated with precision during lung organogenesis. During very early lung development RA signaling is ubiquitously activated in the primary buds when they first invade into the splanchnic mesenchyme. However, once this initial period of development passes, RA signaling is attenuated so that further branching events may proceed (94, 95). This was demonstrated in experiments using constitutively activated RARA and RARB receptors expressed in the pulmonary epithelium by the SFTPC promoter which demonstrated that continued RA activation in the distal lung epithelium resulted in immaturity of the lungs (96). Constitutively active RARA displayed the more severe phenotype of the two, showing elevated levels of *Sftpc*, *Titf1* and *GATA binding protein 6* (*Gata6*) expression, and a loss of *Sftpa* and *Sftpb* at birth. Detailed analysis of human lungs showing the differential distribution patterns of RA receptor subtypes has added further support for the idea that the proximal-distal effects of RA signaling are spatially mediated through its receptors (97). Evidence from other studies has linked RA signaling to another molecule crucial to pulmonary development, namely FGF10. Using the pan-RAR antagonist BMS493 in foregut explant cultures, a connection between RA signaling and *Fgf10* expression was discovered (98). Induction of *Fgf10* expression was successfully blocked in the mesoderm of the prospective lung field, resulting in failure of initial bud out-growth. However, it is possible that there is not a direct link between these two factors. RA may indirectly stimulate *Fgf10* through maintenance of endodermal cell fates and production of a critical mass of mesenchymal cells in the early lung field, which subsequently will transcribe *Fgf10* (98). RARA has also been linked to the late phase of lung development. Overexpression of a dominant-negative form of RARA during the postnatal period of alveolar development resulted in fewer alveoli that were larger in size than normal, resulting in an overall decrease in alveolar surface area (99). It was also noted that there was a lack of *Sftpb* expression, confirming previous data showing a link between RA and surfactant protein expression (100). This illustrates that one of the critical functions of RA may be to regulate *Sftpb* expression during development of the lung and thereby prepare it for the transition to an air breathing environment (101).

TRANSCRIPTION FACTORS

Early Transcription Factors

The T-box family of transcription factors are defined by a DNA-binding domain of approximately 200 amino acids and have been shown to be crucial to development of different organ systems in both vertebrate and invertebrate embryos. For a review see Smith, 1999 (102). Expression of T-box genes one through five has been found in the developing lung, with *Tbx1* being restricted to the epithelium and the latter four to the developing mesenchyme (103). Specifically, *Tbx4* has been detected throughout both the lung and tracheal mesenchyme, and *Tbx5* limited specifically to the lung mesenchyme with higher levels seen adjacent to the epithelial branches (104). Knockdown experiments using antisense oligonucleotides (AS ODNs) illuminated the importance of these TBX transcription factors during lung development. While knockdown of *Tbx2* or *Tbx3* had no effect, AS ODNs directed at *Tbx4* or *Tbx5* showed dramatic effects on lung branching. Using 11.5 dpc embryonic mouse lung explant cultures, the authors showed that an individual knockdown of either *Tbx4* or *Tbx5* using AS ODNs resulted in a reduction of new lung branches in the explant cultures. However, when both were targeted for knockdown concurrently, the formation of new lung branches was completely abrogated (104). When examined for changes in *Fgf10* gene expression the *Tbx4/5* AS ODNs-treated lungs showed a marked reduction in transcript levels, and a complete loss of detection of *Fgf10* was seen in in situ hybridization attempts, thus suggesting that *Fgf10* expression is dependent on *Tbx4* and *Tbx5*. Since both transcription factors are found localized (but not limited) to the distinct areas of *Fgf10* expression and FGF10 is crucial to normal lung branching, the loss of branching morphogenesis in the *Tbx*4/5 AS ODN-treated mice via a reduction in *Fgf10* expression seems plausible. To further support this idea, the authors supplemented the *Tbx4/5* AS ODN-treated lung explants with exogenous FGF10, which restored the loss of branching morphogenesis. Thus, it seems highly feasible that TBX4 and TBX5 are involved in controlling *Fgf10* expression along with some other factor(s) since the expression domains for the Tbxs are not limited to the specific expression domains of *Fgf10*.

The Gli family of transcription factors are part of the SHH pathway and bring to bear the effects of SHH signaling on the receiving cell. During development, all three *Gli*s are expressed generally but not limited to distal areas of the lung mesenchyme in proximity to the epithelium, with overlapping patterns between the three. Expression patterns detected via in situ hybridization become noticeable early on during the pseudoglandular stage. However, northern blot evidence and the phenotype of the $Gli2^{-/-}$ and $Gli2^{-/-};Gli3^{-/-}$ lungs clearly demonstrate that *Gli*s are active before the pseudoglandular stage of development (80, 105). Mutant analysis of all three *Gli* genes revealed dramatic differences between them with regard to lung development. The *Gli1* null mouse shows no detectable developmental aberrations and, thus, it appears that other factor(s), most likely GLI2, can compensate for a loss of GLI1 function. Indeed, the authors (106) went on to further examine this mutant and generated a combined $Gli1^{-/-};Gli2^{+/-}$ double mutant which resulted in a mouse with a variable lung phenotype showing altered size and shape, unlike that of the $Gli2^{+/-}$ mouse, which has no lung phenotype on its own. These mice die shortly after birth with multiple defects, one of which is smaller lungs that are similar to the *Gli2* null lung but not quite as severe (106). When the full *Gli1/Gli2* double knockout mouse ($Gli1^{-/-};Gli2^{-/-}$) was created it resulted in a phenotype much more detrimental to lung formation than the $Gli1^{-/-};Gli2^{+/-}$ and $Gli2^{-/-}$ mutants, indicating that GLI1 is important to lung development and that the lack of phenotype of the *Gli1* null mouse is the result of compensation by GLI2. As already mentioned, the *Gli2* null mouse has quite a severe phenotype, including dramatic changes in lung and skeletal morphology, eventually succumbing to their mutation late in gestation (107). The *Gli2* null lung is quite hypoplastic in appearance, has defective airway branching and a reduction in left lobe wet weight throughout development and also has a left lobar isomerism similar to the *Shh* null mouse. While the trachea and esophagus still manage to separate, there was approximately a 40% and 25% reduction in cellular proliferation in the mesenchyme and epithelium, respectively; however, no obvious changes in apoptosis were noted. The mesenchyme was thicker and surrounded smaller air sacs compared to wild-type animals of the same gestation. While a reduction in *Ptc* and *Gli1* expression was observed, indicating an attenuated response to SHH signaling, no changes were found in lung relevant *Bmp* or *Fgf* transcripts (108). A natural homozygous deletion mutation for *Gli3* has been discovered and labeled the "extra toes" mutant. These mice although viable have several defects relative to their wild-type siblings and most pertinent to this discussion is a reduction in lung size, with a slightly narrower lung width than normal (80). While this phenotype is relatively mild and no change in expression levels of *Bmp4*, *Wnt2* or other SHH pathway members is detected, GLI3's involvement in lung development becomes apparent when combined with the *Gli2* null mutation. Earlier it was mentioned that FGF10 was perhaps the most upstream regulator of the initiation of lung development; however, the *Gli2/Gli3* double knockout suggests otherwise. $Gli2^{-/-};Gli3^{-/-}$ mice have a severe disruption of normal development, dying early on in gestation around 10.5 dpc. A small number of embryos do manage to survive until 14.5 dpc and these mice show no evidence of any trachea or lung primordia. This is in line with GLI3 having an overlapping function in the lung with GLI2 when comparing the $Gli2^{-/-};Gli3^{-/-}$ mouse to the individual $Gli2$ and $Gli3$ null mice. Further demonstrating the individual requirement for both GLI2 and GLI3 is the fact that the $Gli2^{+/-};Gli3^{+/-}$ mouse shows no pulmonary phenotype, while the $Gli2^{-/-};Gli3^{+/-}$ mouse has a severe lung malformation that is different from the $Gli2$ null mouse alone. The $Gli2^{-/-};Gli3^{+/-}$ combined mutation results in a lung that has a single lung lobe that appears to result from the merging of the right and left primary lung buds due to the formation of an ectopic lung bud between the two (108). Thus it appears that there are overlapping yet distinct effects of each of the GLI proteins on pulmonary development. This most likely is an evolutionary development of the three proteins from their individual homologous ancestor Cubitus interruptus (CI). One final SHH pathway dual mutation that has shown interesting effects is the combined $Shh^{-/-};Gli3^{-/-}$ double null mutant. These mice actually show a developmental recovery over the individual Shh null lung, showing enhanced vasculogenesis and growth potential (109). This appears to result from decreased levels of GLI3 repressor (GLI3R), which is normally kept in check by proper SHH signaling. Since loss of SHH results in an up-regulation of GLI3R levels, removal of $Gli3$ reduces the elevated levels of GLI3R in the SHH null lung, thus mitigating transcriptional repression caused by increased levels of GLI3R. For a more detailed review of the effects of GLI mutations on lung development see Rutter and Post (91).

Another transcription factor crucial to both early and late lung development is TITF1, formally known as TTF1 and NKX2.1. $Titf1$ expression is detected in the developing human pulmonary epithelium of the early lung bud. Expression continues throughout gestation, becoming more limited, but not exclusive, to the distal epithelium with levels decreasing towards birth (110). The $Titf1$ null mutant dies at birth due to respiratory failure with striking defects in the lung, brain and thyroid. While heterozygous mutants show no obvious phenotype, the homozygous mutant is born with a lung lacking parenchyma, showing development of only a basic bronchial tree composed of abnormal epithelium. The knockout model also showed that $Titf1$ is required for proper esophago-tracheal separation (111). Studies performed a year earlier using lung explants and antisense knockdown techniques to attenuate the transcript levels of $Titf1$ also demonstrated the effects of $Titf1$ on lung development (112). In these experiments the authors were able to completely block branching morphogenesis in lung explants and also noticed dysplasia of the embryonic mouse lung epithelium. Also, other lung-pertinent growth factors and differentiation markers specifically of $Bmp4$, $Vegf$, $Sftpb$, $Sftpc$ and $Ccsp$ showed decreased expression in the $Titf1$ null mouse (48). Recent work supports the observation that distal epithelial cells are not developing in the $Titf1$ null mouse lung, affirming that distal lung morphogenesis is closely dependent on the activity of TITF1 while proximal lung formation is not (113).

Like $Titf1$, $Gata6$ is expressed in the early lung endoderm, primarily at the developing tips of the lung buds. As development proceeds, expression becomes distributed throughout the entire epithelium, lining the airways. At 15.5 dpc, expression of $Gata6$ expands to the mesenchyme adjacent to the airways. Finally near the end of gestation, expression is only found in the epithelial cells lining the bronchi and the sacculi (114). Antisense oligonucleotides targeted against $Gata6$ used in explant cultures clearly demonstrated the importance of this transcription factor in controlling branching morphogenesis. This was confirmed with chimeric $Gata6$ null mice which also showed a reduction in pulmonary branching as well as reduced growth. Furthermore, the resulting phenotype of highly chimeric $Gata6$ null lungs showed respiratory insufficiency when delivered via caesarian section. GATA6 appears to play a role not only in branching morphogenesis, but also in epithelial differentiation, as evident by in situ hybridization showing a lack of expression in both $Sftpc$ and $Ccsp$ (114).

In an attempt to investigate the effect of the proto-oncogene NMYC on embryological development, Moens and colleagues (115) generated a mouse with a hypomorphic *Nmyc* mutation that revealed a lethal lung phenotype. Upon closer inspection, it was noticed that mice homozygous for the hypomorphic allele suffered from a severe reduction in lung branching morphogenesis, leading to respiratory failure at birth (116). More recent evidence reveals that NMYC exerts potent effects on cell proliferation, differentiation and apoptosis (117). *Nmyc* transcripts are detected at their highest levels of expression at 11.5 dpc, with levels steadily decreasing throughout fetal development, with higher protein levels preferentially localized to the distal epithelium. Immunostaining showed that areas containing high levels of NMYC expression overlap with cells in the S phase of the cell cycle as evident via increased Cyclin D1 (CCND1) and BrdU expression. To further investigate the function of NMYC during lung development, the SFTPC promoter was used to express *Nmyc* fusion construct tagged with a fluorescent marker. *Nmyc* overexpression resulted in increased proliferation and apoptosis as well as reduced cellular differentiation marked by lower levels of *Sftpa*, *Sftpb* and *Aquaporin 5* (*Aqp5*). The authors then generated a lung-specific knockout for *Nmyc* which resulted in a severely abnormal lung. Both the heterozygous and homozygous *Nmyc* null lungs showed reduced lung branching, high levels of apoptosis and a significant reduction in proliferation (117).

Mid Transcription Factors

The FOX family of proteins comprises a group of transcription factors that have a common winged-helix (forkhead) DNA binding domain and several of these factors have been implicated in controlling gene transcription in the lung. *Fox* transcripts have been located to both the conducting and respiratory epithelium as well as the lung mesenchyme, and regulate lung-specific promoters of such genes as *Sftpb*, *Ccsp* and *Titf1* (118). Forkhead box f1 (FOXF1), also known for historical reasons as HFH8, is expressed early on in embryonic development during gastrulation and later becomes restricted to the splanchnic mesenchyme, where it is presumed to be involved in lung and gut morphogenesis (119). A *Foxf1* null mutant has been generated, which succumbs to mesodermal and cell adhesion defects, dying in utero around mid-gestation (120). But when the Mendelian ratios were examined it was revealed that the heterozygous $Foxf1^{+/-}$ mice were dying within 24 hours after birth. However, the investigators observed there was not 100% heterozygous postpartum mortality, but approximately a 55% mortality during the first day, 5% mortality within 6 weeks of birth and the remaining 40% showed normal life spans (121). The large group of pups dying shortly after birth showed signs of severe respiratory distress, which was corroborated by the appearance of lung hemorrhage. On closer inspection it was noticed that the level of severity correlated with the observed reduction in *Foxf1* mRNA levels. Those mice heterozygous for *Foxf1* which had only a minor loss of transcript levels appeared normal in comparison with the mice with a dramatic reduction in mRNA levels relative to their wild-type littermates. This was confirmed on the molecular level through several methods showing disrupted vasculogenesis, angiogenesis, tight cell junctions, and changes in many gene transcript levels in the mice with severely reduced levels of *Foxf1*, compared to both the slightly transcript attenuated *Foxf1* heterozygous and wild-type mice (121). At the same time, another group demonstrated that on a different genetic background the effects of the heterozygous *Foxf1* mutation on murine pulmonary development became even more apparent (122). In these CD1 genetic background mice (previous experiments were performed on 129-J/Black Swiss and Balb/c mice (121)) there was a perinatal mortality rate of 90% and a variable lung phenotype including such anomalies as lung immaturity, hypoplasia, right lobar fusions and a variety of esophagus and trachea defects. Interestingly, in some of the heterozygous mice they did not see evidence of aberrant proximal-distal epithelial differentiation and the expression pattern for endothelial cell markers showed no major alterations in the lung vasculature. They concluded that in general the *Foxf1* mutants suffer from delayed maturation, hypoplasia and defective branching morphogenesis. This phenotype showed similarities to those seen in *Shh*-deficient mice and, combined with the fact that the peak levels of *Shh* and *Foxf1* expression are the opposites of each other across the epithelial-mesenchymal border, led the authors to further investigate this relationship. Results from cell culture experiments demonstrated that extracellular SHH could activate transcription of *Foxf1*. This mechanism was confirmed through observation that *Foxf1* transcripts are clearly absent from areas of normal expression in *Shh* null lungs when examined by in situ hybridization. Also interesting was the reduction of *Foxf1* expression from the area surrounding BMP4 soaked beads implanted into wild-type lung mesenchyme. Thus suggests a potential role of epithelial expressed BMP4 to inhibit the adjacent mesenchymal *Foxf1* expression. The authors also investigated whether FGF7 and FGF10 which are natively expressed in the mesenchyme could affect *Foxf1* expression. Indeed, both factors reduced *Foxf1* transcript levels although with slightly different outcomes. FGF10 was more selective, only resulting in a down-regulation of *Foxf1* in the distal subepithelial mesenchyme, possibly due to a secondary mechanism via increased *Bmp4* expression. In contrast FGF7 reduced *Foxf1* mRNA expression in a broad area around the beads regardless of proximal-distal location; however, it also caused a decrease in *Shh*. These data together suggest that *Foxf1* is regulated by FGF10 and FGF7 indirectly via BMP4 and SHH, respectively (122). Furthermore, the effects seen in BMP4 and SHH mutant experiments may be at least in part due to changes in *Foxf1* regulation. However, to add confusion to the issue, other work has demonstrated that there is altered expression of *Fgf10*, *Bmp4* and *Gli3* in *Foxf1*$^{+/-}$ lungs based on whole mount in situ hybridization and RNase protection assays (123). This begs the question: which came first, the chicken or the egg? There may not be a clear answer here, and more likely these factors are involved in an intricate balance of epithelial-mesenchymal cross-talk, with multiple layers of signaling and feedback mechanisms in play.

The implications of this theory connecting SHH and BMP4 to *Foxf1* have profound significance for many other factors during development, as demonstrated by recent gene array data showing changes in multiple transcription factors, cell cycle regulators, receptors, signaling proteins and ECM molecules (124). The array data revealed a correlation between *Foxf1* and *Notch2* mRNA levels associated with the lung hemorrhage phenotype seen in the *Foxf1*$^{+/-}$ mutant. Hopefully, future investigations into the relationships between *Foxf1* and other major signaling molecules during pulmonary development will provide a clearer picture of these vital molecular interactions.

Other FOX family members involved in lung development include *Foxp1* and *Foxp2*, a more recently discovered subfamily (118). Expressed as early as 12.5 dpc, *Foxp1* is located in both the epithelium and the surrounding mesenchyme, with expression continuing to at least 16.5 dpc, perhaps longer. Although expressed in the same developmental time-frame, *Foxp2* is epithelial-specific, becoming restricted to the distal epithelium as development proceeds, thus marking it as a putative target involved in epithelial differentiation. Indeed, both *Foxp1* and *Foxp2* have the ability to repress the promoters of CCSP and SFTPC as evident by in vitro reporter assays (118). The idea that *Fox* genes control lung cell specification is not a new concept, as it has also been previously demonstrated with *Foxj1*. In the *Foxj1* null mouse, a mouse model for left-right axis formation (discussed later) there are no ciliated cells present (125). However, when overexpressed in the pulmonary epithelium of mice using the SFTPC promoter it results in the abnormal appearance of ciliated epithelial cells in the respiratory airways. These mice also lacked several markers of differentiation, including SFTPB, SFTPC and CCSP (126). *Foxa1* and *Foxa2* comprise another subfamily of *Fox* genes that are expressed in the epithelium during lung development (127). The *Foxa1* null mouse has been generated and this mouse will survive to birth, but dies shortly after with no obvious morphological lung aberrations (128, 129). On closer inspection, it was noticed that these mice suffer from delayed maturation of the lung in both differentiation and morphogenesis at earlier developmental time points that appears to be compensated later in development (130). *Foxa2* null mice on the other hand develop severe defects in the node and notochord, succumbing to these deficiencies before the onset of lung development (131, 132). To further investigate the potential function of *Foxa2* in lung development, Zhou and colleagues (133) used the SFTPC promoter to ectopically express the transcription factor in the distal epithelium. The resulting phenotype showed disrupted airway branching and vasculogenesis, as well as arrested differentiation of respiratory epithelial cells. A conditional knockout for *Foxa2* has been generated that demonstrates that *Foxa2* is required for alveolarization and differentiation; however, no branching defects were evident (134). Combining the *Foxa1* null mutant with the lung-specific *Foxa2* null mouse revealed that these two factors share compensatory roles with one another. These double knockout lungs showed branching defects, as well as an inhibition of cellular proliferation and differentiation. Enlarged cystic bronchial tubules with a lack of functional terminal saccules were present at birth as well as a lack of epithelial SFTPB, proSFTPC, CCSP, and FOXJ1 expression. Most notable was a reduction in expression of *Shh* transcripts which correlated with a decline of other HH-related factors such as *Hhip*, *Myocd*, and ACTA2. Interestingly, *Foxa1* and *Foxa2* are not reduced in the $Shh^{-/-}$ lung (135). This research adds further evidence supporting a relationship between the FOX family of transcription factors and the SHH signaling network, both of which create similar yet distinct phenotypes upon targeted null mutation.

Another group of genes discovered to play a role in mid to late lung morphogenesis is the HOX family of transcription factors, a large group of DNA-binding proteins identified by a conserved homeodomain. HOX transcription factors are expressed throughout development along the anterior-posterior embryonic axis in separate yet overlapping domains. Of the 39 known mammalian *Hox* genes about half have been detected in adult human and mouse lungs, as well as in the newborn rat (136). While not all of these are seen during embryonic development, expression of 16 of these homeobox genes has been confirmed and their expression patterns seem to be dynamically regulated throughout lung formation (137). However, not much is known about their specific contributions to pulmonary development. For the purposes of this review we will limit discussion to those *Hox* genes demonstrating substantial influence on lung formation. A double mutant mouse has been generated that lacks both *Hoxa1* and *Hoxb1* expression, resulting in a lung phenotype showing differing levels of lung hypoplasia and a variable loss in the number of right secondary bronchi formed (138). Previous studies have shown the potent effects of RA on the expression profiles of *Hox* genes in the lung (139). More recent studies have shown not only that *Hoxa2*, *Hoxa4* and *Hoxb6* expression is up-regulated by exogenous RA, but also that RA expands their domain of expression in the developing lung (140, 141). One of the most interesting studies into the contribution of *Hox* genes in lung development arose from analysis of the *Hoxa5* null mutant. Originally described for the profound defects present in axial structure and high incidence of perinatal mortality, this mutant quickly became a model of aberrant lung formation (142). On closer examination it was shown that the early mortality seen in the *Hoxa5* null mouse was due to respiratory failure at birth due to severe pulmonary dysmorphogenesis and the lack of surfactant-associated proteins. These defects were also associated with changes in expression of *Titf1*, *Foxa2*, and *Nmyc*. Morphologically these lungs exhibit disorganized formation of the larynx and trachea, a 33% reduction in airway branching during the pseudo-glandular period, thickening of the alveolar walls, and poorly inflated and collapsed alveoli at birth (143).

Although not as expansive as the HOX family of transcription factors, there are a couple of basic helix-loop-helix (bHLH) transcription factors that play an important role in general neurogenesis, as well as in cellular differentiation of PNECs in the developing lung. Identified in studies examining the neuroendocrine phenotype of different types of lung cancers, achaete-scute complex-like 1 (ASCL1), formally known as MASH-1, is a marker for PNEC cells during lung development. When disrupted through gene targeting, it was found that it prevented normal development of PNECs during lung formation (144). This was confirmed by another group demonstrating the same principle, but further they added that another factor, hairy and enhancer of split 1 (HES1), is a negative regulator of *Ascl1* transcription. In *Hes1* null mutants, *Ascl1* gene expression is enhanced, resulting in an increased number of PNECs during fetal lung development (145). HES1 is part of a larger signaling mechanism known as the NOTCH signaling pathway. It is believed that the primary function of NOTCH signaling is to inhibit general differentiation queues between neighboring cells so as to maintain cellular heterogeneity within a cell population (146). Several NOTCH family members have been found in the lung including *Notch1*, *Notch2*, *Notch3* and their associated ligands *Jagged1* and *Jagged2* (147). Antisense knockdown of *Notch1* in murine lung cultures has revealed an important role for *Notch1* in regulating pulmonary neuroendocrine differentiation (147). One mechanism to control NOTCH signaling is believed to occur via extracellular FRINGE proteins, of which there are three mammalian homologues (148–150). Given that ASCL1 and HES1 are important to PNEC development and that transcriptional up-regulation of *Ascl1* is controlled by HES1 through NOTCH activation, it seems likely that FRINGE proteins may play an important role in lung development by influencing NOTCH signaling. To investigate this possibility, *lunatic fringe* (*Lfng*) was ectopically expressed under the SFTPC promoter in mice to investigate changes in lung development (151). Although *Lfng* is natively expressed during the embryonic and pseudoglandular phases of lung development, ectopic overexpression failed to cause changes in expression of *Ascl1* and *Hes1*. Further investigation revealed no changes in mRNA transcripts for *Sftpc* and *Ccsp*, or other lung-related proteins such as TITF1, T1A, CGRP, platelet-endothelial cell adhesion molecule (PECAM1), ACTA2, tubulin beta 6 (TUBB6), and von Willebrand factor (VWF). These results suggest that although *Lnfg* is expressed during lung development, it is not likely that it plays a role in defining epithelial morphogenetic boundaries, nor that it regulates pulmonary neuroendocrine differentiation in the lung (151).

Another bHLH transcription factor found to have profound effects on the middle phase of lung development is transcription factor 21 (TCF21), also known as POD1. Typically, bHLH transcription factors have important roles in influencing cell fate and differentiation in several different organ systems. TCF21 is no exception, as the *Tcf21* null mouse shows severe defects in both the lung and the kidney, succumbing to respiratory failure at birth (152). In the lung, *Tcf21* is expressed in the mesenchyme of the lung bud at 10.5 dpc and continues to be expressed in the mesenchyme at 14.5 dpc. In the *Tcf21* null lung no aberrations are apparent until the lung reaches the pseudoglandular phase of development, where a 57% reduction in airway branching was observed. But the most severe defects due to lack of *Tcf21* were observed during the canalicular and saccular phases of lung development, with no apparent formation of acinar tubules, terminal air sacs or alveoli. A complete lack of functional respiratory epithelium confirmed why all of the homozygous *Tcf21* null mutant mice were dying at birth. Further investigation revealed defective proximal-distal differentiation shown by the lack of *Sftpc*-expressing type II pneumocytes, and an increased number of *Ccsp*-expressing epithelial cells. This suggests that the epithelium lining the distal airways is adopting a more proximal-bronchiolar rather than the appropriate distal-alveolar phenotype. Interestingly, there was a dramatic reduction in *Bmp4* expression in the lung epithelium, indicating that mesenchymally expressed *Tcf21* plays an important role in regulating epithelial-mesenchymal interactions controlling *Bmp4* expression.

Left-Right Asymmetry

When we look at ourselves in the mirror, we see a symmetric being that perfectly reflects itself down the vertical left-right axis. However, on the inside we are quite different, with almost every internal organ showing some sort of asymmetry relative to the whole body. For review see Supp et al. (153). Lung asymmetry is an integral part of body design as it is essential to proper intraabdominal and intrathoracic positioning of other organs, most notably the heart. The most prominent players in laying out the left-right body plan appear to be left-right determination factor 1 (LEFTY1), LEFTY2 and NODAL. These molecules are all expressed on the left side of the mouse embryo, and appear to signal for "leftness" in the developing lung (48). *Lefty1* null mice show a pulmonary left isomerism, and a loss of spatial restriction of *Lefty2*, *Nodal* and *paired-like homeodomain transcription factor 2* (*Pitx2*) to the left side where they are now expressed on both sides of the embryo (Fig. 1-3). PITX2 is a transcription factor normally restricted to the left lateral plate mesoderm and its deletion results in a right pulmonary isomerism, among other defects (154). It has also become apparent that there is a variety of developmental factors that influence left-right asymmetry by altering the expression patterns of the genes mentioned above. Such factors include SHH, FGF8, N-cadherin (CDH2), activin-B, activin receptor IIB (ACVR2B) and FOXJ1. For review see Groenman et al., 2005 (155). When *Foxj1* is knocked-out in the mouse it results in a random left-right asymmetry of the visceral organs, including the lung, as a result of defective ciliary development (125, 156).

PHYSICAL DETERMINANTS OF LUNG DEVELOPMENT

Although not a molecular factor of lung organogenesis, physical forces exerted on and by the lung during gestation are crucial to normal development. There are three main physical factors that aid lung development. For review see Harding (157) and Kotecha (158). First and foremost is the role of lung fluid, as it is believed the other two factors function through force transduction via lung fluid. Lung fluid volume has been shown to have dramatic effects on lung development if it is not properly maintained. This was demonstrated in fetal sheep by Moessinger and colleagues (159), who surgically altered one lobe of the lung to drain lung fluid and the other to retain lung fluid. The lobe that was allowed to drain developed hypoplasia, and the latter that retained too much lung fluid developed hyperplasia. This is believed to result from chronic under/over stretch of the developing lung epithelium due to lung fluid volumes. This finding was confirmed by another group, who further clarified that it was the pressure exerted by the lung fluid, not the volume of fluid, that was responsible for the hypoplasia in the pressure-reduced model (160). These experiments can correlate to human pregnancies which present with oligohydramnios or Potter's syndrome (158). A vast number of experiments have been performed using tracheal occlusion (TO) in developing fetal sheep to demonstrate the potent effect distension has on the developing lung. Lung expansion induced by TO in fetal sheep was found to cause accelerated lung growth and

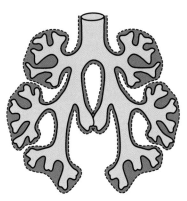 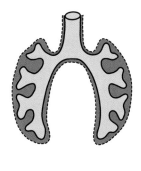

Right lobar isomerism
(Mouse model)

Left lobar isomerism
(Mouse model)

Figure 1-3 Anterior view model diagram illustrating right and left murine pulmonary isomerisms resulting from genetic defects.

was able to reverse fetal lung growth deficit within a relatively short period (161, 162). Further research has started to shed light on the molecular factors mitigating the growth effects caused by TO-induced lung distension. Specifically, increased expression of both *insulin-like growth factor 2* (*Igf2*) and TGFB2 have been documented in the lungs of fetal sheep exposed to TO (163, 164). Interestingly, recent data from experiments using a rat model of TO showed increased levels of CCND1 and possibly Cyclin A (CCNA), suggesting that TO stimulates increased entry into and progression of the cell cycle (165). Lung differentiation is also affected by TO, as there is a dramatic reduction of alveolar type II cells which appear to differentiate into type I cells through an intermediate cell type (166).

The other two physical factors that are critical to normal lung development are both forms of muscle contraction and are responsible for maintaining adequate fluid volume and lung distension, or use fetal lung fluid as the medium to transduce the mechanical forces generated. Fetal breathing movements (FBM) are periodic rhythmic contractions of the diaphragm that maintain lung distension and fluid volume during periods of rest in upper airway contraction (167). The close relationship between FBM and lung growth was clearly shown in experiments that stopped FBM by transecting the spinal cord in fetal rabbits, which resulted in hypoplastic lungs with poorly extended terminal sacs at birth (168). Genetic experiments using a deletion of the myogenin (*Myog*) gene showed that these mice suffered from lung hypoplasia due to lack of FBM (169). Mice with a similar phenotype were also generated using a double knockout of dystrophin (*Dmd*) and myogenic differentiation 1 (*Myod1*), which resulted in insufficient FBM, causing pulmonary hypoplasia via decreased cell proliferation and disturbing the normal TITF1 expression gradient (170). The clinical relevance of FBM to human development has been demonstrated in pregnancies where the lack of FBM has been linked to loss of amniotic fluid, which consequently resulted in lung hypoplasia (171). The second form of muscle contraction required for normal lung growth is peristaltic airway contractions. Similar to those found in the gastrointestinal tract, these smooth muscle contractions create a net movement of fluid into the lung via a repeating wave-like motion. Since there is nowhere for the lung fluid to escape, the net effect is an increase in pressure on the distal lung buds, thus stretching the developing epithelium (172). It was proposed that this mechanism might promote growth of the epithelium out into the surrounding mesenchyme; however, this has yet to be thoroughly demonstrated. Recent work has shed new light into the connection between lung stretch and cellular mechanisms that promote specific differentiation pathways (173). A new group of stretch-responsive molecules called TIPs (tension-induced/inhibited proteins) have been shown to affect chromatin remodeling processes (174). Specifically, TIPs will drive cells towards a myogenic differentiation pathway in the presence of stretch, or an adipogenic differentiation pathway in the absence of stretch. *Tip1* mRNA transcripts were shown to be absent from undifferentiated lung embryonic mesenchymal cells, but *Tip1* expression was mechanically induced after 4 hours of either cyclic or static stretch. Conversely, *Tip3* expression is present in undifferentiated lung embryonic mesenchymal cells but appears unaffected by mechanical stretch. Interestingly, once differentiated, smooth muscle myoblasts show a reduction in native levels of *Tip3* expression. However, upon exposure to static stretch expression levels of *Tip3* are suppressed along with myogenic differentiation. To confirm these observations, expression vectors for *Tip1* and *Tip3* were individually transfected into undifferentiated lung embryonic mesenchymal cells to check for effects on cell differentiation. Indeed, cells transfected with *Tip1* showed increased levels of smooth muscle specific gene expression and suppressed adipogenic gene expression. The *Tip3* transfected cells showed increased adipogenesis, but no change in myogenic markers compared to the non-stretched, non-transfected controls. These studies provide new evidence connecting stretch mechanics to specific molecular effectors which drive cellular differentiation to induce appropriate cell types specific to physical developmental cues.

VASCULAR DEVELOPMENT

As critical to lung development as branching morphogenesis is, it would all be for nothing without the proper vascular network to work in tandem with. These two systems have to coordinate their formation in such a way that the developing respiratory surface area will have an intimately linked vascular capillary bed in close proximity to the gas exchange surface. Also, the lung is distinct from most other organs in that it has a dual vascular system, consisting of both a bronchial system which oxygenates the non-respiratory parts of the lung and a pulmonary system which carries the blood to be oxygenated and transported back to the heart. However, much of the research into lung development thus far has focused primarily on airway branching and not vascular development. With that said, there have been some studies which provide insight into the mechanisms of pulmonary vascular development.

The development of the pulmonary vasculature has traditionally been divided into three distinct processes: proximal development of vessels via angiogenesis, distal vessel formation due to vasculogenesis and then the merging of the two through proximal-distal vessel fusion. Angiogenesis is the formation of new blood vessels from pre-existing ones and vasculogenesis is the formation of new vessels from blood lakes in the peripheral mesenchyme. These two groups of pulmonary vessels are believed to form independently and would then undergo a fusion process linking the two networks together during the pseudoglandular phase of lung development (175). This school of thought has been supported with evidence from several other investigators (176–178). More recently, two other theories on lung vascular development have been put forth. The first shows evidence that both pulmonary arteries and veins are formed by vasculogenesis and that the vessels are created directly from differentiation of the mesenchyme to angioblasts (179, 180). This theory was supported by Schachtner and colleagues (181), who demonstrated early identification of endothelial cell precursors for the future pulmonary vasculature prior to vessel lumen formation, indicating formation of vessels via vasculogenesis not angiogenesis. Furthermore, proximal and distal arteries did not develop separately and undergo a fusion event, but were continuous with each other early on in lung development. A second new theory has recently been published in which the authors show convincing evidence that disputes the other two theories and suggests a distal angiogenesis-driven mechanism for formation of lung vessels. Using the TEK-LacZ mouse to visualize the lung vasculature, it was demonstrated through careful specimen processing and analysis that even the earliest of blood vessels seen in the developing lung are already connected to the embryonic circulation. The pulmonary vascular network starts to form during the first few days of lung development in the mouse and rapidly expands and remodels with the developing airways. The authors further go on to define the "tip zone," which is the distal part of the branching airway that lacks smooth muscle cells and is wrapped in a meshwork of capillaries. Epithelial-endothelial interactions between the capillary plexus and the epithelial bud tip control angiogenesis, ensuring that the vascular network expansion is coordinated with that of the developing airways (182). This model heavily relies on vascular remodeling of the intricate microvasculature at the bud tip into larger proximal vessels as lung development proceeds distally. While they do not completely rule out the process of vasculogenesis, they advocate that it composes a minimal part of pulmonary vessel formation if present at all. The disparity between the three models most likely results from processing techniques and technologies, which result in observational differences due to the physiological sensitivity of analysis.

Molecular Mediators of Vascular Development

Perhaps the most important molecular mediator of vascular development in the lung is the growth factor appropriately named vascular endothelial growth factor (VEGF). This is the generalized name given to VEGFA, which is part of a larger family consisting of VEGFs B through D and placental growth factor (PGF). VEGF (VEGFA) also has four different splice variants, VEGF121, VEGF165, VEGF189 and VEGF206, all deriving from the single genomic copy of VEGF, with VEGF165 representing the most frequent and mitogenic of all the isoforms (183). VEGF has a variety of tasks to perform and is not just limited to being an endothelial growth factor, but also contributes to differentiation, cell survival and a variety of other functions such as nitric oxide (NO) and prostacyclin synthesis which affect vascular properties (184). Another crucial function of VEGF is its role in vascular permeability, which initially led to its being named vascular permeability factor (185). VEGF and its two high-affinity receptors, FLT1 (VEGFR1) and FLK1 (VEGFR2), have had a lot of attention directed towards their roles in angiogenesis in the past few years as they are not only important for development, but also appear to play a crucial role in cancer biology. For review see Ferrara, 2004 (186). In the lung, VEGF isoforms are expressed early on in lung development, with increasing expression towards birth. The relative distribution and levels of transcripts vary by isoform and are expressed in both epithelial and endothelial cells of the developing lung (187). Healy and colleagues (188) demonstrated that VEGF becomes restricted to the branching tips of the developing airways and state that matrix-associated VEGF stimulates neovascularization at the leading edge of the branching airways, thereby linking branching morphogenesis with blood vessel formation.

Several null mutants have been used to investigate VEGF and its receptors and all have led to the same conclusion, supporting the finding that VEGF signaling is absolutely crucial to normal vascular development. The *Flk1*-deficient mouse was generated using homologous recombination in embryonic stem cells and the resulting mouse dies in utero only 9.5 days after conception. This is the same time-frame in which lung formation starts, and therefore no insight was provided into pulmonary development. However, these mice suffered from severe defects in vasculogenesis, which suggests that lung formation, if it did start, would succumb to the same defect (189). The *Flt1* null mouse has also been generated and suffers a similar early embryonic death, showing abnormal vascular channels, most likely due to failure to regulate normal endothelial cell interactions during development (190). The developmental relevance of these two experiments was confirmed in a third mouse study which generated a *Vegf* null mutant to knockout and examine the specific effects of VEGF signaling to these two receptors, since it was known that PGF can bind FLT1 as well. The resulting mouse was quite interesting as it showed that even removal of one allele of *Vegf* resulted in a lethal phenotype, demonstrating the importance of dose-dependent regulation of VEGF. Both the heterozygous and homozygous *Vegf* null mice die early on in gestation around 9.5 dpc with a variety of vascular defects (187, 191). Interestingly, a mouse generated which only expresses the VEGF120 isoform survives to birth, but suffers from severe vascular defects, including pulmonary microvascular and epithelial branching abnormalities, suggesting a link between vascular formation and branching morphogenesis (192). Indeed this concept was also demonstrated in experiments grafting heparin-bound VEGF164 beads onto lung explants, which resulted in an increased neovascular response. Moreover, matrix-associated VEGF stimulates neovascularization at the leading edge of branching airways, linking airway branching and vascular formation (188). Additional support was also provided by van Tuyl and colleagues (193) in antisense knockdown experiments in which *Vegf* transcripts were attenuated in lung explant cultures, which resulted in decreased epithelial branching morphogenesis (193).

Like other potent developmental factors, an elegant system of control has been developed to control *Vegf* expression. The control region for *Vegf* contains elements that respond to oncoproteins, growth factor activators and hypoxia via a hypoxia response element (HRE) (194–196). Control of *Vegf* during lung development is primarily believed to occur through the HRE, as the lung is relatively hypoxic both on the epithelial surface and in the interstitium due to the low oxygen concentration in the amniotic fluid and the shunting of systemic fetal blood away from the lung via the ductus arteriosus and foramen ovale. Oxygen-dependent gene transcription regulation is controlled by a family of proteins called hypoxia inducible factors (HIF) that form a transcriptional activating complex in low oxygen concentrations. This binary complex consists of an oxygen-regulated alpha subunit, of which there are three members, HIF1A, HIF2A, and HIF3A, and one constitutively expressed beta subunit called aryl hydrocarbon nuclear translocator (ARNT), previously known as HIF1B. Under normoxic conditions, HIF alpha units are degraded by hydroxylation via proline hydroxylase which targets the alpha subunits for proteosome-mediated degradation (197). Alternatively under hypoxic conditions HIF alpha units are stabilized, can bind to ARNT and recognize HREs and initiate transcription of hypoxia inducible genes (196). Studies exemplifying this phenomenon in vitro have demonstrated that lung explant cultures grown under low oxygen conditions show enhanced pulmonary vascularization (193). The authors also demonstrated that the opposite effect is obtained when *Hif1a* transcripts are reduced using antisense *Hif1a* oligonucleotides. An even more severe example of lack of *Hif1a* expression has been created by generating a *Hif1a* null mouse. While the heterozygous *Hif1a*$^{+/-}$ mouse appears normal, the homozygous knockout mouse shows severe cardiac and neural crest migratory defects, dying in utero around 10 dpc (198). However, transcript levels for *Vegf* were unaffected, indicating another compensatory mechanism for up-regulating *Vegf* expression exists. A *Hif2a* knockout mouse was generated by removing the DNA binding domain in the second exon. While no defects were apparent in the early phases of lung development, there was impaired thinning of the alveolar septa at birth due to defective differentiation of the epithelial cells. Ultimately the delayed differentiation resulted in lethal respiratory distress syndrome (RDS) in neonatal mice due to insufficient surfactant production by the immature alveolar type II cells at birth (199).

Surprisingly no major vascular malformations were detected other than minor defects in vascularization of the alveolar septa. This occurred at the time point when native *Hif2a* is up-regulated in alveolar epithelial cells, indicating its importance during final microcapillary formation and remodeling.

Another important growth factor regulated by HIF1A is midkine (MDK), an RA-responsive heparin-binding growth factor. Originally linked to lung development through gene array analysis of glucocorticoid receptor (GR) knockout mice, MDK was found to be dynamically regulated during normal lung development (200). The authors also demonstrated that MDK is down-regulated by GC treatment and up-regulated by RA exposure in cultured day 21 fetal rat lung cells. Later experiments using in situ hybridization were able to provide a more detailed analysis of *Mdk* expression patterns. At 13.0 dpc there was a uniform distribution of *Mdk* transcripts throughout the lung mesenchyme and tubules which continued into the canalicular stage at 15.5 dpc. There was a slight drop in *Mdk* expression in late lung development just prior to birth; however, higher expression levels resumed during the final stages of alveolar and microvascular maturation from postnatal days 5 to 12. After lung development completes, *Mdk* transcripts appear not to be required for regular lung maintenance, as they are completely absent from the adult mouse lung (201). During the postnatal period of lung maturation, MDK expression co-localized with PECAM1, linking it to vascular growth and remodeling in the final phases of lung formation. This supports earlier findings connecting MDK to increased vascular density and endothelial proliferation in tumor models (202). Interestingly, in the *Titf1* null mouse there was a complete absence of MDK from the developing epithelium and mesenchyme of the lung; however, expression of MDK in other non-pulmonary tissues was still present. Further support was added through use of an in vitro reporter system using the MDK promoter. In this model the *Titf1* expression vector co-transfected with the MDK reporter construct was able to activate the promoter in a dose-dependent manner, thus demonstrating that TITF1 is a critical factor governing expression of *Mdk* in the developing lung (201). As mentioned earlier, HIF1A has also been identified as a factor capable of inducing *Mdk* expression. As evidence of the involvement of MDK in angiogenesis and vascular remodeling accumulated, the question arose whether its effect could be mediated by ambient oxygen levels like other known vascular growth factors. A link between MDK and oxygen levels was found in examination of two strains of inbred mice, of which one is sensitive to hypoxic conditions and the other is not. Potent activation of MDK expression was noticed in the hypoxia-sensitive mouse strain exposed to low oxygen levels in a time-sensitive manner, while in the other hypoxia-resistant strain it was not. Increasing levels of MDK were also correlated with increased mRNA transcript and protein levels of ACTA2. As in the case of many other hypoxia-inducible factors, HIF1A became the immediate suspect for mediating this hypoxia-induced response of MDK. Indeed reporter assay analysis confirmed this suspicion, and it was also shown that *Titf1* functioned in an additive manner when co-transfected with *Hif1a* (203). To help elucidate the morphological repercussions of increased levels of MDK as seen in situations of chronic hypoxia, an inducible expression system using the SFTPC promoter to localize expression of *Mdk* to the distal lung epithelium was used. The authors noted that while chronic ectopic expression of *Mdk* did not induce increased blood vessel formation or alveolar architecture, it did cause vascular remodeling and increased vascular muscularization during postnatal morphogenesis. This correlated with an observed increase in expression of *Myocd*, which encodes a protein known to activate smooth muscle cell differentiation (203). These experiments collectively point out MDK as an important factor influencing development of the lung vasculature during the alveolar and microvasculature maturation phases of lung development.

Recent work has discovered another key player in lung vascular development which was already known to have a significant role in blood vessel homeostasis. Nitric oxide synthase 3 (NOS3), also known as endothelial nitric oxide synthase (eNOS), has more recently come to light as an important regulator of postnatal angiogenesis (204). There are currently three known nitric oxide synthases (NOS), which includes inducible NOS (NOS2A), neuronal NOS (NOS1), and NOS3, of which the latter two are known to be expressed during lung development and appear to have a role in branching morphogenesis (205). Other experiments investigating blood vessel growth in other tissue systems including tumors have shown that NO has potent effects on stimulating angiogenesis. It appears that NO is a powerful downstream control element of VEGF, which already has been shown to be an important regulator of lung growth and vascular development (206). However, the exact relationship between NO and VEGF still requires further investigation as it appears that NO may also act upstream of VEGF by enhancing the stability of HIF1A (207). While there is a great amount of excitement and discussion about the therapeutic value of NO delivery during neonatal ventilation, NO has more recently been demonstrated to have an important effect on fetal lung development. *Nos3* transcripts were detected as early on as 13 dpc in the developing mouse lung, with expression levels increasing towards birth and located to both the airway epithelial and vascular endothelial cells (208). Mice which carry a homozygous *Nos3* null mutation have been generated and many of the null mutants show signs of severe respiratory distress at birth. Han and colleagues (208) also demonstrated that these lungs exhibit thicker septa, vascular fragility, misalignment of the pulmonary veins, and a severe reduction of distal arterioles, culminating in a lack of vascularized gas-exchange surface. These mice show a number of regulatory defects in other genes, specifically the failure to up-regulate a number of angiogenic genes during later stages of lung development. The authors suggest that the lung phenotype of the *Nos3*-deficient mouse is most likely the result of failure of proper pulmonary vasculature formation and surfactant production, mediated through defective NO/VEGF signaling, leading to respiratory distress at birth (208).

Another important group of cytokines known to have significant effects on development and stability of the vascular system are the angiopoietins 1 and 2 (ANGPT1 and ANGPT2). *Angpt1* has been demonstrated to have a role in the later stages of vascular remodeling and also to increase angiogenesis when overexpressed in the skin (209). When *Angpt1* was co-expressed with *Vegf*, it resulted in increased angiogenesis and improved vessel integrity (210). The effects of ANGPT1 are antagonized by its close relative ANGPT2 through competitive binding to their common receptor TEK (211). *Tek* encodes a receptor tyrosine kinase that, along with its other family member *Tie1*, is expressed throughout the developing vascular system (212). Null mutants for *Tie1* and *Tek* have been generated which highlight their unique roles during blood-vessel formation. *Tie1*-deficient mice have severe defects in vascular integrity and suffer from edema and localized hemorrhage. *Tek* null mice on the other hand suffer from defects in angiogenesis, failing to properly establish endothelial vascular networks (213). Interestingly, work by Pola and colleagues (214) demonstrated a link between SHH and angiogenesis, through stimulation of *Angpt1* and *Angpt2* expression. This finding motivated investigation into the relationship between SHH deficiency and *Angpt1* and *Angpt2* expression in the developing lung. It was noticed that *Angpt1* expression was dramatically decreased in the *Shh* null lung; however, *Angpt2* and *Tek* transcripts appeared to be unaffected. It was theorized that the balance between ANGPT1 and ANGPT2 is crucial in regulating the activity of TEK, and thus in the *Shh* null lung the lower expression of *Angpt1* disrupted the balance, leading to vascular destabilization and deterioration of the pulmonary vasculature (van Tuyl: personal communication). Furthermore, it appears that SHH induces *Angpt1* through activation of NR2F2 (formerly COUP-TFII), a mesenchymally located ligand-activated transcription factor (215, 216). *Angpt1* mRNA is down-regulated in whole mount in situ hybridization analysis of *Nr2f2* null mice (217).

While many of the recently discussed factors are crucial to normal vascular growth and stabilization, it is also important to note those vascular control elements that negatively regulate vessel growth. Small inducible cytokine subfamily E, member 1 (SCYE1), formerly known as endothelial monocyte activating polypeptide II (EMAP II), was first discovered in tumor genesis studies as a potential proinflammatory cytokine (218). Further investigation revealed that it is also a potent anti-angiogenic mediator able to induce apoptosis in endothelial cells (219). Interested in the effect of SCYE1 on lung development, Schwarz and colleagues (220) demonstrated that there is an inverse correlation between SCYE1 expression and vascular formation in the lung. They were successful in demonstrating that both the mRNA transcripts and the protein levels correlated with this observation and furthermore that SCYE1 expression overlapped with other known developmental vascular regulators. They noticed a 5-fold decrease in protein levels from 14 dpc to 18 dpc, a time-frame of rapid vascular growth in the lung. Interestingly, there was a significant increase in postnatal SCYE1 expression during the microvascular maturation phase of lung development, suggesting it may have an important contribution to the remodeling of the pulmonary vasculature. In other experiments by the same group, it was shown that SCYE1-treated lung allografts had a 56% reduction in lung vessel density as well as defects in airway morphogenesis and epithelial cell differentiation. The opposite effect was observed in lung transplants treated with an SCYE1-blocking antibody (221). This further supports the concept mentioned earlier in work by Healy et al. (188) and van Tuyl et al. (193), whereby vascular development influences and perhaps even guides the process of epithelial branching morphogenesis.

FINAL REMARKS

The adult human lung is capable of providing the body with oxygenated blood ranging from 4 L/min at resting state up to 40 L/min at peak exercise. At this point the body can be consuming upwards of 5.5 L/min of oxygen to fuel itself. This level of blood transport and oxygen intake requires that a large surface for gas exchange be intricately linked to a vascular network capable of moving such large volumes of blood. However, for gas exchange to be efficient, the blood must come in very close proximity to the inhaled supply of oxygen. The lung accomplishes this goal by squeezing the blood through a vast network of microcapillaries that sit a mere 0.1 μm from the outside air. This physiological diffusion distance coupled with the overall size of the gas-exchange surface of the adult lung, which is around 70 m^2, enables the lung to meet the systemic oxygen consumption demands of the adult human (48). Like many other organic systems in which large diffusion surfaces are required to couple the exchange of specific molecules between two different mediums (i.e., oxygen and carbon dioxide between air and blood in this case), nature has come up with a solution that we have labeled branching morphogenesis. In its most simplistic form, branching morphogenesis in the lung is the process of laying out hollow tubes inside the body space that are continuous with the outside environment, to allow inhaled air to come in close proximity with the vascular system to allow for gas exchange. However, in practice, this is a very complicated process. The lung is not just a sack of randomly generated tubes, but an organ that contains a vast system of airways carefully constructed to achieve maximal surface area in a confined space, which forms in close proximity to the bronchial and pulmonary vascular systems. These airways, which grow out into the body like a tree towards the sky, require careful guidance from many developmental factors such as

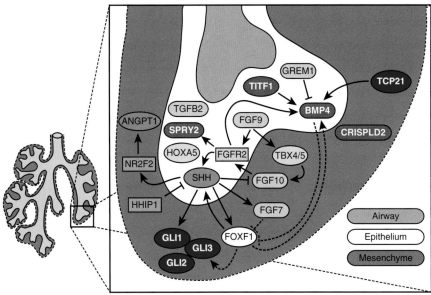

Figure 1-4 Schematic diagram illustrating putative molecular interactions across the epithelial-mesenchymal border of the developing lung. Positive (upregulation) interactions are shown with arrow heads and negative (inhibitory) interactions are shown with a blunt ended line. Those with less substantial evidence are shown by a dashed line. Not all interactions may occur directly as shown but may function through intermediate effectors.

transcriptional regulators, growth factors, morphogens and extracellular matrix molecules. We have explored a variety of factors in this chapter that have been demonstrated to have important contributions to pulmonary development, and have shown that they must be carefully controlled in both time and space in order for proper lung development to occur (Fig. 1-4). When mutations in the genes that control these factors occur lung aberrations develop and can lead to severe morbidity or mortality at birth due to respiratory failure. Further investigation into the processes controlling lung formation will provide us with the knowledge we need to hopefully one day provide better treatments and interventions to prevent the loss of quality of life in these patients and even the loss of life itself.

REFERENCES

1. Maina JN, West JB. Thin and strong! The bioengineering dilemma in the structural and functional design of the blood-gas barrier. Physiol Rev 2005; 85:811.
2. Burri P. Lung development and pulmonary angiogenesis. In: Gaultier CBJ, Post M, eds. Lung development. New York: Oxford University Press; 1999.
3. Perl AK, Whitsett JA. Molecular mechanisms controlling lung morphogenesis. Clin Genet 1999; 56:14.
4. Hogan BL. Morphogenesis. Cell 1999; 96:225.
5. Cutz E. Neuroendocrine cells of the lung. An overview of morphologic characteristics and development. Exp Lung Res 1982; 3:185.
6. Ten Have-Opbroek AA. Lung development in the mouse embryo. Exp Lung Res 1991; 17:111.
7. Alescio T, Cassini A. Induction in vitro of tracheal buds by pulmonary mesenchyme grafted on tracheal epithelium. J Exp Zool 1962; 150:83.
8. Wessells NK. Mammalian lung development: interactions in formation and morphogenesis of tracheal buds. J Exp Zool 1970; 175:455.
9. Shannon JM. Induction of alveolar type ii cell differentiation in fetal tracheal epithelium by grafted distal lung mesenchyme. Dev Biol 1994; 166:600.
10. Goldfarb M. Functions of fibroblast growth factors in vertebrate development. Cytokine Growth Factor Rev 1996; 7:311.
11. Min H, Danilenko DM, Scully SA, et al. Fgf-10 is required for both limb and lung development and exhibits striking functional similarity to drosophila branchless. Genes Dev 1998; 12:3156.
12. Sekine K, Ohuchi H, Fujiwara M, et al. Fgf10 is essential for limb and lung formation. Nat Genet 1999; 21:138.

13. Yamasaki M, Miyake A, Tagashira S, et al. Structure and expression of the rat mrna encoding a novel member of the fibroblast growth factor family. J Biol Chem 1996; 271:15918.
14. Bellusci S, Grindley J, Emoto H, et al. Fibroblast growth factor 10 (fgf10) and branching morphogenesis in the embryonic mouse lung. Development 1997; 124:4867.
15. Orr-Urtreger A, Bedford MT, Burakova T, et al. Developmental localization of the splicing alternatives of fibroblast growth factor receptor-2 (fgfr2). Dev Biol 1993; 158:475.
16. Igarashi M, Finch PW, Aaronson SA. Characterization of recombinant human fibroblast growth factor (fgf)-10 reveals functional similarities with keratinocyte growth factor (fgf-7). J Biol Chem 1998; 273:13230.
17. Peters K, Werner S, Liao X, et al. Targeted expression of a dominant negative fgf receptor blocks branching morphogenesis and epithelial differentiation of the mouse lung. EMBO J 1994; 13:3296.
18. Korfhagen TR, Glasser SW, Wert SE, et al. Cis-acting sequences from a human surfactant protein gene confer pulmonary-specific gene expression in transgenic mice. Proc Natl Acad Sci USA 1990; 87:6122.
19. Wert SE, Glasser SW, Korfhagen TR, et al. Transcriptional elements from the human sp-c gene direct expression in the primordial respiratory epithelium of transgenic mice. Dev Biol 1993; 156:426.
20. Xu X, Weinstein M, Li C, et al. Fibroblast growth factor receptor 2 (fgfr2)-mediated reciprocal regulation loop between fgf8 and fgf10 is essential for limb induction. Development 1998; 125:753.
21. Arman E, Haffner-Krausz R, Gorivodsky M, et al. Fgfr2 is required for limb outgrowth and lung-branching morphogenesis. Proc Natl Acad Sci USA 1999; 96:11895.
22. De Moerlooze L, Spencer-Dene B, Revest J, et al. An important role for the iiib isoform of fibroblast growth factor receptor 2 (fgfr2) in mesenchymal-epithelial signalling during mouse organogenesis. Development 2000; 127:483.
23. Del Moral PM, De Langhe SP, Sala FG, et al. Differential role of fgf9 on epithelium and mesenchyme in mouse embryonic lung. Dev Biol 2006; 293:77.
24. Colvin JS, Feldman B, Nadeau JH, et al. Genomic organization and embryonic expression of the mouse fibroblast growth factor 9 gene. Dev Dyn 1999; 216:72.
25. Colvin JS, White AC, Pratt SJ, et al. Lung hypoplasia and neonatal death in fgf9-null mice identify this gene as an essential regulator of lung mesenchyme. Development 2001; 128:2095.
26. White AC, Xu J, Yin Y, et al. Fgf9 and shh signaling coordinate lung growth and development through regulation of distinct mesenchymal domains. Development 2006; 133:1507.
27. Hacohen N, Kramer S, Sutherland D, et al. Sprouty encodes a novel antagonist of fgf signaling that patterns apical branching of the drosophila airways. Cell 1998; 92:253.
28. Tefft JD, Lee M, Smith S, et al. Conserved function of mspry-2, a murine homolog of drosophila sprouty, which negatively modulates respiratory organogenesis. Curr Biol 1999; 9:219.
29. Mailleux AA, Tefft D, Ndiaye D, et al. Evidence that sprouty2 functions as an inhibitor of mouse embryonic lung growth and morphogenesis. Mech Dev 2001; 102:81.
30. Perl AK, Hokuto I, Impagnatiello MA, et al. Temporal effects of sprouty on lung morphogenesis. Dev Biol 2003; 258:154.
31. Jena N, Martin-Seisdedos C, McCue P, et al. Bmp7 null mutation in mice: Developmental defects in skeleton, kidney, and eye. Exp Cell Res 1997; 230:28.
32. King JA, Marker PC, Seung KJ, et al. Bmp5 and the molecular, skeletal, and soft-tissue alterations in short ear mice. Dev Biol 1994; 166:112.
33. Bellusci S, Henderson R, Winnier G, et al. Evidence from normal expression and targeted misexpression that bone morphogenetic protein (bmp-4) plays a role in mouse embryonic lung morphogenesis. Development 1996; 122:1693.
34. Winnier G, Blessing M, Labosky PA, et al. Bone morphogenetic protein-4 is required for mesoderm formation and patterning in the mouse. Genes Dev 1995; 9:2105.
35. Weaver M, Yingling JM, Dunn NR, et al. Bmp signaling regulates proximal-distal differentiation of endoderm in mouse lung development. Development 1999; 126:4005.
36. Pearce JJ, Penny G, Rossant J. A mouse cerberus/dan-related gene family. Dev Biol 1999; 209:98.
37. Shi W, Zhao J, Anderson KD, et al. Gremlin negatively modulates bmp-4 induction of embryonic mouse lung branching morphogenesis. Am J Physiol Lung Cell Mol Physiol 2001; 280:L1030.
38. Lu MM, Yang H, Zhang L, et al. The bone morphogenic protein antagonist gremlin regulates proximal-distal patterning of the lung. Dev Dyn 2001; 222:667.
39. Nogawa H, Ito T. Branching morphogenesis of embryonic mouse lung epithelium in mesenchyme-free culture. Development 1995; 121:1015.
40. Cardoso WV, Itoh A, Nogawa H, et al. Fgf-1 and fgf-7 induce distinct patterns of growth and differentiation in embryonic lung epithelium. Dev Dyn 1997; 208:398.
41. Nogawa H, Morita K, Cardoso WV. Bud formation precedes the appearance of differential cell proliferation during branching morphogenesis of mouse lung epithelium in vitro. Dev Dyn 1998; 213:228.
42. Cardoso WV. Molecular regulation of lung development. Annu Rev Physiol 2001; 63:471.
43. Mason IJ, Fuller-Pace F, Smith R, et al. Fgf-7 (keratinocyte growth factor) expression during mouse development suggests roles in myogenesis, forebrain regionalisation and epithelial-mesenchymal interactions. Mech Dev 1994; 45:15.
44. Post M, Souza P, Liu J, et al. Keratinocyte growth factor and its receptor are involved in regulating early lung branching. Development 1996; 122:3107.
45. Simonet WS, DeRose ML, Bucay N, et al. Pulmonary malformation in transgenic mice expressing human keratinocyte growth factor in the lung. Proc Natl Acad Sci USA 1995; 92:12461.

46. Guo L, Degenstein L, Fuchs E. Keratinocyte growth factor is required for hair development but not for wound healing. Genes Dev 1996; 10:165.

47. Muglia LJ, Bae DS, Brown TT, et al. Proliferation and differentiation defects during lung development in corticotropin-releasing hormone-deficient mice. Am J Respir Cell Mol Biol 1999; 20:181.

48. Warburton D, Schwarz M, Tefft D, et al. The molecular basis of lung morphogenesis. Mech Dev 2000; 92:55.

49. Serra R, Pelton RW, Moses HL. Tgf beta 1 inhibits branching morphogenesis and n-myc expression in lung bud organ cultures. Development 1994; 120:2153.

50. Zhou L, Dey CR, Wert SE, et al. Arrested lung morphogenesis in transgenic mice bearing an sp-c-tgf-beta 1 chimeric gene. Dev Biol 1996; 175:227.

51. Liu J, Tseu I, Wang J, et al. Transforming growth factor beta2, but not beta1 and beta3, is critical for early rat lung branching. Dev Dyn 2000; 217:343.

52. Kulkarni AB, Huh CG, Becker D, et al. Transforming growth factor beta 1 null mutation in mice causes excessive inflammatory response and early death. Proc Natl Acad Sci USA 1993; 90:770.

53. Shull MM, Ormsby I, Kier AB, et al. Targeted disruption of the mouse transforming growth factor-beta 1 gene results in multifocal inflammatory disease. Nature 1992; 359:693.

54. Sanford LP, Ormsby I, Gittenberger-de Groot AC, et al. Tgfbeta2 knockout mice have multiple developmental defects that are non-overlapping with other tgfbeta knockout phenotypes. Development 1997; 124:2659.

55. Cheng HL, Schneider SL, Kane CM, et al. Tgf-beta 2 gene and protein expression in maternal and fetal tissues at various stages of murine development. J Reprod Immunol 1993; 25:133.

56. Kaartinen V, Voncken JW, Shuler C, et al. Abnormal lung development and cleft palate in mice lacking tgf-beta 3 indicates defects of epithelial-mesenchymal interaction. Nat Genet 1995; 11:415.

57. Wang J, Kuliszewski M, Yee W, et al. Cloning and expression of glucocorticoid-induced genes in fetal rat lung fibroblasts. Transforming growth factor-beta 3. J Biol Chem 1995; 270:2722.

58. Yee W, Wang J, Liu J, et al. Glucocorticoid-induced tropoelastin expression is mediated via transforming growth factor-beta 3. Am J Physiol 1996; 270:L992.

59. Shi W, Heisterkamp N, Groffen J, et al. Tgf-beta3-null mutation does not abrogate fetal lung maturation in vivo by glucocorticoids. Am J Physiol 1999; 277:L1205.

60. Zhao J, Lee M, Smith S, et al. Abrogation of smad3 and smad2 or of smad4 gene expression positively regulates murine embryonic lung branching morphogenesis in culture. Dev Biol 1998; 194:182.

61. Zhao J, Shi W, Chen H, et al. Smad7 and smad6 differentially modulate transforming growth factor beta-induced inhibition of embryonic lung morphogenesis. J Biol Chem 2000; 275:23992.

62. Colvin JS, Bohne BA, Harding GW, et al. Skeletal overgrowth and deafness in mice lacking fibroblast growth factor receptor 3. Nat Genet 1996; 12:390.

63. Weinstein M, Xu X, Ohyama K, et al. Fgfr-3 and fgfr-4 function cooperatively to direct alveogenesis in the murine lung. Development 1998; 125:3615.

64. Howie S, Fisher C. Introduction. In: Howie S, Fisher C, eds. Shh and gli signaling and development. Georgetown: Landes Bioscience; 2005.

65. Bale AE. Hedgehog signaling and human disease. Annu Rev Genomics Hum Genet 2002; 3:47.

66. Cohen MM Jr. The hedgehog signaling network. Am J Med Genet A 2003; 123:5.

67. Hammerschmidt M, Brook A, McMahon AP. The world according to hedgehog. Trends Genet 1997; 13:14.

68. Ingham PW, McMahon AP. Hedgehog signaling in animal development: Paradigms and principles. Genes Dev 2001; 15:3059.

69. Nybakken K, Perrimon N. Hedgehog signal transduction: recent findings. Curr Opin Genet Dev 2002; 12:503.

70. Bitgood MJ, McMahon AP. Hedgehog and bmp genes are coexpressed at many diverse sites of cell-cell interaction in the mouse embryo. Dev Biol 1995; 172:126.

71. Litingtung Y, Lei L, Westphal H, et al. Sonic hedgehog is essential to foregut development. Nat Genet 1998; 20:58.

72. Urase K, Mukasa T, Igarashi H, et al. Spatial expression of sonic hedgehog in the lung epithelium during branching morphogenesis. Biochem Biophys Res Commun 1996; 225:161.

73. Miller LA, Wert SE, Whitsett JA. Immunolocalization of sonic hedgehog (shh) in developing mouse lung. J Histochem Cytochem 2001; 49:1593.

74. Chiang C, Litingtung Y, Lee E, et al. Cyclopia and defective axial patterning in mice lacking sonic hedgehog gene function. Nature 1996; 383:407.

75. Pepicelli CV, Lewis PM, McMahon AP. Sonic hedgehog regulates branching morphogenesis in the mammalian lung. Curr Biol 1998; 8:1083.

76. van Tuyl M, Post M. From fruitflies to mammals: mechanisms of signalling via the sonic hedgehog pathway in lung development. Respir Res 2000; 1:30.

77. Miller LA, Wert SE, Clark JC, et al. Role of sonic hedgehog in patterning of tracheal-bronchial cartilage and the peripheral lung. Dev Dyn 2004; 231:57.

78. Bellusci S, Furuta Y, Rush MG, et al. Involvement of sonic hedgehog (shh) in mouse embryonic lung growth and morphogenesis. Development 1997; 124:53.

79. Goodrich LV, Johnson RL, Milenkovic L, et al. Conservation of the hedgehog/patched signaling pathway from flies to mice: induction of a mouse patched gene by hedgehog. Genes Dev 1996; 10:301.

80. Grindley JC, Bellusci S, Perkins D, et al. Evidence for the involvement of the gli gene family in embryonic mouse lung development. Dev Biol 1997; 188:337.

81. Chuang PT, McMahon AP. Vertebrate hedgehog signalling modulated by induction of a hedgehog-binding protein. Nature 1999; 397:617.

82. Chuang PT, Kawcak T, McMahon AP. Feedback control of mammalian hedgehog signaling by the hedgehog-binding protein, hip1, modulates fgf signaling during branching morphogenesis of the lung. Genes Dev 2003; 17:342.

83. Kaplan F, Ledoux P, Kassamali FQ, et al. A novel developmentally regulated gene in lung mesenchyme: homology to a tumor-derived trypsin inhibitor. Am J Physiol 1999; 276:L1027.

84. Oyewumi L, Kaplan F, Gagnon S, et al. Antisense oligodeoxynucleotides decrease lgl1 mrna and protein levels and inhibit branching morphogenesis in fetal rat lung. Am J Respir Cell Mol Biol 2003; 28:232.

85. Oyewumi L, Kaplan F, Sweezey NB. Lgl1, a mesenchymal modulator of early lung branching morphogenesis, is a secreted glycoprotein imported by late gestation lung epithelial cells. Biochem J 2003; 376:61.

86. Takabatake T, Ogawa M, Takahashi TC, et al. Hedgehog and patched gene expression in adult ocular tissues. FEBS Lett 1997; 410:485.

87. Goodrich LV, Milenkovic L, Higgins KM, et al. Altered neural cell fates and medulloblastoma in mouse patched mutants. Science 1997; 277:1109.

88. Bergstein I, Leopold PL, Sato N, et al. In vivo enhanced expression of patched dampens the sonic hedgehog pathway. Mol Ther 2002; 6:258.

89. Briscoe J, Chen Y, Jessell TM, et al. A hedgehog-insensitive form of patched provides evidence for direct long-range morphogen activity of sonic hedgehog in the neural tube. Mol Cell 2001; 7:1279.

90. Chen Y, Struhl G. Dual roles for patched in sequestering and transducing hedgehog. Cell 1996; 87:553.

91. Rutter M, Post M. Shh/gli signaling during murine lung development. In: Howie S, Fisher C, eds. Shh and gli signaling and development. Georgetown: Landes Bioscience; 2005.

92. Zile MH. Function of vitamin a in vertebrate embryonic development. J Nutr 2001; 131:705.

93. Mendelsohn C, Lohnes D, Decimo D, et al. Function of the retinoic acid receptors (rars) during development (ii). Multiple abnormalities at various stages of organogenesis in rar double mutants. Development 1994; 120:2749.

94. Malpel S, Mendelsohn C, Cardoso WV. Regulation of retinoic acid signaling during lung morphogenesis. Development 2000; 127:3057.

95. Mollard R, Ghyselinck NB, Wendling O, et al. Stage-dependent responses of the developing lung to retinoic acid signaling. Int J Dev Biol 2000; 44:457.

96. Wongtrakool C, Malpel S, Gorenstein J, et al. Down-regulation of retinoic acid receptor alpha signaling is required for sacculation and type i cell formation in the developing lung. J Biol Chem 2003; 278:46911.

97. Kimura Y, Suzuki T, Kaneko C, et al. Retinoid receptors in the developing human lung. Clin Sci (Lond) 2002; 103:613.

98. Desai TJ, Malpel S, Flentke GR, et al. Retinoic acid selectively regulates fgf10 expression and maintains cell identity in the prospective lung field of the developing foregut. Dev Biol 2004; 273:402.

99. Yang L, Naltner A, Yan C. Overexpression of dominant negative retinoic acid receptor alpha causes alveolar abnormality in transgenic neonatal lungs. Endocrinology 2003; 144:3004.

100. George TN, Snyder JM. Regulation of surfactant protein gene expression by retinoic acid metabolites. Pediatr Res 1997; 41:692.

101. Klein JM, Thompson MW, Snyder JM, et al. Transient surfactant protein b deficiency in a term infant with severe respiratory failure. J Pediatr 1998; 132:244.

102. Smith J. T-box genes: What they do and how they do it. Trends Genet 1999; 15:154.

103. Chapman DL, Garvey N, Hancock S, et al. Expression of the t-box family genes, tbx1-tbx5, during early mouse development. Dev Dyn 1996; 206:379.

104. Cebra-Thomas JA, Bromer J, Gardner R, et al. T-box gene products are required for mesenchymal induction of epithelial branching in the embryonic mouse lung. Dev Dyn 2003; 226:82.

105. Hui CC, Slusarski D, Platt KA, et al. Expression of three mouse homologs of the drosophila segment polarity gene cubitus interruptus, gli, gli-2, and gli-3, in ectoderm- and mesoderm-derived tissues suggests multiple roles during postimplantation development. Dev Biol 1994; 162:402.

106. Park HL, Bai C, Platt KA, et al. Mouse gli1 mutants are viable but have defects in shh signaling in combination with a gli2 mutation. Development 2000; 127:1593.

107. Mo R, Freer AM, Zinyk DL, et al. Specific and redundant functions of gli2 and gli3 zinc finger genes in skeletal patterning and development. Development 1997; 124:113.

108. Motoyama J, Liu J, Mo R, et al. Essential function of gli2 and gli3 in the formation of lung, trachea and oesophagus. Nat Genet 1998; 20:54.

109. Li Y, Zhang H, Choi SC, et al. Sonic hedgehog signaling regulates gli3 processing, mesenchymal proliferation, and differentiation during mouse lung organogenesis. Dev Biol 2004; 270:214.

110. Stahlman MT, Gray ME, Whitsett JA. Expression of thyroid transcription factor-1(ttf-1) in fetal and neonatal human lung. J Histochem Cytochem 1996; 44:673.

111. Kimura S, Hara Y, Pineau T, et al. The t/ebp null mouse: Thyroid-specific enhancer-binding protein is essential for the organogenesis of the thyroid, lung, ventral forebrain, and pituitary. Genes Dev 1996; 10:60.

112. Minoo P, Hamdan H, Bu D, et al. Ttf-1 regulates lung epithelial morphogenesis. Dev Biol 1995; 172:694.

113. Yuan B, Li C, Kimura S, et al. Inhibition of distal lung morphogenesis in nkx2.1(-/-) embryos. Dev Dyn 2000; 217:180.

114. Keijzer R, van Tuyl M, Meijers C, et al. The transcription factor gata6 is essential for branching morphogenesis and epithelial cell differentiation during fetal pulmonary development. Development 2001; 128:503.

115. Moens CB, Auerbach AB, Conlon RA, et al. A targeted mutation reveals a role for n-myc in branching morphogenesis in the embryonic mouse lung. Genes Dev 1992; 6:691.

116. Moens CB, Stanton BR, Parada LF, et al. Defects in heart and lung development in compound heterozygotes for two different targeted mutations at the n-myc locus. Development 1993; 119:485.

117. Okubo T, Knoepfler PS, Eisenman RN, et al. Nmyc plays an essential role during lung development as a dosage-sensitive regulator of progenitor cell proliferation and differentiation. Development 2005; 132:1363.

118. Shu W, Yang H, Zhang L, et al. Characterization of a new subfamily of winged-helix/forkhead (fox) genes that are expressed in the lung and act as transcriptional repressors. J Biol Chem 2001; 276:27488.

119. Peterson RS, Lim L, Ye H, et al. The winged helix transcriptional activator hfh-8 is expressed in the mesoderm of the primitive streak stage of mouse embryos and its cellular derivatives. Mech Dev 1997; 69:53.

120. Mahlapuu M, Ormestad M, Enerback S, et al. The forkhead transcription factor foxf1 is required for differentiation of extra-embryonic and lateral plate mesoderm. Development 2001; 128:155.

121. Kalinichenko VV, Lim L, Stolz DB, et al. Defects in pulmonary vasculature and perinatal lung hemorrhage in mice heterozygous null for the forkhead box f1 transcription factor. Dev Biol 2001; 235:489.

122. Mahlapuu M, Enerback S, Carlsson P. Haploinsufficiency of the forkhead gene foxf1, a target for sonic hedgehog signaling, causes lung and foregut malformations. Development 2001; 128:2397.

123. Lim L, Kalinichenko VV, Whitsett JA, et al. Fusion of lung lobes and vessels in mouse embryos heterozygous for the forkhead box f1 targeted allele. Am J Physiol Lung Cell Mol Physiol 2002; 282:L1012.

124. Kalinichenko VV, Gusarova GA, Kim IM, et al. Foxf1 haploinsufficiency reduces notch-2 signaling during mouse lung development. Am J Physiol Lung Cell Mol Physiol 2004; 286:L521.

125. Chen J, Knowles HJ, Hebert JL, et al. Mutation of the mouse hepatocyte nuclear factor/forkhead homologue 4 gene results in an absence of cilia and random left-right asymmetry. J Clin Invest 1998; 102:1077.

126. Tichelaar JW, Lim L, Costa RH, et al. Hnf-3/forkhead homologue-4 influences lung morphogenesis and respiratory epithelial cell differentiation in vivo. Dev Biol 1999; 213:405.

127. Monaghan AP, Kaestner KH, Grau E, et al. Postimplantation expression patterns indicate a role for the mouse forkhead/hnf-3 alpha, beta and gamma genes in determination of the definitive endoderm, chordamesoderm and neuroectoderm. Development 1993; 119:567.

128. Kaestner KH, Katz J, Liu Y, et al. Inactivation of the winged helix transcription factor hnf3alpha affects glucose homeostasis and islet glucagon gene expression in vivo. Genes Dev 1999; 13:495.

129. Shih DQ, Navas MA, Kuwajima S, et al. Impaired glucose homeostasis and neonatal mortality in hepatocyte nuclear factor 3alpha-deficient mice. Proc Natl Acad Sci USA 1999; 96:10152.

130. Besnard V, Wert SE, Kaestner KH, et al. Stage-specific regulation of respiratory epithelial cell differentiation by foxa1. Am J Physiol Lung Cell Mol Physiol 2005; 289:L750.

131. Ang SL, Rossant J. Hnf-3 beta is essential for node and notochord formation in mouse development. Cell 1994; 78:561.

132. Weinstein DC, Ruiz i Altaba A, Chen WS, et al. The winged-helix transcription factor hnf-3 beta is required for notochord development in the mouse embryo. Cell 1994; 78:575.

133. Zhou L, Dey CR, Wert SE, et al. Hepatocyte nuclear factor-3beta limits cellular diversity in the developing respiratory epithelium and alters lung morphogenesis in vivo. Dev Dyn 1997; 210:305.

134. Wan H, Kaestner KH, Ang SL, et al. Foxa2 regulates alveolarization and goblet cell hyperplasia. Development 2004; 131:953.

135. Wan H, Dingle S, Xu Y, et al. Compensatory roles of foxa1 and foxa2 during lung morphogenesis. J Biol Chem 2005; 280:13809.

136. Kappen C. Hox genes in the lung. Am J Respir Cell Mol Biol 1996; 15:156.

137. Golpon HA, Geraci MW, Moore MD, et al. Hox genes in human lung: altered expression in primary pulmonary hypertension and emphysema. Am J Pathol 2001; 158:955.

138. Rossel M, Capecchi MR. Mice mutant for both hoxa1 and hoxb1 show extensive remodeling of the hindbrain and defects in craniofacial development. Development 1999; 126:5027.

139. Bogue CW, Gross I, Vasavada H, et al. Identification of hox genes in newborn lung and effects of gestational age and retinoic acid on their expression. Am J Physiol 1994; 266:L448.

140. Cardoso WV, Mitsialis SA, Brody JS, et al. Retinoic acid alters the expression of pattern-related genes in the developing rat lung. Dev Dyn 1996; 207:47.

141. Packer AI, Mailutha KG, Ambrozewicz LA, et al. Regulation of the hoxa4 and hoxa5 genes in the embryonic mouse lung by retinoic acid and tgfbeta1: implications for lung development and patterning. Dev Dyn 2000; 217:62.

142. Jeannotte L, Lemieux M, Charron J, et al. Specification of axial identity in the mouse: role of the hoxa-5 (hox1.3) gene. Genes Dev 1993; 7:2085.

143. Aubin J, Lemieux M, Tremblay M, et al. Early postnatal lethality in hoxa-5 mutant mice is attributable to respiratory tract defects. Dev Biol 1997; 192:432.

144. Borges M, Linnoila RI, van de Velde HJ, et al. An achaete-scute homologue essential for neuroendocrine differentiation in the lung. Nature 1997; 386:852.

145. Ito T, Udaka N, Yazawa T, et al. Basic helix-loop-helix transcription factors regulate the neuroendocrine differentiation of fetal mouse pulmonary epithelium. Development 2000; 127:3913.

146. Artavanis-Tsakonas S, Rand MD, Lake RJ. Notch signaling: cell fate control and signal integration in development. Science 1999; 284:770.

147. Kong Y, Glickman J, Subramaniam M, et al. Functional diversity of notch family genes in fetal lung development. Am J Physiol Lung Cell Mol Physiol 2004; 286:L1075.

148. Johnston SH, Rauskolb C, Wilson R, et al. A family of mammalian fringe genes implicated in boundary determination and the notch pathway. Development 1997; 124:2245.

149. Panin VM, Papayannopoulos V, Wilson R, et al. Fringe modulates notch-ligand interactions. Nature 1997; 387:908.

150. Wu JY, Rao Y. Fringe: defining borders by regulating the notch pathway. Curr Opin Neurobiol 1999; 9:537.

151. van Tuyl M, Groenman F, Kuliszewski M, et al. Overexpression of lunatic fringe does not affect epithelial cell differentiation in the developing mouse lung. Am J Physiol Lung Cell Mol Physiol 2005; 288:L672.

152. Quaggin SE, Schwartz L, Cui S, et al. The basic-helix-loop-helix protein pod1 is critically important for kidney and lung organogenesis. Development 1999; 126:5771.

153. Supp DM, Brueckner M, Potter SS. Handed asymmetry in the mouse: understanding how things go right (or left) by studying how they go wrong. Semin Cell Dev Biol 1998; 9:77.

154. Lin CR, Kioussi C, O'Connell S, et al. Pitx2 regulates lung asymmetry, cardiac positioning and pituitary and tooth morphogenesis. Nature 1999; 401:279.

155. Groenman F, Unger S, Post M. The molecular basis for abnormal human lung development. Biol Neonate 2005; 87:164.

156. Tamakoshi T, Itakura T, Chandra A, et al. Roles of the foxj1 and inv genes in the left-right determination of internal organs in mice. Biochem Biophys Res Commun 2006; 339:932.

157. Harding R. Fetal pulmonary development: the role of respiratory movements. Equine Vet J 1997; Suppl 32.

158. Kotecha S. Lung growth for beginners. Paediatr Respir Rev 2000; 1:308.

159. Moessinger AC, Harding R, Adamson TM, et al. Role of lung fluid volume in growth and maturation of the fetal sheep lung. J Clin Invest 1990; 86:1270.

160. Kizilcan F, Tanyel FC, Cakar N, et al. The effect of low amniotic pressure without oligohydramnios on fetal lung development in a rabbit model. Am J Obstet Gynecol 1995; 173:36.

161. Nardo L, Hooper SB, Harding R. Lung hypoplasia can be reversed by short-term obstruction of the trachea in fetal sheep. Pediatr Res 1995; 38:690.

162. Nardo L, Hooper SB, Harding R. Stimulation of lung growth by tracheal obstruction in fetal sheep: relation to luminal pressure and lung liquid volume. Pediatr Res 1998; 43:184.

163. Hooper SB, Han VK, Harding R. Changes in lung expansion alter pulmonary DNA synthesis and igf-ii gene expression in fetal sheep. Am J Physiol 1993; 265:L403.

164. Quinn TM, Sylvester KG, Kitano Y, et al. Tgf-beta2 is increased after fetal tracheal occlusion. J Pediatr Surg 1999; 34:701.

165. Yoshizawa J, Chapin CJ, Sbragia L, et al. Tracheal occlusion stimulates cell cycle progression and type i cell differentiation in lungs of fetal rats. Am J Physiol Lung Cell Mol Physiol 2003; 285:L344.

166. Flecknoe S, Harding R, Maritz G, et al. Increased lung expansion alters the proportions of type i and type ii alveolar epithelial cells in fetal sheep. Am J Physiol Lung Cell Mol Physiol 2000; 278:L1180.

167. Hooper SB, Harding R. Fetal lung liquid: a major determinant of the growth and functional development of the fetal lung. Clin Exp Pharmacol Physiol 1995; 22:235.

168. Wigglesworth JS, Desai R. Effect on lung growth of cervical cord section in the rabbit fetus. Early Hum Dev 1979; 3:51.

169. Tseng BS, Cavin ST, Booth FW, et al. Pulmonary hypoplasia in the myogenin null mouse embryo. Am J Respir Cell Mol Biol 2000; 22:304.

170. Inanlou MR, Kablar B. Abnormal development of the diaphragm in mdx:Myod-/-(9th) embryos leads to pulmonary hypoplasia. Int J Dev Biol 2003; 47:363.

171. Roberts AB, Mitchell J. Pulmonary hypoplasia and fetal breathing in preterm premature rupture of membranes. Early Hum Dev 1995; 41:27.

172. Schittny JC, Miserocchi G, Sparrow MP. Spontaneous peristaltic airway contractions propel lung liquid through the bronchial tree of intact and fetal lung explants. Am J Respir Cell Mol Biol 2000; 23:11.

173. Jakkaraju S, Zhe X, Schuger L. Role of stretch in activation of smooth muscle cell lineage. Trends Cardiovasc Med 2003; 13:330.

174. Jakkaraju S, Zhe X, Pan D, et al. Tips are tension-responsive proteins involved in myogenic versus adipogenic differentiation. Dev Cell 2005; 9:39.

175. deMello DE, Sawyer D, Galvin N, et al. Early fetal development of lung vasculature. Am J Respir Cell Mol Biol 1997; 16:568.

176. deMello DE, Reid LM. Embryonic and early fetal development of human lung vasculature and its functional implications. Pediatr Dev Pathol 2000; 3:439.

177. Han RN, Post M, Tanswell AK, et al. Insulin-like growth factor-i receptor-mediated vasculogenesis/angiogenesis in human lung development. Am J Respir Cell Mol Biol 2003; 28:159.

178. Maeda S, Suzuki S, Suzuki T, et al. Analysis of intrapulmonary vessels and epithelial-endothelial interactions in the human developing lung. Lab Invest 2002; 82:293.

179. Hall SM, Hislop AA, Haworth SG. Origin, differentiation, and maturation of human pulmonary veins. Am J Respir Cell Mol Biol 2002; 26:333.

180. Hall SM, Hislop AA, Pierce CM, et al. Prenatal origins of human intrapulmonary arteries: formation and smooth muscle maturation. Am J Respir Cell Mol Biol 2000; 23:194.

181. Schachtner SK, Wang Y, Scott Baldwin H. Qualitative and quantitative analysis of embryonic pulmonary vessel formation. Am J Respir Cell Mol Biol 2000; 22:157.

182. Parera MC, van Dooren M, van Kempen M, et al. Distal angiogenesis: a new concept for lung vascular morphogenesis. Am J Physiol Lung Cell Mol Physiol 2005; 288:L141.

183. Voelkel NF, Vandivier RW, Tuder RM. Vascular endothelial growth factor in the lung. Am J Physiol Lung Cell Mol Physiol 2006; 290:L209.

184. Ku DD, Zaleski JK, Liu S, et al. Vascular endothelial growth factor induces edrf-dependent relaxation in coronary arteries. Am J Physiol 1993; 265:H586.

185. Senger DR, Galli SJ, Dvorak AM, et al. Tumor cells secrete a vascular permeability factor that promotes accumulation of ascites fluid. Science 1983; 219:983.

186. Ferrara N. Vascular endothelial growth factor: basic science and clinical progress. Endocr Rev 2004; 25:581.

187. Ferrara N, Carver-Moore K, Chen H, et al. Heterozygous embryonic lethality induced by targeted inactivation of the vegf gene. Nature 1996; 380:439.

188. Healy AM, Morgenthau L, Zhu X, et al. Vegf is deposited in the subepithelial matrix at the leading edge of branching airways and stimulates neovascularization in the murine embryonic lung. Dev Dyn 2000; 219:341.

189. Shalaby F, Rossant J, Yamaguchi TP, et al. Failure of blood-island formation and vasculogenesis in flk-1-deficient mice. Nature 1995; 376:62.

190. Fong GH, Rossant J, Gertsenstein M, et al. Role of the flt-1 receptor tyrosine kinase in regulating the assembly of vascular endothelium. Nature 1995; 376:66.

191. Carmeliet P, Ferreira V, Breier G, et al. Abnormal blood vessel development and lethality in embryos lacking a single vegf allele. Nature 1996; 380:435.

192. Carmeliet P, Ng YS, Nuyens D, et al. Impaired myocardial angiogenesis and ischemic cardiomyopathy in mice lacking the vascular endothelial growth factor isoforms vegf164 and vegf188. Nat Med 1999; 5:495.

193. van Tuyl M, Liu J, Wang J, et al. Role of oxygen and vascular development in epithelial branching morphogenesis of the developing mouse lung. Am J Physiol Lung Cell Mol Physiol 2005; 288:L167.

194. Josko J, Mazurek M. Transcription factors having impact on vascular endothelial growth factor (vegf) gene expression in angiogenesis. Med Sci Monit 2004; 10:RA89.

195. Mezquita P, Parghi SS, Brandvold KA, et al. Myc regulates vegf production in b cells by stimulating initiation of vegf mrna translation. Oncogene 2005; 24:889.

196. Wenger RH. Cellular adaptation to hypoxia: O_2-sensing protein hydroxylases, hypoxia-inducible transcription factors, and O_2-regulated gene expression. Faseb J 2002; 16:1151.

197. Levy AP, Levy NS, Iliopoulos O, et al. Regulation of vascular endothelial growth factor by hypoxia and its modulation by the von Hippel-Lindau tumor suppressor gene. Kidney Int 1997; 51:575.

198. Compernolle V, Brusselmans K, Franco D, et al. Cardia bifida, defective heart development and abnormal neural crest migration in embryos lacking hypoxia-inducible factor-1alpha. Cardiovasc Res 2003; 60:569.

199. Compernolle V, Brusselmans K, Acker T, et al. Loss of hif-$_2$alpha and inhibition of vegf impair fetal lung maturation, whereas treatment with vegf prevents fatal respiratory distress in premature mice. Nat Med 2002; 8:702.

200. Kaplan F, Comber J, Sladek R, et al. The growth factor midkine is modulated by both glucocorticoid and retinoid in fetal lung development. Am J Respir Cell Mol Biol 2003; 28:33.

201. Reynolds PR, Mucenski ML, Whitsett JA. Thyroid transcription factor (ttf)-1 regulates the expression of midkine (mk) during lung morphogenesis. Dev Dyn 2003; 227:227.

202. Choudhuri R, Zhang HT, Donnini S, et al. An angiogenic role for the neurokines midkine and pleiotrophin in tumorigenesis. Cancer Res 1997; 57:1814.

203. Reynolds PR, Mucenski ML, Le Cras TD, et al. Midkine is regulated by hypoxia and causes pulmonary vascular remodeling. J Biol Chem 2004; 279:37124.

204. Aicher A, Heeschen C, Mildner-Rihm C, et al. Essential role of endothelial nitric oxide synthase for mobilization of stem and progenitor cells. Nat Med 2003; 9:1370.

205. Young SL, Evans K, Eu JP. Nitric oxide modulates branching morphogenesis in fetal rat lung explants. Am J Physiol Lung Cell Mol Physiol 2002; 282:L379.

206. Ziche M, Morbidelli L, Choudhuri R, et al. Nitric oxide synthase lies downstream from vascular endothelial growth factor-induced but not basic fibroblast growth factor-induced angiogenesis. J Clin Invest 1997; 99:2625.

207. Dulak J, Jozkowicz A. Regulation of vascular endothelial growth factor synthesis by nitric oxide: facts and controversies. Antioxid Redox Signal 2003; 5:123.

208. Han RN, Babaei S, Robb M, et al. Defective lung vascular development and fatal respiratory distress in endothelial NO synthase-deficient mice: A model of alveolar capillary dysplasia? Circ Res 2004; 94:1115.

209. Suri C, McClain J, Thurston G, et al. Increased vascularization in mice overexpressing angiopoietin-1. Science 1998; 282:468.

210. Thurston G, Suri C, Smith K, et al. Leakage-resistant blood vessels in mice transgenically over-expressing angiopoietin-1. Science 1999; 286:2511.

211. Maisonpierre PC, Suri C, Jones PF, et al. Angiopoietin-2, a natural antagonist for tie2 that disrupts in vivo angiogenesis. Science 1997; 277:55.

212. Sato TN, Qin Y, Kozak CA, et al. Tie-1 and tie-2 define another class of putative receptor tyrosine kinase genes expressed in early embryonic vascular system. Proc Natl Acad Sci USA 1993; 90:9355.

213. Sato TN, Tozawa Y, Deutsch U, et al. Distinct roles of the receptor tyrosine kinases tie-1 and tie-2 in blood vessel formation. Nature 1995; 376:70.

214. Pola R, Ling LE, Silver M, et al. The morphogen sonic hedgehog is an indirect angiogenic agent upregulating two families of angiogenic growth factors. Nat Med 2001; 7:706.

215. Krishnan V, Pereira FA, Qiu Y, et al. Mediation of sonic hedgehog-induced expression of coup-tfii by a protein phosphatase. Science 1997; 278:1947.

216. Pereira FA, Tsai MJ, Tsai SY. Coup-tf orphan nuclear receptors in development and differentiation. Cell Mol Life Sci 2000; 57:1388.

217. Pereira FA, Qiu Y, Zhou G, et al. The orphan nuclear receptor coup-tfii is required for angiogenesis and heart development. Genes Dev 1999; 13:1037.

218. Kao J, Ryan J, Brett G, et al. Endothelial monocyte-activating polypeptide ii. A novel tumor-derived polypeptide that activates host-response mechanisms. J Biol Chem 1992; 267:20239.

219. Tas MP, Murray JC. Endothelial-monocyte-activating polypeptide ii. Int J Biochem Cell Biol 1996; 28:837.

220. Schwarz M, Lee M, Zhang F, et al. Emap ii: a modulator of neovascularization in the developing lung. Am J Physiol 1999; 276:L365.

221. Schwarz MA, Zhang F, Gebb S, et al. Endothelial monocyte activating polypeptide ii inhibits lung neovascularization and airway epithelial morphogenesis. Mech Dev 2000; 95:123.

Chapter 2

Hereditary Disorders of Alveolar Homeostasis in the Newborn

Jeffrey A. Whitsett MD • Timothy E. Weaver PhD

Lung Maturation and Surfactant Homeostasis

Components of the Surfactant System in the Alveolus

Roles of the Surfactant Proteins

Inherited Disorders of Surfactant Homeostasis: SP-B, SP-C, and ABCA3

Clinical Perspectives

Pulmonary surfactant lipids and proteins serve important roles in reducing surface tension in the alveolus, in the regulation of surfactant structure and metabolism, and in the innate host defense of the lung against microbial pathogens. Genes controlling various aspects of surfactant homeostasis, including transcription factors critical for pulmonary maturation and their transcriptional targets, surfactant proteins B, C, and ABCA3, are required for perinatal respiratory adaptation. Mutations in these genes cause lethal and chronic respiratory disease in neonates. Analysis of the structure and function of the surfactant proteins and associated genes has provided insight into the pathogenesis of both acute and chronic lung disease in infants. The diagnosis of inborn errors of surfactant homeostasis should be considered in full-term infants with acute and chronic lung disease that is refractory to conventional therapies.

LUNG MATURATION AND SURFACTANT HOMEOSTASIS

Lung maturation is a complex process requiring establishment of highly branched tubes that lead to a gas exchange area capable of supporting respiration following birth (1, 2). By 24 weeks gestation, during the canalicular-saccular transition of lung morphogenesis, respiratory epithelial cells in the lung periphery begin to undergo differentiation marked by accumulation and then utilization of glycogen stores for lipid synthesis. During the saccular stage of development, structural and biochemical maturation of the lung proceeds, associated with increasing vascularization of peripheral airspaces and thinning of the pulmonary mesenchyme. Interactions between mesenchymal fibroblasts and the epithelium result in the differentiation of type II epithelial cells, with their characteristic lamellar body inclusions, a storage granule for pulmonary surfactant. Type II cells differentiate to produce the highly differentiated squamous type I epithelial cells that form an increasing proportion of the saccular-alveolar surface of the lung with advancing gestation. In the normal lung, differentiation of the type II epithelial cell begins at 24–26 weeks gestation and can be precociously induced by infection or hormonal stimulation with glucocorticoids (3). Lack of pulmonary surfactant in preterm infants causes respiratory distress syndrome (RDS), a major cause of neonatal morbidity and mortality.

The biochemical maturation of type II epithelial cells is marked by increased synthesis and storage of surfactant lipids highly enriched in phosphatidylcholine and phosphatidylglycerol. The enzymes regulating surfactant lipid synthesis, including fatty acid synthase, cytidylyltransferase, acyltransferase, and steroyl coA-desaturase, increase with advancing gestation and probably play important roles in the induction of surfactant lipid synthesis that occurs prior to birth (4). At the ultrastructural level, particulate glycogen becomes dispersed and is used as substrate for surfactant lipid synthesis. Lamellar bodies, the storage organelle of pulmonary surfactant, increase in number and size, being initially observed within the pools of particulate glycogen at early stages of development. These intracellular inclusions become an increasingly prominent feature of type II epithelial cells with advancing gestation as lung phospholipid content increases prior to birth. Lamellar bodies are multilamellated intracellular inclusions that are enriched in the surfactant lipids and the surfactant proteins, SP-B and SP-C. Prior to birth, lamellar body contents are secreted into the airways and can be measured in amniotic fluid. Surfactant secretion is induced during labor and with initiation of ventilation following birth.

COMPONENTS OF THE SURFACTANT SYSTEM IN THE ALVEOLUS

Surfactant lipids and proteins are secreted by the type II epithelial cells into the airways of the fetal lung and can be measured in the amniotic fluid, serving as useful clinical indicators of pulmonary maturation. The L/S ratio (lecithin/sphingomyelin), DPPC (dipalmitoylphosphatidlycholine), SatPC (saturated phosphatidylcholine), and the surfactant proteins A and B have been measured in amniotic fluid or lung aspirates to predict lung maturation and therefore the risk of RDS in preterm infants. After birth, lamellar bodies are secreted into the alveoli and unravel to form extended tubes and sheets characterized by the formation of tubular myelin, the predominant pool of large aggregate surfactant in the postnatal lung. SP-A, SP-B, and the surfactant lipids are required for the formation of tubular myelin. The surfactant film, consisting of multilayers formed by sheets of lipids and proteins, creates a hydrophobic interface that reduces surface tension at the air-liquid interface established with the initiation of ventilation (Fig. 2-1).

Surfactant spreads and is dynamically compressed during the respiratory cycle, but respreads rapidly to maintain low surface tension, preventing alveolar collapse. The surfactant film consists primarily of phospholipids whose spreading and stability requires the surfactant proteins SP-B and SP-C (5). Absence of surfactant is associated with pulmonary immaturity in the preterm infant. Loss or inactivation of surfactant in mature infants, as occurs with pulmonary hemorrhage, edema, meconium aspiration, and/or infection, can also cause respiratory distress. Loss of surfactant in neonates or older individuals causes atelectasis and pulmonary dysfunction typical of RDS and adult respiratory distress syndrome (ARDS). Surfactant lipids and proteins are recycled and catabolized by the respiratory epithelium. A fraction of surfactant lipids and proteins are taken up by type II cells, degraded, and/or recycled. A small amount of surfactant is cleared by alveolar macrophages in a process controlled by granulocyte-macrophage colony stimulating factor (GM-CSF). Remarkably, defects in GM-CSF signaling, whether caused by auto-antibodies against GM-CSF or defects in the GM-CSF receptor (common ß-chain), cause the accumulation of surfactant in alveolar spaces, as is typical of adult pulmonary alveolar proteinosis (PAP). Auto-antibodies against GM-CSF have been shown to be the cause of idiopathic pulmonary alveolar proteinosis in adult patients (6 for review).

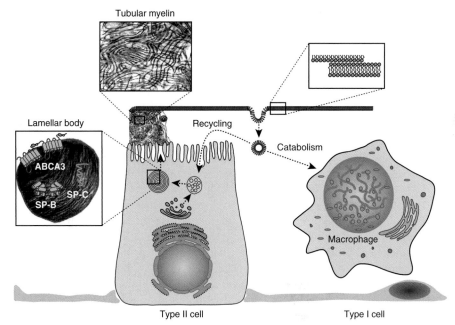

Figure 2-1 Surfactant homeostasis. Surfactant lipids and proteins are synthesized by type II alveolar cells, routed through the ER and Golgi to the lamellar bodies. Lamellar bodies are secreted into the airspace forming tubular myelin and the surface active lipid layers. Surfactant is reutilized by type II cells and catabolized by alveolar macrophages.

Surfactant homeostasis is therefore a complex process that requires the regulated expression of proteins involved in the uptake, metabolism, biosynthesis, routing and packaging of surfactant lipids, the expression, routing, and processing of surfactant proteins, and the formation of lamellar bodies, tubular myelin, and surfactant films required to reduce surface tension. Levels of surfactant proteins and lipids are tightly controlled by processes involved in their expression, reuptake and recycling, and catabolism that are regulated in an integrated fashion to maintain surfactant homeostasis before and after birth (Fig. 2-1).

ROLES OF THE SURFACTANT PROTEINS

Four surfactant proteins, SP-A, SP-B, SP-C, and SP-D, have been identified that each play distinct and important roles in alveolar homeostasis in the mammalian lung. Surfactant proteins A and D (SP-A and SP-D) are structurally related members of the collectin family of host defense proteins that are expressed selectively in the lung (7, 8). The SP-A and SP-D genes are found in close association on human chromosome 10. These pulmonary collectins share similar globular C-terminal lectin domains (termed CRDs or carbohydrate recognition domains) that bind to carbohydrate-rich surfaces on various pulmonary pathogens. They also share an NH_2-terminal domain, consisting of an extended GlyXYGly repeat motif that forms rigid, collagen-like trimeric structures cross-linked near the NH_2-terminus by sulfhydryl bonds. SP-A is synthesized by alveolar type II epithelial cells, non-ciliated cells in conducting airways, and by epithelial cells in tracheal-bronchial glands. SP-A is enriched in tubular myelin in dense, large aggregate forms of surfactant where it is tightly associated with phosphatidylcholine. SP-A-deficient mice lack tubular myelin, but survive normally after birth, indicating that tubular myelin is not required for lung function. Surfactant lipid content and metabolism are not substantially altered in SP-A-deficient mice. In contrast, SP-A-deficient mice are highly susceptible to infection and lung inflammation following intratracheal administration of various pulmonary pathogens, including bacteria, group B *Streptococcus*, fungus, endotoxin, and various respiratory viruses. At present, SP-A is thought likely to play a critical role in the formation of tubular myelin that acts as a host defense barrier. SP-A does not play a critical role in surfactant function or homeostasis in the mouse. Genetic disorders caused by mutations in *SFTPA* genes have not been described in humans at present.

SP-D is expressed in respiratory epithelial cells, but has also been detected in non-pulmonary tissues (9, 10). SP-D is weakly associated with surfactant lipids in the alveolus where it is enriched in small aggregate lipids, and in the soluble phase after organic solvent extraction of bronchoalveolar lavage fluids. SP-D plays an important role in host defense, surfactant homeostasis, and in the regulation of lung inflammation. SP-D binds endotoxin, the surfaces of various fungi and bacteria, as well as viral pathogens including RSV and influenza A (7, 8). SP-D enhances the uptake and clearance of pulmonary pathogens by alveolar macrophages in the lung. Unlike SP-A, SP-D also plays a critical role in the regulation of surfactant lipid pool sizes and is required for the maintenance of normal, large to small surfactant lipid aggregate forms, and surfactant uptake by type II epithelial cells. Surfactant lipid ultrastructure is abnormal and lipid pool sizes are increased 3–4-fold in $Sftpd^{-/-}$ mice, demonstrating a critical role for SP-D in determining the structural forms of surfactant and its metabolism (11).

Allelic heterogeneity in both SP-A and SP-D genes has been described and associated with acute and chronic lung diseases (13). These associations are relatively weak and non-diagnostic, and the structure and functional basis for the proposed susceptibility of individuals expressing certain SP-A and SP-D isoforms remain to be clarified at present. Defects related to mutations in either SP-A or SP-D (*SFTPA* or *SFTPD*) have not been recognized in the clinical setting to date.

INHERITED DISORDERS OF SURFACTANT HOMEOSTASIS: SP-B, SP-C, AND ABCA3

Hereditable disorders of surfactant homeostasis were initially recognized in term newborn infants with clinical features of respiratory distress syndrome (RDS) who do not respond to conventional therapies (14) and in infants with chronic lung diseases, generally termed as Congenital Alveolar Proteinosis (CAP) or Chronic Pneumonitis of Infancy (CPI). In older individuals and children, these disorders have been associated with idiopathic pulmonary fibrosis, often termed non-specific interstitial pneumonitis or usual interstitial pneumonitis. Pathological findings in the lungs of infants with these disorders are similar (Fig. 2-2). Together, mutations in SP-B, SP-C, and ABCA3 represent a relatively rare cause of respiratory failure or chronic lung disease in infants, but should be considered in full-term infants with acute RDS and chronic interstitial lung disease who fail to improve in spite of conventional supportive therapies.

Hereditary SP-B Deficiency

SP-B is a 79-amino-acid amphipathic peptide that is tightly associated with surfactant lipids (PC and PG) in lamellar bodies and in pulmonary surfactant (15). SP-B is selectively expressed in the lungs, where it is produced by proteolytic processing of a 381-amino-acid precursor by type II epithelial cells in the alveolus. Levels of expression of SP-B increase with advancing gestation in association with increasing surfactant lipids and other surfactant proteins (SP-A, SP-D, and SP-C). Deletion of SP-B in mice ($Sftpb^{-/-}$ mice) and mutations in *SFTPB* cause respiratory failure that presents at birth (16, 17). Studies in $Sftpb^{-/-}$ mice, and human infants, demonstrated that SP-B is required for (i) surfactant activity, (ii) formation of lamellar

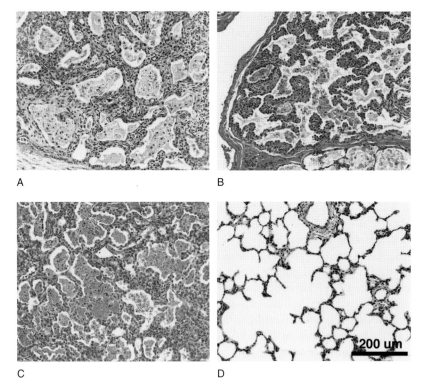

Figure 2-2 Lung histology associated with hereditary disorders of surfactant metabolism. Lung histology of infants with (A) hereditary SP-B deficiency, (B) hereditary SP-C deficiency, (C) ABCA3 deficiency, and (D) normal lung of near-term infant. Adapted from: Whitsett JA, Wert SE, Trapnell BC. Genetic disorders influencing lung formation and function at birth. Hum Mol Genet 2004; 13:R207.

bodies and tubular myelin, (iii) processing of proSP-C, and (iv) the reuptake of surfactant proteins and lipids by type II cells (18 for review). Lack of SP-B (or proSP-B) profoundly disrupts intracellular and extracellular surfactant homeostasis. Since proSP-B and SP-B are required for normal intracellular surfactant homeostasis, hereditary SP-B deficiency has not been successfully treated with surfactant replacement. Partial reduction of SP-B in mice and in patients with ARDS, RDS, and BPD is associated with susceptibility to respiratory failure during lung injury and infection (19-21).

Mutations in *SFTPB* have been associated with respiratory distress in term infants and are inherited as an autosomal recessive disorder (17, 22). SP-B mutations (25 distinct mutations) have been associated with lethal disease in approximately 75 term infants. Infants generally present within hours after birth with respiratory distress, cyanosis, and a chest X-ray compatible with atelectasis, and the diffuse reticulo-granular opacifications more commonly seen in preterm infants with RDS. The active SP-B peptide is generally lacking in BAL fluid from these infants. When *SFTPB* mutations result in the lack of synthesis of proSP-B, immunohistochemical staining of lung tissue reveals the lack of proSP-B and SP-B staining. When mutations cause the synthesis of a mutant proSP-B peptide, abnormal cellular staining and aberrantly sized proSP-B peptides can be detected by Western blot analysis or immunohistochemistry. At the ultrastructural level, lamellar bodies and tubular myelin are absent in lung tissues from patients with hereditary SP-B deficiency. Mutations in *SFTPB* affect mRNA and protein structure in multiple ways, including missense, stop codon, nonsense, deletion mutations, etc. that are identified by nucleotide sequence analysis of the gene.

Hereditary SP-B-associated disease is relatively rare, with a carrier rate estimated to be 1:2000 (23). While heterozygous SP-B-deficient ($Sftpb^{+/-}$) mice are susceptible to lung injury, no clinical findings have been associated with heterozygous carriers of *SFTPB* mutations. Definitive diagnosis of hereditary SP-B deficiency is made by identification of mutations in the *SFTPB* gene. Such analysis is currently available at Johns Hopkins University website (http://www.hopkinsmedicine.org/dnadiagnostic/services.htm). Respiratory failure associated with hereditary SP-B deficiency is refractory to conventional therapies, including surfactant replacement, assisted ventilation and ECMO. Survival of infants with *SFTPB*-related disease has been extended by lung transplantation in a small number of infants to date (24).

Hereditary SP-C Deficiency

SP-C is encoded by the *SFTPC* gene located on human chromosome 8. SP-C is produced from a precursor protein of 191 amino acids that is selectively expressed and processed by type II epithelial cells into a 35-amino-acid, hydrophobic peptide that is closely associated with surfactant lipids in lamellar bodies and in the alveolus (15). SP-C is highly hydrophobic and inserts into the surfactant lipid membranes where it alters lipid packing. Like other surfactant proteins, SP-C is synthesized by the lung in increasing amounts with advancing gestation. Deletion of the *Sftpc* gene in mice perturbed surfactant function, and caused severe chronic pulmonary disorders in some strains of mice (25). Consistent with these findings, mutations in *SFTPC* in humans are associated with acute respiratory failure in newborn infants, with features similar to that seen in *SFTPB* deficiency and in chronic interstitial lung diseases in infants and children (26). This disorder is generally inherited as an autosomal dominant gene caused by the production of an abnormal proSP-C protein and the lack of synthesis of the active SP-C peptide. Lung histology is generally described as Chronic Pneumonitis of Infancy (CPI) or Non-Specific Interstitial Pneumonitis (NSIP). Severe airspace loss and remodeling, mesenchymal thickening, fibrosis, epithelial cell hyperplasia, and accumulations of abnormal alveolar macrophages (often termed desquamating interstitial pneumonitis) are frequently reported in biopsies and pathological reports associated with this disorder. A number of mutations in the *SFTPC* gene have been identified, and approximately 50% of these patients have de novo mutations. An abnormally folded mutant SP-C propeptide interacts with the product of the normal *Sftpc* allele, resulting in the misrouting, degradation or misfolding of both proproteins, and failure to secrete normal SP-C. The intracellular proteins accumulate within type II epithelial cells, causing cellular stress responses that result in lung injury, inflammation, and remodeling. SP-C-related lung disease may be exacerbated by viral infections or other pulmonary stresses that put further stress on pathways involved in folding of proteins and their clearance.

Mutations in *SFTPC* should be suspected in infants with or without a family history of neonatal or chronic lung disease who present with acute RDS or chronic lung disease in infancy that fails to resolve with standard therapies. SP-C is generally associated with the pathologic diagnosis of interstitial lung disease (Fig. 2-2). The SP-C active peptide is generally absent from BALF and proSP-C (or abnormally sized proSP-C fragments) can be detected by immunohistochemistry or Western blot analysis of lung tissue. Mutations have been reported throughout the *SFTPC* gene, most commonly observed in the C-terminal domains of SP-C, resulting in missense, nonsense, and stop mutations. Diagnosis of *SFTPC*-related lung disease should be considered in full-term infants with RDS or infants or children with chronic interstitial lung disease. Definitive diagnosis is made by identification of *SFTPC* mutations.

Infants with lung disease caused by *SFTPC* usually present with interstitial lung disease that may be exacerbated by pulmonary infections. A recent report suggests that hydroxychloroquine might be useful in its therapy, although this is a single case report (27). Respiratory failure has been managed by lung transplantation in some infants. Although the precise incidence of this disorder is unknown at present, hereditary SP-C deficiency is a rare cause of both acute and chronic lung disease in infants, children, and adults.

ABCA3, a Disorder of Lamellar Body Formation

ABCA3 is a 1704-amino-acid polypeptide that is a member of a family of transport proteins that share the Walker domains characteristic of other ABC transport proteins. ABCA3 is present in limiting membranes of lamellar bodies in type II epithelial cells in the alveolus (28). ABCA3 expression increases in a manner similar to surfactant proteins and lipids, increasing in late gestation. ABCA3 induces the formation of the lamellar body-like organelles when transfected into cells in vitro where it regulates lipid transport. ABCA3-related lung disease was recognized in full-term infants with severe lung disease inherited as an autosomal recessive gene (29). A large number of mutations in the *ABCA3* gene have been identified, and most are associated with severe respiratory distress, presenting in the first hours of life with cyanosis, respiratory failure, and refractory to conventional therapies. Light microscopy generally shows acute or chronic lung disease, "desquamating interstitial pneumonitis," and congenital alveolar proteinosis, which is similar to that seen in *SFTPB* and *SFTPC* related disease (Fig. 2-2). While the surfactant proteins A, B, C, and D are expressed and processed in patients with *ABCA3* mutations, initial studies demonstrate abnormalities in surfactant lipid content, a finding that is not diagnostic of ABCA3 deficiency. Electronmicroscopy is useful for the diagnosis of ABCA3-related disease. Lamellar bodies are absent, and small, abnormal vesicles with electron-dense inclusions are strongly suggestive of ABCA3 deficiency (29). As seen in *SFTPB* mutations, tubular myelin is absent in the alveolar spaces in ABCA3 deficiency. The definitive diagnosis is made by identification of the mutations in the *ABCA3* gene. Unfortunately, the large size of the gene and allelic heterogeneity make the diagnosis of ABCA3-associated lung disease difficult. ABCA3 is the most common hereditary disorder of surfactant metabolism, causing respiratory failure in newborn infants, representing approximately 30–40% of such infants.

CLINICAL PERSPECTIVES

Hereditary disorders of surfactant homeostasis should be suspected in full-term infants presenting with unexplained respiratory failure associated with clinical and radiographic findings typical of surfactant deficiency, and in infants with severe chronic lung disease (chronic pneumonitis of infancy). Definitive diagnosis of *ABCA3*-, *SFTPC*-, and *SFTPB*-related lung disease is useful for clinical decision-making, genetic testing, and counseling. Clinical care decisions can be guided by careful assessment of pulmonary function, lung histology/ultrastructure, surfactant lipid and protein content, immunohistochemistry and surfactant analysis. Definitive diagnosis requires identification of the mutations in the genes encoding these proteins. At present, therapy has been supportive. Lung transplantation has been helpful in improving quality of life, and extending survival in a number of infants with these severe lung diseases. In the USA, a number of laboratories are helpful in the diagnosis of diseases of surfactant homeostasis, and can be reached using the following email accessions: 1. lnogee@jhmi.edu, 2. hamvas@wustl.edu, 3. jeff.whitsett@cchmc.org.

Considerable progress has been made in understanding the genetic basis of inherited disorders of surfactant metabolism that cause severe lung disease in newborns. It is highly likely that a number of other genes will be discovered that contribute to this syndrome of "inborn errors of surfactant metabolism."

REFERENCES

1. Burri, PH. Structural aspects of prenatal and postnatal development and growth of the lung. In: McDonald JA, ed. Lung growth and development. New York: Marcel Dekker; 1997: 1–35.
2. Langston C, Kida K, Reed M, et al. Human lung growth in late gestation and in the neonate. Am Rev Respir Dis 1984; 129:607.
3. Ballard PL. Hormonal regulation of pulmonary surfactant. Endocr Rev 1989; 10:165.
4. Rooney SA, Young SL, Mendelson CR. Molecular and cellular processing of lung surfactant. FASEB J 1994; 8:957.
5. Possmayer F. Physico-chemical aspects of pulmonary surfactant. In: Polin RA, Fox WW, Abman S, eds. Fetal and Neonatal Physiology, 3rd edn. Philadelphia: WB Saunders; 2004: 1014–1034.
6. Trapnell BC, Whitsett JA, Nakata K. Pulmonary alveolar proteinosis. N Engl J Med 2003; 349:2527.
7. McCormack FX, Whitsett JA. The pulmonary collectins, SP-A and SP-D, orchestrate innate immunity in the lung. J Clin Invest 2002; 109:707.
8. Wright JR. Immunoregulatory functions of surfactant proteins. Nat Rev Immunol 2005; 5:58.
9. Madsen J, Kliem A, Tornøe I, et al. Localization of lung surfactant protein D on mucosal surfaces in human tissues 1. J Immunol 2000; 164:5866.
10. Stahlman MT, Gray ME, Hull WM, et al. Immunolocalization of surfactant protein-D (SP-D) in human fetal, newborn, and adult tissues. J Histochem Cytochem 2002; 50:651.
11. Korfhagen TR, Sheftelyevich V, Burhans MS, et al. Surfactant protein-D regulates surfactant phospholipid homeostasis in vivo. J Biol Chem 1998; 273:28438.
12. Ramet M, Haataja R, Marttila R, et al. Association between the surfactant protein A (SP-A) gene locus and respiratory-distress syndrome in the Finnish population. Am J Hum Genet 2000; 66:1569.
13. Haataja R, Hallman M. Surfactant proteins as genetic determinants of multifactorial pulmonary diseases. Ann Med 2002; 34:324.
14. Nogee LM. Alterations in SP-B and SP-C expression in neonatal lung disease. Annu Rev Physiol 2004; 66:601.
15. Weaver TE, Conkright JJ. Functions of surfactant proteins B and C. Annu Rev Physiol 2001; 63:555.
16. Clark JC, Wert SE, Bachurski CJ, et al. Targeted disruption of the surfactant protein B gene disrupts surfactant homeostasis, causing respiratory failure in newborn mice. Proc Natl Acad Sci USA 1995; 92:7794.
17. Nogee LM, Garnier G, Dietz HC, et al. A mutation in the surfactant protein B gene responsible for fatal neonatal respiratory disease in multiple kindreds. J Clin Invest 1994; 93:1860.
18. Whitsett JA, Weaver TE. Hydrophobic surfactant proteins in lung function and disease. N Engl J Med 2002; 347:2141.
19. Melton KR, Nesslein LL, Ikegami M, et al. SP-B deficiency causes respiratory failure in adult mice. Am J Physiol 2003; 285:L543.
20. Ballard PL, Nogee LM, Beers MF, et al. Partial deficiency of surfactant protein B in an infant with chronic lung disease. Pediatrics 1995; 96:1046.
21. Gregory TJ, Longmore WJ, Moxley MA, et al. Surfactant chemical composition and biophysical activity in acute respiratory distress syndrome. J Clin Invest 1991; 88:1976.
22. Nogee LM, Wert SE, Proffit SA, et al. Allelic heterogeneity in hereditary surfactant protein B (SP-B) deficiency. Am J Respir Crit Care Med 2000; 161:973.
23. Cole FS, Hamvas A, Rubinstein P, et al. Population-based estimates of surfactant protein B deficiency. Pediatrics 2000; 105:538.
24. Hamvas A, Nogee LM, Mallory GB Jr, et al. Lung transplantation for treatment of infants with surfactant protein B deficiency. J Pediatr 1997; 130:231.
25. Glasser SW, Detmer EA, Ikegami M, et al. Pneumonitis and emphysema in sp-C gene targeted mice. J Biol Chem 2003; 278:14291.
26. Nogee LM, Dunbar AE, Wert SE, et al. A mutation in the surfactant protein C gene associated with familial interstitial lung disease. N Engl J Med 2001; 344:573.
27. Rosen DM, Waltz DA. Hydroxychloroquine and surfactant protein C deficiency. N Engl J Med 2005; 352:207.
28. Mulugeta S, Gray JM, Notarfrancesco KL, et al. Identification of LBM180, a lamellar body limiting membrane protein of alveolar type II cells, as the ABC transporter protein ABCA3. J Biol Chem 2002; 277:22147.
29. Shulenin S, Nogee LM, Annilo T, et al. ABCA3 gene mutations in newborns with fatal surfactant deficiency. N Engl J Med 2004; 350:1296.

Chapter 3

Growth and Development of the Lung Circulation: Mechanisms and Clinical Implications

Steven H. Abman MD • Christopher Baker MD • Vivek Balasubramaniam MD

Anatomy of the Postnatal Pulmonary Circulation

Stages of Vascular Growth in the Developing Lung

Regulation of Lung Vascular Growth during Development

Potential Role of Endothelial Progenitor Cells

Clinical Implications: Disruption of Lung Vascular Development in BPD

Conclusions

Not only is normal lung development critical for successful adaptation at birth, but ongoing growth and remodeling remain essential throughout postnatal life. The ability of the lung to successfully achieve normal gas exchange requires the growth and maintenance of an intricate system of airways and vessels, including the establishment of a thin yet vast blood-gas interface. Insights into basic mechanisms that regulate lung growth and maturation continue to provide new understanding of lung diseases and their treatment, in newborns and adults alike.

Lung branching morphogenesis and epithelial differentiation have been studied extensively in past decades; however, studies of mechanisms that regulate development of the pulmonary circulation have been relatively limited. Until recently, most of the information regarding pulmonary vascular development has been largely descriptive in nature. Vascular growth in the lung is not only important regarding the risk for pulmonary hypertension, but normal vascular growth and structure are absolutely necessary for establishing sufficient surface area for gas exchange.

Recent observations have challenged older notions that the development of the blood vessels in the lung passively follows that of the airways. Increasing evidence suggests that lung blood vessels actively promote normal alveolar growth during development and contribute to the maintenance of alveolar structures throughout postnatal life. Disruption of angiogenesis during lung development can impair alveolarization, and preservation of vascular growth and endothelial survival may promote lung growth and structure of the distal airspace. Understanding how alveoli and the underlying capillary network develop, and how these mechanisms are disrupted in disease states, is critical for developing efficient therapies for lung diseases characterized by impaired alveolar structure.

To better understand abnormalities of the pulmonary circulation in neonatal diseases, insights into basic cellular, molecular, and genetic mechanisms of vessel development are needed. Advances in vascular biology have contributed to growing knowledge of how blood vessels are assembled during early embryonic and fetal development. Developmental abnormalities of the pulmonary circulation contribute to the pathophysiology of diverse diseases, including persistent pulmonary hypertension of the newborn, lung hypoplasia, congenital diaphragmatic hernia, congenital heart disease, and others.

There has been a growing recognition of the importance of understanding basic mechanisms of lung vascular growth in the context of premature birth and the risk for bronchopulmonary dysplasia (BPD). BPD is characterized by arrested lung growth, with decreased alveolarization and a dysmorphic vasculature. Recent studies suggest that disruption of normal lung vascular growth may play a central role in the pathogenesis of BPD; however, little is known about basic mechanisms of pulmonary vascular injury in the immature lung and the impact of this injury on subsequent lung vascular growth and function. Experimental data further suggest a potential therapeutic role for modulation of angiogenesis for lung diseases that are characterized by arrested alveolar growth, such as BPD. Furthermore, advances in stem cell biology suggest at least potential roles for endothelial progenitor cells (EPCs) in the pathogenesis or treatment of lung vascular disease.

This chapter provides a brief overview of pulmonary vascular development in the context of understanding how lung vascular growth and thus lung structure are impaired in BPD, with the hope that insights into such mechanisms may lead to new therapies for BPD and related conditions.

ANATOMY OF THE POSTNATAL PULMONARY CIRCULATION

The postnatal lung has a dual vascular system that includes the bronchial and pulmonary circulations, which function and develop in distinct fashions (1). The bronchial system provides nutrients to the lung and perfusion of the capillary bed within the bronchial wall, perihilar structures (such as lymph nodes), and the vascular wall of elastic and large muscular pulmonary vessels. Bronchial vessels develop late and their walls reflect their origin from the systemic circulation. Pulmonary arteries perfuse respiratory units and ultimately regulate gas exchange. Pulmonary arteries branch with the airways but do not break into a capillary bed until they reach the respiratory bronchioles and alveoli. Pulmonary arteries generally split into capillaries surrounding the walls of bronchioles and adjacent alveolar walls. Intrapulmonary vessels from both systems mostly drain to pulmonary veins, whereas hilar vessels drain to the bronchial veins and the azygos system.

The pulmonary artery accompanies the airways but gives off many more branches than the airway. At least two main types of pulmonary arteries have been described: (i) "conventional" arteries, which run with an airway, dividing as the airway divides and distributes to the capillary bed beyond the level of the terminal bronchioles; and (ii) "supernumerary" arteries, which are additional branches that arise from the pulmonary artery between the conventional branches, run a short course and supply the capillary bed of alveoli immediately around the pulmonary artery. Supernumerary arteries are thought to be a very prominent component of the mature lung, with the ratio of "conventional" to "supernumerary" vessels of the order of 1:2 in the prelobular region to 1:13 in the pre- and intra-acinar region (2). In addition to differences in location, functional differences between supernumerary and conventional arteries have been described. For example, supernumerary vessels are far more reactive to serotonin-induced vasoconstriction than conventional vessels, which may have important implications regarding the regional distribution of pulmonary blood flow (3). It has been suggested that plexiform lesions of severe pulmonary hypertension may selectively develop in supernumerary vessels (4).

As reflected in the pulmonary arterial tree, two types of vein have also been identified (2, 5, 6). "Conventional" veins sprout from the points of division of an airway, travel to the periphery of a given lung unit, and combine to form increasingly large venules. Branches of pulmonary veins also arise from the pleura and connective tissue septa. Within the lung, the anatomic distribution of arteries and veins is characteristic. The bronchovascular bundle includes the airway with the bronchial artery capillary bed, the adjacent pulmonary artery and lymphatic vessels, all within a single adventitial sheath. Veins travel at the periphery of any unit, whether it is the acinus, lobule, or segment. At the hilum, veins merge into superior and inferior veins, which drain to the left atrium.

The bronchial circulation includes vessels that arise from the descending aorta, and the intercostal, subclavian or internal mammary arteries. Bronchial arteries have been classified as extra- or intra-pulmonary. Extrapulmonary bronchial arteries provide small branches to the esophagus, mediastinal tissues, hilar lymph nodes and the lobar bronchus. These vessels drain into extrapulmonary bronchial veins connecting to the azygos or hemiazygos veins, which ultimately drain to the right atrium. Intrapulmonary bronchial arteries distribute to the supporting tissue and structures within intralobar bronchi, the pleura, regional lymph nodes, walls of pulmonary arteries and veins and nerves. Intrapulmonary bronchial arteries drain into intrapulmonary bronchial veins and pulmonary veins, which then connect to the left atrium. Bronchial arteries on the walls of the pulmonary artery and vein subserve the vasa vasorum, and may provide an important conduit for circulating inflammatory or bone-marrow-derived cells, which may play critical roles in development or postnatal pulmonary vascular disorders (7). Ongoing studies have demonstrated the important role of the bronchial circulation in asthma, acute lung injury and other disease, but its role during lung development is poorly understood.

The pulmonary and bronchial circulations are distinct and generally have different responses to injury, but the exact relationship between these systems and mechanisms contributing to cross-communication are unclear (5, 6). For example, intrauterine hypertrophy of the bronchial circulation and collaterals is prominent in newborns with congenital heart disease, such as pulmonary atresia and transposition of the great vessels. Experimentally, ligation of pulmonary arteries can enhance growth of the bronchial circulation, which increases pre-capillary anastomoses and the development of altered blood flow patterns (8–10). Clinically, chronic pulmonary thromboembolic disease stimulates proliferation of bronchial vessels in and around obstructed pulmonary arteries. Marked hypertrophy and proliferation of bronchial arteries is also noted in bronchiectasis (as in cystic fibrosis). In adults with emphysema, disruption of alveolar capillary networks can be associated with prominent bronchial arteries. Prominent bronchial or collateral vessels have also been observed in many infants with severe BPD, which may contribute to persistent lung edema or impaired gas exchange (11).

In addition to the pulmonary and bronchial circulations, the lung's lymphatic system forms as a distinct circuit and has unique roles in fluid exchange, as well as in host defense and in clearing solid particles and cells from the lung. Lymph vessels form a closed circulatory system lined by endothelium. Lymphatics are evident at the level of the alveolar ducts (none is observed in direct relation to alveoli) and extend proximally. Interestingly, the caliber of lymph vessels does not necessarily increase as they move toward the central lung, with lymph capillaries sometimes being larger than collecting lymph vessels. Primary developmental defects of the lung lymphatics, as in pulmonary lymphangiectasia, lead to severe respiratory disease (12). In patients who survive, some develop chronic interstitial lung disease with pulmonary hypertension and cor pulmonale. Mechanisms underlying lymphatic differentiation, growth and function during lung development remain poorly understood.

STAGES OF VASCULAR GROWTH IN THE DEVELOPING LUNG

Lung development is classically divided into five overlapping stages on the basis of histological features (5). Although largely descriptive, changes in lung structure across these stages provide a clear sequence of events that occurs in stereotypical fashion, and allow for subsequent molecular or interventional studies to subsequently examine specific mechanisms. The first four stages, termed the *embryonic, pseudoglandular, canalicular,* and *saccular stages*, occur during gestation. At the end of the saccular stage (at about 36 weeks), lungs have formed alveolar ducts and saccules. Alveolarization, in the final stage of lung development, primarily occurs postnatally, during the first 2–3 years of life, and may continue at a slower rate beyond childhood (2, 5). Distinct anatomic changes in the lung circulation have been well described, although underlying mechanisms regulating structural changes are less clear (Table 3-1). Changes in lung vasculature during each stage and the relative roles of vasculogenesis and angiogenesis during each stage are described below:

Embryonic Period

During *the embryonic period* (weeks 3–7 in humans), the most proximal part of the pulmonary circulation, the pulmonary trunk, is derived from the truncus arteriosus, which becomes divided into the aorta and pulmonary trunk by 8 weeks of gestation in humans by growth of the spiral aorticopulmonary septum (13). The pulmonary trunk connects to the pulmonary arch arteries, which are derived from the 6th brachial arch arteries, the most caudal of the brachial arteries, by 7 weeks gestation in humans. Recent work suggests that these pulmonary arch arteries originate from a strand of endothelial precursors that connect the ventral wall of the dorsal aorta to the pulmonary trunk (14, 15). These strands develop a lumen initially at the sites of connection between the pulmonary trunk and dorsal aorta.

Table 3-1	**Stages of Vascular Growth During Lung Development**	
Stage	**Events**	
Embryonic	<6 wk	Vasculogenesis within immature mesenchyme; pulmonary arteries branch form 6th aortic arches; veins as outgrowths from left atrium
Pseudoglandular	<16 wk	Parallel branching of large pulmonary arteries with central airways; lymphatics appear
Canalicular	<24 wk	Increased vessel proliferation and organization into capillary network around airspaces
Saccular	<36 wk	Marked vascular expansion with thinning and condensation of mesenchyme; thin air-blood barrier; double capillary network in septae
Alveolar	<2–3 yrs	Accelerated vascular growth, fusion of the double capillary network with thinning of septae
Postnatal maturation	3 years to adulthood	Marked vessel growth + remodeling, as surface area increases > 20-fold

The origin of intrapulmonary arteries has been variously described as endothelial sprouts from either the aortic sac or from the dorsal aorta, or as originating from a network of capillaries around the foregut. The latter observation comes closest to the results of more recent studies suggesting that the pulmonary artery and vein develop in situ within the splanchnic mesoderm surrounding the foregut via at least two processes that probably occur concurrently; (i) *vasculogenesis*, in which new blood vessels form in situ from angioblasts, and (ii) *angiogenesis*, which involves sprouting of new vessels from existing vessels (as described below).

Vascular Morphogenesis

Blood vessel morphogenesis involves discrete steps that occur in a continuum, which are regulated by specific signaling pathways that involve soluble effectors, cytokines and their receptors, proteases and extracellular matrix (ECM) components. These various pathways control integral events that contribute to the formation of a functional vasculature, including endothelial and mural cell (pericyte and smooth muscle) differentiation, cell proliferation and migration and the specification of arterial, venous and lymphatic fates. Disruption of these processes may not only result in neonatal pulmonary hypertension but may also contribute to abnormalities of lung structure.

Formation of the pulmonary circulation has been primarily described as dependent on two basic processes: *vasculogenesis* and *angiogenesis*. *Vasculogenesis* is the de novo formation of blood vessels from angioblasts or endothelial precursor cells that migrate and differentiate in response to local cues (such as growth factors and ECM) to form vascular tubes. *Angiogenesis* is the formation of new blood vessels from preexisting ones. It has generally been accepted that the distal vasculature arises by vasculogenesis, and the proximal vasculature by angiogenesis, but this remains controversial (16–19). Vasculogenesis results in the blood vessel formation from blood islands present within the mesenchyme of the embryonic lung (embryonic day 9, or E9) in the mouse. Angiogenesis starts around E12 when arteries and veins begin to sprout from the central pulmonary vascular trunks. Around E14, peripheral sinusoids and central vessel sprouts connect and establish a vascular network. This union of peripheral and central vascular structures is accompanied by extensive branching of the arteries, which follow the branching pattern of the airways.

The origin of blood vessels de novo within the mesoderm surrounding the protruding endoderm was originally suggested by Chang (20). Recent studies using molecular markers of endothelial progenitor cells (EPCs) as well as differentiation markers support this concept (21–23). These studies describe mesodermal cells expressing primitive endothelial markers at stages of lung development that precede evidence of any connection of blood flow with the established circulatory system (16–18). These studies further establish that lung vascular development begins during the embryonic stages of lung development, continues throughout fetal life, and is dependent on epithelial-mesenchymal cross-talk. Molecular evidence is supported by studies combining electron microscopy utilizing vascular casts of the developing lung. These findings suggest that the large pulmonary arteries develop by angiogenesis from central vessels, that distal vessels probably form via vasculogenic mechanisms within the mesenchyme, and that a third process, *vascular fusion*, is necessary to ultimately connect the angiogenic and vasculogenic vessels (16–18).

Studies in human fetal lung suggest that airways act as a template for pulmonary artery development. Endothelial tubes form around the terminal buds of the airways, suggesting an inductive influence of the epithelium. More recently, Parera, et al. suggested distal angiogenesis as a new mechanism for lung vascular morphogenesis, based on morphological analysis from the onset of lung development (E9.5) until the pseudoglandular stage (E13.5) in Tie2-LacZ transgenic mice (24). In their model, capillary networks surrounding the terminal buds exist from the first morphological sign of lung development and then expand by formation of new capillaries from preexisting vessels as the lung bud grows.

Multiple stimuli contribute to alveolar and vascular growth and development, and in part, involve "cross-talk" of paracrine signals between epithelium and mesenchyme (25). For example, vascular endothelial growth factor (VEGF) is expressed in developing lung epithelium, whereas VEGF receptor-2 (VEGFR-2) is localized to angioblasts within the embryonic mesenchyme (26–29). Diffusion of VEGF to precursors of vascular endothelial cells within the mesenchyme leads to angiogenesis by stimulating endothelial proliferation, a key step in vessel development (see below).

These mechanisms may also apply to human lung vascular development. In her studies of human embryos, deMello reported evidence to support the idea that both vasculogenesis and angiogenesis operate cooperatively to form the pulmonary vessels (18). Hall, et al. also proposed that vasculogenesis is a primary mechanism for intrapulmonary vascular development (19). These investigators also suggested that the venous circulation develops in similar fashion to arteries and may actually precede development of early arteries.

Alternatively, this concept has been challenged by studies suggesting that the lung vasculature is formed by "distal angiogenesis," a process in which the formation of new capillaries from preexisting vessels occurs at the periphery of the lung (24). In this model, epithelial and endothelial interactions are necessary to induce angiogenesis and to coordinate expansion of a vascular network as branching proceeds.

Fetal Period

The *pseudoglandular period* (weeks 5–16) is primarily characterized by extensive branching morphogenesis of the airway, in which epithelial buds undergo multiple dichotomous branching. Shannon demonstrated that epithelial-mesenchymal interactions play a critical role in this process (21, 25). Early cross-talk determines the sites, frequency and timing of airway branching, but epithelial-mesenchymal communication further dictates early vascular development within the mesenchyme, which is reflected by the close proximity of vascular growth with airway branching. The formation of these conventional arteries appears to be followed by the development of smaller, supernumerary arteries between these regions. At the end of the pseudoglandular period, all pre-acinar bronchi are present and accompanied by pulmonary and bronchial arteries.

The *canalicular stage* (weeks 17–26) is a period of expansive organ growth and differentiation of epithelium into type II (surfactant production) and type I cells (key for air-blood barrier). The canalicular stage (17–26 weeks) encompasses the early development of the pulmonary parenchyma during which the number of lung capillaries markedly increases within the immature mesenchyme. The lung appears "canalized" as capillaries begin to arrange themselves around the air spaces and come into close apposition with the overlying epithelium. At sites of apposition, thinning of the epithelium occurs to form the first sites of the air-blood barriers.

During the *saccular stage* (24–36 weeks), clusters of thin-walled saccules appear in the distal lung and have formed alveolar ducts, the last generation of airways prior to the development of alveoli. Capillaries form a bilayer ("double capillary network") within the relatively broad and cellular inter-saccular septae at this stage. The interstitium between air spaces contains the capillary network and numerous interstitial cells, but only a thin network of collagen fibers. During this stage, elastic fibers are deposited within the interstitium, which lays the foundation for subsequent formation of alveoli.

Postnatal Period

The *alveolarization stage* is largely a postnatal event, with more than 90% of all alveoli being formed shortly after birth, with the greatest surge in alveolar development between birth and 6 months of age, and continuing during the first 2–3 years in humans. The final step of *microvascular maturation* occurs during this stage (5). Formation of alveoli occurs by the outgrowth of secondary septae that subdivide terminal saccules into anatomic alveoli. Under electron microscopy, the secondary septae show a central layer of connective tissue with numerous cells and very little collagen fibrils, flanked on both sides by capillaries. These capillaries appear to be interconnected over the edge of the crest, and cross-sectioned fibers of elastin can be detected at the tip of the crest or just below the capillary loop. It appears that these new interalveolar walls are formed by the alternate up-folding of one of the two capillary layers on either side of a primary septum. As a result of this process, primary and secondary septae contain double capillary network layers. This contrasts with older infants, children and adults, in which only a single capillary abuts the air space on each side. During the period of alveolarization, thick inter-alveolar septae begin to thin and the double capillary layer that is characteristic of this stage begins to fuse into a single layer to assume the adult form. Secondary septae initially form as low ridges that protrude into primitive airspaces to increase their surface area. Between birth and adulthood, the alveolar and capillary surface areas expand nearly 20-fold and the capillary volume by 35-fold. Further expansion of the capillary network subsequently occurs via two angiogenic mechanisms: *sprouting angiogenesis* from preexisting vessels and *intussusceptive growth* (26, 27, 30, 31). Little is known about intussusceptive microvascular growth in the lung. This novel mode of blood vessel formation and remodeling occurs by internal division of the preexisting capillary plexus (insertion of transcapillary tissue pillars) without sprouting, which may underlie alveolar growth and remodeling throughout adult life and thus be amenable to therapeutic modulation for lung regeneration.

During this time, the lung is undergoing marked microvascular growth and development as well. In addition, the process of septation involves alternate up-folding and growth of capillary layers within primary septa. This mechanism of alveolarization suggests that the failure of capillary network formation and growth, or disruption of the infolding of the double capillary network, could potentially cause failed alveolarization (see below).

Much more needs to be learned about the anatomic events underlying lung vascular development and time-specific mechanisms that regulate growth and function at each stage. Likewise, there is a need for endothelial cell specific surface markers to identify and characterize angioblasts, EPCs and mature endothelial cells, as well as genetic tools allowing better definition of endothelial cell fate and lineage relationships in the embryonic and the postnatal lung.

The Bronchial Circulation

Less is known of the mechanisms contributing to development of the bronchial circulation. However, molecular marker studies suggest that intrapulmonary bronchial arteries also form in situ from the mesenchyme surrounding the epithelial buds (14, 15). Early in development (12 weeks in humans) connections between bronchial arteries within the lung and the systemic circulation are made. However, how the bronchial circulation develops in distinction from the pulmonary circulation is uncertain. This question is especially interesting in light of the striking differences in structure and function between the bronchial and pulmonary circulations, and the potential roles of genetic programming versus environmental stimuli in causing these differences.

REGULATION OF LUNG VASCULAR GROWTH DURING DEVELOPMENT

Genetic Factors

Advances in our understanding of basic mechanisms of blood vessel formation in the embryo, fetus and adult have led to new insights into the biology and pathobiology of vascular growth during normal development and in diverse diseases, including tumor angiogenesis and peripheral ischemic disease. Many of the molecules involved seem to be highly conserved both across species and among various organs. However, there may be subtle differences, and a complete understanding of the signaling pathways that regulate and coordinate vessel development and differentiation in a cell-specific fashion in the lung will be critical to understanding the unique functions and responses that the pulmonary and bronchial circulations exhibit in response to many pathophysiologic stimuli. Molecular programs important for the development of the lung vasculature have only recently begun to be elucidated, and a partial list is provided below.

Although numerous and diverse growth and transcription factors modulate blood vessel formation, we will briefly discuss only a few ligand-receptor signals to illustrate potential mechanisms, including VEGF-VEGF receptor, angiopoietin-Tie, notch-jagged, Wnt and TGF-ß signaling.

VEGF (VEGF-A) is one of the most potent and critical regulators of lung vascular growth, development and maintenance throughout embryonic, fetal and postnatal life (26–29). VEGF-R2 (Flk-1) appears within lung mesenchyme during the embryonic stage, and is the earliest known marker for endothelial cells and endothelial progenitors. Beginning in the embryonic period, VEGF is strongly expressed in the developing epithelium. Studies of genetic mouse models have provided unequivocal evidence for the critical role of VEGF and VEGF receptors for embryonic vascular development. Targeted disruption of the VEGF-A gene causes severe defects in the formation of blood vessels, and loss of a single VEGF allele results in early embryonic death with a marked reduction in endothelial cells, prior to embryonic day 9.5 (32, 33). VEGF-A acts through two distinct tyrosine kinase receptors, VEGFR-1 and VEGFR-2, which are both important for embryonic vascular development. Targeted inactivation of either gene is lethal due to defective vascular development, including the absence of vasculature in mice without VEGFR-2 and increased endothelial cell number but a lack of normal tubular networks in VEGFR-1 null mice (34, 35). Lung epithelium and mesenchyme express ligand and receptor, respectively, from the embryonic stage of development and beyond. Because loss of VEGF-A causes early embryonic death, few studies have examined the roles of VEGF signaling during distinct stages of lung development. Inhibition of VEGF signaling during the pseudoglandular stage markedly disrupts vessel formation and leads to the loss of lung architecture in rat fetal lung explants (Fig. 3-1).

VEGF-A exists as three predominant isoforms, VEGF-120, -164 and -188. Each isoform has differing properties, including affinity for the heparin sulfate component of the extracellular matrix, as well as for VEGF-R1 and VEGF-R2 binding. Each isoform is present in alveolar type II cells in the developing mouse lung, with expression peaking during the canalicular stage, when most of the vessel growth occurs in the lung, then decreases towards term until day 10 postnatal (P10), when it increases to levels that are maintained through adulthood (36).

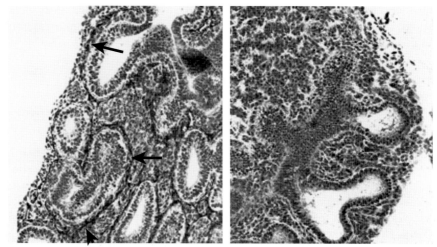

Figure 3-1 Role of VEGF signaling during lung vascular development in fetal rat lung explants. In comparison with controls (left panel), treatment of fetal rat lung explants with SU 5416, a VEGF receptor inhibitor, disrupts vascular structure, as noted by the loss of endothelial cells identified by immunostaining for endothelial nitric oxide synthase (as noted in the normal lung by arrows on left panel) (figures provided by Sarah Gebb).

VEGF-120 is highly diffusible because of lack of binding to heparin sulfate and probably serves a key early role in vascular formation through driving endothelial commitment and expansion. The importance of VEGF-164 and -188 isoforms was demonstrated in mice engineered to express only the VEGF-120 isoform. VEGF-120-only animals had fewer air-blood barriers and decreased airspace-to-parenchyma ratios compared to wild-type litter mates. Thus, as development proceeds, the pattern of VEGF isoform expression becomes more restrictive and the VEGF isoforms serve different roles (37).

VEGF has other family members, including VEGF-C and D. These VEGFs have different affinities for specific VEGF receptors, with both VEGF-C and D demonstrating an ability to bind to VEGF-R3. It is now recognized that this is probably crucial for development of the lymphatic vascular system (38). Recent studies have evaluated the temporal and spatial pattern of VEGF-D expression during mouse lung development (39). The pattern of expression is distinct from that of VEGF-A, suggesting a unique function for each VEGF during lung development. In addition, the finding of VEGF-D expression in the mesenchyme by cells distinctly different from endothelial cells and smooth muscle cells, perhaps fibroblasts, suggests that mesenchymal cells can influence endothelial phenotype during lung development through expression of either VEGF-A or VEGF-D.

Thus, the temporal and spatial pattern of expression of VEGF during development is crucial for normal growth and patterning of the lung circulation. Findings that pharmacologic inhibition of VEGF signaling impairs alveolar architecture in newborn and adult animals (features encountered in clinical BPD and emphysema) suggest that VEGF is required not only for the formation but also for the maintenance of the pulmonary vasculature and alveolar structures throughout life (as discussed below; Fig. 3-2).

The *angiopoietins* (*Ang*) are angiogenic growth factors that specifically act on vascular endothelium (40–44). Their endothelial specificity is due to their unique expression of the Ang receptors Tie 1 and Tie 2 (tyrosine kinase with immunoglobulin and EGF-like domains). Ang-Tie signaling is critical for normal vascular development, as Ang 1−/− or Tie 2−/− mice are embryonically unviable due to the failure of vascular integrity (42–44). Null mutation of the Tie-1 receptor gene causes perinatal death due to respiratory distress, with lung

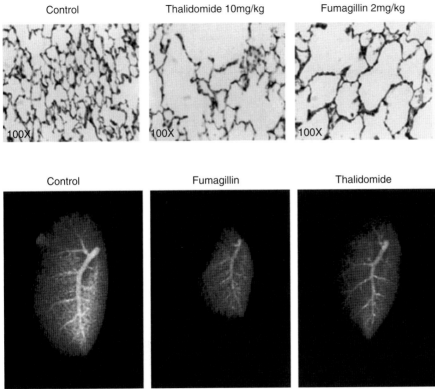

Figure 3-2 Disruption of angiogenesis in neonatal rats impairs lung alveolar and vascular growth. In comparison with controls, neonatal treatment with anti-angiogenesis inhibitor agents (thalidomide and fumagillin) causes alveolar simplification (upper panel), and reduces lung vessel growth (lower panel) in rats (as adapted from Jakkula et al. (108)).

hemorrhage and edema (43). Ang 2 −/− mice lacked embryonic vascular defects, but lymphatic development was impaired (45). Ang 1 is produced by lung mesenchyme and smooth muscle, whereas Tie 2, its receptor, is restricted to endothelial expression. Ang 1 binding to Tie 2 causes receptor tyrosine phosphorylation and downstream signals for endothelial cell survival through PI3kK/ Akt signaling (46). Angiogenic actions of ang-1 require endothelium-derived NO (47). Ang 1 promotes interactions between endothelial cells, extracellular matrix and pericytes that are required for vessel maturation. Ang 1–VEGF interactions are critical for normal vascular maturation, but their interactive effects are complex and dependent upon multiple factors. In some settings, Ang-1 treatment attenuates VEGF-induced angiogenesis by increasing intercellular endothelial cell junctions, but Ang 1 also makes vessels resistant to VEGF withdrawal (48, 49). Ang 2 also binds Tie 2, but blocks the function of Ang 1. Ang 2 is expressed only at sites of vessel remodeling, where it destabilizes vessels, perhaps via Ang 1 inhibition, which may increase endothelial cell responses to VEGF. The combination of low Ang 1 and low VEGF may enhance endothelial cell death. Low Ang 1 to Ang 1 ratios favor decreased Tie 2 phosphorylation, leading to weaker endothelial connections and perhaps increased responsiveness VEGF.

Little is known about Ang expression during development, especially in models of lung hypoplasia, but it is increased in the nitrofen model of congenital diaphragmatic hernia (50). In addition, the role of Ang 1 in pulmonary hypertension has been extremely controversial (51). Overexpression of Ang-1 causes severe pulmonary hypertension and is increased in lungs from human patients with pulmonary hypertension (52). However, cell-based gene transfer studies with Ang 1 protected against experimental pulmonary hypertension due to monocrotaline (53). These differences may be related to the mixed effects of Ang 1 on isolated cells: Ang 1 stimulates smooth muscle cell proliferation, but inhibits endothelial cell apoptosis, and may stimulate pericyte recruitment to stabilize the developing vascular wall (see below).

Notch signaling regulates cell fate through cell-cell interactions, and has been implicated in the development of vasculature (54). Mice homozygous for a targeted null deletion of Jagged, the Notch receptor, died at E10.5 with defects in vascular structure leading to hemorrhage, suggesting that the role of Notch/jagged signaling may be especially important in angiogenic remodeling. Notch ligands and receptors are expressed in the developing lung, in epithelium and mesenchyme, including endothelial cells, but its precise role during lung vascular development is uncertain. Notch-1 and jagged-1 appeared initially on larger vessels within the embryonic lung and were progressively expressed on smaller developing vascular networks (55). Notch signaling may act in part through the forkhead box (Fox) protein transcription factor, Foxf1 (56). Fox proteins regulate cell cycle, cell survival, differentiation and metabolism. Importantly, heterozygous mice with low Foxf1 levels had impaired lung vascular development, including a reduction in the number of distal lung capillaries and hemorrhage (56). Interestingly, lung VEGF expression was reduced in these lungs, suggesting that Foxf1 may be an important regulator of lung vascular growth through regulation of VEGF.

The *Wnt family* of proteins is another paracrine pathway that is important in lung vascular development. Wnt proteins are homologs of the Drosophila wingless gene and have been shown to play important roles in regulating cell differentiation, proliferation and polarity (57). Wnt proteins act largely through binding to receptors of the Frizzled family, and most Wnt ligands act through the canonical pathway involving beta-catenin, which mediates transcription of Wnt target genes (58, 59). Several Wnt genes are expressed in the developing lung, including Wnt-2, Wnt-2B, Wnt-7B, Wnt-5A, and Wnt-11. Wnt-7B expression is especially strong in the developing airway epithelium during early lung development. WNT-7B^{lacz} knock-in mice exhibit severe pulmonary hypoplasia and lung-specific vascular defects, including dilatation of large blood vessels in the lung with subsequent cell death and degradation of the vascular SMC layer leading to pulmonary hemorrhage. Defects in the lungs of Wnt-7B$^{lacz -/-}$ embryos, including early defects in mesodermal proliferation, suggest that Wnt-7B is required for lung mesodermal development. It has been demonstrated that the transcription factor Fox-f2, which is expressed in the developing lung mesoderm, is downregulated in Wnt-7B$^{lacz -/-}$ lung tissue. Since Fox-f2 is related to Fox-f1, which as mentioned above has been shown through loss-of-function experiments to regulate lung vascular development, this suggests that Wnt signaling through forkhead box transcription factors is critical for development of vascular smooth muscle cells from the lung mesoderm and for mesodermal thickening. These studies are among the first to specifically evaluate the factors involved in smooth muscle cell differentiation during lung vascular development.

Upon recruitment to the endothelial tube, newly recruited mesenchymal progenitor cells are induced toward a smooth muscle fate. This process seems to be mediated at least in part by the activation of *transforming growth factor-ß* (TGF-β). Although the exact mechanisms of how TGF-ß is activated and causes mural cell differentiation remain unknown, it is clear that this signaling system plays a critical role in vascular development. TGF-ß control elements have been identified in the promoter regions of smooth muscle cell genes such as SM-α-actin, SM-22 and calponin. TGF-β can also induce differentiation via the upregulation of the transcription factor serum response factor (SRF) (60). SRF binds the serum response elements in the promoter regions of mural cell specific genes including SM-α-actin,

SM-γ-actin, SM22α and calponin and induces their coordinated expression. The acquisition of differentiated contractile SM or SM-like cells is critical to not only stabilize and maintain the integrity of the developing endothelial tubes but also to control blood flow through these tubes. Mechanisms involved in this mural cell/endothelial cell interaction during lung development remain to be elucidated.

Normal vascular development requires expression of angiostatic molecules as well. Schwartz, et al. first described *endothelial monocyte activating peptide*-2 (EMAP-2), a potent angiostatic protein that is expressed in the lung (61). EMAP causes endothelial cell apoptosis, which may account for its anti-angiogenic properties. Over-expression of EMAP-2 inhibits neovascularization, as well as alveolar type II cell development. Other angiostatic proteins, including Ang-2, monokine induced by interferon-γ (MIG) and interferon-γ-inducible protein (IP-1), have been identified, and can attenuate VEGF-induced angiogenesis. The roles of these chemokines in normal lung vascular development or in disease states are uncertain.

Epigenetic Factors: Roles of O_2 Tension and Hemodynamic Forces

O_2 tension modulates lung development, as hyperoxia impairs lung growth and hypoxia is known to enhance vasculogenesis and angiogenesis. Since normal fetal O_2 tension is about 25 torr, it is not surprising that in vitro studies show that mammalian development appears optimal at low oxygen tension (3%) and that even short exposures to room air conditions can be detrimental to embryonic development due to relative hyperoxia. Recent work with mammalian fetal lung explants has provided evidence that branching morphogenesis is O_2-dependent (62). At lower PO_2 values that mimic fetal life, lung explants show a marked increase in airway branches and better maintenance of the mesenchyme (64). Interestingly, the increases in branching morphogenesis appear to be confined to the periphery in lung explant cultures, suggesting that hypoxia dependence is strong within the region of active airway bifurcation and vascular cell proliferation (65). Thus, O_2 tension may modulate both physiologic and structural characteristics of lung vascular and airway development.

Studies have begun to elucidate signaling pathways through which hypoxia acts to modulate vascular growth and development. Null mutations of HIF-1α in mice do not affect the fetus until E 9, an age which coincides with the initiation of lung development and vasculogenesis (63). Consequently, HIF-1α −/− mice display enlarged vascular structures, have impaired early lung morphogenesis and die by E10.5. Impaired expression of such HIF-regulated genes, such as VEGF, may account for at least part of these findings, since hypoxia upregulates VEGF and VEGFR-2 and inhibition of VEGF signaling mimics the effects of hyperoxia (Fig. 3-1). Several other O_2-sensitive genes appear to be involved in this process, including expression of Ang 1 and Ang 2, PDGF-B, FGF-9 and FGF-10, C/EBP-β, hepatocyte nuclear factor family (HNF), TGF family genes, erythropoietin, and others may also play important regulatory roles in vascular growth in this setting.

Thus, low O_2 tension activates unique cellular signaling pathways that are critical for growth and differentiation of cells within the pulmonary vasculature. Studies in the future need to be directed at utilizing the effects of oxygen to study lung vascular development. Such studies will provide better understanding regarding the response of the premature lung that is removed from its normal "hypoxic" environment and placed into relative or absolute hyperoxia, at a vulnerable period of lung development. That this transition can inhibit lung development as well as vascularization often leading to significant cardiopulmonary dysfunction is clear.

Hemodynamic Forces

In vivo and in vitro studies have demonstrated that hemodynamic forces, including shear (tangential) or stretch (pressure) stress, are major epigenetic determinants of vascular morphogenesis (64). Endothelial cells in vitro align in the direction of blood flow, and alter their morphology, mechanical properties and patterns of gene expression in response to shear stress (65). Mechanisms in which altered blood flow or pressure lead to diverse cellular responses are uncertain. The endothelial cell clearly provides a unique interface between intravascular forces and the vessel wall, and appears to serve as a "mechanotransducer," triggering changes in membrane function, intercellular junctions, and others. A change in local hemodynamics markedly alters production of vasoactive mediators, including nitric oxide (from shear stress), and endothelin-1 or PDGF-B (due to stretch or shear stress), which rapidly change vascular tone. Over time, sustained changes in hemodynamic forces and mediators alter vascular structure, as reflected by increases in pulmonary artery smooth muscle cell hyperplasia when exposed to hypertensive stimuli.

Recent studies suggest that chronic changes in pulmonary hemodynamics can influence lung vascular growth and distal airspace structure in late-gestation fetal sheep (66, 67). Intrauterine pulmonary hypertension, caused by surgical compression of the ductus arteriosus, inhibits angiogenesis, resulting in reduced vascular density, lung weight, and alveolarization in near-term fetal sheep (66) (Fig. 3-3). These effects may be at least partly mediated by impaired VEGF signaling, as chronic hypertension reduces lung VEGF protein expression by 75%, and treatment

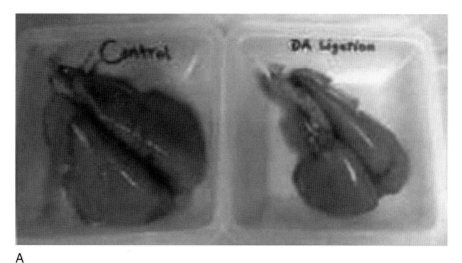

A

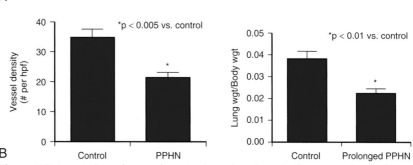

B

Figure 3-3 Intrauterine pulmonary hypertension reduces lung size (upper panel), vascular growth (lower panel, left). lung weight (lower panel, right) and alveolarization (not shown here) in fetal sheep (as adapted from Grover et al. (66)).

with recombinant human VEGF protein protects the lung from these changes (66, 67). These findings suggest a striking effect of hemodynamic stress on vascular growth during late gestation, and in light of the reduction in lung size and alveolarization, suggest a novel mechanism linking pulmonary hypertension and lung hypoplasia, as observed in neonatal lung diseases such as congenital diaphragmatic hernia, lung hypoplasia, BPD and others (see below).

POTENTIAL ROLE OF ENDOTHELIAL PROGENITOR CELLS (EPCS)

Until recently, lung vasculogenesis, the de novo formation of new blood vessels, was thought to result exclusively from local angioblasts or precursor cells within the lung mesenchyme. The discovery of bone-marrow derived EPCs in the blood of normal adults and in patients with diverse cardiopulmonary disorders raises new questions regarding the potential role of EPCs in maintaining vascular function and structure, or in repair after lung vascular injury. EPCs proliferate to form adherent colonies in vitro, which stain positive for endothelial markers, such as von Willebrand Factor, endothelial NO synthase, KDR (VEGFR-2), and VE-cadherin. Classically defined circulating EPCs express a known profile of surface antigens: CD34, CD133, and KDR (68, 69). CD34, a marker of immature hematopoietic cells, participates in the regulation of hematopoietic cell adhesion within the bone marrow stroma (70). CD133, another marker of hematopoietic immaturity, is also present on the surface of EPCs but its function is not known (71). VEGFR-2, or KDR, is expressed on EPCs and mature endothelial cells. EPCs are negative or dimly positive for the hematopoietic marker, CD45 (68, 72–74). Successful isolation of EPCs utilizes flow cytometry and immunomagnetic bead techniques, which select for cells expressing the above antigens. When cultured on collagen-coated plates, Ficoll-separated mononuclear cell isolates can differentiate into colonies of endothelial-like cells. Isolated colonies can be cloned and expanded to develop endothelial cell lines. These cell lines demonstrate self-renewing behavior (75). The potential role of EPCs in lung vasculogenesis is unknown.

There exists little information on the role of circulating EPCs during lung injury and repair. Lipopolysaccharide (LPS)-induced murine lung injury causes a rapid release of EPCs into the circulation which contributes, together with other bone marrow-derived progenitor cells, to lung repair (76). In elastase-induced emphysema, cells derived from the bone marrow develop characteristics of endothelial cells and contribute to repair of the alveolar capillary wall (77, 78). Patients with acute lung injury have a 2-fold higher number of circulating EPCs than healthy control subjects (79), suggesting some biological role for the mobilization of these cells in lung disease. Likewise, the number of circulating EPCs increases significantly in patients with pneumonia and patients with low EPC counts tend to have persistent fibrotic changes in their lungs even after recovery from pneumonia (80). Finally, reduction in circulating EPC number in adults correlates with restrictive and chronic lung disease (81). Mobilization of EPCs from the bone marrow follows increases in multiple growth factors, including VEGF, erythropoietin, hepatocyte growth factor (HGF), granulocyte colony stimulating factor (G-CSF), and granulocyte macrophage colony stimulating factor (GM-CSF) (78).

In BPD, abnormal vascular growth leads to impaired alveolarization. Reduction of lung VEGF in the lungs of human infants with BPD and in animal models of BPD may contribute to impaired EPC mobilization and recruitment. Recent findings suggest that circulating, lung and bone marrow EPC levels are reduced in an experimental model of BPD in hyperoxic neonatal mice (82). These observations support the hypothesis that EPCs migrate from the bone marrow to the peripheral circulation and the lung where they contribute to the repair of injured endothelium and help restore lung integrity. The consistency of these observations with the beneficial effect of angiogenic growth factors in experimental BPD underscores the therapeutic potential of promoting lung vascular growth in the repair of the lung.

CLINICAL IMPLICATIONS: DISRUPTION OF LUNG VASCULAR DEVELOPMENT IN BPD

Altered growth of the pulmonary circulation contributes to clinical disease in several settings, including congenital diaphragmatic hernia, lung hypoplasia, neonatal congenital heart disease and others. Perhaps the most striking example of how disruption of lung vascular development contributes to human disease lies in the clinical problem of BPD.

Pulmonary Vascular Disease in BPD

BPD is the chronic lung disease of infancy that follows mechanical ventilation and oxygen therapy for acute respiratory distress after birth in premature newborns (83–85). BPD has traditionally been defined by the presence of persistent respiratory signs and symptoms, the need for supplemental oxygen to treat hypoxemia, and an abnormal chest radiograph at 36 weeks corrected age. There continues a growing recognition that infants with chronic lung disease after premature birth have a different clinical course and pathology than was traditionally observed in infants dying with BPD during this "pre-surfactant era" (86, 87). The classic progressive stages that first characterized BPD are often absent due to changes in clinical management. Clearly BPD continues to change from being predominantly defined by the severity of acute lung injury to its current characterization, which is primarily defined by a disruption of distal lung growth.

In contrast with "classic BPD," the "new BPD" develops in preterm newborns that generally require minimal ventilator support and relatively low FiO_2 during the early postnatal days. Pathologic signs of severe lung injury with striking fibroproliferative changes have become rare. At autopsy, lung histology now displays more uniform and milder regions of injury with prominent signs of impaired alveolar and vascular growth. These features include a pattern of alveolar simplification with enlarged distal airspaces, reduced growth of the capillary bed, and vessels that are often described as "dysmorphic" due to their centralized location in the thickened mesenchyme. Thus, the so-called "new BPD" of the post-surfactant period represents inhibition of lung development with altered lung structure, growth and function of the distal airspaces and vasculature. Physiologically, these findings suggest that a marked reduction in alveolar-capillary surface area contributes to impaired gas exchange resulting in an increased risk of exercise intolerance, pulmonary hypertension and poor tolerance of acute respiratory infections (88–92).

In addition to adverse effects on the airway, acute lung injury impairs growth, structure and function of the developing pulmonary circulation after premature birth (88, 93–99; Fig. 3-4). Endothelial cells demonstrate particular susceptibility to oxidant injury due to hyperoxia or inflammation (100). The media of small pulmonary arteries may also undergo striking changes, including smooth muscle cell proliferation, precocious maturation of immature mesenchymal cells into mature smooth muscle cells, and incorporation of fibroblasts/myofibroblasts into the vessel wall (101). These structural changes in the lung vasculature contribute to high pulmonary vascular resistance (PVR) due to narrowing of the vessel diameter and decreased vascular compliance. In addition to these structural changes, the pulmonary circulation is further characterized by abnormal vasoreactivity, which also increases PVR. Finally, decreased angiogenesis may limit vascular surface area,

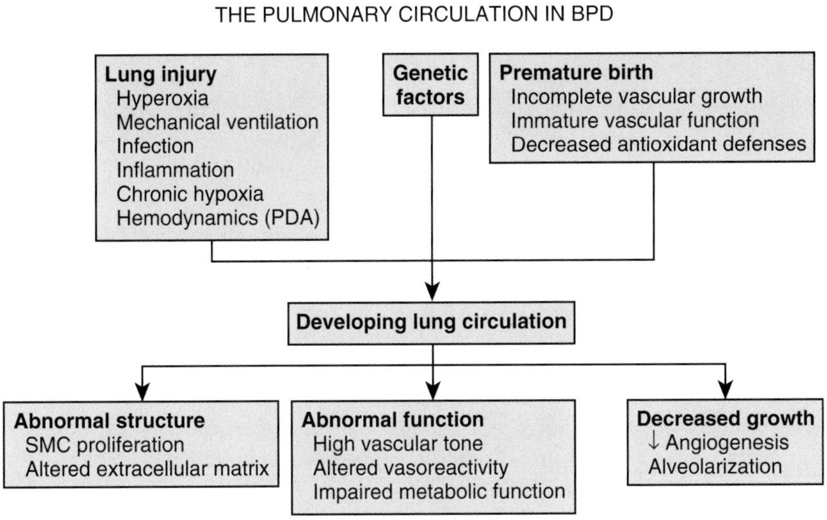

Lung injury	Genetic factors	Premature birth
Hyperoxia Mechanical ventilation Infection Inflammation Chronic hypoxia Hemodynamics (PDA)		Incomplete vascular growth Immature vascular function Decreased antioxidant defenses

Developing lung circulation

Abnormal structure	Abnormal function	Decreased growth
SMC proliferation Altered extracellular matrix	High vascular tone Altered vasoreactivity Impaired metabolic function	↓ Angiogenesis Alveolarization

Figure 3-4 Schematic illustrating abnormalities of the pulmonary circulation in BPD.

causing further elevations of PVR, especially in response to high cardiac output with exercise or stress.

Early injury to the lung circulation leads to the rapid development of pulmonary hypertension, which contributes to the morbidity and mortality of severe BPD. Even the earliest reports of BPD demonstrated a recognition of the association of pulmonary hypertension and cor pulmonale with high mortality (94, 95). Although pulmonary hypertension is a marker of more advanced BPD, elevated PVR also causes poor right ventricular function, impaired cardiac output, limited oxygen delivery, increased pulmonary edema and perhaps a higher risk for sudden death.

Physiologic abnormalities of the pulmonary circulation in BPD include elevated PVR and abnormal vasoreactivity, evidenced by the marked vasoconstrictor response to acute hypoxia (94, 97, 102). Cardiac catheterization studies show that mild hypoxia causes marked elevations in pulmonary artery pressure, even in infants with modest basal levels of pulmonary hypertension. Treatment levels of oxygen saturations above 92–94% effectively lower pulmonary artery pressure (97, 102). Strategies to lower pulmonary artery pressure or limit injury to the pulmonary vasculature, such as early ligation of the patent ductus arteriosus, may limit the subsequent development of pulmonary hypertension in BPD. Recent data suggest that high pulmonary vascular tone continues to elevate PVR in older patients with BPD, as demonstrated by responsiveness to altered oxygen tension and inhaled nitric oxide (102).

Prominent bronchial or other systemic-to-pulmonary collateral vessels noted in early morphometric studies of infants with BPD can be readily identified in many infants during cardiac catheterization (11, 88, 99). Although generally small in size, other large collaterals may contribute to significant shunting of blood flow to the lung, causing edema and need for higher FiO_2. Interestingly, this enlargement of the bronchial circulation shares similarities with descriptions of changes observed in adults with emphysema, chronic atelectasis and/or high PVR, continuing to support the notion that obstruction to blood flow in the pulmonary circulation remains a significant stimulus for growth of the bronchial circulation (see above). The presence of collateral vessels shares an association with high mortality in some patients with severe BPD who also have severe pulmonary hypertension. Some infants have improved after embolization of large collateral vessels, as reflected by a reduced need for supplemental oxygen, ventilator support or diuretics. However, neither the actual contribution of systemic collateral vessels to the pathophysiology of BPD nor the cellular mechanisms driving their enlargement is known.

Finally, pulmonary hypertension and right heart function remain a major clinical concern in infants with BPD. However, it is now clear that pulmonary vascular disease in BPD also includes reduced pulmonary artery density due to impaired growth, which contributes to physiologic abnormalities of impaired gas exchange, as well as to the actual pathogenesis of BPD (103, 104). As discussed below, experimental data support the hypothesis that impaired angiogenesis can impede alveolarization (67, 68), and that strategies that preserve and enhance endothelial cell survival, growth and function may provide new therapeutic approaches for the prevention of BPD.

Abnormal Vascular Growth and Impaired Alveolarization in BPD

Multiple growth factors and signaling systems have been shown to play important roles in normal lung vascular growth (105, 106). Several studies have examined how premature delivery and changes in oxygen tension, inflammatory cytokines and other signals alter normal growth factor expression and signaling and thus lung/lung vascular development. The majority of studies have focused on VEGF. As first suggested through studies in experimental models, impaired VEGF signaling was subsequently associated with the pathogenesis of BPD in the clinical setting (103, 104, 107–111). Bhatt and coworkers first demonstrated decreased lung expression VEGF and VEGFR-1 in the lungs of premature infants who died with BPD (103). In another study, VEGF was found to be lower in tracheal fluid samples from premature neonates who subsequently develop BPD than from those who do not develop chronic lung disease (104). Experimentally, hyperoxia down-regulates lung VEGF expression, and pharmacologic inhibition of VEGF signaling in newborn rats impairs lung vascular growth and inhibits alveolarization (107–112). Thus, the biologic basis for impaired VEGF signaling leading to decreased vascular growth and impaired alveolarization is well established. Additionally, lung VEGF expression is impaired in primate and ovine models of BPD induced by mechanical ventilation after premature birth, further supporting the hypothesis that impaired VEGF signaling contributes to the pathogenesis of BPD (113).

To determine whether angiogenesis is necessary for alveolarization, the effects of the anti-angiogenesis agents thalidomide and fumagillin on lung growth in the newborn and infant rat were studied (108). In comparison with vehicle-treated controls, postnatal treatment with these inhibitors of angiogenesis reduced lung vascular density, alveolarization and lung weight (Fig. 3–2). These findings suggest that angiogenesis is necessary for alveolarization during lung development, and that mechanisms which injure and inhibit lung vascular growth may impede alveolar growth after premature birth. Since VEGF has potent angiogenic effects during lung development and may synchronize vascular growth with neighboring epithelium, the effects of SU 5416, a selective VEGF receptor inhibitor, on alveolarization during early postnatal life were examined (108, 112). Treatment of neonatal rats with a single injection of SU5416 caused pulmonary hypertension, reduced lung vascular density, and reduced alveolarization in infant rats (108, 112). Thus, inhibition of lung vascular growth during a critical period of postnatal lung growth impairs alveolarization, suggesting that endothelial-epithelial cross-talk, especially via VEGF signaling, is critical for normal lung growth following birth.

Administration of an anti-PECAM-1 antibody that inhibits endothelial cell migration, but not proliferation or survival in vitro, also impairs septation in neonatal rats, without reducing endothelial cell content (114). Overall, these data suggest that the loss of PECAM-1 function compromises postnatal lung development and provide evidence that inhibition of endothelial cell function, in contrast to loss of viable endothelial cells, inhibits alveolarization.

The mechanisms through which impaired VEGF signaling inhibits vascular growth and alveolarization are uncertain, but may in part be mediated by altered

NO production. Past in vitro and in vivo studies have shown that VEGF stimulates endothelial NO synthase (eNOS) expression in isolated endothelial cells from the systemic circulation (115), but whether VEGF is an important regulator of lung eNOS expression especially during development and the role of NO on lung growth are incompletely understood. In addition to its effects on vascular tone, NO can alter angiogenesis, but data are conflicting on its effects. Although NO inhibits endothelial cell proliferation in some models, most studies have shown that NO mediates the angiogenic effects of VEGF via activation of VEGFR-2 and stimulation of the Akt-PI3K pathway. Proliferating bovine aortic endothelial cells express greater eNOS mRNA and protein than confluent cells, but NOS inhibition does not apparently affect their rate of proliferation. Studies with the eNOS−/− fetal mouse model suggest that NO plays a critical role in vascular and alveolar growth in utero, and those eNOS−/−newborns are more susceptible to hypoxia-induced inhibition of alveolarization (116–119). Interestingly, lung eNOS expression is down-regulated in primate and ovine models of BPD (120, 121). More recently, treatment of newborn rats with SU5416, the VEGF receptor antagonist, was shown to decrease eNOS expression and NO production during infancy, and that pro-longed treatment with inhaled NO prevented the development of pulmonary hypertension, improved vascular growth, and enhanced alveolarization (122).

The data above form the rationale to test the therapeutic potential for angio-genic growth factor modulation in experimental lung diseases characterized by alveolar damage. Recombinant human VEGF (rhVEGF) treatment of newborn rats during or after exposure to hyperoxia enhances vessel growth and improves alveolarization (123, 124). Similarly, postnatal intratracheal adenovirus-mediated VEGF gene therapy improves survival, promotes lung capillary formation, preserves alveolar development and regenerates new alveoli in this same model of irreversible lung injury (125). In both animal studies, VEGF induced immature and leaky capillaries and lung edema. Indeed, despite its central role in vascular formation, VEGF works in concert with other factors, notably angiopoietins. Angiopoietin-1 is required to stabilize the vessel wall by maximizing interactions between endothelial cells and their surrounding support cells and matrix (126). Accordingly, combined lung VEGF and Ang-1 gene transfer preserves alveolarization and enhances angio-genesis with more mature capillaries that are less permeable, reducing the vascular leakage seen in VEGF-induced capillaries (125).

A recent post-mortem study of newborns dying after short and prolonged durations of mechanical ventilation quantified lung microvascular growth (127). This study confirmed the reduction in vascular branching arteries, but interestingly, although lung PECAM-1 protein content (a marker of endothelial cells) was decreased in infants dying after brief ventilation, it was increased after prolonged ventilation. These findings suggest a transient decrease in endothelial proliferation, followed by a brisk proliferative response, despite a reduction in vessel number. This observation suggests that dysmorphic lung vascular growth in BPD may not nec-essarily result from a reduction of endothelial cells, suggesting the need to better discern distinct mechanisms regulating endothelial cell survival, proliferation, migration, vessel formation and maturation, especially in response to injury. There may be interesting parallels with similar time-specific events which alter the vascular response to hyperoxic injury to the developing retina and lead to retinopathy of prematurity (128).

Previous studies have shown that inhaled NO attenuates hyperoxia-induced acute lung injury (129–131), which may enhance subsequent vascular and lung growth. These studies suggest that decreased VEGF signaling downregulates lung eNOS expression, and that impaired NO production may contribute to abnormal lung growth during development (122). Importantly, a recent randomized single-center study has shown that inhaled NO treatment reduced the combined endpoint of BPD and death in human premature newborns with moderate RDS (132). Recent multicenter clinical trials suggest that early treatment with inhaled NO may attenuate the risk of BPD in premature infants with birth weights above 1000 g (133), and in older infants who require mechanical ventilation beyond the first week of life (134). However, mechanisms through which inhaled NO improved outcomes in these clinical studies are uncertain.

CONCLUSIONS

In summary, lung vascular growth and development is a dynamic process that includes critical changes throughout development, beginning in the embryonic period and continuing throughout gestation and during postnatal life. Production of pro-angiogenic growth factors, such as VEGF and NO, maintains pulmonary vascular structure in normal and disease states, perhaps due to enhanced endothelial cell differentiation, survival and function. Angiogenesis is closely linked with alveolarization in several models of lung development, and clinical and experimental studies suggest that disruption of vascular growth and signaling may contribute to impaired alveolar development in BPD. Future work is needed to better define basic mechanisms of lung vascular growth and development, which is likely to lead to novel therapeutic approaches to diseases associated with impaired vascular growth or pulmonary hypertension. Further studies are needed to clarify the physiology and pathobiology of EPCs, which may lead to cell therapy using EPCs or transfected EPCs for gene therapy in the treatment of sick newborns.

REFERENCES

1. West JB. Thoughts on the pulmonary blood-gas barrier. Am J Physiol 2003; 285:L501.
2. deMello DE, Reid LM. Prenatal and postnatal development of the pulmonary circulation. In: Haddad CG, Abman SH, Chernick VC, eds. Basic mechanisms of pediatric respiratory disease. Hamilton, Ontario: Decker; 2002; 77–101.
3. Shaw AM, Bunton DC, Brown T, et al. Regulation of sensitivity to 5-HT in pulmonary supernumerary but not conventional arteries by a 5-HT(1D)-like receptor. Eur J Pharmacol 2000; 408:69.
4. Ogata T, Iijima T. Structure and pathogenesis of plexiform lesions in pulmonary hypertension. Chin Med J 1993; 106:45–58.
5. Burri PH. Lung development and pulmonary angiogenesis. In: C Gaultier, Bourbon JR, Post M, eds. Lung development. New York: Oxford University Press; 1999; 122–151.
6. Nagaishi C. Functional anatomy and histology of the lung. Tokyo: Univ. Park Press; 1972.
7. Fisher KA, Summer RS. Stem and progenitor cells in the formation of the pulmonary vasculature. Curr Top Dev Biol 2006; 74:117–131.
8. Liebow AA, Hales MR, Bloomer WE, et al. Studies on the lung after ligation of the pulmonary artery. Am J Pathol 1950; 26:177.
9. Liebow AA, Hales MR, Bloomer WE. Relation of bronchial to pulmonary vascular tree. In Pulmonary circulation. New York: Grune and Stratton; 1959; 79–98.
10. Liebow AA, Hales MR, Lindskog GE. Enlargement of the bronchial arteries and their anastomoses with the pulmonary arteries in bronchiectasis. Am J Pathol 1949; 25:211.
11. Ascher DP, Rosen P, Null DM, et al. Systemic to pulmonary collaterals mimicking patent ductus arteriosus in neonates with prolonged ventilator courses. J Pediatr 1985; 101:282–284.
12. Noonan JA, Walters LR, Reeves JT. Congenital pulmonary lymphangiectasia. Am J Dis Child 1970; 120:314–319.
13. Boyd JD. Development of the heart. In: Hamilton WF, Dow P, eds. Handbook of physiology: a critical comprehensive presentation of physiologic knowledge and concepts: Section 2: Circulation. Washington DC: Am Physiol Soc; 1965; 2511–2544.
14. DeRuiter MC, Gittenberger-deGroot AC, Poelmann RE, et al. Development of the pharyngeal arch system related to the pulmonary and bronchial vessels in the avian embryo. With a concept on systemic-pulmonary artery collateral formation. Circulation 1993; 87:1306–1319.
15. DeRuiter MC, Gittenberger-deGroot AC, Ramos S, et al. The special status of the pulmonary arch artery in the branchial arch system of the rat. Anat Embryol 1989; 179:319–325.
16. deMello DE, Sawyer D, Galvin N, Reid LM. Early fetal development of lung vasculature. Am J Respir Cell Mol Biol 1997; 16(5):568–581.
17. Hislop AA. Airway and blood vessel interaction during lung development. J Anat 2002; 201:325–334.

18. deMello DE, Reid LM. Embryonic and early fetal development of human lung vasculature and its functional implications. Pediatr Dev Pathol 2002; 3:439–449.

19. Hall SM, Hislop AA, Pierce CM, Haworth SG. Prenatal origins for human intrapulmonary arteries: formation and smooth muscle maturation. Am J Respir Cell Mol Biol 2000; 23:194–203.

20. Chang C. On the origins of the pulmonary vein. Anat Rec 1931; 50:1–8.

21. Gebb SA, Shannon JM. Tissue interactions mediate early events in pulmonary vasculogenesis. Dev Dyn 2000; 217:159–169.

22. Shachtner SK, Wang Y, Baldwin HS. Qualitative and quantitative analysis of embryonic pulmonary vessel formation. Am J Respir Cell Mol Biol 2000; 22:157–165.

23. Maeda A, Suzuki S, Suzuki T, et al. Analysis of intrapulmonary vessels and epithelial-endothelial interactions in the human developing lung. Lab Invest 2002; 82:293–301.

24. Parera MC, Van Dooren M, Van Kempen M, et al. Distal angiogenesis: a new concept for lung vasculogenesis. Am J Physiol Lung 2005; 288:L141–L146.

25. Shannon JM, Deterding RM. Epithelial-mesenchymal interactions in lung development. In: JA McDonald (ed). Lung growth and development. NY: Decker; 1997; 81–118.

26. Ferrara N, Gerber HP, LeCouter J. The biology of VEGF and its receptors. Nat Med 2003; 9:669–672.

27. Flamme I, Breier G, Risau W. VEGF and VEGF receptor 2 are expressed during vasculogenesis and vascular differentiation in the quail embryo. Dev Biol 1995; 169:699–712.

28. Millauer B, Wizigmann-Voos S, Schnurch H, et al. High affinity VEGF binding and developmental expression suggest Flk-1 as a major regulator of vasculogenesis and angiogenesis. Cell 1993; 72:835–846.

28. Akeson AL, Greenberg JM, Cameron JE, et al. Temporal and spatial regulation of VEGF-A controls vascular patterning in the embryonic lung. Dev Dyn 2003; 264:443–455.

29. Terman BI, Dougher-Vermazen M, Carrion ME, et al. Identification of the KDR tyrosine kinase as a receptor for VEGF. Biochem Biophys Res Commun 1992; 187:1579–1586.

30. Djonov V, Schmid M, Tschanz SA, Burri PH. Intussusceptive angiogenesis: its role in embryonic vascular network formation. Circ Res 2000; 86(3):286–292.

31. Patan S, Alvarez MJ, Schittny JC, Burri PH. Intussusceptive microvascular growth: a common alternative to capillary sprouting. Arch Histol Cytol 1992; 55:65–75.

32. Carmeliet P, Ferreira V, Brier G, et al. Abnormal blood vessel development and lethality in embryos lacking a single VEGF allele. Nature 1996; 380:435–439.

33. Ferrara N, Carver-Moore K, Chen H, et al. Heterozygous embryonic lethality induced by targeted inactivation of the VEGF gene. Nature 1992; 380:439–442.

34. Fong G, Rossant H, Gertsenstein M, Breitman ML. Role of the Flt-1 receptor tyrosine kinase in regulating the assembly of vascular endothelium. Nature 1995; 376(6535):66–70.

35. Shalaby F, Rossant J, Yamaguchi TP, et al. Failure of blood-island formation and vasculogenesis in Flk-1-deficient mice. Nature 1995; 376(6535):62–66.

36. Ng Y, Rohan R, Sunday ME, et al. Differential expression of VEGF isoforms in mouse during development and in the adult. Dev Dyn 2001; 220:112.

37. Galumbos C, Ng YS, Ali A, et al. Defective pulmonary development in the absence of heparin-binding VEGF isoforms. Am J Respir Cell Mol Biol 2002; 27:194–203.

38. Lohela M, Saaristo A, Veikkola T, Alitalo K. Lymphangiogenic growth factors, receptors and therapies. Thromb Haemost 2003; 90:167–184.

39. Greenberg JM, Thompson FY, Brooks SK, et al. Mesenchymal expression of VEGF D and A defines vascular patterning in developing lung. Dev Dyn 2002; 224:144–153.

40. Davis S, Yancopoulos GD. The angiopoietins: yin and yang in angiogenesis. Curr Top Microbiol Immunol 1999; 237:173–185.

41. Loughna S, Sato TM. Angiopoietin and Tie signaling pathways in vascular development. Matrix Biol 2001; 20:319–325.

42. Dumont DJ, Gradwohl G, Fong GH, et al. Dominant negative and targeted null mutations in the endothelial receptor tyrosine kinase, tek, reveal a critical role in vasculogenesis in the embryo. Genes Dev 1994; 8:1897–1909.

43. Sato TN, Tozawa Y, Deutsch U, et al. Distinct roles of the receptor tyrosine kinases Tie-1 and Tie-2 in blood vessel formation. Am J Respir Cell Mol Biol 2000; 22:157–165.

44. Suri C, Jones PF, Patan S, et al. Requisite role of angiopoietin-1, a ligand for the Tie 2 receptor during embryonic angiogenesis. Cell 1996; 87:1171–1180.

45. Gale NW, Thurston G, Hackett SF, et al. Angiopoietin -2 is required for postnatal angiogenesis and lymphatic patterning and only the latter role is rescued by angiopoietin 1. Dev Cell 2002; 3:411–423.

46. Kim I, Kim JH, Moon So, et al. Angiopoietin-2 at high concentrations can enhance endothelial cell survival through the PI3K/Akt signal transduction pathway. Oncogene 2000; 19:4549–4552.

47. Babei S, Teichert-Kuliszewska K, Zhang Q, et al. Angiogenic actions of Ang 1 requires endothelium derived NO. Am J Pathol 2003; 162:1927–1936.

48. Visconti RP, Richardson CD, Sato TN. Orchestration of angiogenesis and arteriovenous contribution by angiopoietins and VEGF. Proc Natl Acad Sci USA 2002; 99:8219–8224.

49. Papatrepopoulos A, Garcia-Caardena G, Douiglas TJ, et al. Direct actions of ang-1 on human endothelium: evidence for network stabilization, cell survival and interaction with other angiogenic growth factors. Lab Invest 1999; 79:213–223.

50. Chinoy MR, Graybill MM, Miller SA, et al. Ang 1 and VEGF in vascular development and angiogenesis in hypoplastic lungs. Am J Physiol Lung 2002; 283:L60–L66.

51. Rudge JS, Thurston G, Yancopoulos GD. Angiopoietin 1 and pulmonary hypertension: cause or cure? Circ Res 2003; 92:947–949.

52. Du L, Sullivan CC, Chu D, et al. Signaling molecules in nonfamilial pulmonary hypertension. N Engl J Med 2003; 348:500–509.
53. Zhao YD, Campbell AIM, Robb M, et al. Protective role of Ang-1 in experimental pulmonary hypertension. Circ Res 2003; 92:984–991.
54. Artavanis-Tsakonas S, Rand MD, Lake RJ. Notch signaling: cell fate control and signal integration in development. Science 1999; 284:770–776.
55. Taichman DB, Loomes KM, Schachtner SK, et al. Notch 1 and Jagged expression by the developing pulmonary vasculature. Dev Dyn 2002; 225:166–175.
56. Kalinichenko VV, Gusarova GA, Kim IM, et al. Foxf1 haploinsufficiency reduces Notch-2 signaling during mouse lung development. Am J Physiol Lung 2004; 286:L521–L530.
57. Cadigan KM, Nusse R. Wnt signaling: a common theme in animal development. Genes Dev 1997; 11:3286–3305.
58. Willert K, Nusse R. Beta-catenin: a key mediator of Wnt signaling. Curr Opin Genet Dev 1998; 8:95–102.
59. Wodarz A, Nusse R. Mechanisms of Wnt signaling in development. Annu Rev Cell Dev Biol 1997; 14:59–88.
60. Hirschi KK, Lai L, Belaguli NS, et al. TGF-ß induction of smooth muscle cell phenotype requires transcriptional and post-transcriptional control of serum response factor. J Biol Chem 2001; 277:6287–6295.
61. Schwarz MA, Zhang F, Gebb S, et al. Endothelial monocyte activating polypeptide II inhibits lung neovascularization and airway epithelial morphogenesis. Mech Dev 2000; 95:123–132.
62. Gebb SA, Jones PL. Hypoxia and lung branching morphogenesis. Adv Exp Med Biol 2003; 543:117–125.
63. Kotch LE, Iyer NV, Laughner E, Semenza GL. Defective vascularization of HIF-1α-null embryos is not associated with VEGF deficiency, but with mesenchymal cell death. Dev Biol 1999; 209:254–267.
64. Davies PF. Flow-mediated endothelial mechanotransduction. Physiol Rev 1995; 75:519.
65. Topper JN, Gimbrone MA. Blood flow and vascular gene expression fluid shear stress as a modulator of endothelial phenotype. Mol Med Today 1999; 5:40.
66. Grover TR, Parker TA, Balasubramaniam V, et al. Pulmonary hypertension impairs alveolarization and lung growth in the ovine fetus. Am J Physiol LCMP 2005; 288:648–654.
67. Grover TR, Parker TA, Hunt-Peacock C, et al. rhVEGF treatment improves pulmonary vasoreactivity and structure in an experimental model of pulmonary hypertension in fetal sheep. Am J Physiol LCMP 2005; 289:L529–L535.
68. Asahara T, Murohara T, Sullivan A, et al. Isolation of putative progenitor endothelial cells for angiogenesis. Science 1997; 275(5302):964–967.
69. Peichev M, Naiyer AJ, Pereira D, et al. Expression of VEGFR-2 and AC133 by circulating human CD34(+) cells identifies a population of functional endothelial precursors. Blood 2000; 95(3):952–958.
70. Healy L, May G, Gale K, et al. The stem cell antigen CD34 functions as a regulator of hemopoietic cell adhesion. Proc Natl Acad Sci USA 1995; 92(26):12240–12244.
71. Bonanno G, Perillo A, Rutella S, et al. Clinical isolation and functional characterization of cord blood CD133 + hematopoietic progenitor cells. Transfusion 2004; 44(7):1087–1097.
72. Khakoo AY, Finkel T. Endothelial progenitor cells. Annu Rev Med 2005; 56:79–101.
73. Yin AH, Miraglia S, Zanjani ED, et al. AC133, a novel marker for human hematopoietic stem and progenitor cells. Blood 1997; 90(12):5002–5012.
74. Ingram DA, Caplice NM, Yoder MC. Unresolved questions, changing definitions, and novel paradigms for defining endothelial progenitor cells. Blood 2005; 106(5):1525–1531.
75. Ingram DA, Mead LE, Tanaka H, et al. Identification of a novel hierarchy of endothelial progenitor cells using human peripheral and umbilical cord blood. Blood 2004; 104(9):2752–2760.
76. Yamada M, Kubo H, Kobayashi S, et al. Bone marrow-derived progenitor cells are important for lung repair after lipopolysaccharide-induced lung injury. J Immunol 2004; 172(2):1266–1272.
77. Ishizawa K, Kubo Yamada M, et al. Bone marrow-derived cells contribute to lung regeneration after elastase-induced pulmonary emphysema. FEBS Lett 2004; 556(1–3):249–252.
78. Ishizawa K, Kubo H, Yamada M, et al. Hepatocyte growth factor induces angiogenesis in injured lungs through mobilizing endothelial progenitor cells. Biochem Biophys Res Commun 2004; 324(1):276–280.
79. Burnham EL, Taylor WR, Quyyumi AA, et al. Increased circulating endothelial progenitor cells are associated with survival in acute lung injury. Am J Respir Crit Care Med 2005; 172(7):854–860.
80. Yamada M, Kubo H, Ishizawa K, et al. Increased circulating endothelial progenitor cells in patients with bacterial pneumonia: evidence that bone marrow derived cells contribute to lung repair. Thorax 2005; 60(5):410–413.
81. Fadini GP, Schiavon M, Cantini M, et al. Circulating progenitor cells are reduced in patients with severe lung disease. Stem Cells 2006; 24(7):1806–1813.
82. Balasubramaniam V, Mervis C, Maxey AM, et al. Neoantal hyperoxia reduces circulating, bone marrow, and lung EPCs in neonatal mice: implications for the pathogenesis of BPD. Am J Physiol. 2007; 292: L1073–L1084.
83. Northway WH Jr, Rosan RC, Porter DY. Pulmonary disease following respirator therapy of hyaline-membrane disease. N Engl J Med 1967; 276:357–368.
84. Jobe AH, Bancalari E. Bronchopulmonary dysplasia. Am J Resp Crit Care Med 2001; 163:1723–1729.
85. Jobe AH. The new BPD: an arrest of lung development. Pediatr Res 1999; 46:641–643.

86. Hussain AN, Siddiqui NH, Stocker JT. Pathology of arrested acinar development in postsurfactant BPD. Hum Pathol 1998; 29:710–717.

87. Coalson JJ. Pathology of chronic lung disease of early infancy. In: Bland RD, Coalson JJ, eds. Chronic lung disease of early infancy. New York: Marcel Dekker; 2000; 85–124.

88. Abman SH. Pulmonary hypertension in chronic lung disease of infancy. Pathogenesis, pathophysiology and treatment. In: Bland RD, Coalson JJ, eds. Chronic lung disease of infancy. New York: Marcel Dekker; 2000; 619–668.

89. Mitchell SH, Teague G. Reduced gas transfer at rest and during exercise in school age survivors of BPD. Am J Resp Crit Care Med 1998; 157:1406–1412.

90. Slavin JD, Mathews J, Spencer RP. Pulmonary ventilation/perfusion and reverse mismatches in an infant. Acta Radiol Diagn 1986; 27:708.

91. Hakulinen AL, Järvenpaa, Turpeinan M, Sorijavi A. Diffusing capacity of the lung in school-age children born very preterm with and without BPD. Pediatr Pulmonol 1996; 21:353.

92. Subcommittee of the Assembly of Pediatrics, American Thoracic Society. Statement on the care of the child with chronic lung disease of infancy and childhood. Am J Respir Crit Care Med 2003; 168:356–396.

93. Hislop AA, Haworth SG. Pulmonary vascular damage and the development of cor pulmonale following hyaline membrane disease. Pediatr Pulmonol 1990; 9:152–161.

94. Halliday HL, Dumpit FM, Brady JP. Effects of inspired oxygen on echocardiographic assessment of pulmonary vascular resistance and myocardial contractility in BPD. Pediatrics 1980; 65:536–540.

95. Fouron JC, LeGuennec JC, Villemont D, et al. Value of echocardiography in assessing the outcome of BPD. Pediatrics 1980; 65:529–535.

96. Tomashefski JF, Opperman HC, Vawter GF. BPD: a morphometric study with emphasis on the pulmonary vasculature. Pediatr Pathol 1984; 2:469–487.

97. Abman SH, Wolfe RR, Accurso FJ, et al. Pulmonary vascular response to oxygen in infants with severe BPD. Pediatrics 1985; 75:80–84.

98. Walther FJ, Bender FJ, Leighton JO. Persistent pulmonary hypertension in premature neonates with severe RDS. Pediatrics 1992; 90:899–904.

99. Goodman G, Perkin R, Anas N. Pulmonary hypertension in infants with BPD. J Pediatr 1988; 112:67–72.

100. Roberts RJ, Weesner KM, Bucher JR. Oxygen induced alterations in lung vascular development in the newborn rat. Pediatr Res 1983; 17:368–375.

101. Jones R, Zapol WM, Reid LM. Pulmonary artery remodeling and pulmonary hypertension after exposure to hyperoxia for 7 days. Am J Pathol 1984; 117:273–285.

102. Mourani PM, Ivy DD, Gao D, Abman SH. Pulmonary vascular effects of inhaled NO and oxygen tension in BPD. Am J Respir Crit Care Med 2004; 170:1006–1013.

103. Bhatt AJ, Pryhuber GS, Huyck H, et al. Disrupted pulmonary vasculature and decreased VEGF, flt-1, and Tie 2 in human infants dying with BPD. Am J Resp Crit Care Med 2000; 164:1971–1980.

104. Lassus P, Turanlahti M, Heikkila P, et al. Pulmonary vascular endothelial growth factor and Flt-1 in fetuses, in acute and chronic lung disease, and in persistent pulmonary hypertension of the newborn. Am J Respir Crit Care Med 2001; 164:1981–1987.

105. D'Angio CT, Maniscalco WM. Role of vascular growth factors in hyperoxia-induced injury to the developing lung. Frontiers in Biosciences 2002; 7:1609–1623.

106. Kumar VH, Ryan RM. Growth factors in fetal and neonatal lung disease. Frontiers in Biosciences 2004; 9:464–480.

107. Abman SH. BPD: a vascular hypothesis. Am J Respir Crit Care Med 2001; 164:1755–1756.

108. Jakkula M, Le Cras TD, Gebb S, et al. Inhibition of angiogenesis decreases alveolarization in the developing rat lung. Am J Physiol Lung Cell Mol Physiol 2000; 279:L600–L607.

109. Klekamp JG, Jarzecka K, Perkett EA. Exposure to hyperoxia decreases the expression of vascular endothelial growth factor and its receptors in adult rat lungs. Am J Pathol 1999; 154:823–831.

110. Maniscalco WM, Watkins RH, D'Angio CT, Ryan RM. Hyperoxic injury decreases alveolar epithelial cell expression of vascular endothelial growth factor (VEGF) in neonatal rabbit lung. Am J Respir Cell Mol Biol 1997; 16:557–567.

111. Maniscalco WM, Watkins RH, Finkelstein JN, et al. VEGF mRNA increases in alveolar epithelial cells during recovery from oxygen injury. Am J Respir Cell Mol Biol 1995; 13:377–386.

112. Le Cras TD, Markham NE, Tuder RM, et al. Treatment of newborn rats with a VEGF receptor inhibitor causes pulmonary hypertension and abnormal lung structure. Am J Physiol Lung Cell Mol Physiol 2002; 283:L555–L562.

113. Maniscalco WM, Watkins RH, Pryhuber GS, et al. Angiogenic factors and the alveolar vasculature: development and alterations by injury in very premature baboons. Am J Physiol 2002; 282:L811–L823.

114. DeLisser HM, Helmke BP, Cao G, et al. Loss of PECAM-1 function impairs alveolarization. J Biol Chem 2006; 281(13):8724–8731.

115. Ziche M, Morbidelli L, Choudhuri R, et al. NO synthase lies downstream from vascular endothelial growth factor-induced but not basic fibroblast growth factor-induced angiogenesis. J Clin Invest 1997; 99:2625–2634.

116. Balasubramaniam V, Tang JR, Maxey A, et al. Mild hypoxia impairs alveolarization in the endothelial nitric oxide synthase-deficient mouse. Am J Physiol Lung Cell Mol Physiol 2003; 284:L964–L971.

117. Leuwerke SM, Kaza AK, Tribble CG, et al. Inhibition of compensatory lung growth in endothelial nitric oxide synthase-deficient mice. Am J Physiol Lung Cell Mol Physiol 2002; 282:L1272–L1278.

118. Young SL, Evans K, Eu JP. Nitric oxide modulates branching morphogenesis in fetal rat lung explants. Am J Physiol Lung Cell Mol Physiol 2002; 282:L379–L385.
119. Han RN, Babei S, Robb M, et al. Defective lung vascular development and fatal respiratory distress in eNOS deficient mice: a model of alveolar capillary dysplasia. Circ Res 2004; 94:1115–1123.
120. Afshar S, Gibson LL, Yuhanna IS, et al. Pulmonary NO synthase expression is attenuated in a fetal baboon model of chronic lung disease. Am J Physiol Lung Cell Mol Physiol 2003; 284:L749–L758.
121. MacRitchie AN, Albertine KH, Sun J, et al. Reduced endothelial nitric oxide synthase in lungs of chronically ventilated preterm lambs. Am J Physiol Lung Cell Mol Physiol 2001; 281:L1011–L1020.
122. Tang JR, Markham NE, Lin YJ, et al. Inhaled NO attenuates pulmonary hypertension and improves lung growth in infant rats after neonatal treatment with a VEGF receptor inhibitor. Am J Physiol Lung Cell Mol Physiol 2004; 287:L344–L351.
123. Kunig AM, Balasubramaniam V, Markham NE, et al. Recombinant human VEGF treatment transiently increases lung edema but enhances lung structure after neonatal hyperoxia. Am J Physiol Lung Cell Mol Physiol 2006; 291:L1068–L1078.
124. Kunig AM, Balasubramaniam V, Markham NE, et al. Recombinant human VEGF treatment enhances alveolarization after hyperoxic lung injury in neonatal rats. Am J Physiol Lung Cell Mol Physiol 2005; 289(4):L529–L535.
125. Thebaud B, Ladha F, Michelakis ED, et al. VEGF gene therapy increases survival, promotes lung angiogenesis, and prevents alveolar damage in hyperoxia-induced lung injury: evidence that angiogenesis participates in alveolarization. Circulation 2005; 112(16):2477–2486.
126. Thurston G, Suri C, Smith K, et al. Leakage-resistant blood vessels in mice transgenically over-expressing angiopoietin-1. Science 1999; 286(5449):2511–2514.
127. De Paepe ME, Mao Q, Powell J, et al. Growth of pulmonary microvasculature in ventilated preterm infants. Am J Respir Crit Care Med 2006; 173(2):204–211.
128. Csak K, Szabo V, Szabo A, et al. Pathogenesis and genetic basis for retinopathy of prematurity. Front Biosci 2006; 11:908–920.
129. Howlett CE, Hutchison JS, Veinot JP, et al. Inhaled nitric oxide protects against hyperoxia-induced apoptosis in rat lungs. Am J Physiol 1999; 277:L596–L605.
130. McElroy MC, Wiener-Kronish JP, Miyazaki H, et al. Nitric oxide attenuates lung endothelial injury caused by sublethal hyperoxia in rats. Am J Physiol 1997; 272:L631–L638.
131. Nelin LD, Welty SE, Morrisey JF, et al. Nitric oxide increases the survival of rats with a high oxygen exposure. Pediatr Res 1998; 43:727–732.
132. Schreiber MD, Gin-Mestan K, Marks JD, et al. Inhaled NO in premature infants with respiratory distress syndrome. N Engl J Med 2003; 349:2099–2107.
133. Kinsella JP, Cutter GR, Walsh WF, et al. Early inhaled nitric oxide therapy in premature newborns with respiratory failure. N Engl J Med 2006; 355(4):354–364.
134. Ballard RA, Truog WE, Canaan A, et al. Inhaled nitric oxide in preterm infants undergoing mechanical ventilation. N Engl J Med 2006; 355(4):343–353.

Chapter 4

Surfactant: The Basis for Clinical Treatment Strategies

Alan H. Jobe MD PhD

Surfactant During Normal Fetal Lung Development

Surfactant Composition and Metabolism

The Controversy about what is RDS

Factors that Influence Surfactant in the Preterm Lung

Meconium Aspiration Syndrome

Bronchopulmonary Dysplasia

Surfactant for Sepsis/Pneumonia Syndromes

Which Surfactant Should be Used to Treat RDS or Other Lung Injury Syndromes?

Surfactant therapy for RDS is standard of care for preterm infants, based on numerous randomized controlled trials and epidemiologic data demonstrating decreased mortality following the introduction of surfactant treatments for RDS in the United States in 1990 (1–3). However, a number of questions and controversies remain about how to best use this very effective therapy and in which populations of infants. The basis for understanding how to optimally use surfactant is the experimental literature about surfactant function and its effects on the developing lung (4, 5). This chapter will review important concepts about surfactant and current clinical controversies about surfactant treatment. The following questions will be addressed: When should infants at risk for RDS be treated? How should surfactant be given? Do surfactant treatments help in diseases such as BPD and meconium aspiration syndrome? Which surfactant should be used?

SURFACTANT DURING NORMAL FETAL LUNG DEVELOPMENT

An Overview

The fetal human lung has undergone primary septation to form about 20 binary airway branches before 20 weeks gestation (6). The distal airway branches become saccules that divide and vascularize between about 22 and 36 weeks gestation. Secondary septation (alveolarization) normally begins at about 32–34 weeks in the human lung (7). Despite the immature saccular structure of the lung when survival is possible after about 23 weeks gestation, the type II cells that make and secrete surfactant are remarkably inducible. Surfactant is a complex aggregate of phospholipids and surfactant-specific proteins that can be characterized by its

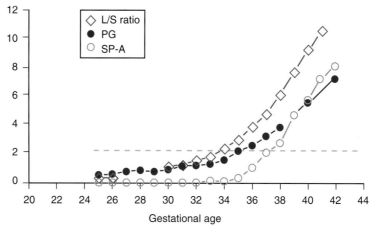

Figure 4-1 Measurements of lung maturity using amniotic fluid. The values are expressed as a ratio of lecithin to sphingomyelin (the L/S ratio), as% phosphatidylglycerol (PG) relative to other phospholipids, and as μg/ml SP-A in amniotic fluid. An L/S ratio of 2.0 indicates lung maturation, which normally occurs at about 35 weeks gestation when PG appears. Data from Gluck et al. (10), Kulovich et al. (8) and Pryhuber et al. (9).

composition or its biophysical functions. The major biophysically active lipid components of surfactant are the saturated phosphatidylcholines, which can be measured in amniotic fluid relative to sphingomyelin to evaluate lung maturation clinically – the L/S ratio (Fig. 4-1) (8, 9). Lung maturation normally is assured only if the L/S ratio is > 2 and phosphatidylglycerol is present in the amniotic fluids. In the normal fetal lung, surfactant is not secreted in sufficient amounts to prevent RDS until after about 35 weeks gestation (10). However, RDS is infrequent at 35 weeks following spontaneous labor, and RDS may not occur at very early gestational ages because surfactant (and perhaps lung structural maturation) can be induced at very early gestational ages. To begin to understand the relationships between surfactant and prematurity, and RDS and treatment responses, the complex metabolism and interactions of surfactant with the preterm lung must be appreciated.

SURFACTANT COMPOSITION AND METABOLISM

Surfactant from adult animals and humans is a macroaggregate of highly organized lipids and surfactant-specific proteins. The lipid and protein components of surfactant are preserved across species. The major components that confer the unique ability of surfactant to lower the surface tension on an air-water interface to very low values are the saturated phosphatidylcholine species, surfactant protein B and surfactant protein C. The preterm with RDS has low amounts of surfactant that contain a lower percent of saturated phosphatidylcholine species, less phosphatidylglycerol and less of all the surfactant proteins than surfactant from a mature lung (11). Minimal surface tensions are higher for surfactant from preterm than term infants. The surfactant from the preterm is intrinsically "immature" in composition and biophysical function (12).

The lipids and proteins in surfactant are synthesized by the type II cells in the epithelium of the saccule (13) (Fig. 4-2). The surfactant components are packaged in lamellar bodies for constitutive secretion or secretion in response to stimulators such as beta agonists, puringergic agonists or lung stretch. The secreted lamellar bodies contribute to the surfactant pool in the fluid hypophase that lines the saccules and distal airways of the preterm lung, resulting in low surface tensions.

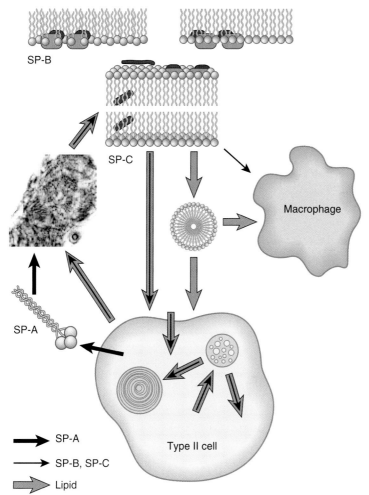

SP-B

SP-C

Macrophage

SP-A

Type II cell

→ SP-A

→ SP-B, SP-C

⟹ Lipid

Figure 4-2 Pathways for surfactant metabolism. Surfactant is synthesized in type II cells, stored in lamellar bodies and secreted into the alveoli where it forms a surface film. It is cleared from the airspaces by macrophages for catabolism or is taken back into type II cells where it is reprocessed and resecreted – a recycling pathway. The pathways for the lipids and proteins are qualitatively similar.

Surfactant normally is taken up by macrophages for catabolism or recycled back into type II cells for either reprocessing into new surfactant for secretion or catabolism. Surfactant metabolism is critical to the persistence of treatment responses, a concept that will be developed below. Thus, surfactant is a multicomponent lipid and protein aggregate that has striking biophysical properties at an air-water interface and a complex metabolism.

Based on measurements in adult, newborn and preterm animals, and more recently in preterm infants, we know that the synthesis of surfactant lipids and proteins from precursors by type II cells is rapid. However, surfactant processing to storage in lamellar bodies and then secretion to the airspaces occurs over many hours. The time from synthesis to peak labeling of surfactant in airway samples is about 3 days in preterm infants with RDS (14, 15) (Fig. 4-3). This time is prolonged above the 1 to 2 days measured in preterm lambs because the stable isotopes used to label the surfactant are given to infants as an infusion over 24 h and the "alveolar pool" is sampled by tracheal suction and not by lavage of the distal lung (16). The alveolar pool of surfactant does not increase very much for several days in ventilated preterm monkeys with RDS (17). The conclusion is that it will take the infant with

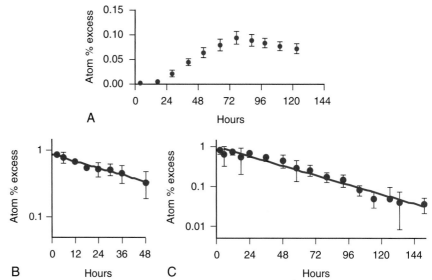

Figure 4-3 Time course of surfactant phospholipid labeling in airway samples of ventilated preterm infants with RDS. (A) Phosphatidylcholine was labeled with a 24-h infusion of ^{13}C-glucose and the appearance of that label in airway samples was measured. There was an initial delay in labeling, and peak labeling did not occur until about 72 h. Data redrawn from Bunt et al. (14). (B) Recovery in airway samples following surfactant treatment with ^{13}C-dipalmitoylphosphatidylcholine from ventilated preterm infants. The specific activity (atom% excess ^{13}C) decreased exponentially. (C) A second dose of ^{13}C-labeled surfactant given at about 2 days of age had a similar slow decrease in specific activity. Redrawn from Torresin et al. (15).

RDS several days to increase the surfactant pool from endogenous synthesis and secretion.

Catabolism and clearance of surfactant can be measured from the lung and airspaces in animals and from the airspaces using tracheal samples in infants with RDS (15). The consistent result from measurements in multiple animal models and infants with RDS is that both the endogenous and exogenous surfactant components have long half-life values in the airspaces – about 3 days for infants with RDS. The lipids also remain in the lung compartment (airspaces, type II cells, lung tissue) for many days. The conclusion is that while synthesis and secretion are slow, catabolism and clearance are also slow. The net balance is for the preterm lung to accumulate a large amount of surfactant over many days.

Surfactant components are recycled from the airspaces back to type II cells where the lipids are, in part, diverted into lamellar bodies for resecretion. The process can be directly measured in animals, because radiolabeled surfactant component recoveries can be measured in subcellular fractions of lung tissue. This recycling has been modeled using stable isotopes in infants with RDS (18). In general, recycling is more efficient in the preterm than the adult lung, and recycling rates as high as 80–90% have been measured in the newborn. The very long biological half-life values for airspace surfactant are explained by continued reuptake and resecretion of surfactant. Surfactant treatment quickly increases the alveolar pool, and the exogenous surfactant becomes part of the endogenous metabolic pools (19). The treatment surfactant becomes substrate for endogenous surfactant metabolism.

THE CONTROVERSY ABOUT WHAT IS RDS

The diagnosis of RDS until the 1980s was based on the presence of progressive respiratory distress after preterm delivery and a typical hazy and granular

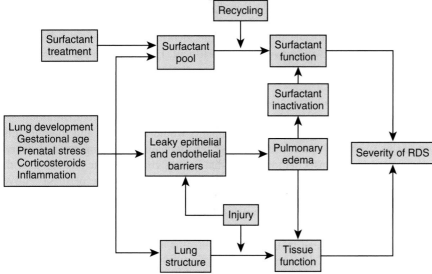

Figure 4-4 Major components in the pathophysiology of RDS. The two main factors contributing to the severity of RDS are lung structural immaturity and the surfactant pool, which both are determined by the stage of development of the lung. Secondary factors such as surfactant treatment and lung injury then modulate the severity of RDS.

chest film. In the 1980s this disease was known to result from inadequate surfactant function, which caused lung injury with pulmonary edema in the preterm lung (Fig. 4-4). Infants who died of RDS had surfactant pool sizes of 0–10 mg/kg (5), and the surfactant present in the airways of infants with RDS was inactivated by the proteinaceous pulmonary edema that entered the saccules and airways (20) (Fig. 4-5). The edema resulted from endothelial and epithelial injury caused by spontaneous or mechanical ventilation of the delicate surfactant-deficient preterm lung (21). Surfactant treatments in the delivery room to "prophylactically" treat

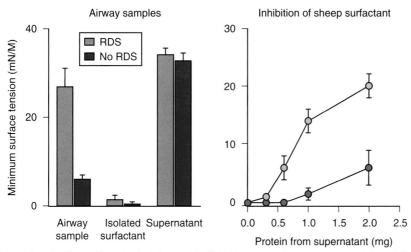

Figure 4-5 Surfactant function in infants with RDS. Airway samples were recovered from infants with RDS just after intubation for respiratory failure. Samples were also collected from control infants without RDS. The surfactant in the airway samples from infants with RDS had high minimum surface tension values. However, surfactant with good function could be recovered by centrifugation. The supernatants from the airway samples had high minimum surface tensions and high protein contents. The supernatants from the infants with RDS (upper line) were more inhibitory to sheep surfactant than supernatants from control infants (lower line). Data from Ikegami et al. (20).

infants at risk of RDS certainly decreased the incidence of clinical RDS (22). Thus, some infants did not get RDS because of very early treatment – the disease was prevented. This remarkable result masks the identification of infants who would have developed RDS without surfactant treatment. However, very early treatments did not prevent RDS in many infants, demonstrating that other factors contribute to the diagnosis.

The diagnosis and presentation of RDS can change when different strategies to assist respiratory transition after birth are used. Until recently, two assumptions of many clinicians were that most VLBW infants would have RDS and these infants would be unable to successfully initiate spontaneous breathing after delivery. European neonatologists demonstrated that infants could breathe after birth with continuous positive airway pressure (CPAP) support and some of these VLBW infants did not develop RDS (23). Two recent reports demonstrate the effectiveness of CPAP for assisting respiratory transition in preterm infants and the effects of that intervention on the use of surfactant treatments for RDS (24, 25). Independent of size or gestational age, all infants who will breathe after delivery are tried on nasal CPAP at Columbia (24) (Fig. 4-6). For infants born between 26 and 28 weeks gestation, 78% required no intubation and could be managed with CPAP alone. Such management was possible for 93% of infants born at gestational ages of 29–31 weeks. Although management with CPAP was less successful in the very premature infants, 69% of infants born at gestations of 23–25 weeks could be managed initially with CPAP and 31% never needed surfactant or intubation. Although many of the infants managed with CPAP had some RDS, surfactant treatments were given to just 17% of infants with birth weights of less than 1250 g. In contrast, about 80% of infants in the Vermont-Oxford database with birth weights less than 1500 g received surfactant (26). In a second clinical experience from George Washington University, nasal CPAP was tried whenever possible in the delivery room for VLBW infants (25). Of 234 infants, 65% could be initially managed with CPAP, and 50% did not require intubation within the next 7 d. Only 27% of the population received surfactant. Infants who required intubation had lower gestational ages and lower Apgar scores, and success increased with staff experience with the use of CPAP in the delivery room.

These clinical experiences suggest that the diagnosis of RDS can be decreased by allowing a preterm infant to transition with CPAP. How is this possible if

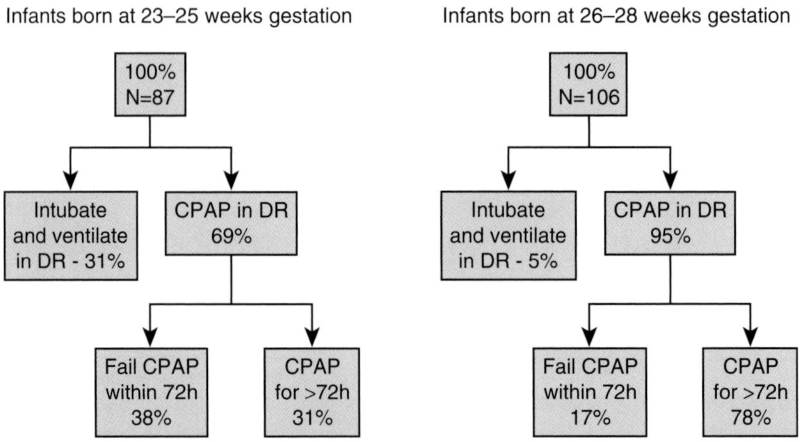

Figure 4-6 Clinical outcomes of infants managed from delivery with early CPAP therapy at Columbia University between 1999 and 2002. The percentages of infants successfully managed with CPAP defined as at least 72 h without intubation are given for infants born at 23–25 weeks gestation and for infants born at 26–28 weeks gestation. Most of the infants initially tolerated CPAP, but more of the earlier gestational age infants needed intubation. Data from Ammari et al. (24).

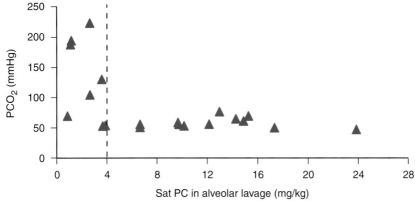

Figure 4-7 Relationship between endogenous surfactant pool size and respiratory failure in preterm lambs supported with 5 cmH₂O CPAP from birth. Preterm lambs with a mean gestational age of 133 days were given CPAP from birth. Lambs with surfactant pool sizes greater than about 4 mg/kg in alveolar lavages maintained reasonable PCO₂ values at 2 h of age. Data redrawn from Mulrooney et al. (27).

surfactant deficiency is the primary cause of RDS? Clinically, many infants who develop RDS have a "honeymoon" period before the progressive respiratory failure, demonstrating that they initially have sufficient surfactant to establish relatively normal ventilation. Recent observations with preterm lambs demonstrate just how little surfactant is required for the preterm to transition to breathing with CPAP (27) (Fig. 4-7). Surfactant amounts above about 4 mg/kg are sufficient for preterm lambs to breathe successfully. Mechanical ventilation of these animals can increase injury and inactivate the small amounts of surfactant, causing more severe RDS. The incidence of RDS and the numbers of infants needing surfactant treatment can be decreased by management approaches to the delivery room care that may decrease lung injury. Other strategies also contribute to a decrease in the diagnosis of RDS. Infants today are different from previous eras because of the more consistent use of antenatal corticosteroids, for example.

FACTORS THAT INFLUENCE SURFACTANT IN THE PRETERM LUNG

The preterm lung changes in multiple ways between first viability at about 23 weeks gestation and a low risk of RDS after about 34 weeks. Those changes include lung structural maturation, improved epithelial barrier function, and increased ability to clear fluid from the airways. These changes influence how surfactant treatment will interact with the lung to acutely improve lung mechanics and how those improvements change with time. Factors that modify surfactant function are: the inactivation and activation of surfactant, effects of antenatal corticosteroids, and the gestational age or stage of lung development (Table 4-1).

Inactivation of Surfactant

The honeymoon period before the development of RDS in some preterm infants suggests that surfactant function is transiently sufficient to allow gas exchange. As illustrated in Fig. 4-5 (20), surfactant function is inadequate as respiratory failure becomes progressive because its function is inhibited. In vitro, surfactant function is inhibited by plasma and other products of lung injury that accumulate in the airspaces. Surfactant function can be degraded by multiple mechanisms

Table 4–1	Factors that Modify Surfactant Function

Inactivation – commonly by lung injury
Activation – by interaction of lung with surfactant
Antenatal steroids
  Increase activation
  Decrease inhibition
  Improve dose-response curve for surfactant
Increase in gestational age
  Increase in lung gas volume
  Lung less easily injured
  Endogenous surfactant less sensitive to inactivation
  More activation of treatment surfactant

(28) (Table 4-2). In RDS, injury and oxidant damage can interfere with surfactant production by type II cells. Hyaline membranes are clots of epithelial debris and plasma proteins that sequester surfactant within the clot. The function of surfactant also is easily inhibited by other substances with surface-active properties such as proteins and bilirubin. The net effect is decreased surfactant function for a given amount of surfactant.

The importance of surfactant to oxygenation is demonstrated by the inverse relationship between PO_2 and surface tension in preterm lambs that had lung injury as a result of mechanical ventilation (29) (Fig. 4-8A). In similar experiments with preterm rabbits, the dose-response curve for surfactant treatment is much less favorable following 30 min of ventilation than for treatment at birth because of the inhibition of the surfactant primarily by proteins (30) (Fig. 4-8B). Because the dose of surfactant used clinically is large and the metabolism of that surfactant is slow, a single dose of surfactant should be adequate treatment for an infant with RDS. Empirically, the majority of infants require only one dose of surfactant. Infants who require more than one dose or who respond poorly to surfactant have lung injury syndromes that result in inactivation of the surfactant used for treatment. The state of lung maturation at a given gestational age is an important variable. The more immature the lung, the more susceptible is the endogenous surfactant to inhibition (12), probably because the surfactant contains less of the surfactant proteins.

Surfactant Activation

Surfactant treatment responses can be divided into three stages: an acute biophysical effect on the surfactant-deficient lung, illustrated by the improvement in PO_2 (Fig. 4-8), a more prolonged effect over hours which further improves compliance and oxygenation, and a prolonged effect of the surfactant as substrate for surfactant metabolism that may persist for days or weeks (Fig. 4-9). Surfactant activation may

Table 4–2	Mechanisms of Surfactant Inactivation

Decreased surfactant in airspace pool
  Injury to type II cells – less synthesis
  Sequestration of surfactant in clots or hyaline membranes
  Increased conversion from surface-active large aggregates to inactive small vesicles
Inhibition of surfactant function/film formation
  Decreased SP-B and SP-C
  Degradation of surfactant – protease, lipase, oxidation
  Competition for surface – plasma proteins, hemoglobin, others

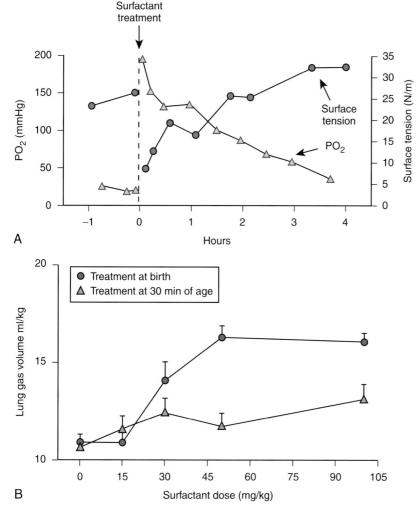

Figure 4-8 Relationship between PO$_2$ and surface tension after treatment of preterm lambs with surfactant, and dose-response curves for treatment of preterm rabbits at birth or at 30 min of age with surfactant. (A) Preterm lambs were ventilated for about 1 h without surfactant treatment. The treatment dose of surfactant caused a rapid increase in PO$_2$, but the improved oxygenation did not persist. Minimal surface tensions in airway samples decreased when PO$_2$ increased but again increased as PO$_2$ decreased. The high surface tensions were caused by protein inhibition of surfactant function. Redrawn from Ikegami et al. (29). (B) Treatment of preterm rabbits at birth resulted in a greater improvement in lung gas volumes at a lower surfactant dose than did surfactant treatment after 30 min of ventilation. Redrawn from Seidner et al. (30).

be the phenomenon most responsible for the continued improvements over the first hours and day after surfactant treatment. The surfactants used for treatment are not equivalent to endogenous surfactant because of differences in lipid composition, surfactant protein content and the lipoprotein organization. The preterm lung has low intracellular as well as alveolar surfactant pool sizes, and that surfactant will contain low amounts of the surfactant proteins and the biophysically critical phospholipids. In experimental models with preterm lungs, surfactant is very efficiently recycled from the airspaces into type 2 cells with resecretion to the airspaces (31). The lungs of preterm ventilated lambs improve the function of the treatment surfactant, presumably by metabolic processing. Within a few hours of treatment and ventilation, surfactant can be recovered that has better function than the surfactant used for treatment (12) (Fig. 4-10). Very preterm lamb lungs are unable to improve the function of the surfactant used for treatment, while the more

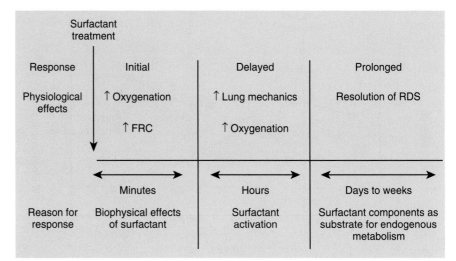

Figure 4-9 The three phases of responses to surfactant treatment. The responses of an infant to surfactant represent a continuum of improved lung function. However, the responses can be divided based on the probable mechanisms contributing to the effects on the lung.

mature lamb lungs can activate surfactant. This improved function depends on metabolism by the preterm lung resulting in alveolar surfactant with increased amounts of surfactant proteins, alterations in lipid composition, and changes in lipoprotein structure.

Antenatal Corticosteroid Effects on Surfactant

Antenatal corticosteroid treatments can decrease the incidence of RDS within 24 h (32). Surfactant is not increased in the fetal sheep for a number of days after maternal betamethasone treatments because of the delay between the synthesis

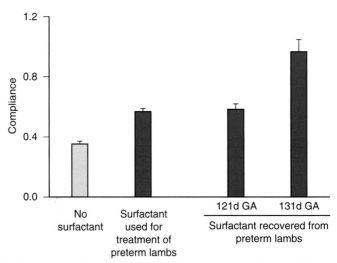

Figure 4-10 Improvement of surfactant function after treatment and recovery from preterm lamb lungs. Preterm lambs at 121 or 131 d gestation were treated at birth with 100 mg/kg Survanta© and gently ventilated for 5 h. Surfactant was recovered by bronchoalveolar lavage. The recovered surfactant from the lambs was used to treat preterm rabbits, and lung function was used as a bioassay for the quality of the surfactant. The lung compliance (ml/cmH₂O/kg) of the preterm rabbits was increased by the surfactant used to treat the lambs. Surfactant recovered from very preterm ventilated lambs was similar to the surfactant used to treat the lambs. However, surfactant from the more mature lambs had improved function. Redrawn from Ueda et al. (12).

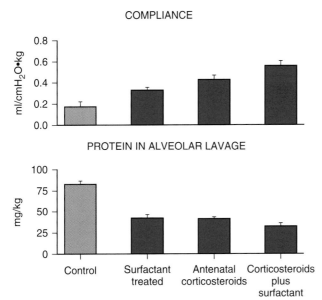

Figure 4-11 Effects of surfactant treatment and antenatal corticosteroid treatment on lung compliance and recovery of protein in alveolar washes from preterm lambs. Both antenatal corticosteroid exposure and postnatal surfactant treatment improved compliance of ventilated preterm lambs. The combination of antenatal corticosteroid and postnatal surfactant further increased lung compliance. The treatments also decreased the amount of protein in alveolar washes, indicating less lung injury. Data from Ikegami et al. (36).

and secretion of surfactant (33). The processing of SP-B from its pro-protein to the mature form also does not occur for several days after maternal corticosteroid treatments. However, lung structure changes within 1 day – the mesenchyme thins, the potential airspace increases, and the epithelium is more resistant to injury and the development of pulmonary edema (34, 35). Therefore, the corticosteroid-exposed preterm lung may be surfactant-deficient and both therapies might have additive effects to improve lung function. Such effects can be demonstrated in experimental models. The interactions between antenatal corticoid treatments and postnatal surfactant treatments are illustrated for protein recovery in alveolar washes and compliance measurements in preterm lambs (36) (Fig. 4-11). Antenatal corticosteroid treatments and postnatal surfactant treatments decrease protein recovery – a measure of lung injury, and increase compliance. Both therapies given to the same lamb qualitatively further decrease protein recovery and increase compliance. The reasons that antenatal corticosteroids improve surfactant responses are multifactorial and complex. The dose-response relationships for endogenous surfactant function during maturation and for treatment with surfactant are altered favorably by antenatal corticosteroid exposure (37, 38) (Fig. 4-12). Corticosteroid-exposed fetuses have larger increases in lung compliances and lower amounts of surfactant are required to achieve those responses. These dose-response effects probably result from the changes in lung structure and decreased surfactant inhibition. The surfactant from the corticosteroid-treated lambs is less sensitive to inhibition by plasma proteins in vitro (39).

The clinical literature also supports the benefits of antenatal corticosteroid treatment followed by surfactant treatments for those infants with RDS. Although antenatal corticosteroids and postnatal surfactant were shown in separate randomized controlled trials to decrease RDS and death, there has not been a trial comparing both treatments with either treatment alone. Such a trial will not be done because both therapies are now considered to be standard of care. In the clinical trials of surfactant, infants who had been exposed to antenatal

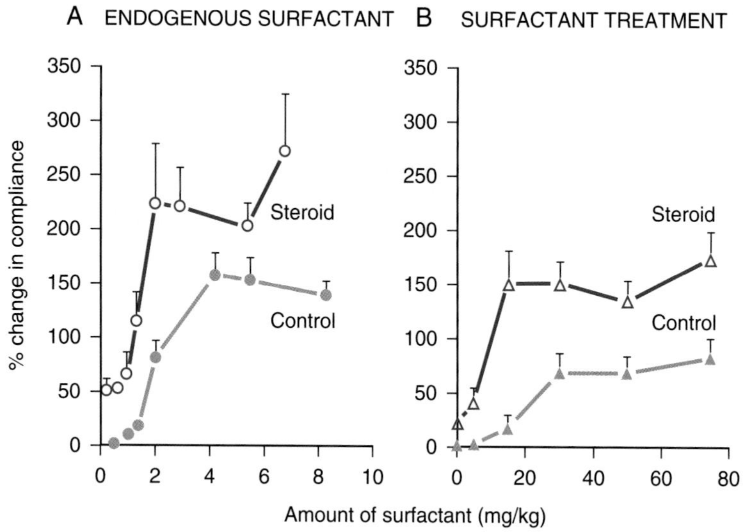

A ENDOGENOUS SURFACTANT **B** SURFACTANT TREATMENT

Figure 4-12 Dose-response curves for endogenous surfactant and surfactant treatment of preterm rabbits: effects of antenatal corticosteroids. (A) Over a narrow range of gestational age, lung compliance increases relative to control animals. Maternal corticosteroid treatment increases the lung compliance at low endogenous surfactant pool sizes relative to controls, and compliance improves more for maternal corticosteroid treated lungs than for control lungs at higher surfactant pool size values. (B) Surfactant treatment of preterm rabbit lungs has less effect on compliance at higher quantities than does lung maturation (curves for controls – A vs. B). Maternal corticosteroid treatment improves the dose-response relationship for surfactant treatment relative to control preterm rabbits. Data redrawn from Ikegami et al. and Seidner et al. (37, 38).

corticosteroids had better outcomes than unexposed infants (40) (Table 4-3). Each therapy is beneficial and the therapies interact to further improve outcomes.

Surfactant Distribution with Treatment

The initial treatment response to surfactant results from the biophysical properties of surfactant and depends on distribution of surfactant rapidly to the distal lung. The surfactants used clinically are very surface-active and when instilled into the lung rapidly adsorb and spread (41). However, the magnitude of the distribution problem is generally not appreciated. The effects of a non-uniform surfactant instillation on aeration of the preterm lung are shown in Figure 4-13 (42). The uninflated lung

Table 4-3 Outcomes of Preterm Infants Treated with Surfactant in Randomized-Controlled Trials Based on Antenatal Corticosteroid Treatments

	MATERNAL CORTICOSTEROIDS		NO MATERNAL CORTICOSTEROIDS	
	+ Surfactant	No surfactant	+ Surfactant	No surfactant
Patient number	57	46	555	566
Air leak	1.7%	13%	11%	23%
Grade – III/IV IVH	7%	11%	25%	23%
28 d mortality	0	15%	18%	25%

Data abstracted from Jobe et al. (40).

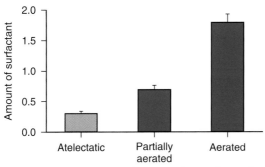

Figure 4-13 Relationship between aeration of preterm lungs after surfactant treatment and recovery of surfactant. Preterm lambs were treated with surfactant and ventilated. The lungs were then cut into multiple pieces and the pieces were scored for amount of aeration visually. The amount of surfactant is expressed relative to a mean value of 1.0 for all lung pieces. The atelectatic lung contained less surfactant than did the aerated lung. Data from Berry et al. (42).

received much less of the surfactant dose than did the lung that was inflated after a period of mechanical ventilation. There are about 20 generations (branch points) from the trachea to the respiratory bronchioles, alveolar ducts, and saccules in the human lung (6). Therefore, there are about 250 000 binary branch points and 500 000 distal airways leading to gas exchange surfaces in the preterm lung. If the distribution is not proportionate to the number of saccules distal to *each* branch point, then surfactant distribution will not be uniform, where uniformity is defined as the same amount of surfactant in each of the perhaps 10 million saccules in the preterm lung prior to 32 weeks gestation. A non-uniformity at a proximal branch point will be amplified at subsequent branch points. Surfactant distribution has been studied in a number of model systems and depends on physical factors during its administration (43) (Table 4-4). Empirically, surfactant distribution is good enough in practice because the lung fields can clear rapidly and oxygenation can improve quickly, indicating minimal atelectasis and intrapulmonary shunt.

However, treatment techniques do matter (44, 45) (Fig. 4-14). Surfactant will distribute to preterm sheep lung more uniformly when given at birth because it will mix with fetal lung fluid, which will increase the volume, and gravity will not be a factor in a fluid-filled lung. In contrast, after a period of mechanical ventilation, the distribution will be less uniform when using four positions for instillation and a volume of 4 ml/kg because the physical variables will influence distribution in the gas-filled lung. An infusion of surfactant into the lungs over 15 min to minimize any acute physiologic changes during treatment will result in a very poor distribution primarily because of the effects of gravity on the slow rate of administration. If an initial dose of surfactant is poorly distributed to the lung, a second dose will distribute similarly to the first dose. The part of the lung that inflates will be the lung containing the most surfactant, and that region of the lung will receive

Table 4–4 Variables that Contribute to the Distribution of Surfactant in the Lungs

Property	Effect
Surface activity	Essential for rapid adsorption and spreading
Gravity	Surfactant distributed with fluid by gravity in large airways
Volume	The higher the volume, the better the distribution
Rate of administration	Rapid administration results in a better distribution
Ventilator settings	Pressure and PEEP push surfactant into distal airways
Fluid volume in lung	Higher volumes of fetal lung fluid or edema fluid may result in a better distribution

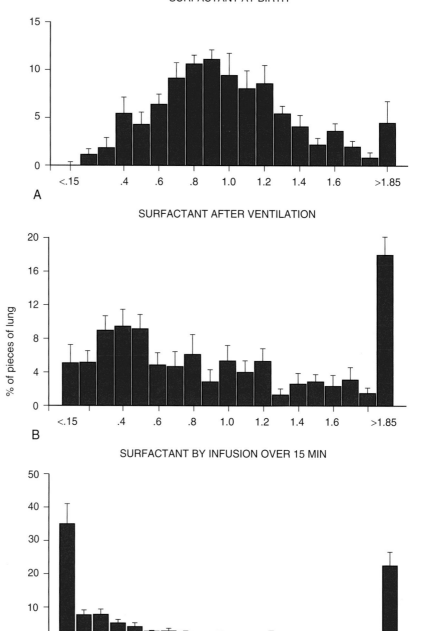

Figure 4-14 Surfactant distributions resulting from different treatment techniques. The distribution of surfactant was measured in the lungs of preterm lambs after treatment with radioactive surfactant and ventilation. Frozen lungs were cut into about 120 pieces and the amount of surfactant/weight of each piece was measured. A mean surfactant amount/piece was calculated and given a value of 1.0. A perfect distribution would be for all pieces to have a value of 1.0. Pieces with distribution intervals < 1 have less surfactant, distribution intervals > 1 indicate pieces of lung with more than the mean amount of surfactant. (A) There was a relatively uniform distribution of surfactant when the surfactant was mixed with fetal lung fluid at birth followed by mechanical ventilation. (B) The surfactant distribution for treatment after birth and ventilation was less uniform. The surfactant was given by the four-position maneuver commonly used clinically. (C) The distribution following a 15 min infusion of surfactant in ventilated lambs was very non-uniform. The surfactant was poorly distributed with 34% of lung pieces receiving less than 15% of the mean amount of surfactant and 25% of the lung pieces receiving large amounts of surfactant. Figure adapted from Jobe et al. (45).

increased pulmonary blood flow because of auto-regulation of blood flow away from unventilated lung to ventilated lung segments, which will tend to mask the severity of the maldistribution of ventilation.

Surfactant delivered to one lobe or one lung will not redistribute between lobes or to the other lung. Aerosolized surfactant distributes proportionately with ventilation, which means it treats the open lung and not the atelectatic or edema-filled lung. Although large volumes of surfactant will improve distribution, there must be a compromise between instillation volume and the infant's tolerance of that volume. More volume will require more pressure and PEEP to distribute the surfactant quickly to minimize acute airway obstruction. While surfactant distribution in practice is not ideal, it is good enough because of the biophysical properties of the surfactant, and the small amount that is needed regionally in the lung for a treatment response. There are no practical ways to improve distribution other than using positioning of the infant to minimize gravity, giving surfactant quickly in a reasonable volume, and giving the infant enough ventilatory support to quickly clear the airways of fluid. It should be remembered that the standard protocol for surfactant treatment in the clinical trials was to increase the oxygen to 100% and the rate to 60 breaths per minute prior to surfactant instillation to avoid cyanosis, and these changes in ventilatory support are seldom done with the general clinical use of surfactant.

The question of how surfactant treatment should be given to infants with RDS can be answered based primarily on this experimental information. Each of the commercial surfactants was tested clinically using somewhat different and quite empirically devised treatment techniques. The treatment techniques described in the package inserts for the different surfactants have not been compared and have been modified by common usage without clinical testing. There is a clinical trial comparing a 4 position, 4 aliquot treatment with a 2 position, 2 aliquot treatment that demonstrated no difference (46). My suggestions, based on the experimental results and clinical experience, are as follows. Gently suction the endotracheal tube and then administer the surfactant using a 5 Fr feeding tube inserted into the ventilation circuit to the end of the endotracheal tube while maintaining the current ventilator settings. A 2 position, 2 aliquot or a 4 position, 4 aliquot technique are probably equivalent. Give each aliquot as fast as it can easily be pushed through the catheter and maintain the infant's position for about 10 s. If bradycardia or desaturation occurs, wait for recovery before the next aliquot is given. If the bradycardia or desaturation persists, increase the peak inspiratory pressure and oxygen concentration. Even with adjustments of the ventilator to a rate of 60 breaths per minute and the oxygen to 100%, bradycardia and desaturations were frequent in the clinical trials (47). Destabilization seems to be more frequent with second or third doses – probably because the infants are on low pressures, low rates and low supplemental oxygen. Surfactants are viscous and volumes are relatively large. For example, a dose of 4 ml/kg translates to the instillation of 280 ml into the trachea of a 70 kg adult male, equivalent to 70% of the contents of a standard 12 oz soft drink can. The preterm infant has less airway and alveolar volume/kg than the adult to accommodate the volume. Some respiratory distress should be anticipated following surfactant treatment, but slow administration is *not* the solution because of its adverse effects on distribution.

When Should Surfactant Be Given?

The first surfactant trials that were done without industry sponsorship demonstrated improved oxygenation and decreased pneumothorax for the treatment of established RDS in ventilated infants (22, 48). Subsequent trials sponsored by industry for approval of surfactant for general clinical use have evaluated two indications for surfactant: prophylactic treatment (synonyms: delivery room treatment, very early treatment), and rescue treatment (synonyms: late treatment, treatment of RDS). I prefer the phrases "early treatment of infants at risk of RDS" and "treatment of infants with RDS" as better descriptors of the goals of the different treatment strategies. The concept for the early treatment of infants at risk of RDS was developed by two of the pioneers in the field of surfactant treatment for RDS – Drs Goran Enhorning and Bengt Robertson (49). Preterm animals ventilated before surfactant treatment rapidly developed severe lung injury and that injury could be minimized by surfactant treatment before mechanical ventilation (50). Surfactant treatment responses were inferior if the preterm animals were ventilated before surfactant treatment (Fig. 4-8B). Several trials were done where spontaneous ventilation of preterm infants was prevented as much as possible before a surfactant treatment after delivery (51). In contrast, most trials defined early treatment as treatment in the delivery room, generally within 15 min of birth, for infants at high risk of developing RDS – less than 28 weeks gestation or less than 1 kg birth weight, for example. The question of "immediate" treatment before the first breath versus early treatment was answered by a large trial reported by Kendig et al. (52). Contrary to the hypothesis and the animal data, treatment before the first breath resulted in more BPD than did early treatment. The likely explanation is that attempts to treat before the infant can breathe can interfere with initial stabilization of the infant. Therefore, attempts to treat before an infant can breathe are not indicated.

That still leaves the larger question of early treatment of infants at risk of RDS versus treatment only of infants who develop RDS. The randomized and controlled trials demonstrated that either treatment strategy decreased deaths and pneumothorax. Comparison trials and meta-analyses of the two-treatment strategies demonstrated benefit for early treatment relative to treatment of established RDS (53). Despite this evidence-based conclusion, Horbar et al. (26) reported that most neonatal units in the Vermont-Oxford Network did not routinely give surfactant in the delivery room and that surfactant treatment was often delayed for infants with gestations of 23 to 29 weeks and birth weights less than 1500 g. Almost 80% of this population of infants was treated at some time with surfactant (data for 2000). These observations stimulated the Vermont-Oxford Network to launch a quality-improvement initiative to promote "evidence-based" early surfactant treatments for 23–29 weeks gestation infants (54). The training intervention decreased the mean time to receive surfactant from 78 min to 21 min, increased the likelihood of delivery room treatment (odds ratio 5.4), and decreased treatments after 2 h of age (odds ratio 0.35). Despite these large improvements toward the evidence-based goals, there was no benefit for the important outcomes of mortality, pneumothorax or BPD (Table 4-5).

What is the explanation for this lack of benefit? The explanation is likely to involve two factors acting together – the quality of the trial evidence and changes in clinical practice. The evidence was based on trials comparing early treatment – within 15 min of age – with late treatment of established RDS – which in many of the trials was randomization after 6 h of age (53). The quality-improvement initiative decreased mean treatment times from 78 min to 21 min, and both mean times resulted in relatively early surfactant treatment. The other factor may be how the infants with delayed treatment were cared for. In the later 1980s, and early 1990s, these infants were frequently intubated and ventilated to PCO_2 values of 30–40 mmHg – aggressively ventilated by today's standards. Today, many of these infants are not intubated in the delivery room and thus these infants may avoid the risk of early lung injury from mechanical ventilation. I previously presented the outcomes for two institutions that manage very low birth weight babies with CPAP (24, 25) (Fig. 4-6). In those clinical experiences, the majority of infants were never intubated and did not receive surfactant, and their outcomes were not very different from those

Table 4–5 **Outcomes of Quality Improvement Initiative to Decrease Time from Birth to Surfactant Treatment for Infants with Birth Gestations of 23–29 Weeks**

	Intervention units	Control units
Number of units	57	57
Average time to surfactant treatment (min)	21	78
Mean birth weight (g)	942	925
Antenatal corticosteroid (%)	77	77
Mortality (%)	17.8	18.2
Pneumothorax (%)	6.6	7.4
BPD – O_2 at 36 weeks	42.1	38.5

Data from Horbar et al. (54).

reported by the Vermont-Oxford Network (Table 4-6). Finer et al. (55) reported an exploratory trial of the randomization of infants to an attempt at the use of CPAP in the delivery room or intubation and surfactant treatment. CPAP was initially successful in 45% of the infants, and Aly demonstrated increased success with experience with the technique (25). There are several randomized controlled trials being performed to ask which approach is best. However, the clinical reality is that trials evaluate populations of patients and do not individualize treatment options.

My view on this question of early versus late surfactant treatment can be summarized by the diagram in Figure 4-15. Ideally the clinician would know which infants would be "good" (mature lungs, no birth depression), marginal, or "bad" (lung immaturity and/or birth depression) before birth. Lung maturation tests can help identify the infants with mature lungs (8), but they are seldom used. Birth depression, sepsis, or other causes of poor transition can be predicted to some degree based on antenatal information. However, for most deliveries, the clinician does not know if an infant will be "good" – breathe and not need surfactant if managed with CPAP or "bad" – require intubation for resuscitation and may or may not have lung immaturity and need surfactant. The changes from the management styles during the era of the surfactant trials are that we now recognize that many very low birth weight infants *will* breathe and *will not* develop severe RDS. These infants do not need resuscitation, but rather gentle assistance to help them with adaptation (56). There is no information about adverse effects of intubation of infants who will breathe spontaneously or to know whether surfactant treatments are safe or harmful for infants who will not develop RDS. The converse is that a delay in resuscitation of a "bad" infant may adversely affect outcome. Ultimately, a quick clinical appraisal followed by the application of selected interventions as indicated by clinical response may benefit more infants than a rigid protocol of either a trial of CPAP or intubation and surfactant treatment. The problem for "evidence-based" decision-making will be the great variability of how these infants

Table 4–6 **Outcomes for 261 Infants with Birth Weights ≤1250 g**

	% of population
Intubated to 72 h of age	33
Treated with surfactant	17.2
Mortality	15.7
Pneumothorax	7.3
BPD – oxygen at 36 weeks	19

Data from Ammari et al. (24).

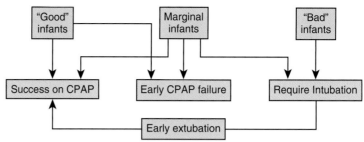

Figure 4-15 Characteristics of infants at delivery and anticipated success with early CPAP. "Good" infants are vigorous and healthy, while "Bad" infants are depressed and require ventilatory resuscitation. Marginal infants can be stimulated to breathe with patience in some cases, but these infants are likely to fail CPAP. Guidance for delivery room management at any gestational age may depend on the distribution of the infants into these three categories.

present, the short time frame for experienced decision-making, and the skills of the personnel for CPAP, intubation and ventilation. I am not optimistic that clinical trials will definitively answer who should receive surfactant and when. In the rush to treat infants at risk for RDS earlier and earlier, it is worth remembering that infants who have RDS and who are not treated for hours or days, for whatever reason, will respond well to surfactant treatments.

Do Infants Need More Than One Dose of Surfactant?

This question has a history from the clinical trials. The initial trials for FDA approval were designed as single-dose trials with the goals of improving oxygenation and decreasing pneumothorax (57). The trials were not powered to demonstrate decreased mortality. Although the single-dose trials did achieve their goals, the FDA requested a demonstration of decreased mortality prior to approval. Repeated-dose protocols were then completed which did show decreased mortality (58). The repeated doses were given after late (by current standards) initial doses and after significant lung injury had already developed. The re-dosing schedules were empirically developed for each surfactant as were the indications for retreatment. We know that a single treatment dose of 100–200 mg/kg surfactant is very large relative to the surfactant pool size of an adult human (perhaps 5 mg/kg) or a preterm animal without RDS (> 4 mg/kg) (59). The slow catabolism and recycling of the treatment dose of surfactant ensures a long persistence of the surfactant in the preterm lung, and mechanisms to preserve and enhance the function of that surfactant also contribute to prolonged effects. Therefore, an infant with an uninjured lung should only require one dose of surfactant. Repetitive doses may be needed to overcome inhibition of surfactant function if lung injury has occurred. However, few infants benefit from more than two doses, and large numbers of doses may be harmful (60). Multiple doses of surfactant are not treating a primary surfactant deficiency. The schedules for retreatment in the surfactant package inserts are based on the trial information collected during a period when ventilator-mediated lung injury was more common than today and may not be relevant to current management approaches. In general, as long as an infant continues to improve (decreased oxygen requirements, decreased ventilator support) after a dose of surfactant, a second dose is not indicated.

Is Surfactant Useful for Diseases Other Than RDS?

Surfactant therapy was developed for RDS because of the understanding that surfactant deficiency was the cardinal element of lung immaturity that limited lung function. However, it was recognized that surfactant function could be inhibited by proteinaceous pulmonary edema and other products of lung injury and result in a secondary surfactant deficiency type syndrome (61). Surfactant treatment improves lung function in multiple experimental models of lung injury. Other than injury caused by mechanical ventilation, the common lung injury syndromes in infants are meconium aspiration syndrome, bronchopulmonary dysplasia and sepsis/pneumonia. As already illustrated in this chapter, lung injury caused by mechanical ventilation results in a less favorable response to surfactant treatment than treatment of the uninjured preterm lung (30) (Fig. 4-8). Surfactant abnormalities in the other lung injury syndromes in newborns have two explanations: inhibition of surfactant function and/or altered surfactant metabolism. Either abnormality might be improved by surfactant treatment.

MECONIUM ASPIRATION SYNDROME

The infants who aspirate meconium are almost all term or post-term and thus do not have surfactant deficiency. In fact, the alveolar pool size of surfactant after term birth exceeds the normal adult levels by more than 10-fold in animals, although values for the human are not available. Meconium is a potent inhibitor of surfactant in vitro and it inactivates surfactant in experimental models (62). Meconium also can degrade lung function by obstruction of airways (complete obstruction causes atelectasis and partial obstruction causes overexpansion) and by induction of inflammation and edema. Mechanical ventilation and exposure of the lung to high oxygen concentrations further promote lung injury, increase inhibitors of surfactant and further inhibit surfactant function. A small randomized trial of surfactant treatment for meconium aspiration and other reports demonstrate that surfactant instillation can improve oxygenation in infants with meconium aspiration (63, 64). Surfactant treatment of term infants with severe respiratory failure also can decrease the need for extracorporeal membrane oxygenation (65). The infants seem to respond to surfactant better if the treatment is given soon after the onset of respiratory failure, and large or repeated doses may be needed. These observations are consistent with the idea that treatment is less effective if injury is already severe.

A poorly documented practice has been "lung lavage" of infants with meconium aspiration with the goal to remove more meconium than could be removed by airway suction at delivery. This technique has been adapted to mixing the saline used for lavage with surfactant. The addition of surfactant might facilitate recovery of particulate meconium, which would relieve airway obstruction. A surfactant suspension also could minimize the depletion of surfactant by the lavage procedure. Surfactant lavage was compared to routine care in several small series and seemed to improve oxygenation (66–68). However, surfactant lavage has not been compared to the more standard surfactant instillation, which may have similar effects and is easier to perform and is less stressful for the infant. Fortunately, severe meconium aspiration is much less frequent today. Less aggressive management (limiting mechanical ventilation, avoiding hyperventilation), with the use of adjunct therapies such as high-frequency oscillation and nitric oxide has decreased the need for extracorporeal membrane oxygenation to salvage infants with severe meconium aspiration. Surfactant instillation is frequently used prior to high-frequency oscillation and nitric oxide to allow the lung to "open" optimally; however, that strategy will probably never be evidence-based because of the complexity of managing these infrequent cases. The use of lavage with surfactant remains experimental.

BRONCHOPULMONARY DYSPLASIA

Surfactant contributes to the abnormalities in the early stages of progression of the preterm lung to BPD. There is good evidence that surfactant metabolism is

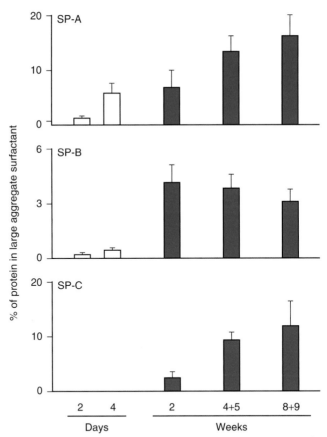

Figure 4-16 Surfactant proteins increase with age after preterm birth. The surfactant proteins SP-A, SP-B and SP-C were measured in the large aggregate (bioactive) surfactant recovered from airway samples of infants with normal surfactant and minimal lung disease. Data redrawn from Ballard et al. (11).

abnormal and that surfactant function often is also abnormal (69). Surfactant from the immature lung is deficient in phosphatidylglycerol, which increases with maturation. Infants developing BPD have a delay in the appearance of phosphatidylglycerol. The surfactant proteins SP-A, SP-B, and SP-C also are very low in surfactant from the preterm with RDS. These proteins increase in surfactant quickly after preterm birth (Fig. 4-16) to achieve concentration ratios similar to surfactant from the mature lung (11). Infants who progress toward BPD continue to have low amounts of the surfactant proteins, and low amounts of the proteins correlate with high minimum surface tension (69) (Table 4-7). The minimum surface tensions of the surfactant recovered from infants developing BPD were high for those samples that contained low amounts of SP-B, and surfactant with less surfactant protein will be more sensitive to inhibition. The samples from infants who had deteriorating respiratory function had higher surface tensions. The net outcome for infants with BPD is that the surfactant protein content of their surfactant is low and that surfactant can be easily inhibited by the inflammatory products of lung injury caused by mechanical ventilation, supplemental oxygen or infection.

The metabolism of the surfactant lipids also is abnormal in BPD. Cogo et al. (70) used dipalmitoylphosphatidylcholine labeled with stable isotope to measure metabolic variables for the phosphatidylcholine compartment of surfactant. They found that relative to control preterm infants of the same birth weight and gestational age, the infants with BPD had only 30% of the surfactant concentration in the airspace fluid, and this surfactant had a shorter half-life (70) (Table 4-8). In contrast, the

Table 4–7   Surfactant in Airway Samples from Infants with BPD

	SURFACTANT FROM INFANTS WITH BPD		
	Surface tension <5 mN/m	Surface tension >5 mN/m	Normal surfactant
Phospholipids (%)			
Phosphatidylcholine	81	80	80
Phosphatidylinositol	1.0	0.4	2
Phosphatidylglycerol	1.6	2.0	7
Proteins (%)			
SP-A	2.6	1.3	5
SP-B	1.0	0.2	1
SP-C	2.1	0.6	2

From Merrill et al. (77).

"apparent lung pool size" of Sat PC was more than double that found in infants without BPD. This combination of a small alveolar pool size together with an increased total pool was replicated in preterm ventilated baboons that were developing BPD. Those animals had small alveolar surfactant pool sizes, large lung tissue pools of Sat PC, and surfactant that had decreased function relative to normal surfactant (30) (Fig. 4-17). The measurements have been made in infants *developing* BPD and not in the chronic stages of the disease beyond 36 weeks gestation. The lungs of infants who have died of BPD have distal saccules lined with dysplastic type II cells with *increased* expression of mRNA for the surfactant proteins (71). Similar findings are seen in preterm baboons developing BPD. Surfactant function and metabolism is abnormal in BPD.

If surfactant is abnormal, then could surfactant treatments be of benefit? Pandit et al. (72) treated 10 infants at a mean age of 13 days who they thought were destined to develop BPD and demonstrated transient improvements in oxygenation. Surfactant treatments could be of long-term benefit if surfactant suppressed ongoing inflammation, overcame inhibition, and allowed the infants to receive less ventilatory support. However, much of the benefit of surfactant treatment for RDS results from the metabolism and reprocessing of the surfactant by the uninjured preterm lung. The BPD lung seems to have *increased* amounts of surfactant lipids and abnormal metabolism. Surfactant treatments might make those metabolic defects worse. Clinical trials to demonstrate a benefit of surfactant therapy for BPD will be difficult because of the variable course of the disease.

SURFACTANT FOR SEPSIS/PNEUMONIA SYNDROMES

Many preterm infants are born after exposure to chorioamnionitis, which causes lung inflammation (73). Although few of these infants have overt pneumonia, the distinction between RDS and RDS with some infection is seldom made. Infants with Group B

Table 4–8   Metabolic Variables for Saturated Phosphatidylcholine (Sat PC) in Control Infants and Infants Developing BPD

	BPD infants	Controls
Sat PC in lung fluid (mg/ml)	2.9 ± 0.6	9.4 ± 3.0
Half-life of sat. PC (h)	19.4 ± 2.8	42.5 ± 6.3
Apparent pool size of sat PC (mg/kg)	136 ± 21	66 ± 16

Data from Cogo et al. (70).

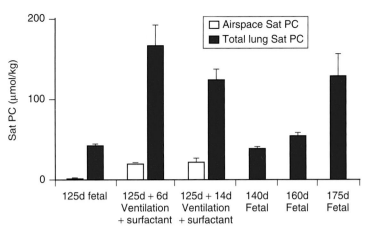

Figure 4-17 Amount of surfactant is increased in lungs of preterm ventilated baboons developing BPD. The amounts of saturated phosphatidylcholine do not increase in the fetal baboon lung until after about 140 days gestation. Baboons that were delivered prematurely at 125 days gestation and treated with surfactant accumulate large amounts of Sat PC in their lung tissue, but airspace Sat PC does not increase between 6 and 14 days of ventilation. Data from Seidner et al. (30).

strep pneumonia/sepsis cannot be easily identified at birth if they are preterm, and some of these infants will have both RDS and infection together. The identification of infection as the cause of respiratory failure is generally much clearer in near-term and term infants. Many infants thought to have RDS were inadvertently treated with surfactant in the clinical trials, and experimental studies in animal models of lung infection demonstrate short-term improvements in lung function (61). Therefore, surfactant treatment might be beneficial for infants with respiratory failure from lung infection. The surfactant therapy will treat any RDS that is present and counteract the inhibition of the endogenous surfactant pool by the inflammatory products and injury. Empirically, infants with pneumonia have been treated and lung function can improve (64). Although no randomized controlled trials are available, Hertig et al. (74) reported the clinical responses and outcomes of 118 preterm infants with Group B sepsis who were treated with surfactant. The infants had initial oxygenation and mean airway pressure responses that were not as large as for infants with RDS. Similar responses have been reported for term infants. Nevertheless, the infants seemed to benefit from surfactant treatment. There appears to be no contraindication to treating an infant with pneumonia with surfactant. However, if the sepsis/pneumonia has caused myocardial depression and low perfusion, then surfactant is unlikely to improve lung function. Surfactant has not been of benefit consistently for adults with the Acute Respiratory Distress Syndrome, which is often caused by sepsis (75).

WHICH SURFACTANT SHOULD BE USED TO TREAT RDS OR OTHER LUNG INJURY SYNDROMES?

The evidence-based answer to this question is confounded by industry efforts to promote different surfactants. There are two general classes of surfactants that have been developed – surfactants extracted in various ways from animal lungs and surfactants that are synthetic. The synthetic surfactants are either a mixture of lipids or the lipids plus proteins or peptides that confer functions similar to the native surfactant proteins SP-B or SP-C. Most clinicians world-wide have used surfactants sourced from animal lungs after the synthetic lipid-only surfactant Colfosceril Palmitate (Exosurf) was no longer available. Synthetic surfactants containing lipid only were not as effective as animal-source surfactants (76). A new synthetic surfactant containing lipids and a synthetic peptide (Lucinactant) is now being tested (69, 77). The clinician needs to be very cautious in accepting claims about small differences in the surfactants that are currently available for the treatment of RDS. Recent reports compare the synthetic surfactant Lucinactant to Colfosceril Palmitate – the lipid-only synthetic surfactant and the animal-sourced surfactant Beractant (Survanta®) (77). In my opinion, the comparison to Colfosceril is not relevant as that surfactant is no longer available. The early treatment trial comparing Lucinactant with Beractant reported unusual primary outcomes – the incidence of RDS at 24 hours and death related to RDS by 14 days of age. Most clinicians would select the relevant primary outcomes as overall death or BPD at 36 weeks. For those outcomes there were no differences, although the death outcome approached significance favoring Lucinactant. The trial did not compare equivalent doses or the same instillation volumes of surfactant, which complicates the interpretation of this and most other trials comparing surfactants. One can ask the question: Do any differences in surfactant result from treatment dose, volume, or treatment technique? A trial comparing Lucinactant with Poractant Alfa (Curosurf®) for the early treatment and the treatment of established RDS demonstrated similar outcomes (78).

Perhaps a useful perspective on surfactant comparison trials can be achieved by reviewing the outcomes of the trials comparing Beractant and Calfactant (Infasurf®) for the early treatment and the treatment of established RDS (79) (Table 4-9). These recent large trials are most relevant to current practice and outcomes. The very low birth weight infants in the early treatment trial received surfactant by about 8 minutes of age. The mean days of intubation was only 3–4 days, only 12% died and very few had severe BPD. For infants treated for RDS, the period of intubation was only 4–5 days, only about 10% died, and 4% had severe BPD. For both studies, other complications were low. I conclude from these trials that the neonatal community is doing a very good job of managing RDS with surfactant. Given the low death and complication rates, it is unlikely that relevant

Table 4–9 **Comparison of Two Surfactants for Early Treatment and Treatment of RDS**

	EARLY TREATMENT		TREATMENT OF RDS	
	Surfactant 1	Surfactant 2	Surfactant 1	Surfactant 2
Characteristics of populations				
Number of infants randomized	375	374	673	688
Gestational age (weeks, mean)	26.6	26.5	28.4	28.4
Birth weight (g, mean)	907	910	1154	1100
Clinical variables				
Age at treatment (minutes)	8	9	159	166
Days intubated (median)	3	4	4	5
≤30% oxygen at 10 days (%)	61	60	68	65
Outcomes				
Died (%)	12	13	10	11
BPD – oxygen at 36 weeks (%)	34	33	31	31
Severe BPD – ventilator at 36 weeks (%)	4	6	4	4
IVH – Grades III or IV (%)	10	14	10	13
Pulmonary interstitial emphysema (%)	5	8	7	6
Pneumothorax	7	5	8	6

Surfactant 1 is Survanta (Beractant) and surfactant 2 is Infasurf (Calfactant).
Data from Bloom et al. (79).

differences in effectiveness between surfactants can be demonstrated. There are differences in the volumes used for treatment, differences in amounts of surfactant, small differences in short-term physiological outcomes, and in the experience of caregivers with the surfactants. However, the important outcomes of death, BPD and the major complications of prematurity are similar. My preference is to use just one surfactant in a neonatal unit to avoid dosing and handling errors and to consider using the least expensive surfactant.

Acknowledgments

This review was supported by Grants HD-12714 and HL-65397 from the National Institutes of Health.

REFERENCES

1. Horbar JD, Wright EC, Onstad L, et al. Decreasing mortality associated with the introduction of surfactant therapy: an observed study of neonates weighing 601 to 1300 grams at birth. Pediatrics 1993; 92.
2. Schwartz RM, Luby AM, Scanlon JW, et al. Effect of surfactant on morbidity, mortality, and resource use in newborn infants weighing 500 to 1500 g. N Engl J Med 1994; 330:1476–1480.
3. Soll RF. Prophylactic natural surfactant extract for preventing morbidity and mortality in preterm infants. Cochrane Database of Systematic Reviews 2001; 3.
4. Jobe AH, Ikegami M. Biology of surfactant. Clin Perinatol 2001; 28:655–669.
5. Jobe A, Ikegami M. Surfactant for the treatment of respiratory distress syndrome. Am Rev Respir Dis 1987; 136:1256–1275.
6. Burri PW. Development and growth of the human lung. In: Fishman AP, Fisher AB, eds. Handbook of physiology: the respiratory system. Bethesda, MD: American Physiologic Society; 1985: 1–46.
7. Hislop AA, Wigglesworth JS, Desai R. Alveolar development in the human fetus and infant. Early Hum Dev 1986; 13:1–11.
8. Kulovich MV, Hallman M, Gluck L. The lung profile: normal pregnancy. Am J Obstet Gynecol 1979; 135:57–63.
9. Pryhuber GS, Hull WM, Fink I, et al. Ontogeny of surfactant protein-A and protein-B in human amniotic fluid as indices of fetal lung maturity. Pediatr Res 1991; 30:597–605.
10. Gluck L, Kulovich M, Borer RC, et al. Diagnosis of the respiratory distress syndrome by amniocentesis. Am J Obstet Gynecol 1971; 109:440–445.
11. Ballard PL, Gonzales LW, Godinez RI, et al. Surfactant composition and function in a primate model of infant chronic lung disease: effects of inhaled nitric oxide. Pediatr Res 2006; 59:157–162.
12. Ueda T, Ikegami M, Jobe AH. Developmental changes of sheep surfactant: in vivo function and in vitro subtype conversion. J Appl Physiol 1994; 76:2701–2706.
13. Whitsett JA, Weaver TE. Hydrophobic surfactant proteins in lung function and disease. N Engl J Med 2002; 347:2141–2148.
14. Bunt JE, Zimmerman LJ, Wattimena D, et al. Endogenous surfactant turnover in preterm infants measured with stable isotope. Am J Respir Crit Care Med 1998; 157:810–814.
15. Torresin M, Zimmermann LJ, Cogo PE, et al. Exogenous surfactant kinetics in infant respiratory distress syndrome: A novel method with stable isotopes. Am J Respir Crit Care Med 2000; 161: 1584–1589.
16. Jobe AH. Surfactant metabolism in newborns – insights from imprecise measurements. Pediatrics 2003; 142:223–224.
17. Jackson JC, Palmer S, Truog WE, et al. Surfactant quantity and composition during recovery from hyaline membrane disease. Pediatr Res 1986; 20:1243–1247.
18. Cogo PE, Toffolo GM, Gucciardi A, et al. Surfactant disaturated phosphatidylcholine kinetics in infants with bronchopulmonary dysplasia measured with stable isotopes and a two-compartment model. J Appl Physiol 2005; 99:323–329.
19. Ikegami M, Jobe A, Yamada T, et al. Surfactant metabolism in surfactant-treated preterm ventilated lambs. J Appl Physiol 1989; 67:429–437.
20. Ikegami M, Jacobs H, Jobe AH. Surfactant function in the respiratory distress syndrome. J Pediatr 1983; 102:443–447.
21. Robertson B, Berry D, Curstedt T, et al. Leakage of protein in the immature rabbit lung; effect of surfactant replacement. Respir Physiol 1985; 61:265–276.
22. Shapiro DL, Notter RH, Morin FCD, et al. Double-blind, randomized trial of a calf lung surfactant extract administered at birth to very premature infants for prevention of respiratory distress syndrome. Pediatrics 1985; 76:593–599.
23. Verder H, Albertsen P, Ebbesen F, et al. Nasal continuous positive airway pressure and early surfactant therapy for respiratory distress syndrome in newborns of less than 30 weeks' gestation. Pediatrics 1999; 103:E24.

24. Ammari A, Suri MS, Milisavljevic V, et al. Variables associated with the early failure of nasal CPAP in very low birth weight infants. J Pediatr 2005; 147:341–347.

25. Aly H, Massaro AN, Patel K, et al. Is it safer to intubate premature infants in the delivery room? Pediatrics 2005; 115:1660–1665.

26. Horbar JD, Carpenter JH, Buzas J, et al. Timing of initial surfactant treatment for infants 23 to 29 weeks' gestation: is routine practice evidence based? Pediatrics 2004; 113:1593–1602.

27. Mulrooney N, Champion Z, Moss TJ, et al. Surfactant and physiological responses of preterm lambs to continuous positive airway pressure. Am J Respir Crit Care Med 2005; 171:488–493.

28. Jobe AH. Surfactant-edema interactions. In: Weir EK, Reeves JT, eds. The pathogenesis and treatment of pulmonary edema. Armonk, NY: Futura Publishing; 1998:113–131.

29. Ikegami M, Jobe A, Glatz T. Surface activity following natural surfactant treatment in premature lambs. Am J Physiol Lung Cell Mol Physiol 1981; 51:L306–L312.

30. Seidner SR, Ikegami M, Yamada T, et al. Decreased surfactant dose-response after delayed administration to preterm rabbits. Am J Respir Crit Care Med 1995; 152:113–120.

31. Jobe AH, Ikegami M, Seidner SR, et al. Surfactant phosphatidylcholine metabolism and surfactant function in preterm, ventilated lambs. Am Rev Respir Dis 1989; 139:352–359.

32. Crowley P. Antenatal corticosteroid therapy: a meta-analysis of the randomized trials – 1972–1994. Am J Obstet Gynecol 1995; 173:322–335.

33. Ballard PL, Ning Y, Polk D, et al. Glucocorticoid regulation of surfactant components in immature lambs. Am J Physiol 1997; 273:L1048–L1057.

34. Ikegami M, Berry D, Elkady T, et al. Corticosteroids and surfactant change lung function and protein leaks in the lungs of ventilated premature rabbits. J Clin Invest 1987; 79:1371–1378.

35. Willet KE, McMenamin P, Pinkerton KE, et al. Lung morphometry and collagen and elastin content: changes during normal development and after prenatal hormone exposure in sheep. Pediatr Res 2000; 45:615–625.

36. Ikegami M, Polk D, Tabor B, et al. Corticosteroid and thyrotropin-releasing hormone effects on preterm sheep lung function. J Appl Physiol 1991; 70:2268–2278.

37. Ikegami M, Jobe AH, Yamada T, et al. Relationship between alveolar saturated phosphatidylcholine pool sizes and compliance of preterm rabbit lungs. The effect of maternal corticosteroid treatment. Am Rev Respir Dis 1989; 139:367–369.

38. Seidner S, Pettenazzo A, Ikegami M, et al. Corticosteroid potentiation of surfactant dose response in preterm rabbits. J Appl Physiol 1988; 64:2366–2371.

39. Rebello CM, Ikegami M, Polk DH, et al. Postnatal lung responses and surfactant function after fetal or maternal corticosteroid treatment of preterm lambs. J Appl Physiol 1996; 80:1674–1680.

40. Jobe AH, Mitchell BR, Gunkel JH. Beneficial effects of the combined use of prenatal corticosteroids and postnatal surfactant on preterm infants. Am J Obstet Gynecol 1993; 168:508–513.

41. Charon A, Taeusch HW, Fitzgibbon C, et al. Factors associated with surfactant treatment response in infants with severe respiratory distress syndrome. Pediatrics 1989; 83:348–354.

42. Berry D, Jobe A, Jacobs H, et al. Distribution of pulmonary blood flow in relation to atelectasis in premature ventilated lambs. Am Rev Respir Dis 1985; 132:500–503.

43. Jobe A. Techniques for administering surfactant. In: Robertson B, ed. Surfactant therapy for lung disease, vol 84. New York: Marcel Dekker; 1995:309–324.

44. Ueda T, Ikegami M, Rider ED, et al. Distribution of surfactant and ventilation in surfactant-treated preterm lambs. J Appl Physiol 1994; 76:45–55.

45. Jobe A, Ikegami M, Jacobs H, et al. Surfactant and pulmonary blood flow distributions following treatment of premature lambs with natural surfactant. J Clin Invest 1984; 73:848–856.

46. Zola EM, Gunkel JH, Chan RK, et al. Comparison of three dosing procedures for administration of bovine surfactant to neonates with respiratory distress syndrome. J Pediatr 1993; 122:453–459.

47. Zola EM, Overbach AM, Gunkel JH, et al. Treatment Investigational New Drug experience with Survanta (beractant). Pediatrics 1993; 91:546–551.

48. Enhorning G, Shennan A, Possmayer F, et al. Prevention of neonatal respiratory distress syndrome by tracheal instillation of surfactant: a randomized clinical trial. Pediatrics 1985; 76:145–153.

49. Enhörning G, Grossman G, Robertson B. Tracheal deposition of surfactant before the first breath. Am Rev Respir Dis 1973; 107:921–927.

50. Robertson D. Pathology and pathophysiology of neonatal surfactant deficiency. In: Robertson B, et al, ed. Pulmonary surfactant. Amsterdam: Elsevier Science Publishers; 1984.

51. Kendig JW, Notter RH, Cox C, et al. Surfactant replacement therapy at birth: final analysis of a clinical trial and comparisons with similar trials. Pediatrics 1988; 82:756–762.

52. Kendig JW, Ryan RM, Sinkin RA, et al. Comparison of two strategies for surfactant prophylaxis in very premature infants: a multicenter randomized trial. Pediatrics 1998; 101:1006–1012.

53. Soll RF, Morley C. Prophylactic versus selective use of surfactant for preventing morbidity and mortality in preterm infants. The Cochrane Library, Issue 2. Oxford: Update Software; 2001.

54. Horbar JD, Carpenter JH, Buzas J, et al. Collaborative quality improvement to promote evidence based surfactant for preterm infants: a cluster randomised trial. Br Med J 2004; 329:1004.

55. Finer NN, Carlo WA, Duara S, et al. Delivery room continuous positive airway pressure/positive end-expiratory pressure in extremely low birth weight infants: a feasibility trial. Pediatrics 2004; 114:651–657.

56. Jobe AH. Transition/Adaptation in the delivery room and less RDS: don't just do something, stand there! J Pediatr 2005; 147:284–286.

57. Soll RF, Hoekstra RE, Fangman JJ, et al. Multicenter trial of single-dose modified bovine surfactant extract (Survanta) for prevention of respiratory distress syndrome. Pediatrics 1990; 85:1092–1102.

58. Soll RF, Merritt TA, Hallman M. Surfactant in the prevention and treatment of respiratory distress syndrome. In: Boynton BR, Carlo WA, Jobe AH, eds. New therapies for neonatal respiratory failure. Cambridge: Cambridge University Press; 1994: 49–80.

59. Jobe AH. Pulmonary surfactant therapy. N Eng J Med 1993; 328:861–868.

60. Early versus delayed neonatal administration of a synthetic surfactant – the judgment of OSIRIS. The OSIRIS Collaborative Group (open study of infants at high risk of or with respiratory insufficiency – the role of surfactant. Lancet 1992; 340:1363–1369.

61. Lewis JF, Jobe AH. Surfactant and the adult respiratory distress syndrome. Am Rev Respir Dis 1993; 147:218–233.

62. Herting E, Rauprich P, Stichtenoth G, et al. Resistance of different surfactant preparations to inactivation by meconium. Pediatr Res 2001; 50:44–49.

63. Findlay RD, Taeusch WH, Walther FJ. Surfactant replacement therapy for meconium aspiration syndrome. Pediatr 1996; 97:48–52.

64. Auten RL, Notter RH, Kendig JW, et al. Surfactant treatment of full-term newborns with respiratory failure. Pediatrics 1991; 87:101–107.

65. Lotze A, Mitchell BR, Bulas DI, et al. Multicenter study of surfactant (beractant) use in the treatment of term infants with severe respiratory failure. Survanta in Term Infants Study Group. J Pediatr 1998; 132:40–47.

66. Wiswell TE, Knight GR, Finer NN, et al. A multicenter, randomized, controlled trial comparing Surfaxin (Lucinactant) lavage with standard care for treatment of meconium aspiration syndrome. Pediatrics 2002; 109:1081–1087.

67. Chinese Collaborative Study Group for Neonatal Respiratory Diseases. Treatment of severe meconium aspiration syndrome with porcine surfactant: a multicentre, randomized, controlled trial. Acta Paediatr 2005; 94:896–902.

68. Szymankiewicz M, Gadzinowski J, Kowalska K. Pulmonary function after surfactant lung lavage followed by surfactant administration in infants with severe meconium aspiration syndrome. J Matern Fetal Neonatal Med 2004; 16:125–130.

69. Merrill JD, Ballard RA, Cnaan A, et al. Dysfunction of pulmonary surfactant in chronically ventilated premature infants. Pediatr Res 2004; 56:918–926.

70. Cogo PE, Zimmermann LJ, Pesavento R, et al. Surfactant kinetics in preterm infants on mechanical ventilation who did and did not develop bronchopulmonary dysplasia. Crit Care Med 2003; 31:1532–1538.

71. Bhatt AJ, Pryhuber GS, Huyck H, et al. Disrupted pulmonary vasculature and decreased vascular endothelial growth factor, Flt-1 and Tie-2 in human infants dying with bronchopulmonary dysplasia. Am J Respir Crit Care Med 2001; 164:1971–1980.

72. Pandit PB, Dunn MS, Kelly EN, et al. Surfactant replacement in neonates with early chronic lung disease. Pediatrics 1995; 95:851–854.

73. Jobe A. Antenatal factors and the development of bronchopulmonary dysplasia. Semin Neonatol 2003; 8:9–17.

74. Herting E, Gefeller O, Land M, et al. Surfactant treatment of neonates with respiratory failure and Group B streptococcal infection. Pediatr 2000; 106:957–964.

75. Spragg RG, Lewis JF, Wurst W, et al. Treatment of acute respiratory distress syndrome with recombinant surfactant protein C surfactant. Am J Respir Crit Care Med 2003; 167:1562–1566.

76. Ainsworth SB, Beresford MW, Milligan DWA, et al. Randomized Controlled Trial of Early Treatment of Respiratory Distress Syndrome with Pumactant (ALEC) or Poractant Alfa (Curosurf) in Infants of 25 to 29 Weeks Gestation. The Lancet 2000; 355:1387–1392.

77. Moya FR, Gadzinowski J, Bancalari E, et al. A multicenter, randomized, masked, comparison trial of lucinactant, colfosceril palmitate, and beractant for the prevention of respiratory distress syndrome among very preterm infants. Pediatrics 2005; 115:1018–1029.

78. Sinha SK, Lacaze-Masmonteil T, Valls i Soler A, et al. A multicenter, randomized, controlled trial of lucinactant versus poractant alfa among very premature infants at high risk for respiratory distress syndrome. Pediatrics 2005; 115:1030–1038.

79. Bloom BT, Clark RH. Comparison of Infasurf (calfactant) and Survanta (beractant) in the prevention and treatment of respiratory distress syndrome. Pediatrics 2005; 116:392–399.

Section II

Injury in the Developing Lung

Chapter 5

Susceptibility of the Immature Lung to Oxidative and Mechanical Injury

Jaques Belik MD FRCPC

Lung Development

Free Radicals

Antioxidants

Lung Oxidative Stress Injury

Other Factors Playing a Role in the Oxidant–Antioxidant Balance

Mechanical Ventilation-Induced Lung Injury

Is the Immature Lung More Susceptible to Oxidative Stress and Mechanical Ventilation-Induced Injury?

The lung, being the internal organ exposed to the highest atmospheric oxygen concentration, is most susceptible to oxidative damage. In mammals the transition from fetal to postnatal life, amongst other changes, involves a switch from a low to higher oxygen environment which is likely to subject the neonate immediately after birth to an oxidant stress. Although the full-term neonate is able to tolerate a certain degree of oxidative stress without tissue injury, premature infants may not be developmentally prepared to protect their lungs from potential injury caused by the therapeutic use of supplemental oxygen and mechanical ventilation.

In this chapter I will review the embryological lung development from fetal to postnatal life focusing on the susceptibility of the prematurely born neonate to iatrogenic lung injury. Oxidative stress, the antioxidant defense system and the factors responsible for lung oxidative damage will be described. Lastly I will discuss the concept of ventilator-induced lung injury (VILI) and the newborn lung susceptibility to this process, emphasizing its significance in the pathogenesis of bronchopulmonary dysplasia (BPD). Given that many aspects of lung injury and clinical modalities commonly utilized in the respiratory therapy of neonates are the focus of other chapters in this book, I will only address certain concepts and their clinical relevance in a limited way.

LUNG DEVELOPMENT

Embryology

In mammals the airways and pulmonary vasculature have a common origin. The lung bud originates from the foregut endoderm and the resulting epithelial tube undergoes branching morphogenesis within the splanchnopleural mesenchyme. Regions of the epithelial tube that cease to branch are surrounded by a sheet of mesenchyme from which smooth muscle and connective tissue forms. The airway acts as a scaffold for the pulmonary arterial tree development and the airway epithelium modulates cell growth and differentiation within the lung from the early stages of development (1).

The human lung embryological development can be divided into five stages. The embryonic is the first, lasting until the 6th week of gestation and is mostly characterized by the growth of the lung bud from the endodermal foregut into the surrounding mesenchyme. During the pseudo-glandular or second stage of development (weeks 6th through 16th) further lung splicings occurs, giving rise to the terminal bronchioles. At this point the lungs resemble an exocrine gland consisting of thick stroma and an almost completely filled lumen. Epithelium formation starts at this point and the tracheae completely separate from the foregut. Division of the terminal bronchioles into two or more respiratory bronchioles, and vascularization of the lungs characterizes the canalicular stage of lung development from 16 through 28 weeks gestation. Differentiation between type-I and type-II pneumocytes slowly progresses during this phase of development, allowing for possible gas exchange from week 22 onwards.

The fourth stage is the saccular one when further division of the respiratory bronchioles into terminal sacs (primitive alveoli) occurs and the capillaries move closer to the terminal sacs until only the basal membrane separates these two structures. Finally maturation of the primitive alveoli starts in the alveolar stage (36 weeks through term gestation) by thinning of the squamous epithelial lining of the sacs, and septal formation occurs. Embryologically the lung is ultimately formed out of endodermal and mesodermal tissue. The mucosal lining and alveoli epithelial cells are derived from the endoderm and the vasculature, muscles and cartilage are of mesodermal origin.

The extent to which in utero oxidative stress impairs fetal lung morphogenesis is unknown, but oxidant/antioxidant imbalance during gestation has been linked to a higher occurrence of congenital malformations (2).

Airway Epithelial Barrier

The fetal airway epithelium actively participates in the lung fluid transport. This is accomplished by dynamic balance between Cl^- ion secretion and Na^+ ion absorption at the epithelial cell level. Prenatally the Cl^--driven liquid secretion predominates creating a positive fluid balance that generates a distending pressure that stretches the lung and stimulates its growth. Near birth the lung exhibits a predominantly Na^+ absorptive capacity that results in a decrease in lung fluid. This allows for adequate gas exchange at birth and postnatally characterizes the absorptive phenotype of the airway epithelial cells (3). The mechanism accounting for the lung lining liquid formation and its volume regulation is not completely understood. Immediately after birth the presence of a large amount of lung fluid leads to respiratory distress and characterizes the so called "transient tachypnea of the newborn." Postnatally the fine control of lung lining fluid ensures adequate diffusion of gas across the alveoli by keeping it to a minimum in the major airways, thus allowing for proper ciliary activity and removal of mucus, debris and pathogens. The amount of this lining fluid is minuscule at the alveoli level and it increases towards the larger airways (4).

The epithelial lining fluid is the first protective barrier against oxidative stress in the lung. It has a filtering role towards toxic gases and other harmful air-mixed pollutants and thus plays an important role towards the mechanical and chemical defenses of the lung. The lung lining fluid contains large amounts of antioxidants (5).

FREE RADICALS

Free radicals and other reactive oxygen, nitrogen or chlorine species are molecules or atoms capable of independent existence that contain one or more unpaired electrons in the outer electron shell. These radicals, by virtue of their unpaired electron(s), are highly reactive. Reactive oxygen species (ROS) are produced endogenously by inflammatory cells as part of the body's defense system, or exogenously following the inhalation of toxic gases such as cigarette smoke, ozone, and nitrogen dioxide, or supplemental oxygen (6). Reactive nitrogen species are oxidants derived from nitric oxide.

When in contact with various cellular components these free radicals induce tissue damage via oxidative stress. Free radical-induced oxidative damage is involved in the pathogenesis of several neonatal disorders coined by Saugstad as "Oxygen Radical Disease of Neonatology" and include BPD, retinopathy of prematurity, necrotizing enterocolitis, patent ductus arteriosus and intraventricular hemorrhage (7).

Table 5-1 lists all the known reactive and non-reactive oxygen/nitrogen/chlorine species known to play a biological role.

Table 5-1	Free and Non-radicals of Oxygen, Nitrogen and Chlorine Species	
Reactive species		**Symbol**
Reactive Oxygen Species (ROS)		
Superoxide		$O_2^{\bullet-}$
Hydroxyl		$OH^{\bullet}$
Alkoxyl		$RO^{\bullet}$
Peroxyl		$RO_2^{\bullet}$
Hydroperoxyl		$HO_2^{\bullet}$
Carbonate		$CO_3^{\bullet-}$
Carbon dioxide		$CO_2^{\bullet-}$
Peroxynitrite		$ONOO^{-}$
Non-radical with potential to generate ROS		
Hydrogen peroxide		H_2O_2
Hypobromous acid		HOBr
Ozone		O_3
Singlet molecular oxygen		$^1O_2$
Organic peroxides		ROOH
Peroxynitrous acid		ONOOH
Reactive Nitrogen Species (RNS)		
Nitric oxide		$NO^{\bullet}$
Nitrogen dioxide		$NO_2^{\bullet}$
Non-radical with potential to generate RNS		
Nitrous acid		HNO_2
Nitrosyl cation		NO^+
Nitroxyl anion		NO^-
Dinitrogen trioxide		N_2O_3
Dinitrogen tetroxide		N_2O_4
Nitronium (nitryl) cation		NO_2^+
Alkyl peroxynitrite		RONOO
Reactive Chloride Species (RCS)		
Atomic chlorine		$Cl^{\bullet}$
Non-radical with potential to generate RCS		
Hypochlorous acid		HOCl
Nitryl (nitronium) chloride		NO_2Cl
Chloramines		
Chlorine gas		Cl_2

Mechanism of free radical production

The main pathways responsible for the cellular production of reactive oxygen species are listed below:

- Mitochondrial respiratory chain
- Enzymatic systems (myeloperoxidase, membrane associated NADPH oxidase, nitric oxide synthase, xanthine oxidase)
- Microsomal and nuclear membrane P-450 enzymes
- Autoxidation of arachidonic acid
- Transition metals

Mitochondrial respiratory chain

It is believed that 1–2% of the oxygen entering the mitochondria results in ROS that "leak" into the cell cytosol compartment. This occurs at the mitochondrial electron transport chain level when oxygen is reduced to water as follows.

$$O_2 \longrightarrow O_2^{\bullet-} \longrightarrow H_2O_2 \longrightarrow OH^{\bullet} \longrightarrow H_2O$$

Electron   −   −   −   −

Also at the mitochondrial level, free oxygen radicals induce a process currently known as the mitochondrial permeability transition (MPT). Such process is characterized by an increase in the mitochondrial Ca^{2+} levels that leads to metabolism disruption and cell death via superoxide anion radical and H_2O_2 formation. Bleomycin-induced lung cytotoxicity is believed to be in part mediated via MPT changes (8).

NAD(P)H

The NADPH is an enzyme that catalyzes the production of superoxide as follows:

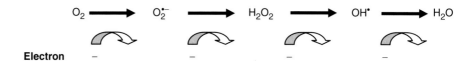

$$NADPH + 2O_2 \xrightarrow{\text{NADPH oxidase}} NADP^+ + H^+ + 2O_2^{\bullet-}$$

NADPH is mostly found in phagocytes (neutrophils, eosinophils, monocytes and macrophages) and in these cells it catalyzes a large amount of superoxide formation as part of their defense mechanism against foreign organisms. Two other groups of NADPH enzymes have been reported, the Nox and Duox systems, and these have mostly a signal transduction role via the formation of small quantities of superoxide.

The Nox systems involve a number of oxidases that promote NADPH-dependent superoxide generation following stimulation of the assembly of several subunits (9). A basal oxidase activity maintained via both NADH and NADPH is present in the vascular tissue (10).

In the lung NADPH via Nox 2 (gp91phox) (11) has an important role in the pathogenesis of chronic hypoxia-induced pulmonary hypertension (12). NADPH is also present in airway epithelial cells (13). In humans the Duox 1 and 2 are the major NADPH oxidases expressed in airway epithelia and appear to have an important role in the production of H_2O_2 as a host defense mechanism (14).

Myeloperoxidase

Infection and/or inflammation induce oxidative stress via either the NAD(P)H system or increased myeloperoxidase activity. Myeloperoxidase is present in neutrophils and participate in the killing of engulfed bacteria via the following reaction:

$$H_2O_2 + Cl^\bullet \xrightarrow{\text{Myeloperoxidase}} HOCL + OH^\bullet$$

Xanthine oxidase

Proteolytic conversion of xanthine dehydrogenase to xanthine oxidase leads to superoxide and H_2O_2 formation. Hypoxia, endotoxin and cytokines induce upregulation of the xanthine oxidase expression and activity in the lung and pharmacological inhibition of this pathway prevents the development of pulmonary edema in animal models of lung injury (15).

Cytochrome P-450 system

Different forms of microsomal and nuclear membrane cytochrome *P*-450 enzymes are involved in a variety of ROS-induced tissue damage (16–19). In the lung different *P*-450 enzymes are expressed in bronchial and bronchiolar epithelium, Clara cells, type II pneumocytes, and alveolar macrophages (20) and appear to be involved in oxidative damage (21)

Arachidonic acid oxidation

The involvement of arachidonic acid in the generation of oxidative stress occurs via its autoxidation in vivo and resultant formation of isoprostanes and other products. This is further discussed below under lipid peroxidation.

Transition metals

Iron, copper, nickel, molybdenum, cobalt, chromium, manganese and vanadium are free radicals because they contain an unpaired electron. Out of all the transition metals, iron is the one present in high concentration in most tissues and neonatal BPD is associated with a higher bronchoalveolar free iron content (22)

Iron is transported across the membrane in a protein-bound manner and utilized by cells for certain metabolic functions. This metal is usually not present in the non-bound form since free iron is rapidly oxidized to ferric ion (Fe^{3+}) by the ferroxidase enzyme. When ferrous iron (Fe^{2+}) interacts with H_2O_2 via the Fenton reaction it generates the toxic hydroxyl radical ($OH^\bullet$) via the following reaction:

$$H_2O_2 + Fe^{2+} \longrightarrow OH^\bullet + OH^- + Fe^{3+}$$

Further recycling of ferric ion (Fe^{3+}) to Fe^{2+} occurs via interaction with antioxidants such as ascorbic acid as follows:

$$Fe^{3+} + \text{ascorbate} \longrightarrow Fe^{2+} + \text{ascorbate}^\bullet$$

Physiological role of oxidative stress

Superoxide and hydrogen peroxide are the main ROS produced by cells even under normal aerobic physiological conditions. Thus, aside from their toxic effects, ROS also have an essential role in cellular functions of many organs (23).

Other examples of the important physiological role of ROS include the dependence on H_2O_2 for thyroxine synthesis and the killing of bacteria by macrophages and neutrophils via the NADPH oxidase or myeloperoxidase enzymes. Lastly the free radical $NO^\bullet$ is produced intracellularly at low levels via nitric oxide synthases and has an important role in the maintenance of a low pulmonary vascular and airway muscle tone.

ANTIOXIDANTS

Antioxidants are defined as any substance that, when present at low concentrations compared with those of an oxidizable substrate, significantly delays or prevents oxidation of that substrate (6). Antioxidants are present in the intra- and extra-cellular compartments and either prevent its formation or scavenge ROS. The biologically active antioxidants are listed below:

- Vitamin C (ascorbate)
- Vitamin E (α-tocopherol)
- Vitamin A
- Urate
- Albumin
- Sulfhydryl groups
- Bilirubin
- Glutathione and glutathione peroxidase (GPx)
- Transferrin
- Ceruloplasmin
- Superoxide dismutase (SOD)
  - Intracellular
    - Copper- and zinc-containing SOD (CuZnSOD)
    - Manganese SOD (MnSOD)
  - Extracellular copper- and zinc-containing SOD EC-SOD
- Catalase (CAT)
- Thioredoxins and peroxiredoxins

Vitamins

Vitamin C scavenges $O_2^{\bullet-}$ and $OH^{\bullet}$, as well as it interacts with vitamin E. It is an important antioxidant at birth, but the levels in the plasma of neonates rapidly fall over the first 2 weeks of life. Plasma ascorbate has a negative correlation with gestational age and, as compared with the full-term infant, its level on the first day of life in premature neonates is high. Yet premature infants requiring supplemental oxygen have a lower plasma ascorbate (24). At high concentrations, vitamin C can induce oxidant stress (25), but data obtained from clinical studies where a high dose of this vitamin was administered to premature neonates do not support this contention (26).

Vitamin E is a major lipophilic antioxidant in mammals, but when compared with later in life its plasma level in the neonatal period is low (27) and directly proportional to the gestational age (28). Vitamin A is a powerful scavenger of singlet oxygen and it inhibits lipid peroxidation. It is the only vitamin proven to be effective in the prevention of BPD in neonates (29).

Urates

Urates are by-products of purines and widely distributed in the extracellular compartment including the lung epithelial lining fluid. In tracheal aspirates uric acid concentrations at birth are high enough to significantly contribute to scavenging free oxygen radicals (30). Following birth uric acid levels increase during the first 24 h of life and within 2 weeks decline to levels comparable to the ones detected in older children. BPD is associated with a significant increase in plasma urate levels (31).

Albumin, Sulfhydryl Groups and Bilirubin

Albumin and sulfhydryl groups containing plasma proteins, as transitional metal binders, are effective antioxidants in the neonatal period (32). Bilirubin has been suggested to have a physiological antioxidant effect in the early period, but this issue remains controversial (33).

Glutathione

Glutathione is present in all animal cells and localized to the cytosol and mitochondria. Although there are two forms of glutathione, namely the reduced and oxidized, under physiological conditions only the former is present in the cells. Glutathione is synthesized via the glutamate cysteine ligase and glutathione synthetase from cysteine, glutamate and glycine. Glutathione plays a critical protective role against lung injury and the glutathione peroxidase activity is higher in neonatal as compared with the adult lung (34). The activity of glutamate cysteine ligase is not developmentally regulated in the lung (35) and oxidative stress induces glutathione synthesis via induction of this enzyme (36). The biosynthesis of glutathione is active in leukocytes from preterm infants (37) and plasma glutathione concentration transiently increases on the first day of life. In contrast, infants with respiratory distress syndrome have a lower mean plasma glutathione concentration when compared with infants without lung disease (38).

Transferrin and Ceruloplasmin

Binding of ferric ions to transferrin reduces their oxidative power, thus conferring an antioxidant effect to this protein. The preterm infant transferrin plasma level at birth is lower than later in life (39). The lung is the predominant extrahepatic site of ceruloplasmin gene expression during fetal development (40). Yet the preterm has a low ceruloplasmin level as compared with the term (24) and the plasma levels continue to rise until adulthood (41, 42).

SOD

Superoxide dismutases are metalloproteins that catalyze the dismutation of superoxide to hydrogen peroxide and oxygen as follows:

$$2O_2^{\bullet-} + 2H^+ \longrightarrow H_2O_2 + O_2$$

There are three types of SODs of biological significance. They are: CuZnSOD, MnSOD, and EC-SOD. The first is localized mainly in the cytoplasm, the second in the mitochondrial matrix and the EC-SOD is mostly found in the extracellular space. In the human neonatal lung MnSOD is predominantly expressed in bronchial epithelium, alveolar epithelium, and macrophages. CuZnSOD is primarily present in the bronchial epithelium, whereas EC-SOD is expressed in bronchial epithelium, vascular endothelium, and the extracellular matrix (43).

Catalase

This enzyme is responsible for the breakdown of H_2O_2 into water and oxygen.

$$2H_2O_2 \longrightarrow H_2O + O_2$$

Amniotic fluid endotoxin exposure increases the catalase expression in premature lambs (44). In the rat the catalase and CuZnSOD activity in the lung progressively increase in the latter part of gestation with a further surge immediately after birth (34). In the newborn lung catalase is expressed in bronchial epithelium and alveolar macrophages (43).

Thioredoxins and Peroxiredoxins

Thioredoxins are a superfamily of proteins that have antioxidant properties by reducing oxidized cysteine groups on proteins and appear to play an important antiinflammatory role in the lung (45). In the human newborn lung these proteins are localized in the bronchial epithelium and alveolar macrophages (43) and oxygen upregulates the lung thioredoxin expression (46).

Peroxiredoxins (also known as thioredoxin peroxidases) are a group of thiol-containing proteins involved in the breakdown of hydrogen peroxide during oxidative stress by using thioredoxin as a source of reducing equivalents (47). In the rat peroxiredoxins VI expression is highest in lung (48) and present in the respiratory airways from the trachea to the distal bronchioles. Its depletions results in a significant decrease in the airway epithelium antioxidant activity (49). Peroxiredoxin I and II expression in rat lung also follows a developmental pattern. Peroxiredoxin I increases during late gestation and fall after birth to adult levels. In contrast peroxiredoxin II protein concentration does not change prenatally, but increase after birth (50). In response to hyperoxia peroxiredoxin I increases in the rat (50) and premature baboon (51), suggesting an important role for these proteins in the physiological response to oxygen exposure during the neonatal period.

Lung Antioxidant Levels in the Preterm Infant

As compared with term, preterm infants, based on the available animal data, appear to have reduced intracellular antioxidant defense levels but in response to oxidative stress in utero the fetus is able to significantly increase the lung antioxidant enzyme activity (44). In the rat, only catalase and copper-zinc superoxide dismutase have increased activity after birth, suggesting that maturation of the antioxidant enzyme system is virtually complete before delivery.

Conflicting data exist regarding the premature lung ability to augment its antioxidant enzyme activity when exposed to supplemental oxygen after birth. In chronic hyperoxic rats the term newborn is more tolerant than the adult, and the prematurely born animals have a greater survival and demonstrate a superior capability of inducing pulmonary antioxidant enzymes SOD, CAT or GPx when compared with the term rats (52). Yet this pattern is not consistent amongst species. The premature rabbit lung does not show an increase in antioxidant enzymes in response to hyperoxia (53) or endotoxin exposure (54).

LUNG OXIDATIVE STRESS INJURY

Oxidative stress is best defined as disturbance in the pro-oxidant and antioxidant balance in favor of the former, leading to tissue damage (6). When the tissue antioxidant defenses are overwhelmed, oxidative stress to its cellular components occurs, inducing inflammatory, adaptive, injurious, and reparative processes (55). Oxidative stress-induced pulmonary inflammation is the result of either excessive production of oxidants, reduced antioxidants tissue levels or the combination of both.

The in utero environment is characterized by low oxygen that may be of importance during lung morphogenesis. At birth the lung is exposed to an oxygen-rich environment that results in transient production of reactive oxygen species. In this context ROS production is physiological and may be critical for the successful transition from fetal to postnatal life (56). Yet, exposure to supplemental oxygen has been shown to induce hydroxyl radical generation in infants (57).

In healthy adults, exposure to as low an FiO_2 as 0.28 for 1 h results in lung oxidative stress (58). The evidence that oxidative stress occurs in the lung of premature infants developing BPD is substantial. 3-Chlorotyrosine a specific biomarker of the neutrophil oxidant hypochlorous acid, in tracheal aspirate is significantly higher in < 1500 g premature infants who developed BPD or who had lung infection (59). Nitrotyrosine (a by-product of the reaction of peroxynitrite with proteins) levels are also higher in premature infants developing BPD (60) and correlate with their respiratory outcome (61)

Lipid Peroxidation

Lipid peroxidation is a natural metabolic process under physiologic conditions. The lung as other tissues contains polyunsaturated fatty acids (PUFAs). PUFA is the main component of membrane lipids and is susceptible to peroxidation as a result of oxidative stress leading to loss of the functional integrity of the cell membranes. Surfactant protein appears to have a lipid peroxidation protective effect (62). In human infants who subsequently develop BPD, lipid peroxidation is present as early as on the first day of life (63).

Isoprostanes are lipid peroxidation by-products mostly derived from arachidonic acid and formed in vivo by non-enzymatic peroxidation of membrane phospholipids by ROS. One of these arachidonic acid products, 8-iso-prostaglandin $F_{2\alpha}$ (8-iso-PG $F_{2\alpha}$), is biologically active and shown to be increased in animal models of oxidant stress tissue injury (64). Aside from their putative role in the process of vascular remodeling, isoprostanes (65, 66) are potent constrictors of pulmonary vessels and airways. Chronic O_2 exposure in the newborn rat results in enhanced lung vascular and airway muscle contraction potential, via a mechanism involving reactive oxygen species (67). The mechanisms responsible for these changes are not fully understood, but there is evidence to support the 8-isoprostane role in this process (68, 69). We have previously shown that compared with air-exposed control animals, 8-iso-PG $F_{2\alpha}$ induced a greater degree of pulmonary arterial muscle contraction and significantly reduced the relaxation of precontracted vessels in the chronically O_2-treated newborn rats (70).

Matrix Metalloproteins

Oxidative stress can damage the lung by increasing collagenase and elastase activity, leading to increased production of extracellular matrix components and remodeling. Matrix metalloproteins (MMPs) together with their inhibitors regulate the extracellular matrix proteins and collagen content. Hyperoxia-induced oxidative stress significantly increases MMP production in the newborn piglet lung (71) and heart (72).

An increase in pulmonary MMP content and/or activity is associated with BPD changes and MMP-9 is also detected in lung tissue of infants subjected to mechanical ventilation (73). MMPs -9 and -2 degrade type-IV collagen, a major constituent of lung basement membrane, and have been found increased in the lung of premature baboons with BPD (74). In human neonates MMP-9 expression and/or content, when expressed as a ratio with tissue inhibitor of matrix metalloproteinase-1 (TIMP-1), increases with decreasing gestation in preterm babies and is higher in babies who developed BPD (75). Reflecting the fact that its role in the pathogenesis of BPD is as much dependent on the content activity of the inhibitor, TIMP-1 protein content in the lung was found to be increased and MMP-9 decreased in newborn rats exposed to hyperoxia (76). Interestingly there is a strong association between chorioamnionitis and changes in MMP bronchoalveolar fluid levels of ventilated premature infants. Bronchoalveolar lavage fluid MMP-9 levels are higher in preterm infants born to women with chorioamnionitis and are directly proportional to the severity of this disease (77). Since infants exposed to chorioamnionitis in utero are more likely to have chronic lung disease, MMPs may play an important role in this association. MMP-8 levels have also been shown to be increased in infants with BPD (78, 79).

Neutrophils and Macrophages

Supplemental oxygen exposure is known to induce a lung inflammatory response involving the recruitment and activation of neutrophils and macrophages. There is mounting evidence that these cells once present in significant numbers are activated, and initiate a process resulting in lung oxidative stress. In newborn rats exposed to 60% O_2 for 14 days (80), or to 95% O_2 for 1 week (81), the presence of an increased number of macrophages appears to be responsible for the production of ROS in the lungs.

Of interest, however, is the fact that the mechanism by which ROS induce BPD is distinct from the pulmonary hypertension in the chronic hyperoxia-exposed newborn rat. Suppression of macrophages with gadolinium in this rat model has a significant attenuating effect on pulmonary macrophage accumulation and the degree of pulmonary hypertension, but no effect on BPD-like morphologic changes (82). Yet inhibition of neutrophil influx using a selective CXC chemokine receptor-2 antagonist attenuates the increased production of ROS and significantly reduces the alveolar growth arrest that characterizes BPD in these newborn rats exposed to chronic hyperoxia (83).

Infection

Aside from supplemental oxygen exposure, infection and/or inflammation induces neutrophil and macrophage recruitment and oxidative stress in the lung, and lung tissue ROS formation is observed in response to lipopolysaccharide toxin via activation of NADPH oxidase (84). Exposure to antenatal glucocorticoids in utero has been shown to decrease alveolarization, which together with chorioamnionitis may significantly impair fetal lung growth (85). Whether oxidant stress is involved in this process is at present unclear, but phagocytosis-induced oxidation can begin prenatally, usually as a result of chorioamnionitis (85). Yet prolonged fetal exposure to intra-amniotic endotoxin does not lead to progressive structural abnormalities in lungs of near-term gestation lambs (86).

Nitric Oxide and Peroxynitrite

Inhaled nitric oxide (iNO) has been shown to have a lung protective as well as oxidant effect on the lung (87). In the newborn rat iNO reduces the degree of alveolar growth arrest following chronic hyperoxia exposure possibly by decreasing oxidative stress (88). In low concentrations, inhaled NO may reduce the prevalence of BPD in ventilated premature infants; however, this issue remains controversial and recent data do not appear to support this claim (89).

Peroxynitrites are formed from the interaction of nitric oxide and superoxide radical as follows

$$NO^{\bullet} + O_2^- \longrightarrow ONOO^-$$

Once formed peroxynitrite promotes nitrotyrosine formation and in vascular tissues it impairs the function of antioxidant enzymes (10).

Peroxynitrite induces surfactant dysfunction (90) and may thus further compromise the respiratory function. In addition peroxynitrites may act on the pulmonary and airway smooth muscle inducing vaso- and bronchoconstriction, respectively. In the newborn, but not adult, rat we have shown that peroxynitrite inhibits lung arterial smooth muscle relaxation and induces pulmonary vasoconstriction (91).

OTHER FACTORS PLAYING A ROLE IN THE OXIDANT–ANTIOXIDANT BALANCE

Blood transfusion

Intraerythrocytic free iron is present in premature infants in a manner inversely proportional to their gestational age (92), and plasma non-transferrin bound iron is significantly increased in preterm infants after blood transfusion (93). Free iron catalyzes the generation of ROS and a higher prevalence of oxidative stress has been documented in premature infant receiving blood transfusions (94).

Maternal Role in Fetal and Neonatal Tissue Oxidative Stress

It is apparent that the lactating woman's dietary habits during pregnancy and lactation impacts on the neonatal antioxidant potential (95). Fetal oxidant stress can occur in association with maternal smoking during pregnancy (96). The antioxidant capacity of neonates is in part dependent on their nutritional intake and for those exclusively breast-fed influenced by the breast milk composition. For micronutrients such as selenium, which is an integral component of the enzymes glutathione peroxidase and iodothyronine deiodinases, a higher dietary intake than the adult requirement has been shown for newborn animals (97).

Possible Interventions to Enhance Antioxidant Defenses and Reduce Oxygen Toxicity in the Preterm Neonate

No safe and effective preventive antioxidant therapy has been identified (98). Yet recent reports of attenuation of hyperoxia-induced lung damage in animal models of BPD suggest possible novel therapeutic approaches to its prevention and/or treatment. The most relevant agents are here reviewed.

SOD is an important antioxidant that catalyzes the dismutation of superoxide to hydrogen peroxide and oxygen. Intratracheal recombinant human SOD administration to premature lambs with surfactant deficiency improves oxygenation and prevents the development of pulmonary hypertension possibly by reducing supplemental oxygen and/or ventilation-induced oxidant stress (99). A recent clinical trial where recombinant human CuZn superoxidase dismutase was administered intratracheally from birth to 1 month of age resulted in a significant reduction in the prevalence of wheezing and need for bronchodilators and/or corticosteroids during the first year of life (100).

Erythropoietin (EPO) is a 30.4-kDa glycoprotein that modulates red blood cell production and is used therapeutically in neonates to prevent and/or treat anemia of prematurity. EPO has been shown to have an antioxidant effect via a decrease in plasma iron concentration and inhibition of lipid peroxidation (101, 102). In the hyperoxia-induced newborn rat model of BPD, EPO has been reported to help preserve alveolar structure, enhance pulmonary vascularity, and diminish lung fibrosis (103).

MECHANICAL VENTILATION-INDUCED LUNG INJURY

Biotrauma, Atelectotrauma, Volutrauma

Premature infants commonly present at birth with lung immaturity requiring mechanical ventilatory support. Although of benefit towards assisting their respiratory needs, ventilation may result in lung injury and BPD (104).

Mechanical ventilation is believed to induce lung injury either by over-stretching, repeated collapse and recruitment of lung units, or by the release of inflammatory mediators. A specific nomenclature addresses these three mechanisms for the ventilation-induced lung injury (VILI):

Volutrauma consists in damage caused by over-distension.

Atelectotrauma occurs as a result of the recruitment and collapse caused by either the use of a level of positive-end-expiratory pressure lower than the low inflection point of the pressure volume curve, or the regional presence of areas of atelectasis in diseases associated with lung disease inhomogeneity.

Biotrauma refers to any mechanical ventilation-related insult that induces the release of lung cytokines and/or other inflammation mediators.

Barotrauma was a commonly utilized term associated with the ventilation-dependent airway pressure-induced lung injury. Considering that pressure only injures lung tissue when associated with cell and/or tissue overstretch, volutrauma is a more appropriate term when referring to VILI related to a high peak inspiratory pressure (PIP).

Growing evidence points to the causative association between intermittent positive pressure ventilation in the premature infant and the development of chronic lung disease (105). With alternative mechanical ventilatory modes such as high-frequency oscillation(106), volume guarantee mode (107), and others (108), although of theoretical benefit in the prevention of lung injury, their impact on the prevalence of BPD in premature infants with respiratory distress is still *controversi*al (109). In fact recent systematic reviews of the available clinical data failed to show an obvious superiority of one particular ventilatory strategy in neonates or older children (110, 111). Avoidance of mechanical ventilatory support by early use of nasal continuous positive airway pressure (nCPAP) has been shown to minimize lung injury in baboons at risk of developing bronchopulmonary dysplasia (112). Similarly, neonatal units with preferential use of early and continuous nCPAP in infants with respiratory distress syndrome have *reported* a lower incidence of BPD (113, 114). Yet to date, the evidence to support the prophylactic use of nCPAP to reduce the BPD morbidity and mortality is still lacking (115).

Mechanical ventilation rapidly induces cytokine production in normal and injured lungs. Interleukins 1, 6 and 8 (IL-1ß, IL-6 and IL-8), tumor necrosis factor (TNF)-alpha and the CXC chemokines have been shown to be involved in this process (116, 117) together with the recruitment of neutrophils (118) and other inflammatory cells (119, 120). There is also evidence that VILI is associated with increased circulating cytokine levels (121), possibly accounting for some of the systemic organ dysfunction seen in mechanically ventilated subjects.

The explanation for the discrepancy between the theoretical advantages of avoidance of volutrauma and atelectotrauma and the limited impact of such strategies on the prevention of lung injury may relate to the rapidity with which the inflammatory process progresses when triggered by VILI. That overdistension of the lungs for a short duration can trigger the inflammatory process is best illustrated by the data recently reported from our laboratory. High tidal volume ventilation of adult rats for 30 min is sufficient to upregulate several genes related to transcription factors, stress proteins, and inflammatory mediators and this occurs before any histological lung changes are recognized (122). Similar observations have been made in the human newborn, where lung inflammatory markers were reported to be present as early as the first day of life in infants developing BPD (123, 124).

When subjected to a high tidal volume (25 ml/kg), ventilation is more injurious to adult than newborn rats (125), as manifested by edema formation, altered lung compliance and histology. A significant maturational difference in the VILI-induced cytokine gene expression was observed in the rat lung. Whereas ventilation of adults for 30 min at 25 ml/kg upregulated the mRNA expression of interleukin IL-1ß, IL-6, IL-10, TNFa and macrophage inflammatory protein-2 (MIP-2), a more prolonged (3 h) and higher tidal volume (40 ml/kg) was necessary to induce upregulation of some of these genes in the newborn lung.

The protective factors accounting for the lesser susceptibility of the newborn rat to VILI are at present unknown. Yet maturational-related differences in the physical characteristics of the lung parenchyma may render the newborn rat a greater tolerance to high tidal volume ventilation-induced lung injury (126). Whether the human newborn is more tolerant than the adult to VILI is difficult to ascertain given the confounding role of factors such as the primary lung disease leading to the requirement for ventilatory support, the general state of the subjects' health and differences in the equipment and strategies of ventilatory support utilized. In the case of premature infants a poor respiratory drive, or the pulmonary complications resulting from a hemodynamically unstable patent ductus arteriosus, often are the primary reason for the prolonged need for mechanical ventilatory support.

Related to the potentially unnecessary use of supplemental oxygen during resuscitation maneuvers at birth (127) is the question of what contribution the inspired gas oxygen concentration has on VILI. In the newborn rat, supplemental oxygen has an additive injurious effect on the lung during high tidal volume ventilation (125). Furthermore, cyclical mechanical strain of pulmonary epithelial cells is associated with an increased production of ROS (13) and an increase in intracellular glutathione (128), suggesting that oxidative stress has an important role in the pathogenesis of VILI. The evidence linking ROS to VILI points to another pathway that could be rapidly and earlier on induced with the initiation of ventilatory support. Supporting this speculation, pharmacological intervention appears to be most successful in BPD prevention when initiated as early as possible in preterm infants requiring ventilatory support (129).

Data from our laboratory addressing the effect of mechanical ventilation on the newborn rat lung compliance also raise important clinical considerations. Ventilation of newborn rats with a low (10 ml/kg) and high (40 ml/kg) tidal volume results in a progressive increase in dynamic compliance of the lung up to 60 min (130). A significant increase in total lung lavage surfactant accounts for the improved lung compliance in these animals. This apparently "beneficial" effect of a slightly higher than physiologic tidal volume ventilation (10 ml/kg) may be operative during the so called "recruitment maneuvers" utilized clinically. Thus, aside from recruiting poorly ventilated areas, a short period of ventilation with higher than physiologic tidal volume may improve lung compliance by transiently increasing the lung surfactant content of neonates.

Lastly, the newborn rat model of VILI has also allowed us to recognize the likely causative association of mechanical ventilation and hypercoagulability. High, but not low, tidal volume ventilation for as little as 15 min significantly reduces plasma clot time and antithrombin, as well as increasing tissue factor, factor Xa and thrombin content in the newborn (131). This volutrauma-induced activation of the clotting cascade is not observed in the adult rat. Given the high prevalence of thrombus formation and stroke in neonates (132, 133), the volutrauma/biotrauma role during resuscitation maneuvers and/or mechanical ventilation warrants further investigation.

IS THE IMMATURE LUNG MORE SUSCEPTIBLE TO OXIDATIVE STRESS AND MECHANICAL VENTILATION-INDUCED INJURY?

The factors predisposing the premature infant lung to oxidative stress include the need for supplemental oxygen to treat respiratory distress, low antioxidant defenses, higher free iron plasma and tissue levels and the common association between preterm birth and chorioamnionitis. Collard et al. found that in ventilated premature infants factors other than antioxidants relate to BPD. These include endotracheal infection, septicemia, and gestational age, as the most powerful predictors of the development of BPD (134).

It is at present unclear as to whether the preterm is more susceptible to mechanical ventilation-induced lung injury than the full-term neonate. Although the lung of a prematurely born neonate is structurally immature, the preterm and term baboon newborn model of BPD appear to exhibit similar changes in lung histology when exposed to prolonged mechanical ventilation and hyperoxia (135, 136). Certain developmental features make lung cells more susceptible to oxidant and ventilator-induced injury. One of these is the p66^{Shc} adapter protein that mediates oxidative stress by antagonizing the mitogen-activated protein kinase. This protein has been shown to be developmentally regulated in the lung during fetal life and is lowest at birth in several animal species and humans. In the premature baboon model of BPD expression of this protein remains high, suggesting that its presence increases susceptibility to oxidative stress in the lung (137). In addition, oxidant stress appears to play a significant role in the respiratory distress of the prematurely born.

In summary, the premature infant in need of respiratory support at birth is more likely than the term neonate to require prolonged mechanical ventilation. In part this greater propensity relates to extrapulmonary factors such as apnea and poor respiratory drive. As illustrated in Figure 5-1, however, higher free iron plasma levels, prenatal infection (chorioamnionitis) and lower antioxidant capacity may make the premature lung more susceptible to oxidative stress and mechanical ventilation-induced injury. Further research utilizing animal models and human data is necessary to assess the immaturity-related predisposition to chronic lung disease.

REFERENCES

1. Caniggia I, Tseu I, Han RN, et al. Spatial and temporal differences in fibroblast behavior in fetal rat lung. Am J Physiol 1991; 261:L424–L433.
2. Martin I, Gibert MJ, Pintos C, et al. Oxidative stress in mothers who have conceived fetus with neural tube defects: the role of aminothiols and selenium. Clin Nutr 2004; 23:507–514.
3. Olver RE, Walters DV, Wilson M. Developmental regulation of lung liquid transport. Annu Rev Physiol 2004; 66:77–101.
4. Walters DV. Lung lining liquid – the hidden depths. The 5th Nils W. Svenningsen memorial lecture. Biol Neonate 81 Suppl 2002; 1:2–5.
5. van der Vliet A, O'Neill CA, Cross CE, et al. Determination of low-molecular-mass antioxidant concentrations in human respiratory tract lining fluids. Am J Physiol 1999; 276:L289–L296.
6. Halliwell B, Whiteman M. Measuring reactive species and oxidative damage in vivo and in cell culture: how should you do it and what do the results mean? Br J Pharmacol 2004; 142:231–255.
7. Saugstad OD. Oxidative stress in the newborn – a 30-year perspective. Biol Neonate 2005; 88:228–236.
8. Hong JS, Ko HH, Han ES, et al. Inhibition of bleomycin-induced cell death in rat alveolar macrophages and human lung epithelial cells by ambroxol. Biochem Pharmacol 2003; 66:1297–1306.
9. Lambeth JD. NOX enzymes and the biology of reactive oxygen. Nat Rev Immunol 2004; 4:181–189.
10. Wolin MS, Ahmad M, Gupte SA. The sources of oxidative stress in the vessel wall. Kidney Int 2005; 67:1659–1661.
11. Liu JQ, Erbynn EM, Folz RJ. Chronic hypoxia-enhanced murine pulmonary vasoconstriction: role of superoxide and gp91phox. Chest 2005; 128:594S–596S.

12. Liu JQ, Zelko IN, Erbynn EM, et al. Hypoxic pulmonary hypertension: role of superoxide and NADPH oxidase (gp91phox). Am J Physiol Lung Cell Mol Physiol 2006; 290:L2–L10.

13. Chapman KE, Sinclair SE, Zhuang D, et al. Cyclic mechanical strain increases reactive oxygen species production in pulmonary epithelial cells. Am J Physiol Lung Cell Mol Physiol 2005; 289:L834–L841.

14. Forteza R, Salathe M, Miot F, et al. Regulated hydrogen peroxide production by Duox in human airway epithelial cells. Am J Respir Cell Mol Biol 2005; 32:462–469.

15. Merker MP, Pitt BR, Choi AM, et al. Lung redox homeostasis: emerging concepts. Am J Physiol Lung Cell Mol Physiol 2000; 279:L413–L417.

16. Jezek P, Hlavata L. Mitochondria in homeostasis of reactive oxygen species in cell, tissues, and organism. Int J Biochem Cell Biol 2005; 37:2478–2503.

17. Jaeschke H, Gores GJ, Cederbaum AI, et al. Mechanisms of hepatotoxicity. Toxicol Sci 2002; 65:166–176.

18. Koop DR. Oxidative and reductive metabolism by cytochrome P450 2E1. FASEB J 1992; 6:724–730.

19. Paine AJ. Excited states of oxygen in biology: their possible involvement in cytochrome P450 linked oxidations as well as in the induction of the P450 system by many diverse compounds. Biochem Pharmacol 1978; 27:1805–1813.

20. Castell JV, Donato MT, Gomez-Lenchon MJ. Metabolism and bioactivation of toxicants in the lung. The in vitro cellular approach. Exp Toxicol Pathol 2005; 57 Supp. 1:189–204.

21. Baulig A, Garlatti M, Bonvallot V, et al. Involvement of reactive oxygen species in the metabolic pathways triggered by diesel exhaust particles in human airway epithelial cells. Am J Physiol Lung Cell Mol Physiol 2003; 285:L671–L679.

22. Gerber CE, Bruchelt G, Stegmann H, et al. Presence of bleomycin-detectable free iron in the alveolar system of preterm infants. Biochem Biophys Res Commun 1999; 257:218–222.

23. Jankov RP, Negus A, Tanswell AK. Antioxidants as therapy in the newborn: some words of caution. Pediatr Res 2001; 50:681–687.

24. Boonsiri P, Panthongviriyakul C, Kiatchoosakun P, et al. Plasma ascorbate and ceruloplasmin levels in Thai premature infants. J Med Assoc Thai 2005; 88:205–213.

25. Berger TM, Polidori MC, Dabbagh A, et al. Antioxidant activity of vitamin C in iron-overloaded human plasma. J Biol Chem 1997; 272:15656–15660.

26. Darlow BA, Buss H, McGill F, et al. Vitamin C supplementation in very preterm infants: a randomised controlled trial. Arch Dis Child Fetal Neonatal Ed 2005; 90:F117–F122.

27. Jain SK, Wise R, Bocchini JJ Jr. Vitamin E and vitamin E-quinone levels in red blood cells and plasma of newborn infants and their mothers. J Am Coll Nutr 1996; 15:44–48.

28. Chan DK, Lim MS, Choo SH, et al. Vitamin E status of infants at birth. J Perinat Med 1999; 27:395–398.

29. Van Marter LJ. Strategies for preventing bronchopulmonary dysplasia. Curr Opin Pediatr 2005; 17:174–180.

30. Schrod L, Neuhaus T, Speer CP, et al. Possible role of uric acid as an antioxidant in premature infants. Biol Neonate 1997; 72:102–111.

31. Schock BC, Sweet DG, Halliday HL, et al. Oxidative stress in lavage fluid of preterm infants at risk of chronic lung disease. Am J Physiol Lung Cell Mol Physiol 2001; 281:L1386–L1391.

32. Dani C, Martelli E, Bertini G, et al. Plasma bilirubin level and oxidative stress in preterm infants. Arch Dis Child Fetal Neonatal Ed 2003; 88:F119–F123.

33. Dani C, Masini E, Bertini G, et al. Role of heme oxygenase and bilirubin in oxidative stress in preterm infants. Pediatr Res 2004; 56:873–877.

34. Tanswell AK, Freeman BA. Pulmonary antioxidant enzyme maturation in the fetal and neonatal rat. I. Developmental profiles. Pediatr Res 1984; 18:584–587.

35. Levonen AL, Lapatto R, Saksela M, et al. Expression of gamma-glutamylcysteine synthetase during development. Pediatr Res 2000; 47:266–270.

36. Rahman I. Regulation of glutathione in inflammation and chronic lung diseases. Mutat Res 2005; 579:58–80.

37. Lavoie JC, Chessex P. Development of glutathione synthesis and gamma-glutamyltranspeptidase activities in tissues from newborn infants. Free Radic Biol Med 1998; 24:994–1001.

38. Ahola T, Levonen AL, Fellman V, et al. Thiol metabolism in preterm infants during the first week of life. Scand J Clin Lab Invest 2004; 64:649–658.

39. Lindeman JH, Lentjes EG, Zoeren-Grobben D, et al. Postnatal changes in plasma ceruloplasmin and transferrin antioxidant activities in preterm babies. Biol Neonate 2000; 78:73–76.

40. Fleming RE, Gitlin JD. Primary structure of rat ceruloplasmin and analysis of tissue-specific gene expression during development. J Biol Chem 1990; 265:7701–7707.

41. Corchia C, Balata A, Soletta G, et al. Increased bilirubin production, ceruloplasmin concentrations and hyperbilirubinaemia in full-term newborn infants. Early Hum Dev 1994; 38:91–96.

42. Berger HM, Mumby S, Gutteridge JM. Ferrous ions detected in iron-overloaded cord blood plasma from preterm and term babies: implications for oxidative stress. Free Radic Res 1995; 22:555–559.

43. Kaarteenaho-Wiik R, Kinnula VL. Distribution of antioxidant enzymes in developing human lung, respiratory distress syndrome, and bronchopulmonary dysplasia. J Histochem Cytochem 2004; 52:1231–1240.

44. Sosenko IR, Jobe AH. Intraamniotic endotoxin increases lung antioxidant enzyme activity in preterm lambs. Pediatr Res 2003; 53:679–683.

45. Nakamura T, Nakamura H, Hoshino T, et al. Redox regulation of lung inflammation by thioredoxin. Antioxid Redox Signal 2005; 7:60–71.

46. Das KC, Guo XL, White CW. Induction of thioredoxin and thioredoxin reductase gene expression in lungs of newborn primates by oxygen. Am J Physiol 1999; 276:L530–L539.

47. Lehtonen ST, Markkanen PM, Peltoniemi M, et al. Variable overoxidation of peroxiredoxins in human lung cells in severe oxidative stress. Am J Physiol Lung Cell Mol Physiol 2005; 288:L997–1001.

48. Fujii T, Fujii J, Taniguchi N. Augmented expression of peroxiredoxin VI in rat lung and kidney after birth implies an antioxidative role. Eur J Biochem 2001; 268:218–225.

49. Chuchalin AG, Novoselov VI, Shifrina ON, et al. Peroxiredoxin VI in human respiratory system. Respir Med 2003; 97:147–151.

50. Kim HS, Kang SW, Rhee SG, et al. Rat lung peroxiredoxins I and II are differentially regulated during development and by hyperoxia. Am J Physiol Lung Cell Mol Physiol 2001; 280:L1212–L1217.

51. Das KC, Pahl PM, Guo XL, et al. Induction of peroxiredoxin gene expression by oxygen in lungs of newborn primates. Am J Respir Cell Mol Biol 2001; 25:226–232.

52. Chen Y, Whitney PL, Frank L. Comparative responses of premature versus full-term newborn rats to prolonged hyperoxia. Pediatr Res 1994; 35:233–237.

53. Frank L, Sosenko IR. Failure of premature rabbits to increase antioxidant enzymes during hyperoxic exposure: increased susceptibility to pulmonary oxygen toxicity compared with term rabbits. Pediatr Res 1991; 29:292–296.

54. Sosenko IR, Chen Y, Price LT, et al. Failure of premature rabbits to increase lung antioxidant enzyme activities after hyperoxic exposure: antioxidant enzyme gene expression and pharmacologic intervention with endotoxin and dexamethasone. Pediatr Res 1995; 37:469–475.

55. Cross CE, Valacchi G, Schock B, et al. Environmental oxidant pollutant effects on biologic systems: a focus on micronutrient antioxidant-oxidant interactions. Am J Respir Crit Care Med 2002; 166:S44–S50.

56. Land SC, Wilson SM. Redox regulation of lung development and perinatal lung epithelial function. Antioxid Redox Signal 2005; 7:92–107.

57. Lubec G, Widness JA, Hayde M, et al. Hydroxyl radical generation in oxygen-treated infants. Pediatrics 1997; 100:700–704.

58. Carpagnano GE, Kharitonov SA, Resta O, et al. 8-Isoprostane, a marker of oxidative stress, is increased in exhaled breath condensate of patients with obstructive sleep apnea after night and is reduced by continuous positive airway pressure therapy. Chest 2003; 124:1386–1392.

59. Buss IH, Senthilmohan R, Darlow BA, et al. 3-Chlorotyrosine as a marker of protein damage by myeloperoxidase in tracheal aspirates from preterm infants: association with adverse respiratory outcome. Pediatr Res 2003; 53:455–462.

60. Banks BA, Ischiropoulos H, McClelland M, et al. Plasma 3-nitrotyrosine is elevated in premature infants who develop bronchopulmonary dysplasia. Pediatrics 1998; 101:870–874.

61. Lorch SA, Banks BA, Christie J, et al. Plasma 3-nitrotyrosine and outcome in neonates with severe bronchopulmonary dysplasia after inhaled nitric oxide. Free Radic Biol Med 2003; 34:1146–1152.

62. Terrasa AM, Guajardo MH, de Armas SE, et al. Pulmonary surfactant protein A inhibits the lipid peroxidation stimulated by linoleic acid hydroperoxide of rat lung mitochondria and microsomes. Biochim Biophys Acta 2005; 1735:101–110.

63. Ogihara T, Hirano K, Morinobu T, et al. Raised concentrations of aldehyde lipid peroxidation products in premature infants with chronic lung disease. Arch Dis Child Fetal Neonatal Ed 1999; 80:F21–F25.

64. Basu S, Helmersson J. Factors regulating isoprostane formation in vivo. Antioxid Redox Signal 2005; 7:221–235.

65. Janssen LJ. Isoprostanes: an overview and putative roles in pulmonary pathophysiology. Am J Physiol Lung Cell Mol Physiol 2001; 280:L1067–L1082.

66. Janssen LJ, Premji M, Netherton S, et al. Vasoconstrictor actions of isoprostanes via tyrosine kinase and Rho kinase in human and canine pulmonary vascular smooth muscles. Br J Pharmacol 2001; 132:127–134.

67. Belik J, Jankov RP, Pan J, et al. Chronic O_2 exposure enhances vascular and airway smooth muscle contraction in the newborn but not adult rat. J Appl Physiol 2003; 94:2303–2312.

68. Jankov RP, Luo X, Cabacungan J, et al. Endothelin-1 and O_2-mediated pulmonary hypertension in neonatal rats: a role for products of lipid peroxidation. Pediatr Res 2000; 48:289–298.

69. Jankov RP, Luo X, Belcastro R, et al. Gadolinium chloride inhibits pulmonary macrophage influx and prevents O_2-induced pulmonary hypertension in the neonatal rat. Pediatr Res 2001; 50:172–183.

70. Belik J, Jankov RP, Pan J, et al. Chronic O_2 exposure in the newborn rat results in decreased pulmonary arterial nitric oxide release and altered smooth muscle response to isoprostane. J Appl Physiol 2004; 96:725–730.

71. Munkeby BH, Borke WB, Bjornland K, et al. Resuscitation of hypoxic piglets with 100% O_2 increases pulmonary metalloproteinases and IL-8. Pediatr Res 2005; 58:542–548.

72. Haase E, Bigam DL, Nakonechny QB, et al. Cardiac function, myocardial glutathione, and matrix metalloproteinase-2 levels in hypoxic newborn pigs reoxygenated by 21%, 50%, or 100% oxygen. Shock 2005; 23:383–389.

73. Tatekawa Y, Kemmotsu H, Joe K, et al. Matrix metalloproteinase-9 expression in congenital diaphragmatic hernia during mechanical ventilation. Surg Today 2005; 35:524–529.

74. Tambunting F, Beharry KD, Hartleroad J, et al. Increased lung matrix metalloproteinase-9 levels in extremely premature baboons with bronchopulmonary dysplasia. Pediatr Pulmonol 2005; 39:5–14.

75. Sweet DG, Curley AE, Chesshyre E, et al. The role of matrix metalloproteinases -9 and -2 in development of neonatal chronic lung disease. Acta Paediatr 2004; 93:791–796.

76. Hosford GE, Fang X, Olson DM. Hyperoxia decreases matrix metalloproteinase-9 and increases tissue inhibitor of matrix metalloproteinase-1 protein in the newborn rat lung: association with arrested alveolarization. Pediatr Res 2004; 56:26–34.

77. Curley AE, Sweet DG, Thornton CM, et al. Chorioamnionitis and increased neonatal lung lavage fluid matrix metalloproteinase-9 levels: implications for antenatal origins of chronic lung disease. Am J Obstet Gynecol 2003; 188:871–875.

78. Cederqvist K, Sorsa T, Tervahartiala T, et al. Matrix metalloproteinases-2, -8, and -9 and TIMP-2 in tracheal aspirates from preterm infants with respiratory distress. Pediatrics 2001; 108:686–692.

79. Sweet DG, McMahon KJ, Curley AE, et al. Type I collagenases in bronchoalveolar lavage fluid from preterm babies at risk of developing chronic lung disease. Arch Dis Child Fetal Neonatal Ed 2001; 84:F168–F171.

80. Jankov RP, Johnstone L, Luo X, et al. Macrophages as a major source of oxygen radicals in the hyperoxic newborn rat lung. Free Radic Biol Med 2003; 35:200–209.

81. Vozzelli MA, Mason SN, Whorton MH, et al. Antimacrophage chemokine treatment prevents neutrophil and macrophage influx in hyperoxia-exposed newborn rat lung. Am J Physiol Lung Cell Mol Physiol 2004; 286:L488–L493.

82. Jankov RP, Luo X, Belcastro R, et al. Gadolinium chloride inhibits pulmonary macrophage influx and prevents O_2-induced pulmonary hypertension in the neonatal rat. Pediatr Res 2001; 50:172–183.

83. Yi M, Jankov RP, Belcastro R, et al. Opposing effects of 60% oxygen and neutrophil influx on alveologenesis in the neonatal rat. Am J Respir Crit Care Med 2004; 170:1188–1196.

84. Sato K, Kadiiska MB, Ghio AJ, et al. In vivo lipid-derived free radical formation by NADPH oxidase in acute lung injury induced by lipopolysaccharide: a model for ARDS. FASEB J 2002; 16:1713–1720.

85. Jobe AH. Antenatal factors and the development of bronchopulmonary dysplasia. Semin Neonatol 2003; 8:9–17.

86. Kallapur SG, Nitsos I, Moss TJ, et al. Chronic endotoxin exposure does not cause sustained structural abnormalities in the fetal sheep lungs. Am J Physiol Lung Cell Mol Physiol 2005; 288:L966–L974.

87. Van Meurs KP, Cohen TL, Yang G, et al. Inhaled NO and markers of oxidant injury in infants with respiratory failure. J Perinatol 2005; 25:463–469.

88. Lin YJ, Markham NE, Balasubramaniam V, et al. Inhaled nitric oxide enhances distal lung growth after exposure to hyperoxia in neonatal rats. Pediatr Res 2005; 58:22–29.

89. Van Meurs KP, Wright LL, Ehrenkranz RA, et al. Inhaled nitric oxide for premature infants with severe respiratory failure. N Engl J Med 2005; 353:13–22.

90. Andersson S, Kheiter A, Merritt TA. Oxidative inactivation of surfactants. Lung 1999; 177:179–189.

91. Belik J, Jankov RP, Pan J, et al. Peroxynitrite inhibits relaxation and induces pulmonary artery muscle contraction in the newborn rat. Free Radic Biol Med 2004; 37:1384–1392.

92. Gazzolo D, Perrone S, Paffetti P, et al. Non protein bound iron concentrations in amniotic fluid. Clin Biochem 2005; 38:674–677.

93. Hirano K, Morinobu T, Kim H, et al. Blood transfusion increases radical promoting non-transferrin bound iron in preterm infants. Arch Dis Child Fetal Neonatal Ed 2001; 84:F188–F193.

94. Collard KJ, Godeck S, Holley JE. Blood transfusion and pulmonary lipid peroxidation in ventilated premature babies. Pediatr Pulmonol 2005; 39:257–261.

95. Alberti-Fidanza A, Burini G, Perriello G. Total antioxidant capacity of colostrum, and transitional and mature human milk. J Matern Fetal Neonatal Med 2002; 11:275–279.

96. Bolisetty S, Naidoo D, Lui K, et al. Postnatal changes in maternal and neonatal plasma antioxidant vitamins and the influence of smoking. Arch Dis Child Fetal Neonatal Ed 2002; 86:F36–F40.

97. Wedekind KJ, Yu S, Combs GF. The selenium requirement of the puppy. J Anim Physiol Anim Nutr (Berl) 2004; 88:340–347.

98. Kinsella JP, Greenough A, Abman SH. Bronchopulmonary dysplasia. Lancet 2006; 367:1421–1431.

99. Kinsella JP, Parker TA, Davis JM, et al. Superoxide dismutase improves gas exchange and pulmonary hemodynamics in premature lambs. Am J Respir Crit Care Med 2005; 172:745–749.

100. Davis JM, Parad RB, Michele T, et al. Pulmonary outcome at 1 year corrected age in premature infants treated at birth with recombinant human CuZn superoxide dismutase. Pediatrics 2003; 111:469–476.

101. Kumral A, Gonenc S, Acikgoz O, et al. Erythropoietin increases glutathione peroxidase enzyme activity and decreases lipid peroxidation levels in hypoxic-ischemic brain injury in neonatal rats. Biol Neonate 2005; 87:15–18.

102. Rao R, Georgieff MK. Neonatal iron nutrition. Semin Neonatol 2001; 6:425–435.

103. Ozer EA, Kumral A, Ozer E, et al. Effects of erythropoietin on hyperoxic lung injury in neonatal rats. Pediatr Res 2005; 58:38–41.

104. Bancalari E, Wilson-Costello D, Iben SC. Management of infants with bronchopulmonary dysplasia in North America. Early Hum Dev 2005; 81:171–179.

105. Bloom R, Yost CC. A consideration of neonatal resuscitation. Pediatr Clin North Am 2004; 51:669–84, ix.

106. Froese AB, Kinsella JP. High-frequency oscillatory ventilation: lessons from the neonatal/pediatric experience. Crit Care Med 2005; 33:S115–S121.

107. Keszler M. Volume-targeted ventilation. J Perinatol 25 Suppl 2005; 2:S19–S22.

108. Donn SM, Sinha SK. Can mechanical ventilation strategies reduce chronic lung disease? Semin Neonatol 2003; 8:441–448.

109. Vento G, Matassa PG, Ameglio F, et al. HFOV in premature neonates: effects on pulmonary mechanics and epithelial lining fluid cytokines. A randomized controlled trial. Intensive Care Med 2005; 31:463–470.

110. Wunsch H, Mapstone J, Takala J. High-frequency ventilation versus conventional ventilation for the treatment of acute lung injury and acute respiratory distress syndrome: a systematic review and Cochrane analysis. Anesth Analg 2005; 100:1765–1772.

111. Ventre KM, Arnold JH. High frequency oscillatory ventilation in acute respiratory failure. Paediatr Respir Rev 2004; 5:323–332.

112. Thomson MA, Yoder BA, Winter VT, et al. Treatment of immature baboons for 28 days with early nasal continuous positive airway pressure. Am J Respir Crit Care Med 2004; 169:1054–1062.

113. Kirchner L, Weninger M, Unterasinger L, et al. Is the use of early nasal CPAP associated with lower rates of chronic lung disease and retinopathy of prematurity? Nine years of experience with the Vermont Oxford Neonatal Network. J Perinat Med 2005; 33:60–66.

114. Polin RA, Sahni R. Newer experience with CPAP. Semin Neonatol 2002; 7:379–389.

115. Subramaniam P, Henderson-Smart DJ, Davis PG. Prophylactic nasal continuous positive airways pressure for preventing morbidity and mortality in very preterm infants. Cochrane Database Syst Rev 2005; CD001243.

116. Tremblay LN, Slutsky AS. Pathogenesis of ventilator-induced lung injury: trials and tribulations. Am J Physiol Lung Cell Mol Physiol 2005; 288:L596–L598.

117. Uhlig S, Ranieri M, Slutsky AS. Biotrauma hypothesis of ventilator-induced lung injury. Am J Respir Crit Care Med 2004; 169:314–315.

118. Choudhury S, Wilson MR, Goddard ME, et al. Mechanisms of early pulmonary neutrophil sequestration in ventilator-induced lung injury in mice. Am J Physiol Lung Cell Mol Physiol 2004; 287:L902–L910.

119. Han B, Lodyga M, Liu M. Ventilator-induced lung injury: role of protein-protein interaction in mechanosensation. Proc Am Thorac Soc 2005; 2:181–187.

120. Kirchner EA, Mols G, Hermle G, et al. Reduced activation of immunomodulatory transcription factors during positive end-expiratory pressure adjustment based on volume-dependent compliance in isolated perfused rabbit lungs. Br J Anaesth 2005; 94:530–535.

121. Parsons PE, Matthay MA, Ware LB, et al. Elevated plasma levels of soluble TNF receptors are associated with morbidity and mortality in patients with acute lung injury. Am J Physiol Lung Cell Mol Physiol 2005; 288:L426–L431.

122. Copland IB, Kavanagh BP, Engelberts D, et al. Early changes in lung gene expression due to high tidal volume. Am J Respir Crit Care Med 2003; 168:1051–1059.

123. Kakkera DK, Siddiq MM, Parton LA. Interleukin-1 balance in the lungs of preterm infants who develop bronchopulmonary dysplasia. Biol Neonate 2005; 87:82–90.

124. Munshi UK, Niu JO, Siddiq MM, et al. Elevation of interleukin-8 and interleukin-6 precedes the influx of neutrophils in tracheal aspirates from preterm infants who develop bronchopulmonary dysplasia. Pediatr Pulmonol 1997; 24:331–336.

125. Copland IB, Martinez F, Kavanagh BP, et al. High tidal volume ventilation causes different inflammatory responses in newborn versus adult lung. Am J Respir Crit Care Med 2004; 169:739–748.

126. Kornecki A, Tsuchida S, Ondiveeran HK, et al. Lung development and susceptibility to ventilator-induced lung injury. Am J Respir Crit Care Med 2005; 171:743–752.

127. Saugstad OD. Oxygen for newborns: how much is too much? J Perinatol 2005; 25 Supp. 2:S45–S49.

128. Jafari B, Ouyang B, Li LF, et al. Intracellular glutathione in stretch-induced cytokine release from alveolar type-2 like cells. Respirology 2004; 9:43–53.

129. Vento G, Matassa PG, Zecca E, et al. Effect of dexamethasone on tracheobronchial aspirate fluid cytology and pulmonary mechanics in preterm infants. Pharmacology 2004; 71:113–119.

130. Martinez F, Lewis J, Copland I, et al. Mechanical ventilation effect on surfactant content, function, and lung compliance in the newborn rat. Pediatr Res 2004; 56:19–25.

131. Chan A, Jayasuriya K, Berry L, et al. Volutrauma activates the clotting cascade in the newborn but not adult rat. Am J Physiol Lung Cell Mol Physiol 2006; 290:L754–L760.

132. Chalmers EA. Perinatal stroke – risk factors and management. Br J Haematol 2005; 130:333–343.

133. Hermansen MC, Hermansen MG. Intravascular catheter complications in the neonatal intensive care unit. Clin Perinatol 2005; 32:141–56, vii.

134. Collard KJ, Godeck S, Holley JE, et al. Pulmonary antioxidant concentrations and oxidative damage in ventilated premature babies. Arch Dis Child Fetal Neonatal Ed 2004; 89:F412–F416.

135. Munson DA, Grubb PH, Kerecman JD, et al. Pulmonary and systemic nitric oxide metabolites in a baboon model of neonatal chronic lung disease. Am J Respir Cell Mol Biol 2005; 33:582–588.

136. Coalson JJ, Winter VT, Gerstmann DR, et al. Pathophysiologic, morphometric, and biochemical studies of the premature baboon with bronchopulmonary dysplasia. Am Rev Respir Dis 1992; 145:872–881.

137. Lee MK, Pryhuber GS, Schwarz MA, et al. Developmental regulation of p66Shc is altered by bronchopulmonary dysplasia in baboons and humans. Am J Respir Crit Care Med 2005; 171:1384–1394.

Chapter 6

Inflammation/Infection: Effects on the Fetal/Newborn Lung

Alan H. Jobe MD PhD ● Suhas Kallapur MD
● Timothy J.M. Moss PhD

Overview of Fetal Inflammation

Diagnosis of Chorioamnionitis: What is it?

How does Chorioamnionitis Occur?

Clinical Associations in the Newborn with Fetal Exposure to Inflammation/ Infection

Experimental Results: The Link Between Fetal Exposure to Inflammation and Lung Maturation

Is Chorioamnionitis Essential for Lung Maturation?

What Mediators can Induce Fetal Lung Responses?

How Early in Gestation can the Fetal Lung Respond to Inflammation?

What is the Mechanism Causing Inflammation-Mediated Lung Maturation?

Do Antenatal Corticosteroid Treatments Interact with Chorioamnionitis Mediated Effects on the Fetal Lungs?

Does Chronic Chorioamnionitis Injure the Fetal Lung?

How Does Chorioamnionitis Increase the Risk of BPD?

OVERVIEW OF FETAL INFLAMMATION

Human fetuses can be exposed to different pathogens, which may initiate an inflammatory process in the placenta, chorioamnion or the fetus. For example, human fetuses are exposed to viral pathogens as a consequence of maternal viremia. The pattern of injury to agents such as varicella and cytomegalovirus depends on the period of gestation during which the infection occurs. Similarly, the fetus can acquire a spirochete infection with syphilis or a parasitic infection with toxoplasmosis secondary to maternal infection and each causes a characteristic syndrome depending on the gestational timing of exposure. These infections are not generally viewed as predominantly inflammatory in nature although the fetal injury and immune responses certainly have inflammatory components. An asphyxial event resulting in fetal tissue injury also will result in inflammation as part of the initial injury and the repair process. Similarly, normal labor is associated with an increase in pro-inflammatory mediators (1). Both innate and acquired inflammatory responses of the fetus are generally considered to be less effective than in the child or adult because the response systems are immature and pregnancy is an immune suppressive environment (2). For example, fetal inflammatory responses to pathogens such as Group B streptococcus and *Listeria monocytogenes* are blunted, resulting in severe infection and often death of the fetus or newborn. Nevertheless, the near-term fetus can make antibody and can mount innate immune responses when challenged by infection.

Although the preterm fetus may be exposed to viral, protozoal or virulent bacterial pathogens (Group B strep, *E. coli*), the most common exposure is to chorioamnionitis, which is the inflammation of the chorioamnion that is frequently associated with preterm labor and delivery (3). This chapter will focus on the questions and controversies about the association of chorioamnionitis with a range of effects on the fetal and newborn lung. Christian Speer will emphasize in his chapter the effects of inflammation on the postnatal lung (see Chapter 8).

DIAGNOSIS OF CHORIOAMNIONITIS: WHAT IS IT?

Chorioamnionitis can be either a clinical syndrome or a silent, indolent process. The clinical diagnosis of chorioamnionitis is made when a pregnant woman has a constellation of findings that include fever, a tender uterus, an elevated blood granulocyte count, bacteria and/or inflammatory cells in amniotic fluid and often preterm or prolonged rupture of membranes. The diagnosis of clinical chorioamnionitis is most frequently made during near-term or term labor and it can be caused by highly virulent organisms. Before 30 weeks gestation, clinical chorioamnionitis is most often diagnosed after attempts to delay preterm delivery or with preterm prolonged rupture of membranes. Another method to diagnose chorioamnionitis is to examine the chorioamnion and the cord after delivery by histopathology for signs of inflammation – to diagnose histologic chorioamnionitis. The amount of infiltration of the chorioamnion by inflammatory cells and the intensity of secondary changes has been used to grade the severity of the fetal exposure to inflammation (4). Inflammation of the cord, called funisitis, is generally considered to indicate a more advanced inflammatory process that involves the fetus (5). Another diagnostic approach is to culture amniotic fluid or fetal membranes for organisms or to assay amniotic fluid for the presence of pro-inflammatory mediators such as TNFα, IL-1 and IL-6 (6). Newer technologies to identify multiple proteins in biological fluids are being adapted to develop proteomic biomarkers for chorioamnionitis in amniotic fluid. These technologies have the potential to rapidly diagnose inflammation and specific organisms (7). The utility of proteomic measurements for clinical practice remains to be demonstrated.

The chorioamnion is fetal tissue and the amniotic fluid surrounding the fetus is in direct contact with the fetal gut and fetal lung. Therefore, the fetus must be exposed to inflammation if there is histologic chorioamnionitis or if the amniotic fluid contains indicators of inflammation. While the distinctions between clinical chorioamnionitis, histologic chorioamnionitis, and an amniotic-fluid-based diagnosis of chorioamnionitis are clear, the clinical implications for the fetal lung are far from clear.

The Venn diagram (Fig. 6-1) illustrates the diagnostic conundrum. Clinical chorioamnionitis does not correlate well with the subsequent diagnosis of histologic chorioamnionitis, and an amniotic fluid diagnosis of infection may or may not predict chorioamnionitis associated with preterm delivery. There are two reports using PCR to survey amniotic fluids collected at 15–19 weeks gestation for genetic amniocentesis that call into question the assumption that fetal colonization with organisms is always abnormal and will cause preterm delivery. The study by Gerber et al. (8) demonstrated that 11% of 254 presumably normal amniotic fluid samples were PCR positive for *Ureaplasma urealyticum* (Table 6-1). While 17 of the 29 *Ureaplasma*-positive pregnancies had preterm labor, only two delivered before

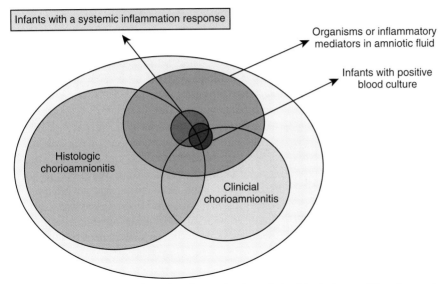

Infants with a systemic inflammation response

Organisms or inflammatory mediators in amniotic fluid

Infants with positive blood culture

Histologic chorioamnionitis

Clinicial chorioamnionitis

Figure 6-1 Venn diagram illustrating the overlapping relationships between different ways to diagnose chorioamnionitis in the preterm and the infant outcomes of sepsis and systemic inflammatory syndromes. The outer circle represents preterm deliveries prior to 30 weeks gestation.

34 weeks gestation. A second report by Perni et al. (9) analyzed 179 amniotic fluid samples and found 13% positive for *Ureaplasma* and 6% positive for *Mycoplasma hominis*. Twenty-eight of the 33 positive pregnancies did not deliver preterm. Recently, Steel et al. (10) used a fluorescent probe for a common 16S rRNA bacterial sequence and identified organisms deep within the membranes of all preterm deliveries and many term deliveries. These startling results suggest that the human pregnancy can tolerate colonization/infection with low pathogenic organisms.

There is at present no clear answer to the question of what is chorioamnionitis. There are multiple ways to make the diagnosis, which are not necessarily congruent. Furthermore, if one accepts that chorioamnionitis results from colonization/infection, then the diagnosis is imprecise in the extreme relative to how infectious diseases are generally diagnosed. The diagnosis of an infection includes the identity of the organism, an estimate of the duration of infection, its intensity and specific sites of involvement. The diagnosis of chorioamnionitis contains none of these elements. Much more clinical research is needed to better define and quantify chorioamnionitis.

HOW DOES CHORIOAMNIONITIS OCCUR?

The best predictor of a preterm delivery is the history of a previous preterm delivery, especially for very preterm births. It is now well recognized that preterm

Table 6-1 **PCR for *Ureaplasma* using Amniotic Fluids Collected at 15–17 Weeks Gestation from Asymptomatic Women**

	Ureaplasma	Negative
Samples (*N* = 254)	11%	89%
Preterm labor	59%	6%
Delivery at < 34 weeks	7%	0%

Of 29 *Ureaplasma*+ samples, 17 had preterm labor but only two delivered before 34 weeks gestation. Data from Gerber et al. (8).

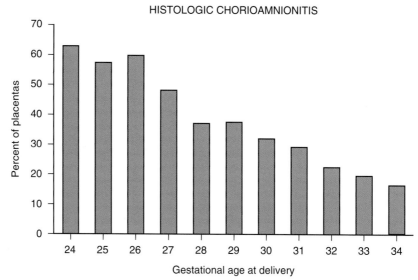

HISTOLOGIC CHORIOAMNIONITIS

Figure 6-2 Relationship between the histopathologic diagnosis of chorioamnionitis and gestational age of delivery at the University of Sydney. The incidence of histologic chorioamnionitis increased as gestational age decreased. Redrawn from Lahra and Jeffrey (11).

deliveries prior to about 30 weeks gestation are commonly associated with histologic chorioamnionitis (11) (Fig. 6-2). Because the majority of these pregnancies are associated with histologic chorioamnionitis, a prediction would be that chorioamnionitis is a recurrent process. Goldenberg et al. (3) make the case in their review of chorioamnionitis that some women may have endometritis prior to pregnancy that evolves into chronic indolent chorioamnionitis. The organisms most commonly associated with chorioamnionitis are primarily vaginal commensal or low pathogenic organisms such as *Ureaplasma urealyticum* and *Mycoplasma hominis*. These organisms are thought to ascend through the cervix to colonize the fetal membranes and to establish a progressive low-grade infection (5). PCR data for *Ureaplasma* in amniotic fluid (Table 6-1) suggest that the colonization need not progress to either overt fetal infection or preterm labor (8). Another inflammatory association with prematurity is periodontal disease (12). These recent observations challenge the commonly held assumption that the fetal compartment normally is sterile and not exposed to inflammation. Research is now linking genetically determined inflammatory response characteristics in the mother and fetus with prematurity (13). The chronic indolent chorioamnionitis associated with prematurity may result from the interaction of the environment and the genetically determined immunomodulatory characteristics of the mother and fetus. A question for the future is how to better diagnose and to understand what makes patients susceptible to chorioamnionitis.

CLINICAL ASSOCIATIONS IN THE NEWBORN WITH FETAL EXPOSURE TO INFLAMMATION/INFECTION

There are inconsistencies in the associations between chorioamnionitis and clinical outcomes for VLBW infants. The link between postnatal inflammation and lung injury from RDS and BPD was made in 1981 (14). However, the source of the inflammation was attributed to lung injury from mechanical ventilation and oxygen exposure. Fetal infection/inflammation before delivery was associated with poor outcomes. For example, the most frequent cause of death just prior to or after

Table 6-2 Preterm Premature Rupture of Membranes (PPROM) Decreases the Incidence of RDS

	PPROM	Intact	P
Number	99	267	
Antenatal steroids	100%	100%	<0.01
Latency after steroids	4.3 days	5.1 days	0.11
Gestational age	30.7 ± 2.9 wks	31.1 ± 2.7 wks	
RDS	17%	39%	
Gr III, IV-IVH	1%	5%	

Data from Sims et al. (21).

preterm delivery was antenatal infection and pneumonia identified at autopsy (15). However, Watterberg et al. (16) reported in 1996 that ventilated preterm infants exposed to histologic chorioamnionitis had a lower incidence of RDS but a higher incidence of BPD than did infants not exposed to chorioamnionitis. Furthermore, the initial tracheal aspirates from infants exposed to chorioamnionitis contained pro-inflammatory mediators such as IL-1, IL-6 and IL-8, indicating that the lung inflammation was of antenatal origin (17, 18). In contrast, Hitti et al. (19) reported that high levels of TNFα in amniotic fluid predicted prolonged postnatal ventilation, suggesting early and persistent lung injury from chorioamnionitis. A decreased incidence of RDS had been associated with preterm prolonged rupture of the membranes, a surrogate marker for chorioamnionitis, as early as 1974 (20). More recent reports continue to support that association (21) (Table 6-2). Clinical chorioamnionitis was associated with decreased death in all infants born at ≤ 26 weeks gestation in the United Kingdom and Ireland in 1995 (22). Hannaford et al. (23) identified *Ureaplasma urealyticum* as an organism of fetal origin that was associated with a decreased risk of RDS (Table 6-3). Recently, there have been many reports associating chorioamnionitis with either improved or poor pulmonary and other outcomes. Examples are the report by Ramsey et al. demonstrating that chorioamnionitis increased neonatal morbidities (24), the report by Choi et al. (25) that chorioamnionitis was associated with BPD in those infants without RDS, and the report by Cheah et al. (26) that histologic chorioamnionitis was associated with activation of NFkB, the intracellular master regulator of inflammation, in leucocytes from preterm infants. Van Marter et al. (27) evaluated the outcomes of both ventilated and non-ventilated VLBW infants and found that chorioamnionitis was associated with a decreased incidence of BPD (odds ratio 0.2). However, BPD was increased if the infant was exposed to chorioamnionitis and was either ventilated for greater than 7 days (odds ratio 3.2) or had postnatal sepsis (odds ratio 2.9). Therefore, chorioamnionitis correlates in the clinical literature with both

Table 6-3 Outcomes of Singleton Infants < 28 weeks Gestational Age with Tracheal Aspirate Cultures Positive for *Ureaplasma urealyticum*

	Culture+	Culture−	P
Number of infants	30	69	
Birth weight (g)	850 ± 161	825 ± 181	NS
RDS	47%	81%	0.001
Surfactant treatment	40%	77%	0.001
Oxygen at 36 weeks	43%	19%	0.03
Death	7%	23%	NS

Data from Hannaford et al. (23).

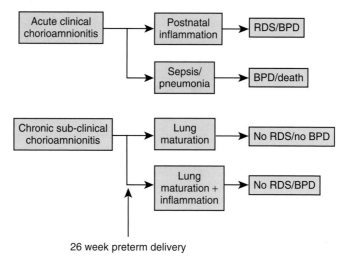

26 week preterm delivery

Figure 6-3 Overview of outcomes following acute clinical or chronic sub-clinical chorioamnionitis. Acute chorioamnionitis with virulent organisms is likely to cause severe lung disease or death. In contrast, chronic chorioamnionitis may improve lung outcomes by inducing lung maturation. However, BPD may occur if the inflammation in the fetal lung is increased by postnatal exposures to oxygen, ventilation or postnatal sepsis.

improved outcomes (less RDS) and bad outcomes (death from infection, more early respiratory failure and BPD).

These inconsistent clinical correlates most likely result from the imprecise diagnosis of chorioamnionitis and its association with different populations of infants. The diagram in Figure 6-3 may help frame the question. A progressive chorioamnionitis caused by a virulent organism may cause severe postnatal lung and systemic inflammation with the outcomes of BPD or sepsis/death. Such outcomes are relatively infrequent in VLBW infants who are not stillborn. Fewer than 2% of VLBW infants have positive blood cultures at birth (28). Chronic, indolent chorioamnionitis caused by organisms such as *Ureaplasma* seems to induce lung maturation (less RDS) in some clinical reports, but that maturation may be associated with more BPD (16). These associations may depend on how the diagnosis of chorioamnionitis is made (clinical, histopathologic, other), the population of infants studied (ventilated only, all VLBW infants, other selected populations), and perhaps patient populations with different racial mixes, exposures and socioeconomic status (periodontal disease is increased in disadvantaged populations, for example). In an attempt to better establish a cause to effect relationship, Viscardi et al. (29) recently correlated the intensity of the inflammatory response to chorioamnionitis in the fetal membranes with the clinical outcome of BPD (Fig. 6-4). More severe chorioamnionitis at delivery predicted an increased incidence and severity of BPD. However, we do not know for how long the chorioamnionitis was present or what organisms were responsible. The fetus will have a graded response to chorioamnionitis based on currently poorly defined variables such as the organism and the duration of fetal exposure. If chorioamnionitis causes a fetal inflammatory response (funisitis, increased IL-6 in cord blood) then neonatal morbidity and mortality will be increased (30).

Another variable that is generally not considered in clinical studies is the influence of postnatal management on the association of chorioamnionitis with clinical outcomes such as the incidence of RDS or BPD. Recent attempts to minimize intubation and ventilation of VLBW infants with strategies such as the early use of CPAP can strikingly change the apparent incidence of a disease such as RDS. An example of the use of delivery-room CPAP on surfactant treatment for RDS and BPD is given in Figure 6-5 (31). In a population of VLBW infants, 62% were not

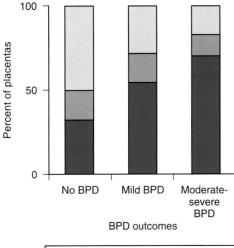

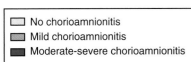

No chorioamnionitis
Mild chorioamnionitis
Moderate-severe chorioamnionitis

Figure 6-4 Relationship of severity of chorioamnionitis by histologic grading with the severity of BPD. Infants with moderate to severe BPD were more likely to have been exposed to more severe histologic chorioamnionitis. [Data from Viscardi et al. (29).]

intubated and ventilated in the delivery room, only 24% of the population received surfactant, and 21% developed BPD. In another recent report of a clinical experience from Columbia University, the early use of CPAP was successful for infants with gestational ages greater than 26 weeks (32) (Table 6-4). If RDS is defined as the need for surfactant treatment in this population of infants with birth weights < 1250 g, then only 16% had RDS. If RDS is defined as the need for ventilation at any time to 72 h, then 47% of infants with birth weights < 1 kg had RDS. These experiences differ strikingly from the data reported in 2000 for the Vermont-Oxford Network, where 80% of infants ≤ 1500 g received surfactant (33). The importance to the present discussion is that an outcome such as RDS depends critically on clinical management and definition. We need to realize that the diagnosis of RDS is as nuanced as the diagnosis of chorioamnionitis. When neither is precise, outcomes are likely to vary in different clinical series.

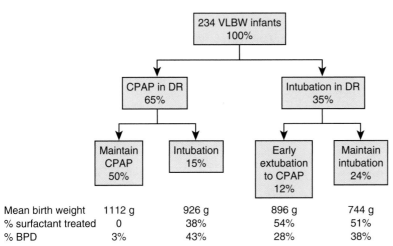

	Maintain CPAP 50%	Intubation 15%	Early extubation to CPAP 12%	Maintain intubation 24%
Mean birth weight	1112 g	926 g	896 g	744 g
% surfactant treated	0	38%	54%	51%
% BPD	3%	43%	28%	38%

Figure 6-5 Outcomes of infants when CPAP was used to avoid intubation in the delivery room (DR). The majority of infants initially tolerated CPAP and 50% of the population were maintained on CPAP for 7 days. The percentages of infants with each treatment outcome who were treated with surfactant and who developed BPD are indicated below the diagram. [Redrawn from Aly et al. (31).]

Table 6-4	Percent of Infants Initially Stabilized with Intubation or CPAP and Outcome at 72 h of Age				
		INITIAL STABILIZATION		OUTCOME AT 72 H*	
Gestational age (weeks)	N	Intubation	CPAP	CPAP fail	CPAP success
23–25	87	31%	69%	38%	31%
26–28	106	5%	95%	17%	78%
29–31	54	0%	100%	7%	93%

CPAP fail is intubation; CPAP success is no therapy other than CPAP for 72 h.
*Percentages calculated for overall population (intubation + CPAP fail + CPAP success = 100%).
Data from Ammari et al. (32).

This problem is compounded for relating an antenatal exposure to a late neonatal outcome such as BPD (Fig. 6-6). The diagnosis of BPD defined as the need for supplemental oxygen or oxygen with respiratory support at 36 weeks is imprecise as it does not include physiologic assessments of lung function or anatomic criteria. In all probability there is a spectrum of injury and developmental abnormalities resulting from the multiple factors that contribute to BPD. BPD is not just one disease. Figure 6-6 emphasizes the distance in time after exposure to chorioamnionitis and the other interventions that contribute to the outcome of BPD. The clinical observations indicating an association between chorioamnionitis and BPD suggest that there may be large effects of chorioamnionitis on the injury sequence that results in BPD. The clinical associations do not provide much information about mechanisms linking fetal exposure to inflammation with RDS or BPD. However, animal models are beginning to explain these clinical observations.

EXPERIMENTAL RESULTS: THE LINK BETWEEN FETAL EXPOSURE TO INFLAMMATION AND LUNG MATURATION

In contrast to the experimental basis for the maturational effects of corticosteroids on the fetal lung first reported in 1969 (34), the first experiment demonstrating that inflammation might induce lung maturation was not reported until 1997 by Bry et al. (35). In studies to evaluate the effects of the pro-inflammatory cytokines on preterm labor in rabbits, intra-amniotic injection of IL-1α caused increased steady-state levels of the surfactant proteins SP-A and SP-B and increased lung compliance. We found that intra-amniotic injection of the pro-inflammatory mediator

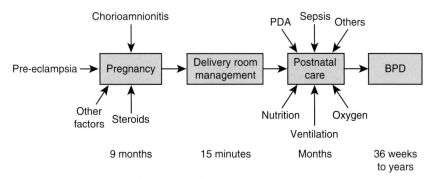

Figure 6-6 Time line for the multiple factors that contribute to the outcome of BPD. Chorioamnionitis is early in the sequence and any effect of chorioamnionitis on the incidence of BPD will be confounded by the multiple other factors contributing to BPD.

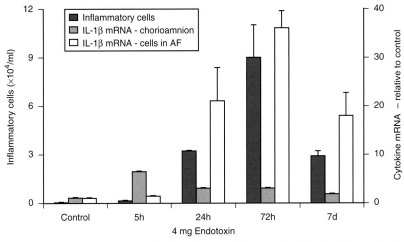

Figure 6-7 Intra-amniotic injection of endotoxin caused chorioamnionitis in fetal sheep. The intra-amniotic injection of endotoxin increased inflammatory cells in amniotic fluid (AF) and IL-1β mRNA in the chorioamnion and in cells in the amniotic fluid. Data from Kramer et al. (37).

endotoxin from *E. coli* caused chorioamnionitis – inflammatory cells and increased IL-1β and IL-6 mRNA expression in the chorioamnion and cells in amniotic fluid and increased IL-8 protein levels in amniotic fluid (36, 37) (Fig. 6-7). The chorioamnionitis was accompanied by inflammation of the fetal lung as demonstrated by expression of heat-shock protein 70 by the airway epithelium within 5 h, recruitment of granulocytes to the fetal lung tissue and airspaces within 24 h, and expression of multiple pro-inflammatory mediators (Fig. 6-8) (38, 39). Apoptosis of lung cells increased at 24 h and proliferation increased at 3 days. This lung inflammation/injury sequence included multiple indicators of lung microvascular

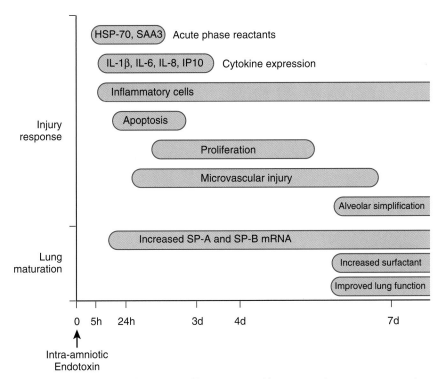

Figure 6-8 Time course in fetal sheep of lung injury and lung maturation responses to an intra-amniotic injection of endotoxin. The lung initially has inflammation followed by lung maturation.

injury – epithelial nitric oxide synthase and vascular endothelial growth factor decreased and medial smooth muscle hypertrophied (39). Thus, intra-amniotic endotoxin causes lung inflammation and an injury sequence.

Inflammation also was associated with the induction of the mRNAs for the surfactant proteins within 12–24 h, persistent elevation of those mRNAs for weeks, and an increase in alveolar surfactant proteins and lipids with improved lung function within 5–7 days (36, 40). The improvement in lung function also was accompanied by a decrease of mesenchymal tissue and an increase in potential gas volume in the fetal lung. The residual effects of the injury at 7 days were increased thickness of the pulmonary microvessels and a decrease in secondary septation of the alveoli (39, 41). However, the net effect was a lung that was easier to ventilate because of improved compliance and that had improved gas exchange (Fig. 6-9). Of note, the lung injury followed by maturation sequence did not result from "fetal stress" because fetal blood cortisol levels did not increase (Fig. 6-9). Therefore, lung inflammation was associated with lung maturation by a mechanism independent of corticosteroids.

IS CHORIOAMNIONITIS ESSENTIAL FOR LUNG MATURATION?

Intra-amniotic endotoxin induced a cascade of inflammatory mediators in the chorioamnion and amniotic fluid. The fetal lung could be signaled by a systemic inflammatory response or by direct contact with endotoxin or mediators from the amniotic fluid. There was a modest fetal systemic response to intra-amniotic endotoxin that included a large increase in the acute-phase reactant serum amyloid A3 in the fetal liver, and modestly increased cytokine mRNA in the liver (38, 42).

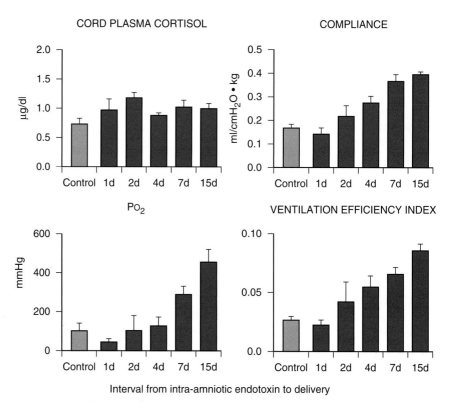

Figure 6-9 Cord plasma cortisol values and lung function following intra-amniotic injections of endotoxin for intervals from 1 day to 15 days before preterm delivery and mechanical ventilation at 125 days gestation. Plasma cortisol did not increase from the low fetal levels. Lung function increased progressively following the intra-amniotic injection of endotoxin. Data redrawn from Jobe et al. (40).

The blood granulocytes decreased at 2 days and granulocytes and platelets increased at 7 days. To test for systemic signaling of the fetal lung, the lung was isolated from the amniotic fluid surgically with collection of the fetal lung fluid in a bag placed in the amniotic cavity (43). Intra-amniotic endotoxin induced chorioamnionitis but not lung inflammation or lung maturation. In contrast, a 24 h tracheal infusion of 10% of the intra-amniotic dose of endotoxin induced both lung inflammation and lung maturation. This same result was achieved using IL-1 as the pro-inflammatory agonist. Therefore, the sequence from fetal lung inflammation to maturation did not result from a lung response to a systemic fetal inflammatory response. Also, new mediators resulting from the chorioamnionitis were not required for the response. Rather direct contact of the fetal lung – presumably the airway epithelium – with endotoxin or IL-1 given by intra-amniotic injection or tracheal infusion induced the lung maturation. The initial inflammatory response is assumed to result from recognition of the mediators by the airway epithelium because the airways express the acute-phase reactants HSP-70 and SAA3 and there are very few monocytes/macrophages present in the fetal lung to initiate an inflammatory response. However, in chronic chorioamnionitis, the inflammatory products of the chorioamnionitis or organisms in the amniotic fluid probably are mediating the responses of the fetal lungs. There is minimal information about how the fetal lung might respond to inflammation.

WHAT MEDIATORS CAN INDUCE FETAL LUNG RESPONSES?

Innate immune responses are signaled by a family of pattern-recognition molecules called the Toll-like receptors (TLR). TLR4 recognizes endotoxin from Gram-negative organisms, TLR2 signals Gram-positive organisms and TLR3 recognizes double-stranded RNA from viral pathogens, for example. There is very little information about the pattern of responses or the expression or location of expression of the TLRs in the human fetus. The chorioamnion does contain TLRs, and chorioamnionitis represents an innate immune response (44). However, the inflammatory cells in the chorioamnion may be of maternal origin when organisms localized between the endometrium and chorioamnion initiate the inflammation (45). The fetal rabbit lung expresses low levels of TLR2 and TLR4, and TLR2, 3 and 4 mRNA levels remain unchanged for the last third of gestation in the fetal sheep (46, 47). Empirically, *E. coli* endotoxin induces a rapid inflammatory response in the fetal sheep lung, as does IL-1, a cytokine that signals inflammation through a receptor that shares receptor elements and the signaling pathways with endotoxin. In recent experiments, we found that a high dose of a TLR2 agonist given by intra-amniotic injection induced less inflammation than did endotoxin and had inconsistent effects on lung maturation. Blood monocytes from preterm sheep also do not respond as well as do monocytes from adult sheep to challenge with TLR agonists (48). This result suggests that the fetus does not respond uniformly to TLR agonists.

Ureaplasma given by intra-amniotic injection can colonize the amniotic fluid and fetal lung as early as 67 days gestation and cause low-grade lung inflammation and lung maturation (49) (Table 6-5). In the fetal sheep the innate inflammatory response to *Ureaplasma* is quite modest, and the organism is not cleared from the fetal lungs. Colonization with *Ureaplasma* also does not cause fetal death or injury, a result similar to the outcomes of human pregnancies that were PCR positive for *Ureaplasma* at 15 to 19 weeks gestation (8, 9). However, the fetal lungs have large increases in surfactant and persistent elevations in the mRNA for surfactant proteins. This model of chronic colonization/infection of the fetal lung with *Ureaplasma* may closely resemble the clinical effects of *Ureaplasma* associated with preterm deliveries in humans.

Table 6-5	Measurements for Sheep Fetuses at 124 days Gestation after Intra-Amniotic Injection of 2×10^7 CFU of *Ureaplasma Parvum* at 67 days Gestation		
		CONTROLS	**UREAPLASMA**
Culture for *Ureaplasma*		Negative	Positive
Plasma cortisol (μg/dl)		0.43 ± 0.05	0.54 ± 0.06
Measurements in bronchiolar lavage			
Inflammatory cells ($\times 10^6$/kg)		0.1 ± 0.06	6.7 ± 1.2
Protein (mg/kg)		34 ± 3	85 ± 21
Saturated phosphatidylcholine (μmol/kg)		0.2 ± 0.1	6.7 ± 3.0
Lung gas volume (ml/kg)		11.2 ± 1.5	28.5 ± 2.8

Values/kg are expressed per kg body weight; all values for the *Ureaplasma* animals are different from controls except plasma cortisol.
Data from Moss et al. (49).

Women with periodontal disease are at increased risk of preterm delivery and their fetuses can develop antibodies to periodontal associated organisms (12). It is not clear how the periodontitis results in transfer of organisms, their products or the maternal response mediators to the placental-fetal unit. Endotoxin-type material isolated from the periodontal associated organism *Porphyromonas gingivalis* caused fetal lethality when given in low dose to fetal sheep by intra-amniotic injection (50). In contrast, endotoxin isolated from an *Actinobaccilus actinomycetemcomitans* caused chorioamnionitis and lung maturation in fetal sheep.

These experiments demonstrate that the fetal sheep can respond to a variety of pro-inflammatory agonists and can be colonized with *Ureaplasma*, which are the organisms most frequently associated with preterm delivery in the human. However, fetal responses do not simply replicate responses in the adult. For example, fetal sheep do not respond to intra-amniotic or intravascular injections of sheep recombinant TNFα and, as noted above, responses to TLR2 agonist were insufficient to consistently induce lung maturation (51). The spectrum of the response potential of the fetus and the fetal lung to the multiple mediators of innate immune responses remains to be studied. Questions relate to receptor expression, the cell localization of that expression, the response potential of the signaling pathways, and the maturity of the integration of innate and acquired immune responses.

HOW EARLY IN GESTATION CAN THE FETAL LUNG RESPOND TO INFLAMMATION?

The interval from fetal exposure to chorioamnionitis and lung inflammation or lung maturation is not known in the human, primarily because of the lack of precision about the diagnosis of chorioamnionitis. In the fetal sheep, significant lung maturation is not detected until 4–7 days after an intra-amniotic injection of endotoxin (40). Lung maturation is striking if the interval between intra-amniotic endotoxin and preterm delivery is 15 days. Intra-amniotic *Ureaplasma* did not induce lung maturation within 7 days but did induce lung maturation when given 14–45 days before preterm delivery (49). Intra-amniotic endotoxin given at 60 days gestation (40% of gestation) to fetal sheep resulted in a doubling of lung-saturated phosphatidylcholine, increased SP-A, SP-B and SP-C mRNA and improved lung function 65 days later with preterm delivery at 125 days gestation (52). This striking result demonstrates that the early-gestation lung does respond to inflammation. These experiments in the sheep demonstrate responses of the fetal lung to intra-amniotic endotoxin/chorioamnionitis across a wide range of gestational ages. The question of how early in gestation an inflammatory stimulus can modulate fetal lung development remains unanswered in the clinical context.

WHAT IS THE MECHANISM CAUSING INFLAMMATION-MEDIATED LUNG MATURATION?

The mechanism(s) responsible for inflammation-induced lung maturation are just beginning to be explored. In the human, chorioamnionitis is associated with an increase in cortisol in cord blood collected at delivery (53) and, of course, glucocorticoids induce lung maturation. The clinical samples are from infants who have been exposed to chorioamnionitis and who have been delivered as a result of preterm labor, which may represent a selected population – as most women colonized with *Ureaplasma* may not deliver prematurely, for example. In fetal sheep, endotoxin, IL-1 or *Ureaplasma* induced chorioamnionitis **does not** induce preterm labor, preterm delivery or an increase in fetal blood cortisol levels sufficient to induce lung maturation.

The minimal amount of *E. coli* endotoxin that will induce lung maturation in the fetal sheep is 1–4 mg and doses as high as 100 mg induce lung maturation without increasing the amount of lung inflammation, or causing fetal injury or preterm delivery (37, 40). Doses of intra-amniotic endotoxin less than 1 mg cause less inflammation and no lung maturation. In general, the amount of lung inflammation induced by chorioamnionitis correlated with the amount of lung maturation. These results indicate that low amounts of lung inflammation will not induce lung maturation and above some minimal level there is a dose-response relationship between lung inflammation and lung maturation. We have initiated experiments to block lung inflammation to directly evaluate the importance of inflammation for lung maturation. A monoclonal antibody to the integrin CD-18 blocked endotoxin-induced lung inflammation and lung maturation (Fig. 6-10) (54). In contrast, inflammation and lung maturation induced by IL-I was not blocked by this anti-CD-18 antibody. This experiment links inflammation to lung maturation and further demonstrates that different pro-inflammatory agonists can recruit inflammatory cells to the fetal lungs by different mechanisms.

This inflammation-maturation relationship was further examined using an IL-1 receptor blocker. IL-1α is a potent inducer of chorioamnionitis, lung inflammation, and lung maturation. IL-1α also induces the expression of IL-1β in the chorioamnion, cells in amniotic fluid and in the fetal lung. When the IL-1 receptor antagonist anakinra (Amgen®) was given into the amniotic fluid and to the fetus to block IL-1 signaling in the fetal compartment, intra-amniotic IL-1α induced neither inflammation nor lung maturation (55). This experiment demonstrates effective blockade of IL-1 signaling. This IL-1 receptor antagonist blocked about 80% of the lung inflammatory response to intra-amniotic endotoxin and decreased lung maturation. These experiments demonstrate that inflammation is essential to the lung maturation response. There is at present no information about what products of lung inflammation signal lung maturation. Presumably mediators produced locally in the distal lung parenchyma, possibly by granulocytes and/or monocytes, induce a signaling cascade resulting in the mesenchymal and type II cell changes that result in lung maturation. Insight into the signaling sequence may provide clues to clinically practical strategies to induce lung maturation.

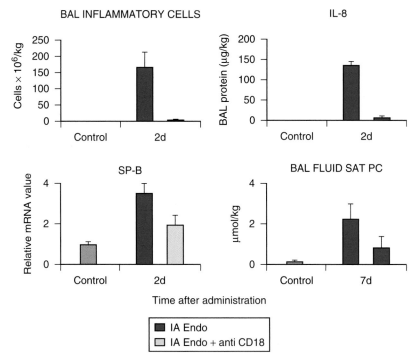

BAL INFLAMMATORY CELLS

IL-8

SP-B

BAL FLUID SAT PC

Time after administration

■ IA Endo
□ IA Endo + anti CD18

Figure 6-10 Anti-CD-18 antibody blocks lung inflammation and maturation in fetal sheep. Fetal sheep given an anti-CD-18 antibody 3 h before intra-amniotic (IA) endotoxin had decreased numbers of inflammatory cells in bronchoalveolar lavage (BAL) and decreased IL-8 in BAL, indicating almost complete blockade of the endotoxin-induced lung inflammation at 2 days. Both the surfactant protein SP-B mRNA and the amount of saturated phosphatidylcholine (Sat PC) are indicators of decreased lung maturation. Data from Kallapu et al. (54).

DO ANTENATAL CORTICOSTEROID TREATMENTS INTERACT WITH CHORIOAMNIONITIS MEDIATED EFFECTS ON THE FETAL LUNGS?

This is a clinically relevant question because antenatal corticosteroids are given to more than 80% of the women at risk of preterm delivery before 30 weeks gestation and the majority of these women will have undiagnosed (histologic) chorioamnionitis (3). The majority of women with preterm rupture of membranes have histologic chorioamnionitis. Even though preterm rupture of membranes is a surrogate marker for chorioamnionitis, the current recommendation is to give antenatal corticosteroids because they decrease the incidence of both RDS and intraventricular hemorrhage (56). In clinical series, antenatal corticosteroids are of benefit for preterm deliveries that in retrospect had associated histologic chorioamnionitis (57) (Table 6-6). Although there is no specific clinical information available about how corticosteroids influence chorioamnionitis, the corticosteroids might suppress inflammation – a potential benefit, or increase the risk of progressive infection – a potential risk.

Both outcomes seem possible based on the small amount of information available from experimental studies. Maternal treatment with betamethasone suppressed the inflammation caused by intra-amniotic endotoxin in the chorioamnion and lungs of fetal sheep (42, 58) (Fig. 6-11). Inflammatory cells and pro-inflammatory cytokine expression were suppressed for about 2 days after the betamethasone treatment, but subsequently inflammation was **increased** in the lungs of lambs exposed to both maternal betamethasone and intra-amniotic endotoxin relative to endotoxin alone 5 and 15 days after the exposures (Fig. 6-12). Lung maturation

Table 6-6 **Antenatal Corticosteroid Effects on Fetal Outcomes for Preterm Infants Exposed to Histologic Chorioamnionitis**

	+Steroids	−Steroids	P
Number of infants	169	358	
RDS	40%	56%	< 0.001
IVH/PVL	22%	37%	< 0.001
NEC	6%	6%	−
PDA	15%	24%	0.02
Neonatal sepsis	18%	14%	−
Death	8%	16%	0.01

Data from Elimian et al. (57).

seemed to be greater in lambs exposed to both betamethasone and endotoxin than to either treatment alone (59) (Fig. 6-13). A surprising result was that growth restriction induced by betamethasone did not occur with concurrent endotoxin exposure. These results with fetal sheep support the clinical observations that betamethasone can decrease RDS in the presence of histologic chorioamnionitis. In fetal sheep, either exposure matures the fetal lung and both exposures when given together tend to further increase the fetal lung maturational response. However, the lung maturational response to endotoxin is larger than is the response to betamethasone. In fetal sheep the response to endotoxin is quite uniform, while animals have more variable responses to maternal betamethasone treatment. A distinct difference in the responses is the rapid improvement in lung function within 15 h with betamethasone and the delay for an improvement in lung function of at least 4 days following intra-amniotic endotoxin (40, 60).

The increased inflammation in the fetal sheep lungs that occurs 5 to 15 days after combined betamethasone and endotoxin exposures is a potential concern. Such effects have not been apparent clinically, but they have not been evaluated. A potential mechanism to explain the increased inflammation is that both betamethasone and the endotoxin "mature" an immature inflammatory system. Blood monocytes isolated from fetal sheep have decreased responses in vitro to endotoxin stimulation relative to monocytes from adult sheep (61) (Fig. 6-14). However, 7 days after the fetal exposures, the monocytes respond to endotoxin in vitro like monocytes from adult sheep. Similarly, maternal betamethasone initially suppress the fetal monocyte, but function is increased 7 days after the maternal

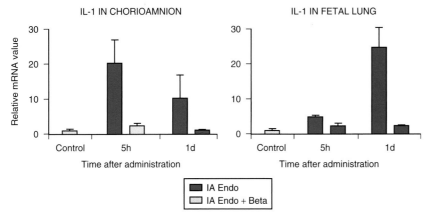

Figure 6-11 Maternal betamethasone suppressed the inflammation induced by intra-amniotic (IA) endotoxin in the chorioamnion and fetal lung. The expression of IL-1β mRNA was decreased to control values by maternal betamethasone given to sheep 3 h before intra-amniotic endotoxin. Data from Newnham et al. (58) and Kallapur et al. (42).

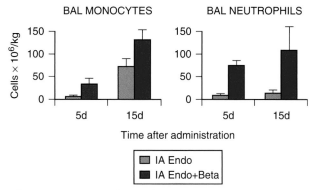

BAL MONOCYTES

BAL NEUTROPHILS

Time after administration

☐ IA Endo
■ IA Endo+Beta

Figure 6-12 Inflammation is increased in the fetal lung by maternal betamethasone 5 days and 15 days after intra-amniotic (IA) endotoxin. The monocytes and neutrophils recovered by broncho-alveolar lavage (BAL) were increased if fetuses were exposed to maternal betamethasone prior to intra-amniotic endotoxin relative to the endotoxin exposure alone. Data from Kallapur et al. (42).

treatment (62). These results illustrate just how complex interactions between exposures may be clinically.

These experiments in fetal sheep describe simultaneous exposures to betamethasone and chorioamnionitis. Clinically, the more likely scenarios are the superposition of maternal betamethasone treatments on chronic, sub-clinical chorioamnionitis or maternal betamethasone treatments followed by the acute onset of chorioamnionitis. There is just no information about how timing of exposures may alter clinical outcomes. Repetitive courses of betamethasone treatments may be a concern particularly when chorioamnionitis is present. The clinical dilemma is that histologic chorioamnionitis is a retrospective diagnosis of a clinically silent process.

DOES CHRONIC CHORIOAMNIONITIS INJURE THE FETAL LUNG?

Although the majority of VLBW infants may be exposed to chronic chorioamnionitis, the duration and the intensity of the inflammatory exposure to the fetus

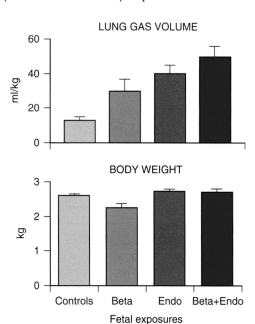

LUNG GAS VOLUME

BODY WEIGHT

Figure 6-13 Lung gas volumes and body weights of fetal sheep 7 days after exposure to maternal betamethasone (Beta), intra-amniotic endotoxin (Endo) or both (Beta+Endo). Maximal lung gas volume measured at 40 cmH$_2$O airway pressure increased with either treatment but was largest with both treatments. Only maternal betamethasone decreased fetal weight, and this effect was prevented by concurrent endotoxin exposure. Data redrawn from Newnham et al. (59).

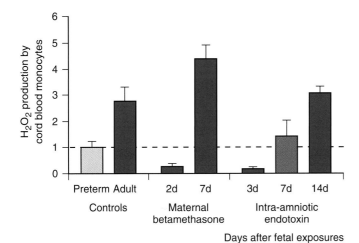

Figure 6-14 Hydrogen peroxide production (H_2O_2) by cord blood monocytes from preterm lambs and blood monocytes from adult sheep on challenge in vitro with endotoxin. The monocytes from the preterm sheep produce less H_2O_2 than the monocytes from adult sheep. Maternal betamethasone suppressed monocyte function at 2 days but enhanced monocyte function at 7 days. Intra-amniotic endotoxin also initially suppressed the enhanced monocyte function. Data from Kramer et al. (62, 71).

remain undefined. A single pro-inflammatory fetal exposure from intra-amniotic injections of mediators caused acute lung inflammation followed by mild micro-vascular injury and an arrest in alveolar septation by 7 days (39, 41). Low-grade inflammation (increased inflammatory cells) persisted for weeks. Live *Ureaplasma* caused very mild inflammation despite prolonged persistence in the fetal lung (49). The clinically relevant question is how does the fetal lung cope with prolonged exposures to inflammatory agonists such as endotoxin. Surprisingly, few VLBW infants seem to have severe pneumonia after preterm birth despite exposure to infection/inflammation. Although intrauterine exposure to endotoxin caused his-tologic changes consistent with a mild BPD phenotype in experimental animals, infants are not born with BPD. The possible exception is the rapid development of the BPD variant described by radiologic changes as the Wilson-Mikity syndrome, which has been associated with chorioamnionitis (63). However, in general, severe lung injury and pneumonia are infrequent after the histologic chorioamnionitis associated with preterm birth.

We have modeled chronic endotoxin-induced chorioamnionitis with repeated weekly doses of endotoxin given by intra-amniotic injection and by placing osmotic pumps that deliver endotoxin continuously over 28 days in the amniotic cavity. A prolonged fetal exposure resulting from a 28-day intra-amniotic infusion of endo-toxin from 53% to 72% of gestation caused striking lung maturation and increases in surfactant at 125 days (83% of gestation) (52). However, the lung had decreased alveolar septation. When the lungs of the fetal sheep were examined at 138 days of gestation, low-grade inflammation persisted 30 days after the end of endotoxin administration and surfactant was increased as a residual effect of the induced lung maturation (64) (Fig. 6-15). Remarkably, all anatomic indicators of the arrest of alveolar septation seen at 125 days gestation had disappeared by 138 days gesta-tion. There also were no biochemical or histologic indicators of microvascular injury.

Weekly intra-amniotic injections with 10 mg endotoxin given at 100 days, 107 days, 114 days and 121 days gestation resulted in the recovery of 3.3×10^7 inflammatory cells per kg body weight by bronchoalveolar lavage at 145 days gestation, just prior to term (64). In contrast, control lungs had $<10^4$ inflammatory cells in bronchoalveolar lavage fluid. At 145 days gestation and after repeated

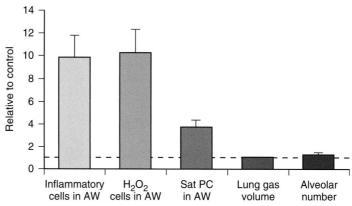

Figure 6-15 Residual effects at 138 days gestation of intra-amniotic infusion of 1 mg/day of endotoxin from 80 to 108 days gestation in fetal sheep. All measurements are expressed relative to the control group, which was normalized to 1.0 (dashed line). Residual indicators of inflammation were the number of inflammatory cells in bronchoalveolar lavage (BAL) and their ability to produce peroxide (H_2O_2). Although the amount of saturated phosphatidylcholine (Sat PC) in the BAL was increased, lung structure was not altered. Data from Kallapur et al. (64).

intra-amniotic endotoxin injections, the mRNA for the pro-inflammatory cytokine IL-1β in lung tissue was higher than control, as was the amount of surfactant, but there were no significant changes in lung architecture or microvasculature (Fig. 6-16). These results demonstrate that the fetal lung can adapt to chronic inflammation and, despite a brief interference with alveolar septation and microvascular development, the fetal lung corrects the deficits and can continue to develop. Although these lungs appear normal after the prolonged endotoxin exposures, there will be alterations in innate immune responses to inflammation. Of note, the fetal lung contains few mature macrophages, and these lungs exposed to endotoxin contain large numbers of histologically mature macrophages.

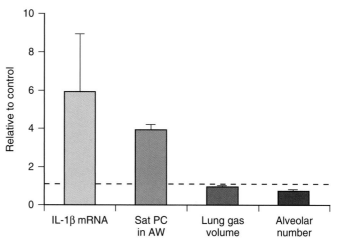

Figure 6-16 Residual effects of weekly intra-amniotic injections of endotoxin on fetal sheep lungs at term. Fetal sheep were exposed to four intra-amniotic injections of 10 mg endotoxin at weekly intervals beginning at 100 days gestation. At delivery 24 days after the final injection, expression of IL-1β mRNA in lung tissue was increased, the amount of saturated phosphatidylcholine (Sat PC) in bronchoalveolar lavage was increased, but lung gas volumes or alveolar numbers were similar to control values. The control values were normalized to 1.0 and are indicated by the dashed line. Data from Kallapur et al. (64).

HOW DOES CHORIOAMNIONITIS INCREASE THE RISK OF BPD?

This question cannot be easily answered with the present experimental or clinical information. However, there are observations that can be tied together into different sequences that could lead to BPD. The present understanding of BPD is that it is primarily an abnormal developmental process associated with an arrest of secondary septation (alveolarization), which is associated with inflammation (65). Inflammation from any source can interfere with postnatal secondary septation in rodents. An antenatal lung inflammatory response resulting from chorioamnionitis can cause an arrest in alveolar septation and interfere with microvascular development (39, 41). This fetal exposure also initiates an inflammation that can persist in the fetal lungs for weeks and matures monocytes to macrophages to generate a population of cells with more inflammatory potential (64).

When preterm delivery occurs, the preterm lung is exposed to oxygen and stretch as a result of ventilation (Fig. 6-6). Mechanical ventilation and perhaps spontaneous ventilation of the normal preterm lung will initiate lung inflammation. The inflammation is increased if preterm lambs are ventilated with high tidal volumes or without positive end-expiratory pressure, and surfactant treatments protect the preterm lungs from injury (65–67). The effects of the initiation of ventilation on the lung injury response will be modulated by the antenatal history of the lung. For example, if lung maturation resulting from antenatal glucocorticoid treatments or chorioamnionitis has occurred, then surfactant will be increased and the initiation of ventilation can occur with less probability of injury. However, the more mature lung will contain more mature macrophages, which may make that lung more able to initiate and sustain an inflammatory response. An example of such an effect is shown in Figure 6-17. In fetal sheep, a single intra-amniotic exposure to endotoxin 30 days before preterm delivery resulted in increased numbers of lymphocytes and granulocytes in the bronchoalveolar lavage after delivery, surfactant treatment and 6 h of ventilation (68). Infants exposed to chorioamnionitis who have a systemic acute inflammatory response at birth (diagnosed by elevated IL-6 levels in cord blood) may have the equivalent of the acute respiratory distress syndrome (ARDS) seen in adults with sepsis (69). The increased permeability of the lungs, aggravated by ventilation, and small pool sizes of surfactant may result in a respiratory problem that is difficult to distinguish from RDS. The reciprocal problem also can occur: if the fetal lungs contain pro-inflammatory mediators, mechanical ventilation will translocate those mediators to the circulation and cause a systemic inflammatory response, as demonstrated in animal models (70).

The pathways from chorioamnionitis to BPD after preterm birth currently are unclear mechanistically – probably because there are multiple potential pathways. In a recent clinical report, Choi et al. (25) correlated the outcome of BPD with histologic chorioamnionitis. Of the infants who developed BPD after RDS, 30% had histologic chorioamnionitis, while 71% of infants with BPD who did not have RDS had histologic chorioamnionitis. More severe chorioamnionitis associated with a systemic inflammatory response may increase the severity of RDS and decrease the effectiveness of surfactant treatments because of an ARDS-like syndrome with pulmonary edema. In contrast, less severe chorioamnionitis causing lung maturation and no RDS may prime the preterm lung to mount a greater and more sustained inflammatory response to postnatal challenges such as ventilation, oxygen and nosocomial infection. The effects of antenatal inflammation as an inducer/modulator of innate inflammatory responses after preterm delivery remain essentially unexplored.

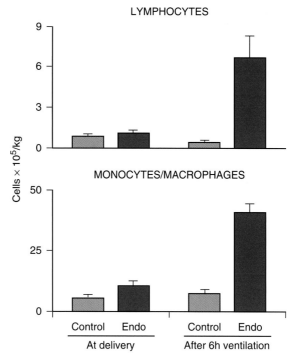

Figure 6-17 Lymphocytes and monocytes in bronchoalveolar lavage from preterm lambs: effects of fetal exposure to intra-amniotic endotoxin. The fetal sheep received intra-amniotic injections of saline or 10 mg endotoxin at 100 days gestation and were delivered at 130 days gestation. The lambs were randomized to sampling at delivery or to 6 h of ventilation after surfactant treatment. The lambs exposed to endotoxin as fetuses had increased numbers of lymphocytes and monocytes in bronchoalveolar lavages after 6 h of ventilation. Data redrawn from Ikegami and Jobe (68).

Acknowledgments

This review was supported by Grants HD-12714 and HL-65397 from the National Institutes of Health.

REFERENCES

1. Stjernholm-Vladic Y, Stygar D, Mansson C, et al. Factors involved in the inflammatory events of cervical ripening in humans. Reprod Biol Endocrinol 2004; 2:74.
2. Marshall-Clarke S, Reen D, Tasker L, Hassan J. Neonatal immunity: how well has it grown up? Immunol Today 2000; 21:35–41.
3. Goldenberg RL, Hauth JC, Andrews WW. Intrauterine infection and preterm delivery. N Engl J Med 2000; 342:1500–1507.
4. Redline RW, Wilson-Costello D, Borawski E, et al. Placental lesions associated with neurologic impairment and cerebral palsy in very low-birth-weight infants. Arch Pathol Lab Med 1998; 122:1091–1098.
5. Romero R, Espinoza J, Chaiworapongsa T, Kalache K. Infection and prematurity and the role of preventive strategies. Semin Neonatol 2002; 7:259–274.
6. Yoon BH, Romero R, Jun JK, et al. Amniotic fluid cytokines (interleukin-6, tumor necrosis factor-alpha, interleukin-1 beta, and interleukin-8) and the risk for the development of bronchopulmonary dysplasia. Am J Obstet Gynecol 1997; 177:825–830.
7. Gravett MG, Novy MJ, Rosenfeld RG, et al. Diagnosis of intra-amniotic infection by proteomic profiling and identification of novel biomarkers. JAMA 2004; 292:462–469.
8. Gerber S, Vial Y, Hohlfeld P, Witkin SS. Detection of Ureaplasma urealyticum in second-trimester amniotic fluid by polymerase chain reaction correlates with subsequent preterm labor and delivery. J Infect Dis 2003; 187:518–521.
9. Perni SC, Vardhana S, Korneeva I, et al. Mycoplasma hominis and Ureaplasma urealyticum in midtrimester amniotic fluid: association with amniotic fluid cytokine levels and pregnancy outcome. Am J Obstet Gynecol 2004; 191:1382–1386.

10. Steel JH, Malatos S, Kennea N, et al. Bacteria and inflammatory cells in fetal membranes do not always cause preterm labor. Pediatr Res 2005; 57:404–411.

11. Lahra MM, Jeffery HE. A fetal response to chorioamnionitis is associated with early survival after preterm birth. Am J Obstet Gynecol 2004; 190:147–151.

12. Boggess KA, Moss K, Madianos P, et al. Fetal immune response to oral pathogens and risk of preterm birth. Am J Obstet Gynecol 2005; 193:1121–1126.

13. Annells MF, Hart PH, Mullighan CG, et al. Interleukins-1, -4, -6, -10, tumor necrosis factor, transforming growth factor-beta, FAS, and mannose-binding protein C gene polymorphisms in Australian women: risk of preterm birth. Am J Obstet Gynecol 2004; 191:2056–2067.

14. Merritt TA, Stuard ID, Puccia J, et al. Newborn tracheal aspirate cytology: classification during respiratory distress syndrome and bronchopulmonary dysplasia. J Pediatr 1981; 98:949–956.

15. Barton L, Hodgman JE, Pavlova Z. Causes of death in the extremely low birth weight infant. Pediatrics 1999; 103:446–451.

16. Watterberg KL, Demers LM, Scott SM, Murphy S. Chorioamnionitis and early lung inflammation in infants in whom bronchopulmonary dysplasia develops. Pediatrics 1996; 97:210–215.

17. Groneck P, Goetze-Speer B, Speer CP. Inflammatory bronchopulmonary response of preterm infants with microbial colonization of the airways at birth. Arch Dis Child 1996; 74:F51–F55.

18. De Dooy J, Colpaert C, Schuerwegh A, et al. Relationship between histologic chorioamnionitis and early inflammatory variables in blood, tracheal aspirates, and endotracheal colonization in preterm infants. Pediatr Res 2003; 54:113–119.

19. Hitti J, Krohn MA, Patton DL, et al. Amniotic fluid tumor necrosis factor-alpha and the risk of respiratory distress syndrome among preterm infants. Am J Obstet Gynecol 1997; 177:50–56.

20. Richardson CJ, Pomerance JJ, Cunningham MD, Gluck L. Acceleration of fetal lung maturation following prolonged rupture of the membranes. Am J Obstet Gynecol 1974; 118:1115–1118.

21. Sims EJ, Vermillion ST, Soper DE. Preterm premature rupture of the membranes is associated with a reduction in neonatal respiratory distress syndrome. Am J Obstet Gynecol 2002; 187:268–272.

22. Costeloe K, Hennessy E, Gibson AT, Marlow N, Wilkinson AR. The EPICure study: outcomes to discharge from hospital for infants born at the threshold of viability. Pediatrics 2000; 106:659–671.

23. Hannaford K, Todd DA, Jeffery H, et al. Role of Ureaplasma urealyticum in lung disease of prematurity. Arch Dis Child Fetal Neonatal Ed 1999; 81:F162–167.

24. Ramsey PS, Lieman JM, Brumfield CG, Carlo W. Chorioamnionitis increases neonatal morbidity in pregnancies complicated by preterm premature rupture of membranes. Am J Obstet Gynecol 2005; 192:1162–1166.

25. Choi CW, Kim BI, Koh YY, et al. Clinical characteristics of chronic lung disease without preceding respiratory distress syndrome in preterm infants. Pediatr Int 2005; 47:72–79.

26. Cheah FC, Winterbourn CC, Darlow BA, et al. Nuclear factor kappaB activation in pulmonary leukocytes from infants with hyaline membrane disease: associations with chorioamnionitis and Ureaplasma urealyticum colonization. Pediatr Res 2005; 57:616–623.

27. Van Marter LJ, Dammann O, Allred EN, et al. Chorioamnionitis, mechanical ventilation, and postnatal sepsis as modulators of chronic lung disease in preterm infants. J Pediatr 2002; 140:171–176.

28. Stoll BJ, Hansen N, Fanaroff AA, et al. Changes in pathogens causing early-onset sepsis in very-low-birth-weight infants. N Engl J Med 2002; 347:240–247.

29. Viscardi RM, Muhumuza CK, Rodriguez A, et al. Inflammatory markers in intrauterine and fetal blood and cerebrospinal fluid compartments are associated with adverse pulmonary and neurologic outcomes in preterm infants. Pediatr Res 2004; 55:1009–1017.

30. Lau J, Magee F, Qiu Z, et al. Chorioamnionitis with a fetal inflammatory response is associated with higher neonatal mortality, morbidity, and resource use than chorioamnionitis displaying a maternal inflammatory response only. Am J Obstet Gynecol 2005; 193:708–713.

31. Aly H, Massaro AN, Patel K, El-Mohandes AA. Is it safer to intubate premature infants in the delivery room? Pediatrics 2005; 115:1660–1665.

32. Ammari A, Suri MS, Milisavljevic V, et al. Variables associated with the early failure of nasal CPAP in very low birth weight infants. J Pediatr 2005; 147:341–347.

33. Horbar JD, Carpenter JH, Buzas J, et al. Timing of initial surfactant treatment for infants 23 to 29 weeks' gestation: is routine practice evidence based? Pediatrics 2004; 113:1593–1602.

34. Liggins GC. Premature delivery of fetal lambs infused with glucocorticoids. J Endocrinol 1969; 45:515–523.

35. Bry K, Lappalainen U, Hallman M. Intraamniotic interleukin-1 accelerates surfactant protein synthesis in fetal rabbits and improves lung stability after premature birth. J Clin Invest 1997; 99:2992–2999.

36. Kallapur SG, Willet KE, Jobe AH, et al. Intra-amniotic endotoxin: Chorioamnionitis precedes lung maturation in preterm lambs. Am J Physiol 2001; 280:L527–L536.

37. Kramer BW, Moss TJ, Willet K, et al. Dose and time response after intra-amniotic endotoxin in preterm lambs. Am J Respir Crit Care Med 2001; 164:982–988.

38. Kramer BW, Kramer S, Ikegami M, Jobe A. Injury, inflammation and remodeling in fetal sheep lung after intra-amniotic endotoxin. Am J Physiol Lung Cell Mol Physiol 2002; 283:L452–L459.

39. Kallapur SG, Bachurski CJ, Le Cras TD, et al. Vascular changes following intra-amniotic endotoxin in preterm lamb lungs. Am J Physiol Lung Cell Mol Physiol 2004; 287:L1178–L1185.

40. Jobe AH, Newnham JP, Willet KE, et al. Endotoxin induced lung maturation in preterm lambs is not mediated by cortisol. Am J Respir Crit Care Med 2000; 162:1656–1661.

41. Willet K, Jobe A, Ikegami M, et al. Antenatal endotoxin and glucocorticoid effects on lung morphometry in preterm lambs. Pediatr Res 2000; 48:782–788.

42. Kallapur SG, Kramer BW, Moss TJ, et al. Maternal glucocorticoids increase endotoxin-induced lung inflammation in preterm lambs. Am J Physiol Lung Cell Mol Physiol 2003; 284:L633–642.

43. Moss TJ, Nitsos I, Kramer BW, et al. Intra-amniotic endotoxin induces lung maturation by direct effects on the developing respiratory tract in preterm sheep. Am J Obstet Gynecol 2002; 187:1059–1065.

44. Kim YM, Romero R, Chaiworapongsa T, et al. Toll-like receptor-2 and -4 in the chorioamniotic membranes in spontaneous labor at term and in preterm parturition that are associated with chorioamnionitis. Am J Obstet Gynecol 2004; 191:1346–1355.

45. Steel JH, O'Donoghue K, Kennea NL, et al. Maternal origin of inflammatory leukocytes in preterm fetal membranes, shown by fluorescence in situ hybridisation. Placenta 2005; 26:672–677.

46. Harju K, Glumoff V, Hallman M. Ontogeny of Toll-like receptors Tlr2 and Tlr4 in mice. Pediatr Res 2001; 49:81–83.

47. Hillman N, Kallapur SG, Moss T, Jobe AH. Toll-like receptors 2, 3 and 4: ontogeny and their differential induction in preterm fetal sheep lung exposure to LPS. Abstract, PAS 2005; www.pas-meeting.org.

48. Kramer BW, Jobe AH. The clever fetus: responding to inflammation to minimize lung injury. Biol Neonate 2005; 88:202–207.

49. Moss T JM, Nitsos I, Ikegami M, Jobe AH, Newnham JP. Experimental intra-uterine Ureaplasma infection in sheep. Am J Obstet Gynecol 2005; 192:1179–1186.

50. Newnham JP, Shub A, Jobe AH, et al. The effects of intra-amniotic injection of periodontopathic lipopolysaccharides in sheep. Am J Obstet Gynecol 2005; 193:313–321.

51. Ikegami M, Moss T JM, Kallapur SG, et al. Minimal lung and systemic responses to TNFα in preterm sheep. Am J Physiol 2003; 285:L121–L129.

52. Moss TM, Newnham J, Willet K, et al. Early gestational intra-amniotic endotoxin: lung function, surfactant and morphometry. Am J Respir Crit Care Med 2002; 165:805–811.

53. Watterberg KL, Scott SM, Naeye RL. Chorioamnionitis, cortisol, and acute lung disease in very low birth weight infants. Pediatrics 1997; 99:E6.

54. Kallapur SG, Moss J TM, Newnham JP, et al. Recruited inflammatory cells mediate endotoxin-induced lung maturation in preterm fetal lambs. Am J Respir Crit Care Med 2005; 172:1315–1321.

55. Kallapur SG, Moss T JM, Ikegami M, et al. IL-1 mediates endotoxin induced lung maturation in preterm lambs. Proc Am Thorac Soc 2005:A275.

56. Harding JE, Pang J, Knight DB, Liggins GC. Do antenatal corticosteroids help in the setting of preterm rupture of membranes? Am J Obstet Gynecol 2001; 184:131–139.

57. Elimian A, Verma U, Beneck D, et al. Histologic chorioamnionitis, antenatal steroids, and perinatal outcomes. Obstet Gynecol 2000; 96:333–336.

58. Newnham J, Kallapur SG, Kramer BW, et al. Betamethasone effects on chorioamnionitis induced by intra-amniotic endotoxin in sheep. Am J Obstet Gynecol 2003; 189:1458–1466.

59. Newnham JP, Moss TJ, Padbury JF, et al. The interactive effects of endotoxin with prenatal glucocorticoids on short-term lung function in sheep. Am J Ob Gyn 2001; 185:190–197.

60. Ikegami M, Polk D, Jobe A. Minimum interval from fetal betamethasone treatment to postnatal lung responses in preterm lambs. Am J Obstet Gynecol 1996; 174:1408–1413.

61. Kramer BW, Ikegami M, Moss T JM, et al. Endotoxin induced chorioamnionitis modulates innate immunity of monocytes in preterm sheep. Am J Respir Crit Care Med 2004; 171:73–77.

62. Kramer BW, Ikegami M, Moss TJ, et al. Antenatal betamethasone changes cord blood monocyte responses to endotoxin in preterm lambs. Pediatr Res 2004; 55:764–768.

63. Hodgman JE. Relationship between Wilson-Mikity syndrome and the new bronchopulmonary dysplasia. Pediatrics 2003; 112:1414–1415.

64. Kallapur SG, Nitsos I, Moss T JM, et al. Chronic endotoxin exposure does not cause sustained structural abnormalities in the fetal sheep lungs. Am J Physiol Lung Cell Mol Physiol 2005; 288:L966–L974.

65. Jobe AH. The New BPD: an arrest of lung development. Pediatr Res 1999; 46:641–643.

66. Wada K, Jobe AH, Ikegami M. Tidal volume effects on surfactant treatment responses with the initiation of ventilation in preterm lambs. J Appl Physiol 1997; 83:1054–1061.

67. Naik AS, Kallapur SG, Bachurski CJ, et al. Effects of ventilation with different positive end-expiratory pressures on cytokine expression in the preterm lamb lung. Am J Respir Crit Care Med 2001; 164:494–498.

68. Ikegami M, Jobe A. Postnatal lung inflammation increased by ventilation of preterm lambs exposed antenatally to E. coli endotoxin. Pediatr Res 2002; 52:356–362.

69. Gomez R, Romero R, Ghezzi F, et al. The fetal inflammatory response syndrome. Am J Obstet Gynecol 1998; 179:194–202.

70. Kramer BW, Ikegami M, Jobe A. Intratracheal endotoxin causes systemic inflammation in ventilated preterm lambs. Am J Respir Crit Care Med 2002; 165:463–469.

71. Kramer BW, Ikegami M, Moss TJ, et al. Endotoxin-induced chorioamnionitis modulates innate immunity of monocytes in preterm sheep. Am J Respir Crit Care Med 2005; 171:73–77.

Chapter 7

Lung Fluid Balance During Development and in Neonatal Lung Disease

Richard D. Bland MD • David P. Carlton MD • Lucky Jain MD MBA

Secretion of Fetal Lung Liquid and its Contribution to Lung Growth

Composition and Dynamics of Fetal Lung Liquid

Decrease of Lung Liquid Before Birth: Effects of Labor

Hormonal Effects on Production and Absorption of Fetal Lung Liquid

Mechanism of Lung Liquid Clearance at Birth: Increased Epithelial Cell Na Transport

Postnatal Clearance of Fetal Lung Liquid

Pathways for Removal of Fetal Lung Liquid

Epilogue on Lung Fluid Balance During Development

Persistent Postnatal Pulmonary Edema

Pulmonary Edema in Neonatal Respiratory Distress Syndromes

Epilogue on Pulmonary Edema After Premature Birth

Curious students of mammalian development recognized more than a century ago that the lungs are filled with liquid during fetal life (1), but the origin of that liquid remained obscure until 1948 when an unexpected discovery by two French scientists dispelled the prevailing view that fetal lung liquid derived from intrauterine inhalation of amniotic fluid. In studies designed to explore the ontogeny of the pituitary-adrenal axis, tracheal ligation of fetal rabbits for 9 days resulted in fluid distension of the lungs (2). This serendipitous finding, subsequently confirmed and embellished by others (3–5), established that the fetal lung itself, rather than the amniotic sac, is the source of the liquid that fills the lung during development. This liquid forms a slowly expanding structural template that prevents collapse and promotes growth of the fetal lung.

Subsequent studies, conducted mostly with sheep, showed that liquid in the lumen of the fetal lung forms as a result of chloride secretion in the respiratory epithelium (6, 7), a process that can be inhibited by diuretics which block Na,K-2Cl co-transport (8, 9). In vitro experiments using cultured explants of lung tissue and monolayers of epithelial cells harvested from human fetal lung have indicated that cation-dependent chloride transport, driven by epithelial cell Na,K-ATPase, is the mechanism responsible for liquid secretion into the lumen of the mammalian lung during fetal life (10–12).

Rapid clearance of liquid from potential air spaces during and soon after birth is essential for establishing the timely switch from placental to pulmonary gas exchange. A sudden gush of fluid from the mouth often punctuates a baby's birth, signaling the start of extrauterine life. This observation helped to promulgate what has come to be known as the "vaginal squeeze," a notion that was introduced nearly half a century ago to explain how liquid might be expelled from the lungs as air breathing starts (13). Since then, however, numerous studies have established that the normal transition from liquid to air inflation is considerably more complex than the characteristic oral gush at delivery might suggest. This chapter will consider some of the experimental work that provides the basis for our current understanding of lung liquid dynamics before, during and after birth, focusing on the various pathways and mechanisms by which this process occurs. For further enlightenment on this important aspect of perinatal adaptation, the reader is referred to a recent comprehensive review (14). The chapter also includes a section describing neonatal respiratory disorders that are associated with abnormal lung fluid balance, conditions that typically develop following premature birth.

SECRETION OF FETAL LUNG LIQUID AND ITS CONTRIBUTION TO LUNG GROWTH

During fetal development, the lung is a secretory organ that exhibits breathing-like movements without contributing to respiratory gas exchange, which is exclusively a placental function in the mammalian fetus. In utero the lungs are filled with liquid and receive less than 10% of the combined ventricular output of blood from the heart (15). In fetal sheep, this scant blood supply is sufficient to deliver to the lung epithelium the substrate needed to make surfactant and secrete up to half a liter of liquid into the lung lumen each day during the last third of gestation (16, 17). Studies performed with cultured explants of human fetal lung indicate that liquid production by the bronchopulmonary epithelium may occur as early as the sixth week of gestation, with resultant expansion of the lung lumen (11). Several studies have shown that the presence of an appropriate volume of secreted liquid within the fetal respiratory tract is essential for normal lung growth and development before birth (3–5). Conditions that interfere with normal production of fetal lung liquid, such as pulmonary artery occlusion (18), diaphragmatic hernia with displacement of abdominal contents into the chest (19), and uterine compression of the fetal thorax from chronic leak of amniotic fluid (20), also inhibit lung growth.

Figure 7-1 is a diagram depicting the fluid compartments of the fetal lung. Potential air spaces are filled with liquid that is rich in Cl (~ 150 mEq/L) and almost free of protein (< 0.03 mg/mL) (21). Studies of water and solute exchange across the pulmonary epithelium and endothelium of fetal sheep, reported by Strang and associates (22–24), showed that the lung epithelium has tight intercellular junctions that provide an effective barrier to macromolecules, including albumin, whereas the vascular endothelium has wider openings that allow passage of large plasma proteins, including globulins and fibrinogen. Consequently, liquid in the interstitial space, which is sampled in fetal sheep by collecting lung lymph, has a protein concentration that is about 100-times greater than the protein concentration of liquid contained in the lung lumen (25). Despite the large trans-epithelial difference in protein osmotic pressure, which tends to inhibit liquid flow out of the interstitium into potential air spaces, active transport of Cl ions across the fetal lung epithelium generates an electrical potential difference that averages about −5 mV, luminal side negative (7). The osmotic force created by this secretory process drives liquid from the pulmonary microcirculation through the interstitium into potential air spaces.

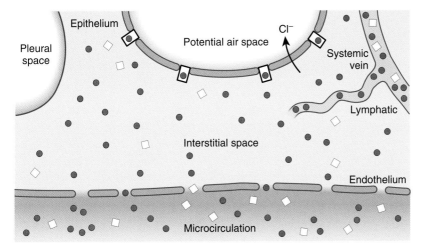

Figure 7-1 Schematic diagram of the fluid compartments in the fetal lung, showing the tight epithelial barrier to protein and the more permeable vascular endothelium, which restricts passage of globulins (open squares) more than it restricts albumin (solid circles). In the fetal mammalian lung, chloride secretion in the respiratory epithelium is responsible for liquid production within potential air spaces. From Bland (159).

Lung epithelial Cl transport, which in fetal sheep begins as early as mid-gestation (26), is inhibited by diuretics that block Na,K-2Cl co-transport (8, 9). Studies of liquid secretion in cultured lung explants harvested from late-gestation fetal mice showed that water content was less in lungs of Na,K-2Cl-null fetuses compared to wild-type fetuses, leading the authors to conclude that Na,K-2Cl-dependent Cl secretion plays an important role in fetal lung liquid production during development (27). These findings support the concept that the driving force for trans-epithelial Cl movement in the fetal lung is similar to the mechanism described for Cl transport across other epithelia. Accordingly, Cl enters the epithelial cell across its basal membrane linked to Na and to K (Fig. 7-2). Na enters the cell down its electrochemical gradient and is subsequently extruded in exchange for K (three Na ions exchanged for two K ions) by the action of Na,K-ATPase located on the basolateral surface of the cell. This energy-dependent process increases the concentration of Cl within the cell so that it exceeds its electrochemical equilibrium. Cl then passively exits the epithelial cell through anion-selective channels, including the cystic fibrosis transmembrane regulator (CFTR) and other chloride channels (CLC) that are located on the apical membrane of the cell. Na also can traverse the epithelium via paracellular pathways, while water can flow either between epithelial cells or through water channels, one of which (aquaporin 5) is abundantly expressed in type I lung epithelial cells (28). Type I cells are highly permeable to water and are well equipped to facilitate liquid removal from the lung lumen (29). The recent observation that type I lung epithelial cells contain detectable CFTR mRNA and protein, and exhibit functional evidence of CFTR channel activity, as assessed by patch-clamp technique, suggests that these cells may contribute to Cl secretion in the fetal lung, just as type II cells do (30).

COMPOSITION AND DYNAMICS OF FETAL LUNG LIQUID

While the Cl concentration of liquid withdrawn from the lung lumen of fetal sheep is about 50% greater than that of plasma (Table 7-1), the Na concentration is virtually identical to that of plasma (6, 21). The concentration of bicarbonate in lung liquid of fetal sheep is < 3 mEq/L, yielding a pH of ~6.3. This finding led to the notion that the lung epithelium of fetal sheep may actively transport

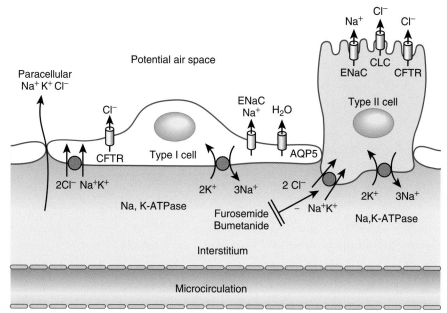

Figure 7-2 Schematic drawing of the fluid compartments of the fetal lung, highlighting the lung epithelium, made up of type I cells that occupy most of the surface area of the lung lumen, and type II cells, which manufacture and secrete surfactant. These cells also secrete Cl by a process that involves Na,K-2Cl co-transport and Na,K-ATPase (Na pump) activity. This energy-dependent process, which can be blocked by loop diuretics, furosemide and bumetanide, increases the concentration of Cl within the cell so that it exceeds its electrochemical equilibrium, with resultant extrusion of Cl through anion-selective channels (cystic fibrosis transmembrane conductance regulator, CFTR; and volume- and voltage-gated chloride channels, CLC) on the apical membrane surface. Sodium (Na) and water follow the movement of Cl into the lung lumen through Na channels (ENaC) and aquaporins (AQP5), respectively, or through paracellular openings.

bicarbonate out of the lung lumen (31). The demonstration that acetazolamide, a carbonic anhydrase inhibitor, blocks secretion of lung liquid in fetal sheep supports this view. Both physiologic and immunohistochemical studies have shown that H^{+}-ATPases are present on the respiratory epithelium of fetal sheep, where they probably provide an important mechanism for acidification of liquid within the lung lumen during development. In vitro electrophysiological studies using fetal rat lung epithelial cells provided evidence that exposure to an acid pH might activate Cl channels and thereby contribute to the production of fetal lung liquid (32). Recent studies have described the transcriptional regulation of this pH-activated Cl channel, ClC-2, which is highly expressed in fetal distal lung epithelial cells and suppressed (33, 34), coincident with the increased alveolar liquid pH (6.99 ± 0.04) measured in newborn lambs (35). In fetal dogs and monkeys, however, the

Table 7–1 Composition of Lung Luminal Liquid, Lymph, Plasma, and Amniotic Liquid of Fetal Lambs Late in Gestation

	Sodium (mEq/L)	Potassium (mEq/L)	Chloride (mEq/L)	Bicarbonate (mEq/L)	pH	Total protein (g/dL)
Luminal liquid	150 ± 1	6.3 ± 0.7	157 ± 4	2.8 ± 0.3	6.27 ± 0.01	0.03 ± 0.002
Lung lymph	147 ± 1	4.8 ± 0.5	107 ± 1	25 ± 1	7.31 ± 0.02	3.27 ± 0.41
Plasma	150 ± 1	4.8 ± 0.2	107 ± 1	24 ± 1	7.34 ± 0.04	4.09 ± 0.26
Amniotic liquid	113 ± 7	7.6 ± 0.8	87 ± 5	19 ± 3	7.02 ± 0.09	0.10 ± 0.01

Values are mean ± SEM and are taken from the work of Adamson et al. (21) and Humphreys et al. (109).

bicarbonate concentration of lung luminal liquid is not significantly different from that of fetal plasma (36). Thus, the importance of lung liquid pH and acidification mechanisms during mammalian lung development in utero remains unclear.

The concentration of K in fetal lung liquid exceeds that of plasma and increases further at the end of gestation as lung epithelial cells release surfactant into potential air spaces (17). Studies done with fetal goats showed that mechanical stretch of the lung caused a decrease in secretion and sometimes led to absorption of luminal liquid, with associated fluxes of Na and Cl in the direction of the interstitium and K toward the lung lumen (37). Direct micro-puncture measurements of Cl concentration in the alveolar lining liquid of lambs before and after birth showed that the large Cl gradient between lung luminal liquid and plasma decreases rapidly with the onset of air breathing (35). This change was accompanied by a 3-fold increase in the calcium concentration of alveolar liquid (38). Studies performed with fetal sheep before and during labor showed that the Cl concentration of lung liquid often decreases during labor, while the K concentration increases as liquid is absorbed from the lungs during labor (39). Increased K flux into the lung lumen might be linked to the increase in lung epithelial cell Na,K-ATPase that occurs in labor (40), as discussed below.

The volume of liquid within the lung lumen of fetal sheep increases from 4 to 6 mL/kg at mid-gestation (26) to between 20 and 30 mL/kg near term (23, 25). The hourly flow rate of lung liquid increases from about 2 mL/kg body weight at mid-gestation (26) to about 5 mL/kg body weight at term (16, 17, 41). Increased production of luminal liquid during development reflects a rapidly expanding pulmonary microvascular and epithelial surface area that occurs with proliferation and growth of lung capillaries and respiratory units (26, 42).

The observation that unilateral pulmonary artery occlusion decreases lung liquid production in fetal sheep by at least 50% (43) shows that the pulmonary circulation, rather than the bronchial circulation, is the major source of fetal lung liquid. Intravenous infusion of isotonic saline at a rate sufficient to increase lung microvascular pressure and lung lymph flow in fetal lambs had no effect on liquid flow across the pulmonary epithelium (44). Thus, trans-epithelial Cl secretion appears to be the major driving force responsible for the production of liquid in the fetal lung lumen. In vitro studies of epithelial ion transport across the fetal airways indicate that the epithelium of the upper respiratory tract also secretes Cl, thereby contributing to lung liquid production (45–47). However, most of this liquid forms in the distal portions of the fetal lung, where total surface area is many times greater than it is in the conducting airways.

DECREASE OF LUNG LIQUID BEFORE BIRTH: EFFECTS OF LABOR

Several studies have demonstrated that both the rate of lung liquid production and the volume of liquid within the lumen of the fetal lung normally decrease before birth, most notably during labor (25, 39, 41, 48, 49). Thus, lung water content is about 25% greater after premature delivery than it is at term, and newborn animals that are delivered by caesarean section without prior labor have considerably more liquid in their lungs than do animals that are delivered either vaginally or operatively after the onset of labor (50, 51). In studies done with fetal sheep, extravascular lung water was 45% less in mature fetuses that were in the midst of labor than in fetuses that did not experience labor, and there was a further 38% decrease in extravascular lung water measured in term lambs that were studied 6 h after a normal vaginal birth (25).

No Labor   Labor

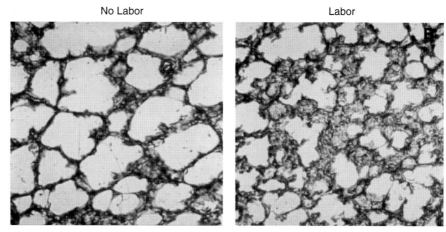

Figure 7-3 Sections of lung obtained from a lamb killed without labor (left) and another lamb killed during labor (right). By a point-counting technique we found that the volume of potential air space relative to the volume of interstitial tissue was significantly greater in lambs killed without labor (2.29 ± 0.12) than it was in lambs killed during labor (0.99 ± 0.25). Magnification $\times 125$ From Bland et al. (25).

Morphometric analysis of sections of frozen lung taken from fetal lambs with and without prior labor showed that the decrease in lung water content that occurs before birth is the result of a decrease in the liquid volume of potential air spaces relative to interstitial tissue volume (Fig. 7-3). These studies showed that reduced secretion, and perhaps absorption, of luminal liquid before birth decreases lung water by about 15 mL/kg body weight, leaving a residual volume of about 6 mL/kg (25) which must be cleared from potential air spaces soon after birth to allow effective pulmonary gas exchange. Subsequent studies performed with late-gestation fetal guinea pigs showed that labor induced by maternal injection of oxytocin yielded changes in lung liquid absorption similar to those observed after spontaneous onset of labor (52).

HORMONAL EFFECTS ON PRODUCTION AND ABSORPTION OF FETAL LUNG LIQUID

Hormonal changes that occur in the fetus just before and during labor may play an important role in reducing secretion of lung liquid and promoting its absorption during labor and after birth. A major focus of research in this area has been on catecholamines, in particular the β-adrenergic effects of epinephrine, in decreasing lung liquid formation in fetal animals. Studies done with fetal sheep late in gestation showed that intravenous infusion of epinephrine or isoproterenol, but not norepinephrine, caused reabsorption of liquid from the lung lumen, an effect that β-adrenergic blockade with propranolol prevented (53). A subsequent report showed that intraluminal administration of amiloride, a Na-transport inhibitor, blocked the effect of epinephrine on absorption of lung liquid (54). This finding indicates that β-adrenergic agonists stimulate Na uptake by the lung epithelium, which drives liquid from the lung lumen into the interstitium, where it can be absorbed into the pulmonary circulation or transported via lung lymphatics to the systemic venous system.

Tracheal instillation of dibutyryl cAMP (db-cAMP) also induces lung liquid absorption in fetal sheep late in gestation (55). The inhibitory effects of both db-cAMP and epinephrine on net production of lung luminal liquid in fetal sheep increase with advancing gestational age, and both responses are attenuated by prior resection of the thyroid gland (56). Replacement therapy with triiodothyronine after thyroidectomy restored the inhibitory effect of epinephrine on lung liquid production in fetal sheep (57). Treatment of preterm fetal sheep with the combination of triiodothyronine and hydrocortisone may stimulate early maturation of epinephrine-induced absorption of lung liquid (58). Another study showed a synergistic effect of terbutaline, a β-adrenergic agonist, and aminophylline, a phosphodiesterase inhibitor, in switching lung liquid secretion to absorption in fetal lambs (59). In these studies, addition of amiloride to the lung liquid prevented its absorption. Likewise, in studies conducted with fetal lambs in spontaneous labor, intrapulmonary delivery of amiloride either slowed or reversed lung liquid absorption (39, 48). These observations are consistent with the view that birth-related events associated with release of cAMP in the lung may stimulate active transport of Na across the epithelium, which causes liquid to be absorbed from the lung lumen into the interstitium.

Studies performed on animals during labor, either spontaneous or induced by oxytocin, have demonstrated an association between increased plasma concentrations of epinephrine and reduced production or absorption of lung liquid during labor (48, 52, 60). The concentration of β-adrenergic receptors in lung tissue increases late in gestation (61, 62), which might render the lungs particularly responsive to the effects of epinephrine during labor. At least two reports have indicated, however, that absorption of lung liquid near birth may not depend on epinephrine. One study showed that irreversible blockade of β-adrenergic receptors in fetal rabbits did not prevent the normal reduction in lung water that occurs during parturition (63). Another study reported that inhibition of β-adrenergic activity with propranolol did not prevent lung liquid absorption in fetal lambs late in labor (39).

A number of other hormones have been shown to inhibit net production of fetal lung liquid. Several studies have indicated that intravenous infusion of arginine vasopressin can reduce liquid formation in the fetal lung, and that this effect can be inhibited by the Na-transport blocker amiloride (64, 65). It is noteworthy, however, that the dose of vasopressin needed to cause lung liquid absorption in these studies yielded plasma concentrations of the hormone that far exceeded those usually detected during labor (66). Nevertheless, there is evidence that release of both epinephrine and vasopressin at birth may be additive in stimulating absorption of lung liquid (67). Studies performed with excised lungs of fetal guinea pigs have shown that epinephrine, cAMP, cortisol and aldosterone each can cause an abrupt decrease in fetal lung liquid formation (68–70). Further studies using a similar experimental model provided evidence that the stimulatory effect of epinephrine on lung liquid clearance is linked to increased postnatal pulmonary expression of amiloride-sensitive sodium channels, which is mediated, at least in part, by a perinatal increase in plasma cortisol concentrations (71). Taken together, these findings indicate that the interaction of multiple hormones of adrenal origin plays a key regulatory role in converting the respiratory epithelium from a predominantly Cl-secreting membrane during fetal development to a predominantly Na-absorbing membrane after birth.

MECHANISM OF LUNG LIQUID CLEARANCE AT BIRTH: INCREASED EPITHELIAL CELL Na TRANSPORT

A broad array of physiological, biochemical and molecular studies conducted over the past 25 years have demonstrated that active Na transport across the respiratory epithelium provides the driving force for lung liquid clearance at birth, as described in several comprehensive reviews (72–76). In vitro electrophysiological studies of cultured alveolar epithelial cells harvested from fetal and adult rats showed that the same cells which secrete surfactant into the air spaces also can pump Na in the opposite direction, thus generating the driving force for absorption of liquid from the lung lumen (77–83). These studies demonstrated that monolayers of cultured distal lung epithelial cells (type II cells), when mounted in an Ussing-type chamber, maintain a trans-epithelial electrical potential difference (luminal side negative) that increases in response to β-adrenergic stimulation and decreases in response to the Na transport inhibitors amiloride and ouabain. Amiloride blocks Na transport pathways on the luminal surface of the epithelium, and ouabain blocks Na,K-ATPase activity on the basolateral surface of the epithelium (Fig. 7-4). Several reports have documented the presence and activity of amiloride-sensitive cation channels in cultured distal lung epithelial cells harvested from fetal rats (84–86). The selectivity of these cation channels for Na appears to vary according to the culture conditions in which the cells are studied, notably the impact on Na specificity induced by exposure to glucocorticoids and air (87).

More than 95% of the surface area of the adult lung is lined by type I alveolar epithelial cells. Recent studies showed that these expansive cells have abundant Na channels (ENaC) and Na,K-ATPase, and that they too can transport Na by a process that is inhibited by both amiloride and ouabain (30, 88–90). Thus, both type I and type II cells are equipped to play a key role in clearing liquid from the lung lumen during and after birth.

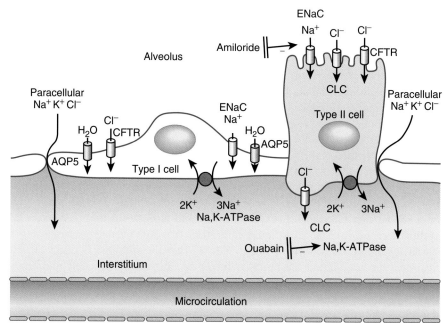

Figure 7-4 Epithelial sodium absorption in the fetal lung near birth. Na enters the cell through the apical surface of both type I and type II lung epithelial cells via amiloride-inhibitable epithelial Na channels (ENaC). Electroneutrality is conserved with chloride movement through anion-selective channels, namely the cystic fibrosis transmembrane conductance regulator (CFTR) or volume- and voltage-gated chloride channels (CLC) in type I and type II lung epithelial cells. Chloride transport also may occur through tight junctions between epithelial cells. The increase in cell Na stimulates Na,K-ATPase activity on the basolateral aspect of the cell membrane, which drives out three Na ions in exchange for two K ions, a process that can be blocked by the cardiac glycoside ouabain. Both type I and type II lung epithelial cells are equipped with the necessary machinery, apical Na channels and basolateral Na pumps, to participate in Na transport and related liquid absorption. Net ion movement from the luminal to the interstitial side of the epithelium creates an osmotic gradient that drives water transport, either via aquaporins (AQP5 is expressed in type I cells) or by diffusion, in the same direction, thereby removing liquid from potential air spaces into the interstitium, where the liquid drains via the pulmonary circulation or lung lymphatics.

Na,K-ATPase activity in distal lung epithelial cells increases around the time of birth (40, 91, 92). Studies done with freshly isolated distal lung epithelial cells from fetal, newborn and adult rabbits showed that Na pump turnover number, an index of Na,K-ATPase enzyme activity, increased 4-fold during labor, followed by a 3-fold increase in the number of Na pumps/cell between newborn and adult stages of lung development (40, 91). Na,K-ATPase activity was not significantly different in newborn and adult lung epithelial cells. Thus, Na pump activity in distal lung epithelium of rabbits increases at birth, and the number of Na pumps/cell increases postnatally. In related studies, Na pump activity was similar in cells harvested from fetal rabbits and from newborn rabbits that had respiratory distress after premature birth (40). These findings suggest that the stress of premature birth and subsequent respiratory distress fails to increase lung epithelial cell Na absorption, an observation that may help to explain the pulmonary edema that is associated with respiratory distress after premature birth (93).

Other studies have shown that mRNA expression of the α_1 and β_1 subunits of Na,K-ATPase in fetal rat lungs increases just before birth (92, 94). These changes are associated with parallel increases in the expression of epithelial Na and water channels in perinatal rat lung (95, 96). There is now considerable evidence that glucocorticoids may up-regulate expression of Na,K-ATPase, epithelial Na channels (ENaC) and aquaporins in the developing rat lung (97–99). Glucocorticoids also were shown to upregulate expression of the α-, β- and γ-subunits of ENaC in explants of human fetal lung (100).

A number of reports also indicate that the increased oxygen tension that occurs around the time of birth (air breathing) may have an important role in signaling the switch from Cl secretion to Na absorption in the lung epithelium near birth (101–104). Two recent studies suggest that exposure to the combination of postnatal oxygen (21%) and glucocorticoids increases Na transport in fetal rat lung epithelial cells, which in turn can drive liquid absorption from the lung lumen into the interstitium, with subsequent drainage via the pulmonary circulation and lymphatics (105, 106).

The observation that early postnatal death from respiratory failure occurs in the absence of functional epithelial Na channels (107) clearly defines the pivotal role of epithelial Na absorption in clearing liquid from potential air spaces and facilitating pulmonary gas exchange at birth. Studies showing that inactivation of the α-subunit of ENaC causes early death in newborn mice provided the first direct in vivo evidence that ENaC is the crucial element in enabling Na absorption in lung epithelial cells, which is an essential step in neonatal adaptation to air breathing. In a related series of studies, lung liquid clearance was slower in newborn mice lacking the γ-subunit of ENaC (108). Lung water content 12 h after birth in these γENaC-null pups, however, was similar to lung water content of control littermates that were γENaC +/+. Newborn mice lacking the γ-subunit of ENaC died as a result of hyperkalemia from renal dysfunction rather than from pulmonary edema.

POSTNATAL CLEARANCE OF FETAL LUNG LIQUID

There are two components of the process by which luminal liquid drains from the lungs during and after birth: transepithelial flow of liquid into the interstitium, as described above, followed by flow of liquid into the bloodstream, either directly into the pulmonary circulation or through lymphatics that empty into the systemic venous system. Development of effective respiratory gas exchange and lung volume soon after birth suggest that the shift of liquid from air spaces into the lung interstitium occurs rapidly, after which there is slower uptake of liquid into the lung vasculature or lymphatics (25, 109). In sheep, liquid absorption from the lung lumen often begins during labor and accelerates immediately after birth (39, 48).

Studies conducted with fetal sheep during and after parturition have demonstrated a decrease in net Cl secretion and a corresponding increase in Na uptake by the respiratory epithelium (35, 39). The fact that Na transport inhibitors reverse lung liquid absorption in fetal sheep during labor and slow the rate of lung liquid clearance in newborn guinea pigs (110, 111) underscores the importance of this change in epithelial Na uptake in hastening liquid removal from the lung lumen near birth.

Studies done with fetal lambs at the start of breathing showed a transient postnatal increase in hydraulic conductivity and small solute permeability of the lung epithelium, which may contribute to increased bulk flow of liquid from potential air spaces into the interstitium (112). Lung inflation with air also reduces hydraulic pressure in the pulmonary interstitium, which may help to drain liquid out of the lung lumen into the interstitial space (113, 114). As plasma protein concentration increases during the few days before birth (25, 51), the resultant increase in plasma protein osmotic pressure also helps to draw liquid from the lung interstitium into the circulation.

Liquid removal from the lungs continues for several hours after birth. Studies done with fetal and newborn rabbits showed that lung blood volume increases with the onset of breathing, whereas lung water content does not begin to decrease postnatally until 30–60 min after birth (115). When breathing starts, air inflation shifts residual liquid from the lung lumen into distensible perivascular spaces around large pulmonary blood vessels and airways (Fig. 7-5). Accumulation of liquid in these connective tissue spaces, which are distant from sites of respiratory gas exchange, allows time for small blood vessels and lymphatics to remove the displaced liquid with little or no adverse effect on lung function. In rabbits born at term gestation, perivascular cuffs of fluid are of maximal size 30 min after birth, at

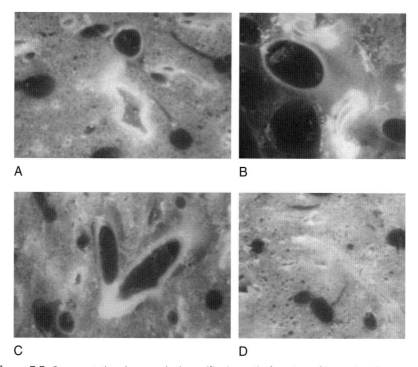

A   B

C   D

Figure 7-5 Representative photographs (magnification ×8) of sections of lung taken from vaginally delivered rabbits that were killed before breathing (A), 30 min after birth (B), 1 h after birth (C), and 6 h after birth (D). Before birth, airways are filled with fluid and there are small cuffs of fluid surrounding pulmonary arteries. By 30 min of age, perivascular and peribronchial cuffs are large, and airways appear compressed in the absence of distending pressure. At 60 min of age, fluid cuffs are smaller, and several hours later they are virtually absent. From Bland et al. (115).

which time they contain up to 75% of the total amount of extravascular water in the lungs. The fluid cuffs normally disappear by about 6 h after birth.

The perinatal pattern of lung liquid clearance is similar in sheep (25). As net production of lung liquid decreases before birth, the volume of liquid within the lung lumen also decreases, with a corresponding reduction in the caliber of potential air spaces. After breathing begins, residual liquid shifts into the interstitium and collects around large blood vessels and airways. Perivascular fluid cuffs progressively decrease in size as aeration of terminal respiratory units improves postnatally. Clearance of fetal lung liquid in sheep is complete by about 6 h after normal vaginal delivery. The process is slower in preterm lambs (93, 116), as it is in preterm rabbits (51).

Studies conducted with human neonates likewise have shown that immaturity of Na transport mechanisms may contribute to impaired clearance of fetal lung liquid, which is manifest as transient neonatal tachypnea (TNT) or respiratory distress syndrome (RDS). One study showed that human infants with TNT had evidence of reduced Na transport in their respiratory epithelium, as assessed by the reduction in electrical potential difference (PD) across the nasal epithelium induced by amiloride (117). Nasal PD (PD = Resistance × Current) is a reliable measure of net electrogenic transport of Na and Cl across the respiratory epithelium, and has been shown to mirror-image ion transport occurring in the lower respiratory tract. Nasal PD was reduced in infants with TNT, suggesting a defect in Na transport, and recovery from TNT was associated with an increase in PD to normal values. Subsequent studies performed on premature infants with RDS showed that maximal nasal PD was reduced compared to measurements made in infants without RDS (118). When the Na transport inhibitor amiloride was applied to the nasal mucosa of premature newborns with RDS on day 1, the change in PD was less than it was in infants without RDS. Nasal PD, both in the presence and absence of amiloride, became normal with resolution of RDS, suggesting that impaired respiratory Na transport may be an important feature of the lung dysfunction that prevails in premature infants with RDS, in whom pulmonary edema is a major pathological finding.

Developmental changes in transepithelial ion and fluid movement in the lung thus can be viewed as occurring in three distinct stages (76). In the *first* (fetal) stage, the lung epithelium is in a secretory mode, exhibiting active Cl secretion via Cl channels, with relatively little reabsorption activity of Na channels. Why the Na channels remain inactive through much of fetal life is unclear. The *second* (transitional) stage involves a reversal in the direction of ion and water movement. Many factors may be involved in this transition, including exposure of epithelial cells to an air–liquid interface and to high concentrations of steroids and cyclic nucleotides. This stage involves not only increased expression of Na channels in the lung epithelia, but possibly a switch from nonselective cation channels to highly selective Na channels. The net increase in Na movement into the cell can cause a change in resting membrane potential that leads to a slowing, and eventually reversal, of the direction of Cl movement through Cl channels. This stage is accompanied by an increase in Na,K-ATPase activity in the lung epithelium, which drives Na absorption and associated liquid movement out of the lung lumen. The *third* and final (postnatal) stage represents lung epithelia with predominantly Na reabsorption through Na channels, and possibly Cl reabsorption through Cl channels, with a fine balance between the activity of ion channels and tight junctions that serve to maintain a thin layer of liquid over the epithelium during postnatal life. Such an arrangement not only helps to ensure adequate wetting of the alveolar surface during air breathing, but its response to various chemical and mechanical stimuli at times of stress can protect the alveolus from flooding in the face of adverse events, such as heart failure or lung injury.

PATHWAYS FOR REMOVAL OF FETAL LUNG LIQUID

Potential routes for drainage of lung liquid at birth include lung lymphatics, the pulmonary circulation, the pleural space, the mediastinum and the upper airway. Studies done with chronically catheterized fetal and newborn lambs showed that the postnatal increase in lung lymph flow is modest and transient, accounting for no more than 15% of the amount of residual liquid that drains from the lung post-natally (25). In these studies, the concentration of protein in lung lymph decreased with the start of ventilation, presumably the result of protein-poor liquid flowing from within the lung lumen into the interstitium. With subsequent uptake of this liquid into the bloodstream, the concentration of protein in lymph returned to its baseline level. These studies showed that lung lymphatics normally drain only a small fraction of liquid in potential air spaces. In preterm lambs with respiratory distress, the postnatal increase in lung lymph flow lasted for several hours and was accompanied by a substantial increase in protein clearance, indicative of increased lung vascular permeability to protein (93).

Other studies from the same laboratory showed that either elevated left atrial pressure or reduced plasma protein concentration slows the rate of liquid clearance from the lungs of healthy, mature lambs (119, 120). These findings support the view that the pulmonary circulation absorbs at least some, and perhaps most, of the residual liquid that drains from the lungs after birth. It is also possible that some liquid enters the bloodstream through the mediastinum and pleural cavity, although other studies indicate that in normal lambs very little luminal liquid drains via the pleural space.

For many years it was thought that much of the liquid contained in the lungs at birth was extruded via the upper airway as a result of the "vaginal squeeze." This concept derived from measurements of intrathoracic pressure that were made during delivery of normal term infants, which led to the inference that chest compression associated with vaginal delivery drives liquid from the lungs into the oropharynx (13). Other studies, however, indicate that increased thoracic pressure during spontaneous birth may have little effect on clearance of fetal lung liquid. Animals that are delivered by caesarean section during labor after tracheal ligation have no more water in their lungs than do animals that are born vaginally (25, 50). Moreover, studies of lung fluid dynamics in near-term fetal sheep showed that late in labor, as luminal liquid is absorbed across the epithelium, little or no liquid could be withdrawn from the trachea (39, 48). Thus, although the conducting airways may serve as an escape route for lung liquid during delivery without prior labor, they probably play a lesser role in clearing liquid from the lungs during the normal birth process.

EPILOGUE ON LUNG FLUID BALANCE DURING DEVELOPMENT

Figure 7-6 is a schematic drawing of the liquid compartments in the fetal lung and the forces that contribute to liquid clearance. Liquid within the lung lumen contains < 0.3 mg of protein/mL, whereas pulmonary interstitial liquid has a protein concentration of ~ 30 mg/mL. This transepithelial difference in protein concentration generates an osmotic pressure difference of > 10 cmH$_2$O, which draws liquid from the lung lumen into the interstitium, as Cl secretion decreases. Increased activity of lung epithelial Na,K-ATPase during labor provides the main driving force for liquid absorption into the lung interstitium. Transpulmonary pressure associated with lung inflation also contributes to bulk flow of liquid from the lung lumen into the interstitium. Together, these forces increase the protein osmotic

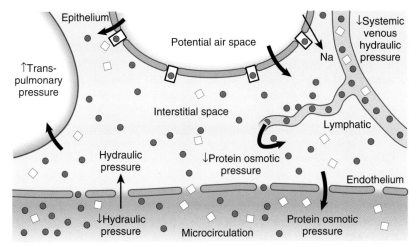

Figure 7-6 Schematic diagram of the fluid compartments in the fetal lung showing the forces that affect liquid removal near birth. Lung epithelial Na absorption, coupled with increased transpulmonary pressure associated with air inflation, drives liquid into the interstitial space. As hydraulic pressure in the microcirculation decreases with air breathing, plasma protein osmotic pressure draws the protein-poor luminal liquid from the interstitial space into the bloodstream. Some liquid also drains from the lung via lymphatics into the systemic venous system. Solid circles represent albumin molecules, open squares represent globulin molecules. From Bland (159).

pressure difference between plasma and interstitial fluid. Air entry into the lungs not only displaces liquid, but also decreases hydraulic pressure in the pulmonary circulation and increases pulmonary blood flow, which in turn increases lung blood volume and effective vascular surface area for fluid uptake. These circulatory changes facilitate absorption of liquid into the lung vascular bed. About 10–15% of the luminal liquid drains from the lungs via lymphatics into the systemic venous system. With spontaneous breathing, the postnatal reduction of intrathoracic pressure decreases systemic venous pressure, which may augment lymphatic drainage, but most of the displaced luminal liquid enters the pulmonary microcirculation or seeps into the mediastinum, with subsequent drainage into the systemic circulation.

PERSISTENT POSTNATAL PULMONARY EDEMA

Clearance of liquid from potential air spaces into the bloodstream, as described above, occurs quickly, usually within a few hours in most newborn infants. Sometimes the process is delayed, however, producing the clinical and radiographic features of a condition that has been called transient tachypnea of the newborn (TNT), or the syndrome of retained fetal lung liquid. As tachypnea is not a consistent finding in this condition, notably in situations associated with respiratory depression, and because some of the liquid may enter the lungs postnatally from the pulmonary circulation, a more appropriate term for this mild form of neonatal respiratory dysfunction is persistent postnatal pulmonary edema. Although this disorder was initially described in infants who were born at term gestation (121), only one of whom was delivered by caesarean section, subsequent reports have noted an association with operative delivery and with premature birth, especially in the absence of prior labor (122, 123).

Premature birth is associated with several conditions that may contribute to delayed removal of fetal lung liquid, including impaired Na-pump activity in lung epithelial cells (40), high filtration pressure in the pulmonary circulation (93), often with persistent patency of the ductus arteriosus (124), reduced microvascular surface area for fluid absorption (125), and a low plasma protein osmotic pressure (126).

Unless the lungs are immature, with resultant atelectasis and respiratory failure, absorption of fetal lung liquid usually is complete within 24 h of birth, and respiratory symptoms disappear accordingly. An increased concentration of inspired oxygen is sometimes needed to maintain a normal partial pressure of oxygen in arterial blood. Usually no other treatment is necessary. As the condition may be aggravated by exogenous fluid overload, fluid and salt intake of infants with persistent pulmonary edema should not exceed their insensible losses. Diuretics offer little or no benefit and may produce complicating abnormalities of serum electrolytes.

PULMONARY EDEMA IN NEONATAL RESPIRATORY DISTRESS SYNDROMES

Pulmonary edema is a consistent pathological feature of both acute and chronic respiratory distress syndromes that occur after premature birth. In acute respiratory distress syndrome (RDS), sometimes called hyaline membrane disease (HMD), the lungs typically are heavy and have a widened interstitium between air spaces and blood vessels, with fluid accumulation in dilated lung lymphatics and connective tissue spaces around large pulmonary blood vessels and airways, and abundant deposits of plasma proteins within the terminal respiratory units (127). These signs of abnormal vascular and epithelial permeability usually disappear as the respiratory distress resolves, either spontaneously or after treatment with surfactant and assisted ventilation. In some cases, however, the need for prolonged mechanical ventilation persists because of continuing respiratory failure, either from residual lung disease, chest wall instability, apnea or infection. Long-term exposure to repetitive lung inflation with positive pressure and supplemental oxygen often leads to chronic lung disease (CLD). This condition was first described by Northway et al. (128) as bronchopulmonary dysplasia (BPD), the pathology of which included lung edema, prominent pulmonary lymphatics, inflammation and subsequent fibrosis (129). The clinical, radiographic and pathological features of this condition have changed considerably in recent years because of major advances in perinatal care, including widespread use of antenatal glucocorticoid therapy, postnatal surfactant replacement and improved respiratory and nutritional support (130). Enhanced survival of extremely premature infants, many of whom require lengthy mechanical ventilation, has led to a persistently high incidence of CLD, in which pulmonary edema is a major pathological element (131, 132).

Factors Favoring Pulmonary Edema after Premature Birth

Several features of the immature lung make it especially vulnerable to postnatal edema (Table 7-2). Because the volume of liquid within the lumen of the fetal lung

Table 7–2	Features of the Immature Lung, Compared to the Mature Lung, Which Make it Vulnerable to Postnatal Edema

- Excess fetal lung liquid per unit lung mass
- Fewer sodium channels and less Na,K-ATPase activity in lung epithelium
- Greater lung vascular filtration pressure
- Increased lung epithelial protein leak associated with postnatal ventilation
- Increased lung vascular protein permeability

normally decreases late in gestation (41, 49, 93), premature birth is often associated with an excess amount of liquid in potential air spaces (51). Reduced numbers of sodium channels, sodium pumps and sodium pump activity on epithelial cells of the immature lung may retard normal clearance of this liquid, thereby contributing to postnatal respiratory distress (40, 91, 111). The burden of this excess retained fetal lung liquid, most of which must drain from the lungs via the pulmonary circulation, may be further complicated by persistent elevation of lung vascular filtration pressure that often prevails after premature birth (93).

Studies conducted with newborn lambs, some of which were delivered prematurely and others at term, have shown that hydraulic pressure in the pulmonary circulation is greater after premature birth than it is at term (Table 7-3) (93, 133–136). This increased fluid filtration pressure is at least partly the result of greater blood flow per kg body weight and per unit lung mass in the immature lung compared to the mature lung (Table 7-3). Greater hydraulic pressure in the pulmonary circulation, coupled with less plasma protein osmotic pressure and a lower interstitial hydraulic pressure (113), causes increased transvascular fluid filtration, detected as increased lung lymph flow, with a low lymph:plasma protein ratio and more extravascular lung water in the preterm lung compared to the term neonatal lung (Table 7-3).

These differences in fluid filtration forces are further accentuated by the presence of severe respiratory failure (93) associated with lung inflammation (137), and by excess pulmonary blood flow through a large patent ductus arteriosus (124), both of which frequently complicate the postnatal course of very premature infants. In the case of respiratory failure from inadequate surfactant in the air spaces, assisted ventilation with high inflation pressures and high concentrations of supplemental oxygen may contribute further to lung edema by increasing both lung vascular and epithelial protein leaks (93, 138–141).

These effects on protein permeability across the pulmonary endothelial-epithelial barrier may be attenuated by immediate postnatal treatment with surfactant (140, 142). Other studies have shown that antenatal glucocorticoid treatment may reduce lung vascular and epithelial protein leaks and reduce vulnerability to air leaks (143, 144). Prenatal glucocortoid therapy also has been shown to increase expression of lung epithelial cell Na channels (98, 100) and Na,K-ATPase in the developing lung (97), in addition to increasing epinephrine-induced absorption of lung liquid in fetal sheep (58), and birth-related absorption of lung liquid in perinatal guinea pigs (71). Thus, the combination of antenatal glucocorticoid treatment and surfactant replacement at birth may have important beneficial effects in hastening postnatal clearance of lung liquid and preventing postnatal protein leaks and fluid accumulation in the lungs after premature birth.

Pulmonary Edema from Increased Lung Protein Permeability in RDS

Animals that are born prematurely often die of respiratory failure from a condition that mimics the clinical, physiological and histological features observed in human infants with RDS (93, 145–147). Studies performed with chronically catheterized lambs that were delivered prematurely by caesarean section at ∼130 days gestation (term = 147 days) showed that respiratory failure developed in six of 10 lambs that were mechanically ventilated with 100% oxygen for 8 h after birth (93). These six lambs required peak inflation pressures that averaged > 50 cmH₂O between 4 and 8 h after birth. They had severe hypoxemia and pulmonary

Table 7–3   Variables Related to Fluid Balance in the Immature and Mature Newborn Lung

Gestation	VASCULAR PRESSURE (mmHg)		Lung interstitial pressure[†] (mmHg)	PROTEIN CONCENTRATION (g/dl)			Pulmonary blood flow ((ml/min) /kg)	Lung lymph flow ((ml/h) /kg)	Extravascular lung water (g/g dry lung)
	Pulmonary artery	Left atrium		Lymph	Plasma	L:P			
Preterm	36 ± 5	4 ± 2	2 ± 1	1.54 ± 0.24	3.22 ± 0.45	0.48 ± 0.02	381 ± 153	0.79 ± 0.29	4.8 ± 0.5
Term	20* ± 3	4* ± 1	6* ± 1	3.59* ± 0.40	5.80* ± 0.30	0.62* ± 0.05	314* ± 40	0.34* ± 0.10	4.3* ± 0.2

Data from references 17, 74, 84, 91, 92, 95.
Numbers are mean ± SD.
[†]Relative to pleural pressure at inflation pressure of 25 cmH₂O.
*Significant difference, term vs. preterm, $P < 0.05$.

hypertension, with a progressive increase in hematocrit and a reduction in plasma protein concentration secondary to generalized protein loss from the circulation. In contrast to earlier studies performed with more mature lambs (25), lung lymph flow and lymph protein flow remained high for the entire study. The postnatal tripling of lymph flow and lymph protein flow clearly showed that lung vascular permeability to protein increased in these preterm lambs with severe RDS (Fig. 7-7). Lung histology and postmortem measurement of extravascular lung water confirmed the presence of severe pulmonary edema (Fig. 7-8). In the four lambs that did not have RDS, lung lymph flow and protein clearance decreased to values that were at or below prenatal values, and postmortem measurements of extravascular lung water were significantly less than they were in lambs that had RDS. Thus, abnormal leakage of protein-rich liquid from the lung microcirculation into the interstitium constitutes a major component in the pathogenesis of RDS in preterm lambs (93). Subsequent studies showed that this lung vascular injury and edema can be inhibited by surfactant administration at birth (142), probably by reducing the need for high inflation pressures to achieve adequate ventilation and oxygenation, and by yielding uniform inflation of distal respiratory units (148).

It is noteworthy that mechanically ventilated preterm lambs with severe RDS had a marked reduction in circulating neutrophils within 30 min of birth, and that this was associated with abundant neutrophils in the lungs. The magnitude of the postnatal reduction in circulating neutrophils correlated with the degree of lung vascular protein leak and pulmonary edema (137). When lambs were rendered neutropenic from prenatal treatment with nitrogen mustard, lung vascular injury and edema did not develop postnatally after premature birth followed by 8 h of mechanical ventilation. These and earlier observations of neutrophil abundance in airway secretions of infants with severe RDS indicate that circulating neutrophils and their secretory products, specifically proteolytic enzymes and toxic oxygen metabolites, may play an important role in the pathogenesis of acute lung vascular protein leak and edema in RDS (137, 149–151). The mechanisms by which neutrophils are recruited into the lungs after premature birth and mechanical ventilation are unclear, but it is likely that several chemoattractants, including macrophage inflammatory protein-1α, and interleukins 6 and 8 (152–154), are released in response to the pulmonary stresses associated with increased blood flow and pressures within the lung circulation, and increased gas flow and pressures within the airways and distal air spaces.

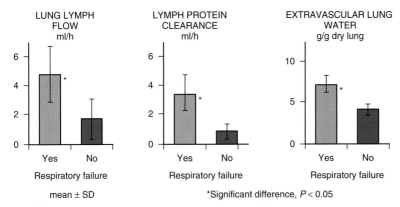

Figure 7-7 Studies of lung vascular protein permeability done with 10 lambs (birth weight 3.6 ± 0.7 kg) that were delivered prematurely by caesarean section at 133 ± 1 days gestation (term = 147 days) and mechanically ventilated for 6 h after birth. Six lambs (light bars) had respiratory failure, as judged by severe hypoxemia in 100% oxygen and need for peak inflation pressures > 50 cmH$_2$O. Four lambs (dark bars) had no respiratory failure. Lung lymph flow and lymph protein flow during the last 2 h of study and postmortem extravascular lung water were significantly greater ($P < 0.05$) in lambs that had respiratory failure compared to those that did not. From Bland et al. (93).

Pulmonary Edema from Increased Lung Vascular Filtration Pressure in CLD

Pulmonary edema is a consistent pathological feature of neonatal CLD, which typically afflicts extremely premature infants who receive prolonged mechanical ventilation because of continuing respiratory failure, either from residual lung disease after initial RDS, or from chest wall instability, apnea or infection, which are frequent complications of premature birth. An ovine model of CLD has yielded a number of insights regarding the pulmonary edema that typically occurs in this condition (131, 155–158). These studies showed that sustained mechanical ventilation of lambs for 3–4 weeks after premature birth leads to a chronic form of lung injury that closely mimics the pathophysiology and histopathology of the "new BPD," including pulmonary vascular dysfunction and edema. Lambs that were delivered by caesarean section at $\sim 80\%$ of term gestation and then mechanically ventilated for up to a month of age had persistent elevation of lung vascular and respiratory tract resistances when compared to control lambs born at term. These physiological abnormalities were associated with increased abundance of smooth muscle and elastin in pulmonary arteries and airways (131, 155). Compared to control lambs born at term, the preterm lambs with CLD had fewer alveoli and lung capillaries, which probably contributed to increased filtration pressure in their pulmonary microcirculation. Thus, studies of lung fluid balance in these animals showed a progressive increase in lung lymph flow and a consistent decrease in the lymph:plasma protein ratio, indicative of increased lung microvascular pressure rather than increased permeability, and postmortem histopathology revealed varying degrees of interstitial pulmonary edema (Fig. 7-9) (131).

Subsequent studies showed evidence of lung vascular dysfunction, with loss of the pulmonary vascular response to inhaled nitric oxide (iNO) that was attributed to diminished abundance of endothelial nitric oxide synthase and soluble guanylate cyclase in the pulmonary circulation (156, 157). Efforts to lower lung vascular and respiratory tract resistances by continuous delivery of low-dose (5–15 ppm) iNO beginning at birth had only a modest effect on the pulmonary circulation, without reducing pulmonary edema (158). Extravascular lung water averaged 6.0 ± 1.0 g/g

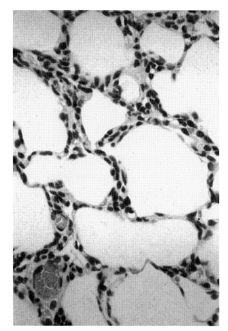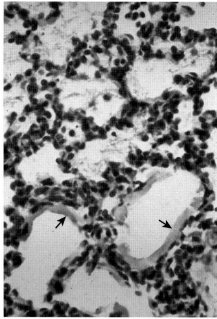

Figure 7-8 Histological sections of lung obtained from lambs that were delivered by caesarean section at 128 days gestation (term = 147 days) and mechanically ventilated for 8 h after birth. The lungs were cross-clamped at the hilum and fixed in 10% formalin at the prevailing peak-inflation pressure. Left panel: lung from a lamb that did not have respiratory failure, showing well-inflated air spaces and thin interstitium. Right panel: lung from a lamb that had respiratory failure, showing non-uniform inflation, atelectasis, proteinaceous fluid within open air spaces (arrows: hyaline membranes) and abundant leukocytes, indicative of inflammation and edema from abnormal lung vascular and epithelial protein permeability. Adapted from Bland et al. (93).

dry lung (mean $\pm$ SD) in lambs with CLD, compared to 4.6 ± 0.4 g/g dry lung in control lambs born at term (significant difference, $P < 0.05$). Lung histology showed fluid accumulation in the interstitium, but rarely within air spaces, suggesting that the barrier function of the lung epithelium, which typically breaks down in RDS, remains intact in most cases of CLD.

Some of these chronically ventilated preterm lambs had episodes of generalized bacterial infection, during which their lung lymph flow and lymph protein concentration increased, indicative of increased pulmonary vascular protein permeability. When their infection resolved in response to appropriate antibiotic therapy, however, lung lymph flow returned to baseline values and lymph protein concentration invariably decreased to low levels, consistent with elevated lung vascular filtration pressure. Thus, the pulmonary edema that typically occurs in CLD after premature birth and prolonged mechanical ventilation appears to be the result of increased lung vascular filtration pressure rather than abnormal protein permeability.

EPILOGUE ON PULMONARY EDEMA AFTER PREMATURE BIRTH

There is abundant experimental work to help explain why infants who are born prematurely have a high incidence of respiratory distress associated with pulmonary edema. Animal studies have shown that the lungs contain more fluid per unit tissue mass after premature birth than after birth at term. In addition, the lung epithelium

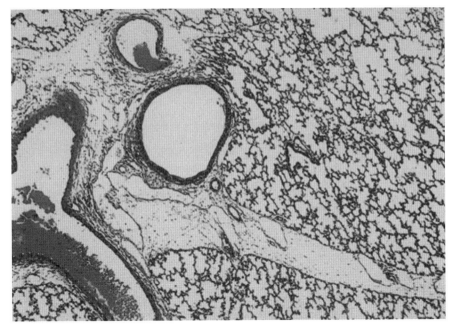

Figure 7-9 Histological section of lung obtained from a lamb that was delivered prematurely at 125 days gestation (term = 147 days) and mechanically ventilated at a rate of 20 breaths/min for 3 weeks after birth. Note the perivascular cuffs of fluid, dilated lymphatics and thickened interlobar fissure, indicative of interstitial edema. Adapted from Bland et al. (131).

has fewer sodium channels, fewer sodium pumps and less Na,K-ATPase activity after preterm compared to term birth, such that postnatal absorption of fetal lung liquid may be slower after premature birth than it is after birth at term. Compared to infants who are born at term, those who are delivered prematurely have greater filtration pressure in their pulmonary circulation, particularly if they experience hypoxia, or if they have increased pulmonary blood flow from persistent patency of the ductus arteriosus. Protein osmotic pressure in their plasma is low, especially if they receive too much fluid and salt, which in turn can contribute to increased lung fluid filtration and development of pulmonary edema. Because the air spaces of their lungs are often unstable from insufficient surfactant, a large transpulmonary pressure often develops, with considerable heterogeneity of lung expansion. Chemoattractants in the lung draw neutrophils from the pulmonary circulation into the air spaces, with subsequent release of inflammatory mediators. These developments may cause leaks in the epithelium and endothelium and reduce interstitial pressure around extra-alveolar vessels, which may contribute to the lung edema observed in infants with RDS.

Infants with RDS often require mechanical ventilation with high concentrations of inspired oxygen, which may injure the lungs, cause release of toxic oxygen metabolites and proteolytic enzymes, and possibly interfere with lymphatic drainage, particularly in the presence of interstitial emphysema or fibrosis. These events may lead to fluid accumulation and an abnormal distribution of protein in the lungs, with impaired respiratory gas exchange. Prolonged mechanical ventilation may be complicated by recurrent episodes of hypoxemia and intermittent infection. This series of events often leads to CLD, which is associated with persistent elevation of pulmonary vascular resistance, increased lung fluid filtration and pulmonary edema. Table 7-4 lists strategies to help prevent or reduce the severity of CLD and associated pulmonary edema.

Table 7–4	**Strategies for Reducing Lung Edema After Premature Birth**

Prenatal glucocorticoid therapy to enhance lung epithelial Na transport and surfactant function

Allowing labor (stress-related hormone release) to begin and progress whenever possible

Postnatal surfactant treatment to reduce the need for oxygen and assisted ventilation

Early application of nasal continuous positive airway pressure (nCPAP) to help avoid mechanical ventilation and lung overdistension

Early closure of the ductus arteriosus to help prevent lung overperfusion and increased vascular filtration pressure

Early treatment of systemic and pulmonary infection to inhibit lung inflammation and associated protein leaks

Restricted salt and fluid intake, and avoidance of rapid intravascular volume infusions to help prevent hypoproteinemia and fluid accumulation in the lungs

Judicious use of diuretics if the above measures fail to prevent or reduce the severity of pulmonary edema

Acknowledgments

Thanks to the National Heart, Lung and Blood Institute of the National Institutes of Health for its longstanding, generous support of much of the research that is described in this review.

Portions of this chapter were published previously by The American Academy of Pediatrics as part of its series of NeoReviews (Vol. 6, No. 6, June 2005); and in a volume entitled Chronic Lung Disease in Early Infancy, edited by RD Bland and JJ Coalson, Chapter 29 (Pulmonary Edema After Premature Birth by RD Bland and DP Carlton), in Vol. 137 of the series on Lung Biology in Health and Disease, executive editor C Lenfant, Marcel Dekker Inc, New York, 2000.

Permission has been granted by the American Academy of Pediatrics and Marcel Dekker Inc to include portions of these publications in this chapter.

REFERENCES

1. Preyer W. Specielle Physiologie des Embryos. Leipzig: Th. Grieben's Verlag; 1885.
2. Jost A, Policard A. Contribution experimentale a l'étude du developement prenatal du poumon chez le lapin. Arch Anat Microsc Morphol Exp 1948; 37:323–332.
3. Alcorn D, Adamson TM, Lambert TF, et al. Morphological effects of chronic tracheal ligation and drainage in the fetal lamb lung. J Anat 1977; 123:649–660.
4. Moessinger AC, Harding R, Adamson TM, et al. Role of lung fluid volume in growth and maturation of the fetal sheep lung. J Clin Invest 90; 86:1270–1277.
5. Harding R, Hooper SB. Regulation of lung expansion and lung growth before birth. J Appl Physiol 1996; 81:209–224.
6. Adams FH, Fujiwara T, Rowshan G. The nature and origin of the fluid in the fetal lamb lung. J Pediatr 1963; 63:881–888.
7. Olver RE, Strang LB. Ion fluxes across the pulmonary epithelium and the secretion of lung liquid in the foetal lamb. J Physiol 1974; 241:327–357.
8. Cassin S, Gause G, Perks AM. The effects of bumetanide and furosemide on lung liquid secretion in fetal sheep. Proc Soc Exp Biol Med 1986; 181:427–431.
9. Carlton DP, Cummings JJ, Chapman DL, Poulain FR, Bland RD. Ion transport regulation of lung liquid secretion in foetal lambs. J Dev Physiol 1992; 17:99–107.
10. McCray PB, Jr., Bettencourt JD, Bastacky J. Secretion of lung fluid by the developing fetal rat alveolar epithelium in organ culture. Am J Respir Cell Mol Biol 1992; 6:609–616.
11. McCray PB, Jr., Bettencourt JD, Bastacky J. Developing bronchopulmonary epithelium of the human fetus secretes fluid. Am J Physiol 1992; 262:L270–L279.
12. Barker PM, Boucher RC, Yankaskas JR. Bioelectric properties of cultured monolayers from epithelium of distal human fetal lung. Am J Physiol 1995; 268:L270–L277.
13. Karlberg P, Adams FH, Geubelle F, Wallgren G. Alteration of the infant's thorax during vaginal delivery. Acta Obstet Gynecol Scand 1962; 41:223–229.
14. Olver RE, Walters DV, S MW. Developmental regulation of lung liquid transport. Annu Rev Physiol 2004; 66:77–101.

15. Rudolph AM, Heymann MA. Circulatory changes during growth in the fetal lamb. Circ Res 1970; 26:289–299.

16. Adamson TM, Brodecky V, Lambert TF, et al. Lung liquid production and composition in the "in utero" foetal lamb. Aust J Exp Biol Med Sci 1975; 53:65–75.

17. Mescher EJ, Platzker ACG, Ballard PL, et al. Ontogeny of tracheal fluid, pulmonary surfactant, and plasma corticoids in the fetal lamb. J Appl Physiol 1975; 39:1017–1021.

18. Wallen LD, Kulisz E, Maloney JE. Main pulmonary artery ligation reduces lung fluid production in fetal sheep. J Dev Physiol 1991; 16:173–179.

19. Harrison MR, Bressack MA, Churg AM, de Lorimier AA. Correction of congenital diaphragmatic hernia in utero. II. Simulated correction permits fetal lung growth survival at birth. Surgery 1980; 88:260–268.

20. Moessinger AC, Singh M, Donnelly DF, et al. The effect of prolonged oligohydramnios on fetal lung development, maturation and ventilatory patterns in the newborn guinea pig. J Dev Physiol 1987; 9:419–427.

21. Adamson TM, Boyd RDH, Platt HS, Strang LB. Composition of alveolar liquid in the foetal lamb. J Physiol 1969; 204:159–163.

22. Boyd RDH, Hill JR, Humphreys PW, et al. Permeability of lung capillaries to macromolecules in fetal and newborn lambs and sheep. J Physiol 1969; 201:567–588.

23. Normand ICS, Reynolds EOR, Strang LB. Passage of macromolecules between alveolar and inter-stitial spaces in foetal and newly ventilated lungs of the lamb. J Physiol 1970; 210:151–164.

24. Normand ICS, Olver RE, Reynolds EOR, Strang LB. Permeability of lung capillaries and alveoli to non-electrolytes in the foetal lamb. J Physiol 1971; 219:303–330.

25. Bland RD, Hansen TN, Haberkern CM, et al. Lung fluid balance in lambs before and after birth. J Appl Physiol 1982; 53:992–1004.

26. Olver RE, Schneeberger EE, Walters DV. Epithelial solute permeability, ion transport and tight junction morphology in the developing lung of the fetal lamb. J Physiol 1981; 315:395–412.

27. Gillie DJ, Pace AJ, Coakley RJ, et al. Liquid and ion transport by fetal airway and lung epithelia of mice deficient in sodium-potassium-2-chloride transporter. Am J Respir Cell Mol Biol 2001; 25:14–20.

28. Borok Z, Lubman RL, Danto SI, et al. Keratinocyte growth factor modulates alveolar epithelial cell phenotype in vitro: expression of aquaporin 5. Am J Respir Cell Mol Biol 1998; 18:554–561.

29. Dobbs LG, Gonzalez R, Matthay MA, et al. Highly water-permeable type I alveolar epithelial cells confer high water permeability between the airspace and vasculature in rat lung. Proc Natl Acad Sci USA 1998; 95:2991–2996.

30. Johnson MD, Bao HF, Helms MN, et al. Functional ion channels in pulmonary alveolar type I cells support a role for type I cells in lung ion transport. Proc Natl Acad Sci USA 2006; 103:4964–4969.

31. Adamson TM, Waxman BP. Carbonate dehydratase (carbonic anhydrase) and the fetal lung. Lung Liquids, Ciba Symposium. London. Amsterdam: Elsevier/North-Holland; 1976: 221–233.

32. Blaisdell CJ, Edmonds RD, Wang XT, et al. pH-regulated chloride secretion in fetal lung epithelia. Am J Physiol Lung Cell Mol Physiol 2000; 278:L1248–L1255.

33. Holmes KW, Hales R, Chu S, et al. Modulation of Sp1 and Sp3 in lung epithelial cells regulates ClC-2 chloride channel expression. Am J Respir Cell Mol Biol 2003; 29:499–505.

34. Vij N, Zeitlin PL. Regulation of the ClC-2 lung epithelial chloride channel by glycosylation of SP1. Am J Respir Cell Mol Biol 2006; 34:754–759.

35. Nielson DW. Changes in the pulmonary alveolar subphase at birth in term and premature lambs. Pediatr Res 1988; 23:418–422.

36. O'Brodovich H, Merritt TA. Bicarbonate concentration in Rhesus monkey and guinea pig fetal lung liquid. Am Rev Resp Dis 1992; 146:1613–1614.

37. Perks AM, Cassin S. The rate of production of lung liquid in fetal goats, and the effect of expansion of the lungs. J Dev Physiol 1985; 7:149–160.

38. Nielson DW, Lewis MB. Calcium increases in pulmonary alveolar fluid in lambs at birth. Pediatr Res 1988; 24:322–325.

39. Chapman DL, Carlton DP, Nielson DW, et al. Changes in lung liquid during spontaneous labor in fetal sheep. J Appl Physiol 1994; 76:523–530.

40. Bland RD, Boyd CAR. Cation transport in lung epithelial cells derived from fetal, newborn and adult rabbits. Influence of birth, labor and postnatal development. J Appl Physiol 1986; 62:507–515.

41. Kitterman JA, Ballard PL, Clements JA, et al. Tracheal fluid in fetal lambs: spontaneous decrease prior to birth. J Appl Physiol 1979; 47:985–989.

42. Schneeberger EE. Plasmalemmal vesicles in pulmonary capillary endothelium of developing fetal lamb lungs. Microvasc Res 1983; 25:40–55.

43. Shermeta DW, Oesch I. Characteristics of fetal lung fluid production. J Pediatr Surg 1981; 16:943–946.

44. Carlton DP, Cummings JJ, Poulain FR, Bland RD. Increased pulmonary vascular filtration pressure does not alter lung liquid secretion in fetal sheep. J Appl Physiol 1992; 72:650–655.

45. Cotton CU, Lawson EE, Boucher RC, Gatzy JT. Bioelectric properties and ion transport of airways excised from adult and fetal sheep. J Appl Physiol 1983; 55:1542–1549.

46. Krochmal EM, Ballard ST, Yankaskas JR, et al. Volume and ion transport by fetal rat alveolar and tracheal epithelia in submersion culture. Am J Physiol 1989; 256:F397–F407.

47. Zeitlin PL, Loughlin GM, Guggino WB. Ion transport in cultured fetal and adult rabbit tracheal epithelia. Am J Physiol 1988; 254:C691–C698.

48. Brown MJ, Olver RE, Ramsden CA, et al. Effects of adrenaline and of spontaneous labour on the secretion and absorption of lung liquid in the fetal lamb. J Physiol 1983; 344:137–152.

49. Dickson KA, Maloney JE, Berger PJ. Decline in lung liquid volume before labor in fetal lambs. J Appl Physiol 1986; 61:2266–2272.

50. Bland RD, Bressack MA, McMillan DD. Labor decreases the lung water content of newborn rabbits. Am J Obstet Gynecol 1979; 135:364–367.

51. Bland RD. Dynamics of pulmonary water before and after birth. Acta Paediatr Scand 1983; Suppl 305:12–20.

52. Norlin A, Folkesson HG. Alveolar fluid clearance in late gestational guinea pigs after labor induction: mechanisms and regulation. Am J Physiol 2001; 280:L606–L616.

53. Walters DV, Olver RE. The role of catecholamines in lung liquid absorption at birth. Pediatr Res 1978; 12:239–242.

54. Olver RE, Ramsden CA, Strang LB, Walters DV. The role of amiloride-blockable sodium transport in adrenaline-induced lung liquid reabsorption in the fetal lamb. J Physiol 1986; 376:321–340.

55. Walters DV, Ramsden CA, Olver RE. Dibutyryl cyclic-AMP induces a gestation-dependent absorption of fetal lung liquid. J Appl Physiol 1990; 68:2054–2059.

56. Barker PM, Brown MJ, Ramsden CA, et al. The effect of thyroidectomy in the fetal sheep on lung liquid reabsorption induced by adrenaline or cyclic AMP. J Physiol 1988; 407:373–383.

57. Barker PM, Walters DV, Strang LB. The role of thyroid hormones in maturation of the adrenaline-sensitive lung-liquid reabsorptive mechanism in the fetal sheep. J Physiol 1990; 424:473–485.

58. Barker PM, Walters DV, Markiewicz M, Strang LB. Development of the lung liquid reabsorptive mechanism in fetal sheep; synergism of triiodothyronine and hydrocortisone. J Physiol 1991; 433:435–449.

59. Chapman DL, Carlton DP, Cummings JJ, et al. Intrapulmonary terbutaline and aminophylline decrease lung liquid in fetal lambs. Pediatr Res 1991; 29:357–361.

60. Finley N, Norlin A, Baines DL, Folkesson HG. Alveolar epithelial fluid clearance is mediated by endogenous catecholamines at birth in guinea pigs. J Clin Invest 1998; 101:972–981.

61. Cheng JB, Goldfein A, Ballard PL, Roberts JM. Glucocorticoids increase pulmonary ß-adrenergic receptors in fetal rabbit. Endocrinol 1980; 107:1646–1648.

62. Whitsett JA, Manton MA, Carovec-Beckerman C, et al. ß-adrenergic receptors in the developing rabbit lung. Am J Physiol 1981; 240:E351–E357.

63. McDonald JV, Gonzales LW, Ballard PL, et al. Lung ß-adrenergic blockade affects perinatal surfactant release but not lung water. J Appl Physiol 1986; 60:1727–1733.

64. Wallace MJ, Hooper SB, Harding R. Regulation of lung liquid secretion by arginine vasopressin in fetal sheep. Am J Physiol 1990; 258:R104–R111.

65. Cassin S, Perks AM. Amiloride inhibits arginine vasopressin-induced decrease in fetal lung liquid secretion. J Appl Physiol 1993; 75:1925–1929.

66. Cummings JJ, Carlton DP, Poulain FR, et al. Vasopressin effects on lung liquid volume in fetal sheep. Pediatr Res 1995; 38:30–35.

67. Perks AM, Cassin S. The effects of arginine vasopressin and epinephrine on lung liquid production in fetal goats. Can J Physiol Pharmacol 1989; 67:491–498.

68. Kindler PM, Chuang DC, Perks AM. Fluid production by in vitro lungs from near-term fetal guinea pigs: effects of cortisol and aldosterone. Acta Endocrinol 1993; 129:169–177.

69. Kindler PM, Ziabakhsh S, Perks AM. Effects of cAMP, its analogues, and forskolin on lung fluid production by in vitro lung preparations from fetal guinea pigs. Can J Physiol Pharmacol 1992; 70:330–337.

70. Woods BA, Doe S, Perks AM. Effects of epinephrine on lung liquid production by in vitro lungs from fetal guinea pigs. Can J Physiol Pharmacol 1997; 75:772–780.

71. Baines DL, Folkesson HG, Norlin A, et al. The influence of mode of delivery, hormonal status and postnatal O_2 environment on epithelial sodium channel (ENaC) expression in perinatal guinea-pig lung. J Physiol 2000; 522:147–157.

72. Strang L. Fetal lung liquid: secretion and reabsorption. Physiol Rev 1991; 71:991–1016.

73. Bland RD, Nielson DW. Developmental changes in lung epithelial ion transport and liquid movement. Annu Rev Physiol 1992; 54:373–394.

74. Bland RD. Loss of liquid from the lung lumen in labor: more than a simple "squeeze." Am J Physiol Lung Cell Mol Physiol 2001; 280:L602–L605.

75. Barker PM, Olver RE. Invited review: clearance of lung liquid during the perinatal period. J Appl Physiol 2002; 93:1542–1548.

76. Jain L, Eaton DC. Physiology of fetal lung fluid clearance and the effect of labor. Semin Perinatol 2006; 30:34–43.

77. Mason RJ, Williams MC, Widdicombe JH, et al. Transepithelial transport by pulmonary alveolar type II cells in primary culture. Proc Natl Acad Sci USA 1982; 79:6033–6037.

78. Cheek JM, Kim KJ, Crandall ED. Tight monolayers of rat alveolar epithelial cells: bioelectric properties and active sodium transport. Am J Physiol 1989; 256:C688–C693.

79. O'Brodovich H, Rafii B, Post M. Bioelectric properties of fetal alveolar epithelial monolayers. Am J Physiol 1990; 258:L201–L206.

80. Rao AK, Cott GR. Ontogeny of ion transport across fetal pulmonary epithelial cells in monolayer culture. Am J Physiol 1991; 261:L178–L187.

81. Barker PM, Stiles AD, Boucher RC, Gatzy JT. Bioelectric properties of cultured epithelial monolayers from distal lung of 18-day fetal rat. Am J Physiol 1992; 262:L628–L636.

82. Pitkänen OM, Tanswell AK, O'Brodovich HM. Fetal lung cell-derived matrix alters distal lung epithelial ion transport. Am J Physiol 1995; 268:L762–L771.

83. Matalon S, Lazrak A, Jain L, Eaton DC. Invited review: biophysical properties of sodium channels in lung alveolar epithelial cells. J Appl Physiol 2002; 93:1852–1859.

84. Orser BA, Bertlik M, Fedorko L, O'Brodovich H. Cation selective channel in fetal alveolar type II epithelium. Biochim Biophys Acta 1991; 1094:19–26.

85. MacGregor GG, Olver RE, Kemp PJ. Amiloride-sensitive Na+ channels in fetal type II pneumocytes are regulated by G proteins. Am J Physiol 1994; 267:L1–8.

86. Marunaka Y. Amiloride-blockable Ca^{2+}-activated Na^+-permeant channels in the fetal distal lung epithelium. Pflugers Arch 1996; 431:748–756.

87. Jain L, Chen XJ, Ramosevac S, et al. Expression of highly selective sodium channels in alveolar type II cells is determined by culture conditions. Am J Physiol Lung Cell Mol Physiol 2001; 280:L646–L658.

88. Johnson MD, Widdicombe JH, Allen L, et al. Alveolar epithelial type I cells contain transport proteins and transport sodium, supporting an active role for type I cells in regulation of lung liquid homeostasis. Proc Natl Acad Sci USA 2002; 99:1966–1971.

89. Borok Z, Liebler JM, Lubman RL, et al. Na transport proteins are expressed by rat alveolar epithelial type I cells. Am J Physiol Lung Cell Mol Physiol 2002; 282:L599–L608.

90. Ridge KM, Olivera WG, Saldias F, et al. Alveolar type 1 cells express the alpha2 Na,K-ATPase, which contributes to lung liquid clearance. Circ Res 2003; 92:453–460.

91. Chapman DL, Widdicombe JH, Bland RD. Developmental differences in rabbit lung epithelial cell Na-K-ATPase. Am J Physiol 1990; 259:L481–L487.

92. Ingbar DH, Weeks CB, Gilmore-Hebert M, et al. Developmental regulation of Na,K-ATPase in rat lung. Am J Physiol 1996; 270:L619–L629.

93. Bland RD, Carlton DP, Scheerer RG, et al. Lung fluid balance in lambs before and after premature birth. J Clin Invest 1989; 84:568–576.

94. O'Brodovich H, Staub O, Rossien BC, et al. Ontogony of a1- and ß1-isoforms of Na+, K+-ATPase in fetal distal rat lung epithelium. Am J Physiol 1993; 264:C1137–C1143.

95. O'Brodovich H, Canessa C, Ueda J, et al. Expression of the epithelial Na+ channel in the developing rat lung. Am J Physiol 1993; 265:C491–C496.

96. Umenishi F, Carter EP, Yang B, et al. Sharp increase in rat lung water channel expression in the perinatal period. Am J Resp Cell Mol Biol 1996; 15:673–679.

97. Celsi G, Wang ZM, Akusjarvi G, Aperia A. Sensitive periods for glucocorticoids' regulation of Na,K-ATPase mRNA in the developing lung and kidney. Pediatr Res 1993; 33:5–9.

98. Tchepichev S, Ueda J, Canessa C, et al. Lung epithelial Na channel subunits are differentially regulated during development and by steroids. Am J Physiol 1995; 269:C805–C812.

99. King LS, Nielsen S, Agre P. Aquaporin-1 water channel protein in lung. J Clin Invest 1996; 97:2183–2191.

100. Venkatesh VC, Katzberg HD. Glucocorticoid regulation of epithelial sodium channel genes in human fetal lung. Am J Physiol 1997; 273:L227–L233.

101. Barker PM, Gatzy JT. Effect of gas composition on liquid secretion by explants of distal lung of fetal rat in submersion culture. Am J Physiol 1993; 265:L512–L517.

102. Pitkänen O, Tanswell AK, Downey G, O'Brodovich H. Increased PO_2 alters the bioelectric properties of fetal distal lung epithelium. Am J Physiol 1996; 270:L1060–L1066.

103. Ramminger SJ, Baines DL, Olver RE, Wilson SM. The effects of PO_2 upon transepithelial ion transport in fetal rat distal lung epithelial cells. J Physiol 2000; 524 Pt 2:539–547.

104. Ramminger SJ, Inglis SK, Olver RE, Wilson SM. Hormonal modulation of Na(+) transport in rat fetal distal lung epithelial cells. J Physiol 2002; 544:567–577.

105. Thome UH, Davis IC, Nguyen SV, et al. Modulation of sodium transport in fetal alveolar epithelial cells by oxygen and corticosterone. Am J Physiol Lung Cell Mol Physiol 2003; 284:L376–385.

106. Otulakowski G, Rafii B, Harris M, O'Brodovich H. Oxygen and glucocorticoids modulate alphaENaC mRNA translation in fetal distal lung epithelium. Am J Respir Cell Mol Biol 2006; 34:204–212.

107. Hummler E, Barker P, Gatzy J, et al. Early death due to defective neonatal lung liquid clearance in aENaC-deficient mice. Nat Genet 1996; 12:325–328.

108. Barker PM, Nguyen MS, Gatzy JT, et al. Role of ENaC subunit in lung liquid clearance and electrolyte balance in newborn mice. Insights into perinatal adaptation and pseudohypoaldosteronism. J Clin Invest 1998; 102:1634–1640.

109. Humphreys PW, Normand ICS, Reynolds EOR, Strang LB. Lymph flow and clearance of liquid from the lungs of the lamb at the start of breathing. J Physiol 1967; 193:1–29.

110. O'Brodovich H, Hannam V, Rafii B. Sodium channel but neither Na^+-H^+ nor Na-glucose symport inhibitors slow neonatal lung water clearance. Am J Resp Cell Mol Biol 1991; 5:377–384.

111. O'Brodovich H, Hannam V, Seear M, Mullen J. Amiloride impairs lung water clearance in newborn guinea pigs. J Appl Physiol 1990; 68:1758–1762.

112. Egan EA, Olver RE, Strang LB. Changes in non-electrolyte permeability of alveoli and the absorption of lung liquid at the start of breathing in the lamb. J Physiol 1975; 244:161–179.

113. Raj JU. Alveolar liquid pressure measured by micropuncture in isolated lungs of mature and immature fetal rabbits. J Clin Invest 1987; 79:1579–1588.

114. Fike CD, Lai-Fook SJ, Bland RD. Alveolar liquid pressures in newborn and adult rabbit lungs. J Appl Physiol 1988; 64:1629–1635.

115. Bland RD, McMillan DD, Bressack MA, Dong LA. Clearance of liquid from lungs of newborn rabbits. J Appl Physiol 1980; 49:171–177.

116. Egan EA, Dillon WP, Zorn S. Fetal lung liquid absorption and alveolar epithelial solute permeability in surfactant deficient, breathing fetal lambs. Pediatr Res 1984; 18:566–570.

117. Gowen CW, Jr, Lawson EE, Gingras J, et al. Electrical potential difference and ion transport across nasal epithelium of term neonates: correlation with mode of delivery, transient tachypnea of the newborn, and respiratory rate. J Pediatr 1988; 113:121–127.

118. Barker PM, Gowen CW, Lawson EE, Knowles MR. Decreased sodium ion absorption across nasal epithelium of very premature infants with respiratory distress syndrome. J Pediatr 1997; 130:373–377.

119. Raj JU, Bland RD. Lung luminal liquid clearance in newborn lambs. Am Rev Resp Dis 1986; 134:305–310.

120. Cummings JJ, Carlton DP, Poulain FR, et al. Hypoproteinemia slows lung liquid clearance in young lambs. J Appl Physiol 1993; 74:153–160.

121. Avery ME, Gatewood OB, Brumley G. Transient tachypnea of newborn. Possible delayed resorption of fluid at birth. Am J Dis Child 1966; 111:380.

122. Malan AF. Neonatal tachypnoea. Aust Paediatr J 1966; 3:159–164.

123. Sundell H, Garrott J, Blankenship WJ, et al. Studies on infants with type II respiratory distress syndrome. J Pediatr 1971; 78:754–764.

124. Alpan G, Scheerer R, Bland R, Clyman R. Patent ductus arteriosus increases lung fluid filtration in preterm lambs. Pediatr Res 1991; 30:616–621.

125. Sundell HW, Harris TR, Cannon JR, et al. Lung water and vascular permeability-surface area in premature newborn lambs with hyaline membrane disease. Circ Res 1987; 60:923–932.

126. Bland RD. Cord-blood total protein level as a screening aid for the idiopathic respiratory distress syndrome. N Engl J Med 1972; 287:9–13.

127. Lauweryns JM. Hyaline membrane disease: a pathological study of 55 infants. Arch Dis Child 1965; 40:618–625.

128. Northway WH, Jr, Rosan RC, Porter DY. Pulmonary disease following respiratory therapy of hyaline membrane disease: bronchopulmonary dysplasia. N Engl J Med 1967; 276:357–368.

129. Bonikos DS, Bensch KG, Northway WH, Jr, Edwards DK. Bronchopulmonary dysplasia: the pulmonary pathologic sequel of necrotizing bronchiolitis and pulmonary fibrosis. Human Pathology 1976; 7:643–666.

130. Jobe AH, Bancalari E. Bronchopulmonary dysplasia. Am J Respir Crit Care Med 2001; 163:1723–1729.

131. Bland RD, Albertine KH, Carlton DP, et al. Chronic lung injury in preterm lambs: abnormalities of the pulmonary circulation and lung fluid balance. Pediatr Res 2000; 48:64–74.

132. Bland RD. Neonatal chronic lung disease in the post-surfactant era. Biol Neonate 2005; 88:181–191.

133. Bland RD, McMillan DD. Lung fluid dynamics in awake newborn lambs. J Clin Invest 1977; 60:1107–1115.

134. Sundell HW, Brigham KL, Harris TR, et al. Lung water and vascular permeability-surface area in newborn lambs delivered by cesarean section compared with the 3–5-day-old lamb and adult sheep. J Dev Physiol 1980; 2:191–204.

135. Bland RD, Hansen TN, Hazinski TA, et al. Studies of lung fluid balance in newborn lambs. Ann NY Acad Sci 1982; 384:126–145.

136. Hazinski TA, Bland RD, Hansen TN, et al. Effect of hypoproteinemia on lung fluid balance in awake newborn lambs. J Appl Physiol 1986; 61:1139–1148.

137. Carlton DP, Albertine KH, Cho SC, et al. Role of neutrophils in lung vascular injury and edema after premature birth in lambs. J Appl Physiol 1997; 83:1307–1317.

138. Bressack MA, McMillan DD, Bland RD. Pulmonary oxygen toxicity: increased microvascular permeability to protein in unanesthetized lambs. Lymphology 1979; 12:133–139.

139. Carlton DP, Cummings JJ, Scheerer RG, et al. Lung overexpansion increases pulmonary microvascular protein permeability in young lambs. J Appl Physiol 1990; 69:577–583.

140. Jobe A, Ikegami M, Jacobs H, et al. Permeability of premature lamb lungs to protein and the effect of surfactant on that permeability. J Appl Physiol 1983; 55:169–176.

141. Jobe A, Jacobs H, Ikegami M, Berry D. Lung protein leaks in ventilated lambs: effect of gestational age. J Appl Physiol 1985; 58:1246–1251.

142. Carlton DP, Cho SC, Davis P, et al. Surfactant treatment at birth reduces lung vascular injury and edema in preterm lambs. Pediatr Res 1995; 37:265–270.

143. Ikegami M, Berry D, Elkady T, et al. Corticosteroids and surfactant change lung function and protein leaks in the lungs of ventilated premature rabbits. J Clin Invest 1987; 79:1371–1378.

144. Elkady T, Jobe A. Corticosteroids and surfactant increase lung volumes and decrease rupture pressures of preterm rabbit lungs. J Appl Physiol 1987; 63:1616–1621.

145. Normand ICS, Reynolds EOR, Strang LB, Wigglesworth JS. Flow and protein concentration of lymph from lungs of lambs developing hyaline membrane disease. Arch Dis Child 1968; 43:334–339.

146. Reynolds EOR, Jacobson HN, Motoyama EK, et al. The effect of immaturity and prenatal asphyxia on the lungs and pulmonary function of newborn lambs: the experimental production of respiratory distress. Pediatrics 1965; 35:382–392.

147. Stahlman M, LeQuire VS, Young WC, et al. Pathophysiology of respiratory distress in newborn lambs. Am J Dis Child 1964; 108:375–393.

148. Carlton DP, Cho S-C, Davis P, Bland RD. Inflation pressure and lung vascular injury in preterm lambs. Chest 1994; 105:115S–116S.

149. Merritt TA, Cochrane CG, Holcomb K, et al. Elastase and alpha 1-proteinase inhibitor activity in tracheal aspirates during respiratory distress syndrome. J Clin Invest 1983; 72:656–666.

150. Ogden BE, Murphy SA, Saunders GC, et al. Neonatal lung neutrophils and elastase/proteinase inhibitor imbalance. Am Rev Resp Dis 1984; 130:817–821.

151. Jackson JC, Chi EY, Wilson CB, et al. Sequence of inflammatory cell migration into lung during recovery from hyaline membrane disease in premature newborn monkeys. Am Rev Resp Dis 1987; 135:937–940.

152. Jones CA, Cayabyab RG, Kwong KY, et al. Undetectable interleukin (IL)-10 and persistent IL-8 expression early in hyaline membrane disease: a possible developmental basis for the predisposition to chronic lung inflammation in preterm newborns. Pediatr Res 1996; 39:966–975.

153. Murch SH, Costeloe K, Klein NJ, MacDonald TT. Early production of macrophage inflammatory protein occurs in respiratory distress syndrome and is associated with poor outcome. Pediatr Res 1996; 40:490–497.

154. Munshi UK, Niu JO, Siddiq MM, Parton LA. Elevation of interleukin-8 and interleukin-6 precedes the influx of neutrophils in tracheal aspirates from preterm infants who develop bronchopulmonary dysplasia. Pediatr Pulmonol 1997; 24:331–336.

155. Albertine KH, Kim BI, Kullama LK, et al. Chronic lung injury in preterm lambs. Disordered respiratory tract development. Am J Respir Crit Care Med 1999; 159:945–958.

156. MacRitchie AN, Albertine KH, Sun J, et al. Reduced endothelial nitric oxide synthase in lungs of chronically ventilated preterm lambs. Am J Physiol Lung Cell Mol Physiol 2001; 281:L1011–L1020.

157. Bland RD, Ling CY, Albertine KH, et al. Pulmonary vascular dysfunction in preterm lambs with chronic lung disease. Am J Physiol Lung Cell Mol Physiol 2003; 285:L76–L85.

158. Bland RD, Albertine KH, Carlton DP, MacRitchie AJ. Inhaled nitric oxide effects on lung structure and function in chronically ventilated preterm lambs. Am J Respir Crit Care Med 2005; 172:899–906.

159. Bland RD. Pathogenesis of pulmonary edema after premature birth. Adv Pediatr 1987; 34:175–222.

Chapter 8

Role of Inflammation in the Pathogenesis of Acute and Chronic Neonatal Lung Disease

Christian P. Speer MD FRCPE

Neutrophils and Macrophages in Airways, Pulmonary Tissue and Systemic Circulation

Adherence and Cellular-Endothelial Interaction

Deformability and Chemotaxis

Chemotactic and Chemokinetic Factors

Pro- and Anti-Inflammatory Cytokines

Proteolytic Damage

Oxidative Damage

Increased Alveolar Capillary Permeability and Systemic Inflammatory Response

Repair Mechanisms and Growth Factors

Factors Inducing Pulmonary Inflammation

Conclusion

The "classic" form of bronchopulmonary dysplasia (BPD), which has mainly affected more mature preterm infants with severe respiratory distress syndrome (RDS), is only rarely observed nowadays. This chronic respiratory disease is characterized by fibroproliferative changes with areas of emphysema and atelectasis and is clearly associated with long-term pulmonary morbidity and neurodevelopmental outcome (1–2). In contrast, a considerable number of very immature infants who initially have minimal or even absent signs of RDS may subsequently develop oxygen dependency and ventilatory needs within the first 2 weeks of life and stay oxygen-dependent for weeks or months (3). Up to 60% of these infants with "new" BPD may have been exposed to chorioamnionitis and may demonstrate signs of a pulmonary or systemic inflammatory response prior to delivery. This topic has been elegantly addressed in one of the previous chapters (see Jobe et al., Chapter 6). Additionally, various post-natal factors have been shown to induce an injurious inflammatory response in the immature airways and the pulmonary interstitium of preterm infants. These risk factors may act individually or additively and may perpetuate or even amplify the intrauterine inflammatory reaction and may subsequently affect normal alveolarization and pulmonary vascular development in preterm infants with "new" BPD (4). This chapter will mainly focus on inflammation-associated events and on the potential role of postnatal risk factors in pulmonary inflammation.

The inflammatory response is characterized by an accumulation of neutrophils and macrophages in the airways and pulmonary tissue of immature infants and, moreover, by an arsenal of proinflammatory mediators which affect the alveolar capillary unit and tissue integrity. The main part of this chapter will follow – whenever possible – the primary cell functions exhibited by circulating neutrophils and macrophages in response to inflammation. In the later part the role of individual postnatal risk factors will be discussed. In general, this article will expand on previously published reviews (3, 5, 6)

NEUTROPHILS AND MACROPHAGES IN AIRWAYS, PULMONARY TISSUE AND SYSTEMIC CIRCULATION

Neutrophils and macrophages have a pivotal and crucial role in acute and chronic stages of pulmonary inflammation. In premature animals, a neutrophil influx into the airways has been observed within minutes after initiation of mechanical ventilation (7) and this influx was associated with a decrease in the number of circulating neutrophils. This phenomenon was shown to correlate with the extent of pulmonary edema formation and increased risk of developing BPD (6, 8). Nearly identical findings have been described in premature infants (9). There is no doubt that circulating neutrophils and monocytes – as reflected by CD11b expression – become activated within 1–3 h after initiation of mechanical ventilation (10). Most likely, activated neutrophils adhere to the endothelium of the pulmonary vascular system and thus initiate a sequence of pathogenetic events. Besides an increased pulmonary "trapping" of neutrophils, a diminished bone marrow storage pool in neonates may be responsible for the rapid decrease in number of circulating phagocytes (11). Preterm infants born before 32 weeks of gestation were found to have a neutrophil cell mass of about 20% compared with term neonates and adults (12). One may speculate that low numbers of circulating neutrophils and monocytes – although increasing the risk of infection – may have a protective effect on the inflammatory response by decreasing the number of phagocytes at the site of inflammation. Several investigators have convincingly demonstrated that preterm infants with various stages of BPD had much higher and persisting numbers of inflammatory cells – both neutrophils and macrophages – in their bronchoalveolar lavage fluid than did infants who recovered from RDS (13–17). The predominant cell identified in the airways at the early phase of inflammation was the neutrophil (13–17).

In lung tissue of preterm infants who died during the early stages of RDS, the interstitial density of CD68-positive macrophages and neutrophils was at least 10–15-fold higher than in stillborn infants of equivalent age (18). During the development of acute lung injury alveolar and pulmonary tissue macrophages play a very important role upon their activation. Activated macrophages secrete numerous cytokines, among them chemoattractants and chemokines which orchestrate the inflammatory response, particularly neutrophil recruitment. Neutrophils and cells of the mononuclear phagocyte system originate in the bone marrow as a common progenitor cell for the granulocyte and the monocyte-macrophage pathways: the colony-forming unit – granulocyte monocyte (CFU-GM). Glycoprotein hormones termed colony-stimulating factors (G-CSF/GM-CSF) induce proliferation, maturation, and differentiation into neutrophils and monocyte-macrophages (19). Affinity, binding, and number of G-CSF receptors and GM-CSF receptors seem to be expressed identically on cord blood phagocytes and adult peripheral cells (20). Production of G-CSF by mononuclear cells, however, has been reported to be significantly less in mid-gestation fetuses and preterm infants than in term newborns or adults (21). Recently, prolonged survival of neonatal neutrophils due to an inappropriate suppression of neutrophil apoptosis has been reported (22–24). Since apoptosis of inflammatory neutrophils and their timely removal by resident macrophages are critical to the resolution of inflammation neonatal neutrophils with prolonged survival may have the functional capacity to perpetuate pulmonary inflammation (24). Neutrophil apoptosis is induced by endogenous ligands such as Fas which engage various death receptors, including Fas receptor (FasR). A decreased expression of FasR was recently observed in neonatal neutrophils when compared with adult phagocytes (23), a finding which could help to explain the prolonged survival of neonatal neutrophils.

ADHERENCE AND CELLULAR-ENDOTHELIAL INTERACTION

Before neutrophils leave the circulation via a one-way exit into the extravascular space, the phagocytic cell must adhere to the vascular endothelium adjacent to a site of inflammation. After activation by systemic or local factors, primed endothelial cells interact with neutrophils through adhesion molecules that include selectins and ß-integrins (Fig. 8-1) (11). The first step in the process of neutrophil emigration is the capture and reversible tethering of cells to endothelium. This initial attachment and "rolling down" is mediated by various types of selectins. Leukocyte selectin (L-selectin) is expressed essentially on the leukocyte as the primary mediator of rolling (25), and is shed by proteolytic cleavage after stimulation with proinflammatory cytokines. This mechanism appears to be a physiologic reaction and may be a mechanism of downregulating adhesion following firm attachment (25). The expression of L-selectin was shown to be reduced on cells of neonates compared with adults (26). However, shedding of L-selectin in term newborns and especially preterm infants was found to be impaired (26–28). Firm adhesion of phagocytes is mediated by $ß_2$-integrins. The most important "adhesion" of this group is complement receptor 3 (CR3; synonym: CD11b/CD18). CR3 recognizes members of the superfamily such as intercellular

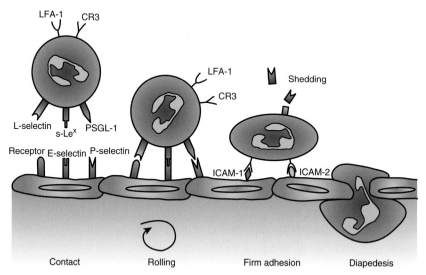

Figure 8-1 Neutrophil and endothelial interaction. First contact and rolling is mediated by selectin receptors (E-, P-, and L-selectin) and their ligands such as sialyl-Lewis X (s-Le^x), P-selectin glycoprotein ligand-1 (PSGL-1) and receptors for L-selectin. Shedding of the L-selectin by proteolytic cleavage, neutrophil activation and upregulation of the ß2-integrins – the lymphocyte function-associated antigen-1 (LFA-1) and complement receptor 3 (CR3) – is inducing neutrophil adhesion to the endothelium. The neutrophils penetrate by moving through the interendothelial-cell junctions into the interstitium. Reproduced with permission from: Urlichs F, Speer CP. Neutrophil function in preterm and term infants. Neo Reviews 2004; 5(10):417–429.

endothelial adhesion molecule 1 (ICAM-1) and ICAM-2 which mediate the firm adhesion of the neutrophil to the endothelium (29, 30)

Resting neonatal neutrophils were shown to have a CR3 expression similar to that of adult neutrophils (26). Stimulation and activation by inflammatory factors induced an upregulation of CR3 complexes in vitro and in vivo (31). Neonatal neutrophils, however, exhibited a significantly lower upregulation of the CR3 complexes than did adult cells (26, 30, 32, 33). Moreover, an abnormal interaction of CR3 with ICAM-1 has been observed in neonatal neutrophils (34). It seems most likely that the diminished transmigration rate of neonatal neutrophils which might also affect subsequent neutrophil function is reflected in the reduced CR3 expression (34). Despite these qualitative deficiencies in cellular-endothelial interactions which might be considered as a protective factor in the sequence of pulmonary inflammation, increased concentrations of various soluble adhesion molecules on neutrophils and endothelium such as selectins and ICAM-1 have been detected in airway secretions and the circulation of infants with BPD, reflecting greater shedding of these molecules in response to inflammation (35–39). These data provide indirect evidence for an effective recruitment of circulating neutrophils into the airways and the pulmonary tissue. Most recently, a strong upregulation of ICAM-1 in endothelial cord cells and increased serum concentrations of soluble ICAM-1 in preterm infants exposed to chorioamnionitis have been reported (40).

DEFORMABILITY AND CHEMOTAXIS

After adhering to the vascular endothelium, the neutrophil must attenuate itself, altering both cell membrane and cytoplasmatic contents, to squeeze through junctions between endothelial cells into the extracellular space. Outside the vessel, phagocytic cells move in a gradient of chemotactic factors and accumulate in the area of highest concentration of chemoattractants. This phenomenon is defined as chemotaxis, a directional locomotion of cells determined by substances in the environment. The ability of phagocytes to undergo chemotaxis implies the possession of a sensory mechanism, including receptors for chemoattractants on the plasma membrane that can detect differences in concentrations of chemotactic molecules. A number of investigators have reported a decreased chemotaxis of neutrophils from preterm and term infants compared to adults (41–47). Besides a reduced upregulation of C5a receptors and other chemotactic receptors, an impaired signal transduction pathway has been identified in neonatal neutrophils (43, 48, 49).

CHEMOTACTIC AND CHEMOKINETIC FACTORS

Airway secretions of infants with BPD have been shown to contain high concentrations of well-defined chemotactic factors which are responsible for the recruitment of neutrophils: C5a, tumor necrosis factor-α (TNF-α), interleukin-1 (IL-1), interleukin-8 (IL-8), interleukin-16 (IL-16), lipoxygenase products, leukotriene B$_4$, elastin fragments, fibronectin and others. Potent ß-chemokines that induce chemotaxis of monocytes and macrophages have been detected in the airway secretions of infants with RDS and BPD: monocyte chemotactic protein, macrophage inflammatory protein and growth-related protein (15, 17, 18, 50–53). High concentrations of macrophage inflammatory protein-1-α in particular were associated with the later development of pulmonary fibrosis (18, 54). Not surprisingly, the chemotactic activity and the concentrations of numerous chemotactic and chemokinetic factors were considerably higher in infants with BPD when compared with babies who recovered from RDS (15) (Fig. 8-2). IL-8, which is involved in the initiation of cellular endothelial interaction, is probably the most important chemotactic factor in the lung. Increased IL-8 levels in bronchoalveolar secretions of infants with

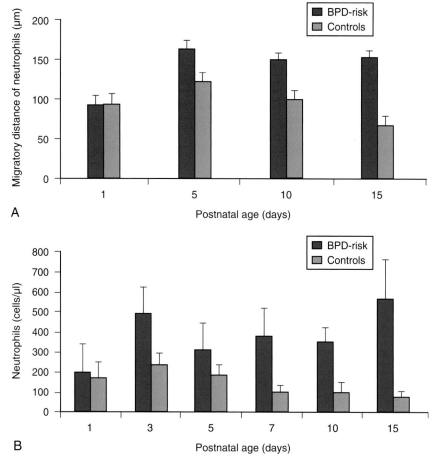

Figure 8-2 Chemotactic activity, expressed as migratory distance of peripheral blood neutrophils exposed to tracheobronchial aspirate fluid (A) and neutrophil count (B) in lung effluent fluid of neonates at risk for bonchopulmonary dysplasia (BPD) and of control neonates. *$P < .05$, **$P < .01$. Reproduced with permission of the publisher from: Groneck P, Goetze-Speer B, Oppermann M, et al. Association of pulmonary inflammation and increased microvascular permeability during the development of bronchopulmonary dysplasia: a sequential analysis of inflammatory mediators in respiratory fluids of high risk preterm infants. Pediatrics 1994; 93: 712–718.

developing BPD clearly preceded the marked neutrophil influx observed in these infants (6). The impaired chemotaxis of neonatal neutrophils seems to be outweighed by numerous potent chemotactic factors present in the airways of preterm infants with BPD. It was recently demonstrated in animals exposed to 60% oxygen that the application of a selective chemokine receptor antagonist completely inhibited neutrophil influx into the lungs. This strategy suppressed pulmonary inflammation and enhanced lung growth (55).

PRO- AND ANTI-INFLAMMATORY CYTOKINES

Besides IL-8, other proinflammatory cytokines such as TNF-α, IL-1 as well as interleukin-6 (IL-6) are important mediators in the early inflammatory response and in the evolution of the inflammatory events. These cytokines are synthesized by alveolar macrophages, airway epithelial cells, fibroblasts, type II pneumocytes and endothelial cells of preterm infants upon stimulation by hypoxia, hyperoxia, nitric oxide (NO), microorganisms, endotoxin, lipopolysaccharide (LPS), other bacterial cell wall constituents and biophysical factors (3, 56, 57) such as baro- and volutrauma of the bronchoalveolar system (Fig. 8-3). It has clearly been shown that proinflammatory

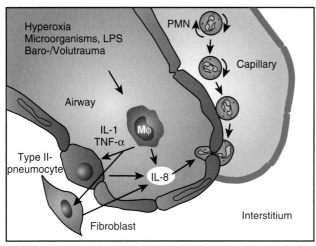

Figure 8-3 Postnatal risk factors such as hyperoxia, microorganisms, LPS and baro-/volutrauma induce the generation and secretion of proinflammatory cytokines by various pulmonary and inflammatory cells which are responsible, in part, for the recruitment and influx of neutrophils into the airways.

cytokines do not cross the placenta (58). As mentioned earlier, increased protein levels and high mRNA expression of these proinflammatory cytokines (TNF-α, IL-1, IL-6, IL-8) have been detected in airway secretions, bronchoalveolar cells and systemic circulation of infants with developing BPD (6, 15, 59–61). A transient overexpression of IL-1 in rat lungs by adenoviral gene transfer has recently been found to be accompanied by a local increase in TNF-α and IL-6 expression and a vigorous acute inflammatory reaction with evidence of profound tissue injury and fibrotic changes (62). In contrast, the treatment of surfactant-depleted rabbits with aerosolized IL-1 receptor antagonists before the induction of experimental lung injury clearly decreased inflammation and lung damage (63).

Recent findings suggest that IL-1 present in the airway fluid of mechanically ventilated preterm infants induced airway epithelial IL-8 expression via a nuclear transcription factor (NF-κB)-dependent pathway (64). NF-κB activation has also been reported in airway neutrophils and macrophages as well as tracheobronchial secretion from infants with RDS (65–67). NF-κB plays a crucial role in the regulation of the inflammatory response of neutrophils activated by lipopolysaccharide (LPS). NF-κB is normally sequestered in the cytoplasm. In response to LPS (64) or proinflammatory cytokines, NF-κB is translocated to the nucleus, where it can bind to the promoter region of the target genes and, thus, induce gene transcription of proinflammatory cytokines. In neonatal neutrophils NF-κB was activated to a higher extent than in adult cells after stimulation with TNF-α (68). This fact may contribute to the increased ability of neonatal neutrophils to synthesize proinflammatory cytokines (69). There is increasing evidence that the LPS-induced cytokine response is controlled by Toll-like receptor 4 (TLR 4), a highly conserved transmembrane protein with an extracellular and a cytoplasmatic domain (70). Coupling of LPS with TLR4 results in its activation of an intracellular signaling cascade, ultimately leading to liberation of NF-κB from the cytoplasm into the nucleolus. Basal mRNA and protein expression of TLR4 in the human neonate was shown to be equivalent to adults (71, 72). Since there are heterogeneous triggers which can initiate the inflammatory response in the neonatal lung one may speculate that distinct mechanisms of NF-κB activation may exist.

In preterm infants who had died of severe RDS the influx of TNF-α-positive macrophages in pulmonary tissue was found to be associated with a striking loss of endothelial basement membrane and a destruction of interstitial glycosaminoglycans (73). A pronounced IL-8 mRNA expression could also be detected in the bronchoalveolar epithelium and in a scattered pattern in the interstitial tissue of post-mortem lung tissue of infants with RDS (74). These findings underline the importance of IL-8 expression and other proinflammatory cytokines in the initiation and perpetuation of injurious events in pulmonary tissue of preterm infants. The increased levels and enhanced mRNA expression of proinflammatory cytokines present in the airways and pulmonary tissue of preterm infants may reflect an inability to regulate inflammation through an adequate expression of the anti-inflammatory cytokines IL-10, IL-4, IL-12 and IL-13, IL-18 or IL-1 receptor antagonist (75–79). Cellular IL-10 mRNA was undetectable in most airway samples of preterm infants with RDS, but it was expressed in all cell samples of term infants with meconium aspiration syndrome (75). Interestingly, lung inflammatory cells of preterm infants exposed to IL-10 in vitro responded with a reduced expression of proinflammatory cytokines (80). An imbalance between proinflammatory and anti-inflammatory cytokines favoring proinflammatory cytokines can be considered as an important feature of lung injury. In this context, substances which exert an anti-inflammatory effect or which interfere with neutrophil influx into the airways or lung tissue may be helpful in downregulating the inflammatory process.

Clara cell protein 10 (CC10) is a small molecule generated by Clara cells in the lung and has various inhibitory in vitro effects on inflammatory responses, including the inhibition of phospholipase A_2. In animal models CC10 deficiency has been associated with high expression of cytokines in the lung and an infiltration of pulmonary tissue by inflammatory cells (81, 82). Most recently, in a pilot study a single dose of CC10 administered to premature infants shortly after birth resulted in lower numbers of neutrophils and a decreased protein concentration in airway secretions when compared with controls (83).

PROTEOLYTIC DAMAGE

Neutrophil intracellular granules serve as a source of proteolytic enzymes, antimicrobial proteins that can be incorporated into and expressed by the plasma membrane (11). The primary granules contain proteinases, such as elastase, myeloperoxidase, lysozyme, defensins, and bacterial permeability increasing protein (BPI). The secondary granules contain membrane receptors (e.g. CR3) as well as collagenase, metalloproteinase, and lactoferrin I. During phagocytosis and upon stimulation, various granule constituents are released sequentially into the extracellular space. Exocytosis of elastase, β-glucoronidase, myeloperoxidase and others was equivalent in neutrophils from newborn and adults (83, 84).

Data from in vitro studies, animal experiments and observations made in preterm infants with BPD clearly indicate that an imbalance between proteases and protease inhibitors may essentially contribute to the pathogenesis of BPD. Besides neutrophils, macrophages present at sites of inflammation release various potent proteases which are thought to play an essential role in the destruction of the alveolar-capillary unit or the extracellular matrix (Fig. 8-4). An imbalance between elastase – a powerful neutral protease stored in neutrophils – and α_1-proteinase inhibitor (α_1-PI) within the airways has clearly been demonstrated in preterm infants with RDS and BPD (5, 85, 86) (Fig. 8-1). α_1-PI is presumably functionally inactivated by oxygen intermediates with the consequence that oxidized α_1-PI is degraded by proteolytic cleavage (85). As a result of elastolytic damage, an increased urinary excretion of desmosine, a degradation product of mature cross-linked elastic fibres, was identified in infants with free elastase activities in their airway secretions. This is of particular concern in the light of animal and human studies showing that alveolar septation is markedly reduced in the lungs of infants with severe BPD (87). In addition, an increased elastin deposition in pulmonary tissue of

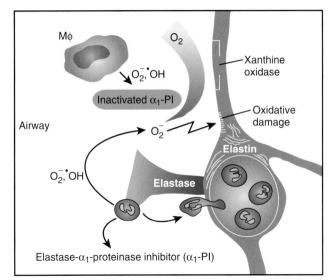

Figure 8-4 Schematic representation of elastolytic and oxidative damage to the alveolar capillary unit. Elastase, a powerful neutral protease stored in the azurophilic granules of neutrophils which have migrated into the airways, is released upon stimulation. Under normal circumstances elastase is rapidly inactivated by α1-proteinase inhibitor (α1-PI). Under conditions in which oxidative inactivation of α1-PI takes place, free elastase may attack pulmonary elastin, the primary substrate of neutrophil elastase. Toxic oxygen radicals O_2 and OH are generated by neutrophils and macrophages as well as by xanthine oxidase and may directly cause oxidative damage by lipid peroxidation. Reproduced with permission from: Speer CP. Inflammation and bronchopulmonary dysplasia: a continuing story. Semin Fetal Neonat Med. 2006; 11(5):354–362.

an animal model with BPD has been reported (88). Moreover, disruption of sulfated glycosaminoglycans, changes in hyaluronan deposition and increased laminin concentrations in airway secretions of infants with BPD have been attributed to elastolytic destruction (89–91). Furthermore, an imbalance between the cystein proteases cathepsins B, H, L and S and their inhibitors, cystatins B and C, has also been recently described in a baboon model of BPD (92). All cathepsins were immunolocalized to macrophages. Similarly, high concentrations of different matrix metalloproteinases which play a significant role in remodeling throughout all stages of lung development have been identified in airway secretions of infants with BPD and, while overexpressed, they cause disruption of the extracellular matrix (93–96). Protective levels of various tissue inhibitors of metalloproteinases were rather low in these infants, a finding which is suggestive of an imbalance within the metalloproteinase system. Since profiles of matrix metalloproteinases and tissue inhibitors of matrix metalloproteinases in tracheal aspirates do not adequately represent the profiles in either trachea and lung, all data obtained from tracheal aspirates should be interpreted for trends rather than actual tissue levels (97). This statement most likely holds true for all cytokines, proteases/antiproteases and other inflammatory mediators. In respiratory epithelium, activation of proteinase-activated receptor-2 (PAR$_2$) by trypsin stimulates the release of inflammatory mediators, such as IL-6, IL-8 and metalloproteinase-9, and induces vascular permeability and infiltration of neutrophils. A high expression of PAR$_2$ has recently been reported (98).

OXIDATIVE DAMAGE

During phagocytosis, there is a dramatic change in cellular oxygen metabolism, characterized by increased oxygen consumption, and production of oxygen metabolites, including superoxide anion ($O_2{}^-$), hydrogen peroxide (H_2O_2), and hydroxyl radical ('OH). These toxic oxygen metabolites appear to be essential for the microbicidal activity of neutrophils and macrophages and are released into the extracellular space. Many studies have explored the possibility of a deficit in the generation of toxic oxygen metabolites in the newborn (11). However, compared with adult values, neonatal neutrophils and monocytes generated identical or nearly identical amounts of toxic oxygen metabolites under normal conditions (11, 99). In contrast, neutrophils of preterm infants with RDS showed a slightly decreased activity of the respiratory burst (100). It seems questionable, however, whether such in vitro findings may have any implications for the inflammatory process in a baby's lung, since toxic oxygen metabolites are generally produced in excess. LPS can further upregulate the generation of oxygen radicals in phagocytic cells by the mechanism of priming (101). Interestingly, neutrophils from newborns could not be upregulated as effectively by LPS compared to cells from adults (102). This may be due to a decreased expression on neonatal phagocytes of CD14, a receptor for LPS, coupled with LPS-binding protein (103, 104). Together with the Toll-like receptor, CD14 plays an essential role in immune cell activation during infection with Gram-negative bacteria or LPS exposure (101). In the light of oxidative tissue damage, a reduced generation of toxic radicals by neonatal neutrophils and macrophages could be beneficial in the process of pulmonary inflammation.

No doubt, exposure to high oxygen concentrations causes direct oxidative cell damage through increased production of reactive oxygen species (105). Oxygen radicals are not only released by neutrophils and macrophages at sites of inflammation, but also generated under hyperoxic conditions by free iron or by the cell-bound xanthine-oxidase system. Reactive oxygen species (ROS) have been shown to cause tissue damage by lipid peroxidation and to contribute to the oxidative inactivation of protective antiprotease systems in the airways and lung tissue (106, 107) and, furthermore, to upregulate the activity of matrix metalloproteinases (93). Free iron was detected in airway secretions in the vast majority of ventilated preterm infants with RDS (108). Interestingly, free elastase, cathepsin G and trypsin stored in neutrophils were shown to prime macrophages for an increased release of toxic oxygen metabolites (109). Moreover, resting and stimulated alveolar macrophages of infants with BPD generated increased amounts of hydrogen peroxide when compared with cells of control infants (5). Animal experiments indicate that oxidative stress as reflected by generation of toxic oxygen radicals is a very early and crucial event in the initiation of pulmonary inflammation (110). The activity of ROS is normally balanced by the antioxidant system (111). However, preterm infants are particularly susceptible to hyperoxia and damage caused by ROS, since the antioxidant system has yet to mature. Following term birth, enzymes such as superoxide dismutase (SOD), catalase and glutathione peroxidase have protective activities against ROS. However, there is insufficient activity of these enzymes in various tissues and cells at lower gestational ages (106, 107). This means that preterm infants will be deficient in antioxidant enzyme activity at the time during which they are receiving high inspiratory oxygen concentrations and are most likely exposed to hyperoxia.

INCREASED ALVEOLAR CAPILLARY PERMEABILITY AND SYSTEMIC INFLAMMATORY RESPONSE

The increased alveolar capillary permeability is pathognomonic for the early stages of pulmonary inflammation, and it is clearly associated with a deterioration of lung function (Fig. 8-5) (5, 6). Several factors may have detrimental effects on microvascular permeability: direct effects of inflammatory cells and mediators on the alveolar and capillary membrane, including cytokines, toxic oxygen radicals,

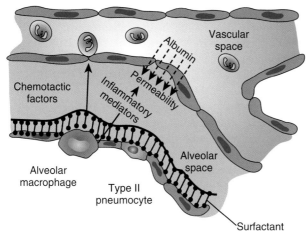

Figure 8-5 Schematic representation of the inflammatory mediators that are thought to be responsible for the increased alveolar capillary permeability during the evolution of BPD. Plasma proteins entering the airways contribute to the inactivation of the surfactant system. Reproduced with permission from: Speer CP. Inflammation and bronchopulmonary dysplasia. Semin Neonatol 2003; 8: 29–38.

inactivation of the surfactant system by various serum proteins, modulation of vascular perfusion in the inflamed area or increased shunting via the ductus arteriosus, microbial colonization and infection of the airways (112). A variety of lipid mediators with well-defined direct effects on microvascular permeability, including leukotrienes, prostacyclin, platelet-derived factor and endothelin-1, have been demonstrated in the airways of infants with BPD (113–117). Protein leakage into the alveoli and airways of preterm infants was shown to take place within 1 h of initiation of mechanical ventilation (8). At a postnatal age of 10–14 days preterm infants who later developed BPD had a drastic increase in albumin concentrations in airway secretions when compared with infants who recovered from RDS (15). Utilizing magnetic resonance imaging it was recently demonstrated that infants with BPD had an increased lung water content and were susceptible to gravity-induced collapse and alveolar flooding of the lung (118).

Furthermore, it has been clearly demonstrated that compounds of the plasma protein system which are activated after the initiation of RDS are able to affect the alveolar capillary membrane directly and indirectly by sequestration of activated neutrophils and platelets in the pulmonary vascular bed. In mechanically ventilated infants with RDS a simultaneous activation of clotting, fibrinolysis, kinin kallikrein, and the complement system was observed (119–121). An early and nearly identical activation of inflammation and the clotting system has also been described in animals conventionally ventilated or treated with high-frequency oscillatory ventilation (122). The activation of plasma protein systems in preterm infants was associated with a stimulation of neutrophils and platelets as indicated by an increased release of cellular constituents. In addition, an increased but transient CD11b expression on neutrophils, reflecting cellular activation, has recently been described in mechanically ventilated preterm infants in the early stages of RDS (10, 123). One may speculate that various factors which induce injury to the pulmonary capillary endothelium may subsequently promote neutrophil and platelet activation, and induce pulmonary as well as systemic inflammation and activation of the clotting system (124).

REPAIR MECHANISMS AND GROWTH FACTORS

Inflammation-induced tissue injury is normally followed by a phase of repair, a complex event which has only partially been studied in BPD. Lung injury and the associated inflammatory process leads to an induction of transforming growth factor-ß (TGF-ß) which limits some of the inflammatory reactions and plays a key role in mediating tissue remodeling and repair (125). However, if the reparative processes are exaggerated normal lung development may be inhibited. Furthermore, overexpression of TGF-ß and of platelet-derived growth factor-BB has been shown to result in severe pulmonary fibrosis (126, 127). In preterm infants with BPD increased concentrations of TGF-ß have been detected in the airway secretions (128–130). Moreover, in preterm animals with inflamed lungs an increased expression of TGF-ß has been recently observed. Interestingly, expression of connective tissue growth factor (CTGF), a second important mediator in the induction of pulmonary fibrosis, was decreased in this model (131). These preliminary findings could add an important step in the understanding of the "new BPD," which is characterized more by arrest of lung and pulmonary vessel formation rather than by fibrosis. One may speculate that overexpression of TGF-ß and the subsequent downregulation of CTGF together with low or suboptimal levels of various pulmonary and vascular growth factors may add to the pathogenetic sequence of the "new BPD." Low airway concentrations of keratinocyte and hepatocyte growth factors which are thought to participate in normal lung development and in tissue repair after lung injury as well as low levels of hypoxia-inducible factors promoting angiogenic response have been found to be associated with BPD (132–134). Similarly, impaired vascular endothelial growth factor (VEGF) and VEGF receptor mRNA expression in lungs from extremely premature baboons developing BPD were shown to contribute to dysmorphic microvasculature and disrupted alveolarization (135). Additionally, in a hyperoxia-induced BPD rat model, air space enlargement and loss of lung capillaries were shown to be associated with decreased lung VEGF and VEGF receptor expression. Postnatal administration of intratracheal adenovirus-mediated VEGF gene therapy improved survival and promoted lung capillary formation. Moreover, alveolar development was preserved in this model of irreversible lung injury (136). These findings underscore the importance of the vasculature in what is traditionally thought of as an airway disease and open new therapeutic avenues for the new BPD that is characterized by an irreversible loss of alveoli and capillaries through the modulation of angiogenic factors (136). VEGF may also be of importance in the early phase of neonatal RDS by contributing to pulmonary maturation and surfactant secretion. Recently, premature infants with higher cord blood levels of VEGF were shown to have a lower risk of developing RDS (137). Since growth and development of the fetal lung normally occurs in a low-oxygen environment, it has been hypothesized that low oxygen tension during fetal life enhances pulmonary artery endothelial cell growth and nitric oxide production (NO) modulates endothelial growth. In fact, data from animal experiments indicate that NO is essential for pulmonary angiogenesis, and impaired NO production as a consequence of increased postnatal oxygen tensions may contribute to abnormalities of angiogenesis observed in infants with BPD (138).

FACTORS INDUCING PULMONARY INFLAMMATION

Chorioamnionitis

In lung tissue of human fetuses exposed to chorioamnionitis, a pronounced inflammatory response reflected by a marked infiltration of inflammatory cells and an increased expression of the proinflammatory cytokine IL-8 mRNA has been demonstrated (74). In addition, intrauterine exposure to proinflammatory cytokines and other mediators during chorioamnionitis resulted in a marked increase in the number of apoptotic airway cells in human fetuses (139). Epidemiological data suggest a strong association between chorioamnionitis and the development of BPD.

Increased concentrations of proinflammatory cytokines in human amniotic fluid and fetal cord blood – indicating a systemic inflammatory response during chorioamnionitis – were shown to be independent risk factors for the development of BPD (140, 141). Although the mechanisms by which a fetal systemic inflammatory response increases the risk of BPD are incompletely understood, the antenatal intrauterine initiation of pulmonary inflammation seems to be a crucial step in the pathogenesis sequence of BPD. Chorioamnionitis, mechanical ventilation and postnatal sepsis have clearly been identified as modulators of BPD (142). The intrauterine mechanisms of pulmonary inflammation are discussed in Chapter 6 (Jobe et al.).

Infection

An association between early-onset systemic bacterial infections and the development of BPD in very low birth weight infants has been described (59, 143). In addition, systemic nosocomial infections have clearly been identified as an individual risk factor of BPD (143–145). Most likely, vasoactive prostaglandin mediators released during septicaemia prevent ductal closure or induce reopening (146). Besides direct effects of systemic infections and inflammatory mediators on endothelial pulmonary and bronchoalveolar cells, hemodynamic changes in the pulmonary vascular bed associated with a persistent ductus arteriosus seem to play an essential role in the development of BPD (112). However, the possible impact of airway colonization or even infection with coagulase-negative staphylococci and Gram-negative bacteria on the development of BPD is less clear and has generated contradictory results. The potential role of *Ureaplasma urealyticum* (Uu) in the pathogenesis of BPD is also controversial (147). Uu is the microorganism most frequently isolated from the amniotic fluid in preterm births and a predominant pathogen detected in the airway secretions immediately after birth (143, 148). The presence of Uu in the respiratory tract of preterm infants – even without clinical or laboratory signs of infection – has been correlated with elevated cellular and molecular markers of inflammation and associated with an increased risk of BPD (59, 149, 150). In baboons colonized antenatally with Uu two different patterns of disease were observed. One group with persistent Uu-positive tracheal cultures manifested continuous elevation of proinflammatory cytokine levels and had significantly worse lung function than control animals. The other group, which cleared Uu from their trachea by 48 h of postnatal age, showed lower airway cytokine levels and white blood cell numbers, and this was associated with significantly better lung function (148). Inherent maternal-fetal immune system responses to antenatal Uu, which are not well understood, most likely determine the pulmonary outcome of Uu-colonized infants (148). During the past decade "innate immunity" has been identified as a collection of factors, both cell-associated and cell-free, that comprises an impressively effective and well-organized system which is capable of immediate recognition of a whole array of microbes and microbial components. The name "innate" implies that the system is present at birth, presumably in a functionally active state. This is particularly crucial for the newborn host, which is devoid of any protection against microbes by products of the adaptive immune system. However, the functional state of the various components of innate immunity at birth is largely unknown. Some studies have been devoted to the cell-bound Toll-like receptors (TLRs), which is understandable, because of the central role of these molecules in the process of pathogen recognition and the activation of the adaptive immunity (151).

Mechanical Ventilation

Initiation of mechanical ventilation in preterm animals has shown that overdistension of the lungs causes disruption of structural elements and the release of proinflammatory mediators, with subsequent leukocyte influx, suggesting that any baro-/volutrauma of the immature lung may be injurious (152–158). However, certain ventilation strategies may cause more damage than others. For example, in an isolated rat lung model, high volume ventilation with zero PEEP (positive end expiratory pressure) caused significantly greater production and release of proinflammatory cytokines than a moderate volume with high PEEP, which allows stabilization of alveoli (152). Selection of the least harmful ventilation strategy is therefore of utmost importance if lung damage is to be minimized. Interestingly, high-frequency ventilation compared to conventional ventilation induced identical proinflammatory responses in preterm infants (156). Recently, the effect of mechanical ventilation on various pro- and anti-inflammatory cytokines in the presence or absence of endotoxin(LPS)-induced sepsis was studied (155). After pre-treatment with LPS, bronchoalveolar lavage fluid concentrations (BALF) of proinflammatory cytokines in isolated, non-perfused lungs were impressively increased even with a "less" injurious ventilation strategy (159). "Priming" of the fetal lung by intrauterine endotoxin or exposure to proinflammatory cytokines generated during chorioamnionitis is most likely a considerable pathogenetic factor in the initiation of the pulmonary inflammatory sequence. As a consequence basically every form of mechanical ventilation and specially a relatively "traumatic" bag-and-mask resuscitation may act as a "second strike" and may amplify the inflammatory reaction in the immature lung. Surprisingly, even the application of continuous positive airway pressure (CPAP) was shown to induce inflammatory changes in rat lungs following the administration of LPS (160). In vitro cyclic cell stretch also provoked an upregulation and release of IL-8 by human alveolar epithelial cells without any evidence of structural cell damage (161). A recent study demonstrated that preterm infants with severe RDS who died of respiratory failure had an increased apoptosis of pulmonary epithelial cells, and the rate of apoptosis was clearly associated with the duration of mechanical ventilation (157).

Hyperoxia

Preterm infants, especially very immature babies, with their reduced antioxidant defense system, may have a high risk of suffering from potential detrimental effects of hyperoxia and hyperoxemia during the first weeks of life (106, 107). In preterm and term animals hyperoxia has clearly been shown to be a strong and independent inducer of various mediators involved in pulmonary inflammation (162, 163). Recently, differential gene expression with DNA microarray analysis in premature rat lungs exposed to prolonged hyperoxia during the saccular stage has been studied; this developmental stage closely resembles the pulmonary development of preterm infants who are at risk for BPD. Oxidative stress affects a complex group of genes involved in inflammation, extracellular matrix turnover, coagulation and other developmental events (164). The majority of proinflammatory genes are considerably upregulated while VEGF receptor-2 is downregulated. These findings are associated with an increased influx of inflammatory cells, especially macrophages in pulmonary tissue. Exposure of premature baboons (162), neonatal mice (163, 165), rats (166–168) and fetal human lung organ culture (169) to hyperoxia results in progressive lung changes which closely resemble BPD. When macrophages obtained from preterm and term rabbits were incubated in 95% oxygen overnight, only "preterm" macrophages showed a significant increase in IL-1 and IL-8 mRNA expression and a higher intracellular oxygen radical content (170). In addition, hyperoxic ventilated premature baboons had increased oxidative DNA damage and decreased VEGF expression. A potential mechanism for the effect of hyperoxia on VEGF expression is an increased induction of p53, a transcription factor that represses VEGF gene transcription (171).

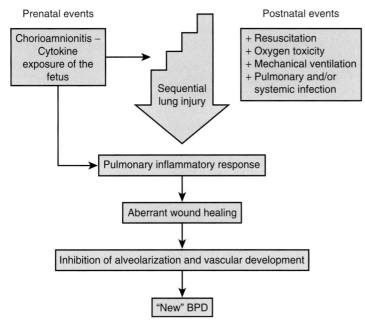

Figure 8-6 Possible pathogenetic sequence of pre- and postnatal events which induce lung injury and pulmonary inflammation in preterm infants with "new" BPD (173).

Hypoxia

Current knowledge about the role of hypoxia in lung inflammation is limited. A recent animal study demonstrated that hypoxia had a substantial effect on LPS-induced pulmonary inflammation by increasing the magnitude of lung injury. The hypoxic damage was characterized by increased expression of inflammatory mediators, excessive neutrophil accumulation and increased vascular permeability (172) and therefore represented a "second hit" injury. Pre- and postnatal factors inducing pulmonary inflammation are summarized in Figure 8-6 (173).

CONCLUSION

Increasing evidence indicates that bronchopulmonary dysplasia (BPD) results – at least in part – from an imbalance between proinflammatory and anti-inflammatory mechanisms, with a persistent imbalance that favors proinflammatory mechanisms. The inflammatory response is characterized by an accumulation of neutrophils and macrophages in the airways and pulmonary tissue of preterm infants and, moreover, by an arsenal of inflammatory mediators which may directly affect the alveolar capillary unit and tissue integrity. Besides inflammatory cells and cytokines, toxic oxygen radicals, various lipid mediators as well as potent proteases may be responsible for acute lung injury. During the last decade it has become evident that there are multiple pre- and postnatal events contributing to the development of BPD in preterm infants. Chorioamnionitis and cytokine exposure in utero, plus sequential lung injury caused by risk factors such as postnatal resuscitation, oxygen toxicity, volu- and barotrauma and infection, all lead to a pulmonary inflammatory response which is most likely associated with aberrant tissue repair. As a consequence normal alveolarization as well as vascular development seems to be inhibited in the immature lungs of very preterm infants, a feature which characterizes the "new BPD."

Despite some well-defined deficits in neutrophil supply and phagocyte function which result in a quantitative and qualitative dysfunction of this first-line inflammatory response, preterm infants are apparently able to mount a considerable and sustained neutrophil response to a variety of inflammatory mediators. The prolonged survival of neonatal neutrophils in areas of inflammation may contribute to the devastating and injurious effects of these cells on pulmonary tissues and airways. Besides neutrophils, pulmonary macrophages seem to be the primary source of various inflammatory mediators which are responsible for the initiation and the perpetuation of the inflammatory response. However, it must be recognized that the exact pathogenetic sequence of acute and chronic pulmonary inflammation is far from clear and has only partially been elucidated. The possible interaction between inflammatory cells and humoral mediators as well as regulatory aspects of inflammation and tissue repair are largely descriptive and speculative since the molecular basis of these events has not been fully defined. Moreover, most of the reported findings reflect associations of experimental clinical observations rather than causal relationships. In addition, numerous factors may have an impact on the results of the various experiments and clinical studies reported. These include the source of inflammatory cells, techniques of cell preparation and recovery of airway fluid, experimental design, differences in the sensitivity of various analytical tests performed and, importantly, a considerable heterogeneity between the babies selected for observational studies. Especially in preterm babies exposed to multiple postnatal risk factors, it becomes extremely difficult to define the importance of an individual event for the inflammatory process. Nevertheless, our current knowledge of the inflammatory mechanisms has opened up new avenues which will permit a deeper understanding of the pathogenesis of BPD in the future.

REFERENCES

1. Bland RD. Neonatal chronic lung disease in the post-surfactant era. Biol Neonate 2005; 88(3):181–191.
2. Vohr BR, Wright LL, Dusick AM, et al. Neurodevelopmental and functional outcomes of extremely low birth weight infants in the National Institute of Child Health and Human Development Neonatal Research Network, 1993–1994. Pediatrics 2000; 105:1216–1226.
3. Speer CP. Inflammation and bronchopulmonary dysplasia: a continuing story. Semin Fetal Neonat Med. 2006; 11(5):354–362.
4. Husain AN, Siddiqui NH, Stocker JT. Pathology of arrested acinar development in postsurfactant bronchopulmonary dysplasia. Hum Pathol 1998; 29:710–717.
5. Speer CP. New insights into the pathogenesis of pulmonary inflammation in preterm infants. Biol Neonate 2001; 79:205–209.
6. Speer CP. Inflammation and bronchopulmonary dysplasia. Semin Neonatol 2003; 8:29–38.
7. Carlton DP, Albertine KH, Cho SC, et al. Role of neutrophils in lung vascular injury and edema after premature birth in lambs. J Appl Physiol 1997; 83:1307–1317.
8. Jaarsma A, Braaksma MA, Geven WB, et al. Activation of the inflammatory reaction within minutes after birth in ventilated preterm lambs with neonatal respiratory distress syndrome. Biol Neonate 2004; 86:1–5.
9. Ferreira PJ, Bunch TJ, Albertine KH, Carlton DP. Circulating neutrophil concentration and respiratory distress in premature infants. J Pediatr 2000; 136:466–472.
10. Turunen R, Nupponen I, Siitonen S, et al. Onset of mechanical ventilation is associated with rapid activation of circulating phagocytes in preterm infants. Pediatrics 117(4, 200; 2):448–456.
11. Urlichs F, Speer CP. Neutrophil function in preterm and term infants. Neo Reviews 2004; 5(10):417–429.
12. Carr R, Huizinga TWJ. Low soluble FcRIII demonstrates reduced neutrophil reserves in preterm neonates. Arch Dis Child, Fetal Neonatal Ed, 2000; 84:F160.
13. Merritt TA, Cochrane CG, Holcomb K, et al. Elastase and α_1-proteinase inhibitor activity in tracheal aspirates during respiratory distress syndrome. J Clin Invest 1983; 72:656–666.
14. Arnon S, Grigg J, Silverman M. Pulmonary inflammatory cells in ventilated preterm infants: Effect of surfactant treatment. Arch Dis Child 1993; 69:44–48.
15. Groneck P, Goetze-Speer B, Oppermann M, et al. Association of pulmonary inflammation and increased microvascular permeability during the development of bronchopulmonary dysplasia: a sequential analysis of inflammatory mediators in respiratory fluids of high risk preterm infants. Pediatrics 1994; 93:712–718.
16. Kotecha S, Chan B, Azam N, et al. Increase in interleukin-8 and soluble intercellular adhesion molecule-1 in bronchoalveolar lavage of premature infants with chronic lung disease. Arch Dis Child 1995; 72:F90–F96.

17. Ogden BE, Murphy SA, Saunders GC, et al. Neonatal lung neutrophils and elastase/proteinase inhibitor imbalance. Am Rev Respir Dis 1984; 130:817–821.
18. Murch SH, Costeloe K, Klein NJ, et al. Early production of macrophage inflammatory protein-1a occurs in respiratory distress syndrome and is associated with poor outcome. Pediatr Res 1996; 40(3):490–497.
19. Speer CP, Johnston RB Jr. Neutrophil function in newborn infants. In: Pollin RA, Fox WW, eds. Fetal and neonatal physiology. Philadelphia: WB Saunders; 1998: 1954–1960.
20. Gessler P, Neu S, Nebe T, Speer CP. G-CSF-receptor expression on neutrophils of term and preterm neonates without sign of infection. Eur J Ped 1999; 158:497–500.
21. Ohls RK, Abdel-Mageed A, Buchanan G Jr, et al. Neutrophil pool sizes and granulocyte colony-stimulating factor production in human mid-trimester fetuses. Pediatr Res 1995; 37:806–811.
22. Kotecha S, Mildner RJ, Prince LR, et al. The role of neutrophil apoptosis in the resolution of acute lung injury in newborn infants. Thorax 2003; 58:961–967.
23. Nazeeh H, Vasquez P, Pham P, et al. Mechanisms underlying reduced apoptosis in neonatal neutrophils. Pediatr Res 2005; 57:56–62.
24. Koenig JM, Stegner JJ, Schmeck AC, et al. Neonatal neutrophils with prolonged survival exhibit enhanced inflammatory and cytotoxic responsiveness. Pediatr Res 2005; 57:424–429.
25. Kansas GS. Selectins and their ligands: current concepts and controversies. Blood 1996; 88:3259–3287.
26. Kim SK, Keeney SE, Alpard SK, Schmalstieg FC. Comparison of L-selectin and CD11b on neutrophils of adults and neonates during the first month of life. Pediatr Res 2003; 53:132–136.
27. Anderson DC, Abbassi O, Kishimoto TK, et al. Diminished lectin-, epidermal growth factor-, complement binding domain-cell adhesion molecule-1 on neonatal neutrophils underlies their impaired CD18-independent adhesion to endothelial cells in vitro. J Immunol 1991; 246:3372–3379.
28. Koenig JM, Simon J, Anderson DC, et al. Diminished soluble and total cellular L-selectin in cord blood associated with its impaired shedding from activated neutrophils. Pediatr Res 1996; 39:616–621.
29. Xia Y, Borland G, Huang J, et al. Function of the lectin domain Mac-1/complement receptor type 3 (CD11b/CD18) in regulating neutrophil adhesion. J Immunol 2002; 169:6417–6426.
30. Bruce MC, Baley JE, Medvik KA, Berger M. Impaired surface membrane expression of C3bi but not C3b receptors on neonatal neutrophils. Pediatr Res 1987; 21(3):306–311.
31. Weirich E, Rabin RL, Maldonado Y, et al. Neutrophil CD11b expression as a diagnostic marker for early onset neonatal infection. J Pediatr 1998; 132:445–451.
32. Abughali N, Beger M, Tosi MF. Deficient total cell content of CR3 (CD11b/CD18) in neonatal neutrophils. Blood 1994; 83:1086–1092.
33. Anderson DC, Becker-Freeman KL, Heerdt B, et al. Abnormal stimulated adherence of neonatal granulocytes impaired induction of surface Mac-1 by chemotactic factors of secretagogues. Blood 1987; 70:740–750.
34. Anderson D, Rothlein R, Marlin SD, et al. Impaired transendothelial migration by neonatal neutrophils; abnormalities of Mac-1 (CD11b/CD18)-dependent adherence reactions. Blood 1990; 76:2613–2621.
35. Little S, Dean T, Bevin S, et al. Role of elevated plasma soluble ICAM-1 and bronchial lavage fluid IL-8 levels as markers of chronic lung disease in premature infants. Thorax 1995; 50:1073–1079.
36. Kotecha S, Silverman M, Shaw RJ, et al. Soluble L-selectin concentrations in bronchoalveolar fluid obtained from infants who develop chronic lung disease. Arch Dis Child 1998; 78:F143–F147.
37. Ramsay PL, O'Brian Smith E, Hegemier S, et al. Early clinical markers for the development of bronchopulmonary dysplasia: soluble E-selectin and ICAM-1. Pediatrics 1998; 102:927–932.
38. Kim BI, Lee HE, Choi CW, et al. Increase in cord blood soluble E-selectin and tracheal aspirate neutrophils at birth and the development of new bronchopulmonary dysplasia. J Perinat Med 2004; 32(3):282–287.
39. Ballabh P, Simm M, Kumari J, et al. Neutrophil and monocyte adhesion molecules in bronchopulmonary dysplasia, and effects of corticosteroids. Arch Dis Child Fetal Neonatal Ed 2004; 89:F76–F83.
40. D'Alquen D, Kramer BW, Seidenspinner S, et al. Activation of umbilical cord endothelial cells and fetal inflammatory response in preterm infants with chorioamnionitis and funisitis. Pediatr Res 2005; 57:263–269.
41. Krause PJ, Herson VC, Boutin-Lebowitz J, et al. Polymorphonuclear leukocyte adherence and chemotaxis in stressed and healthy neonates. Pediatr Res 1986; 20:296–300.
42. Nybo M, Sørensen O, Leslie R, Wang P. Reduced expression of C5a receptors on neutrophils from cord blood. Arch Dis Child, Fetal Neonatal Ed. 1998; 78:F129–F132.
43. Weinberger B, Laskin DL, Mariano TM, et al. Mechanisms underlying reduced responsiveness of neonatal neutrophils to distinct chemoattractants. J Leukocyte Biol 2001; 70:969–976.
44. Bektas S, Goetze B, Speer CP. Decreased adherence, chemotaxis and phagocytic activities of neutrophils from preterm neonates. Acta Paediatr Scand 1990; 79:1031–1038.
45. Pahwa SG, Pahwa R, Grimes E. Cellular and humoral components of monocyte and neutrophil chemotaxis in cord blood. Pediatr Res 1977; 77:677–680.
46. Tono-Oka T, Nakayama M, Uehara H, Matsumoto S. Characteristics of impaired chemotactic function in cord blood leukocytes. Pediatr Res 1979; 13:148–151.
47. Yegin O. Chemotaxis in childhood. Pediatr Res 1983; 17:183–187.
48. Payne NR, Frestedt J, Gehrz R. Cell-surface expression of immunoglobulin G receptors on the polymononuclear leukocytes and monocytes of extremely premature infants. Pediatr Res 1993; 33:452–457.

49. Carr R, Davies JM. Abnormal FcRIII expression by neutrophils from very preterm neonates. Blood 1990; 76:607–611.

50. Clement A, Chadelat K, Sardet A, et al. Alveolar macrophage status in bronchopulmonary dysplasia. Pediatr Res 1988; 23:470–473.

51. Rindfleisch MS, Hasday JD, Taciak V, et al. Potential role of interleukin-1 in the development of bronchopulmonary dysplasia. J Interferon Cytokine Res 1996; 16:365–373.

52. Wang H, Oei J, Lui K, et al. Interleukin-16 in tracheal aspirate fluids of newborn infants. Early Hum Dev 2002; 67:79–86.

53. Inwald DP, Costeloe K, Murch SH. High concentrations of GRO-α and MCP-1 in bronchoalveolar fluid of infants with respiratory distress syndrome after surfactant. Arch Dis Child 1998; 78:F234–F235.

54. Groneck P, Oppermann M, Speer CP. Levels of complement anaphylatoxin C5a in pulmonary effluent fluid of infants at risk for chronic lung disease and effects of dexamethasone treatment. Pediatr Res 1993; 34:586–590.

55. Yi M, Jankov RP, Belcastro R, et al. Opposing effect of 60% oxygen and neutrophil influx on alveologenesis in the neonatal rat. Am J Respir Crit Care Med 2004; 170:1188–1196.

56. Kotecha S. Pathophysiology of chronic lung disease or prematurity. Biol Neonate 2000; 78:233–268.

57. Sparkman L, Boggaram V. Nitric oxide increases interleukin-8 (IL-8) gene transcription and mRNA stability to enhance IL-8 gene expression in lung epithelial cells. Am J Physiol Lung Cell Mol Physiol 2004; 287(4):L764–L773.

58. Aaltonen R, Heikkinen T, Hakala K, et al. Transfer of proinflammatory cytokines across term placenta. Obstet Gynecol 2005; 106:802–807.

59. Groneck P, Schmale J, Soditt V, et al. Bronchoalveolar inflammation following airway infection in preterm infants with chronic lung disease. Pediatr Pulmonol 2001; 31:331–338.

60. An H, Nishimaki S, Ohyama M, et al. Interleukin-6, interleukin-8, and soluble tumor necrosis factor receptor-I in the cord blood as predictors of chronic lung disease in premature infants. Am J Obstet Gynecol 2004; 191(5):1649–1654.

61. Won CC, Il Kim B, Kim HS, et al. Increase of interleukin-6 in tracheal aspirate at birth: a predictor of subsequent bronchopulmonary dysplasia in preterm infants. Acta Paediatr 2006; 95(1):38–43.

62. Kolb M, Margetts PJ, Anthony DC, et al. Transient expression of IL-1ß induces acute lung injury and chronic repair leading to pulmonary fibrosis. J Clin Invest 2001; 107:1529–1536.

63. Narimanbekov IO, Rozyiki HL. Effect of IL-1 blockade on inflammatory manifestations of acute ventilator-induced lung injury in a rabbit model. Exp Lung Res 1995; 21:239–254.

64. Shimotake TK, Izhar FM, Rumilla K, et al. Interleukin (IL)-1ß in tracheal aspirates from premature infants induces airway epithelial cell IL-8 expression via an NF-κB dependent pathway. Pediatr Res 2004; 56:907–913.

65. Cao L, Liu C, Cai B, et al. Nuclear factor-kappa B expression in alveolar macrophages of mechanically ventilated neonates with respiratory distress syndrome. Biol Neonate 2004; 86(2):116–123.

66. Cheah FC, Winterbourn CC, Darlow BA, et al. Nuclear factor KB activation in pulmonary leukocytes from infants with hyaline membrane disease: associations with chorioamnionitis and Ureaplasma urealyticum colonization. Pediatr Res 2005; 57:616–23.

67. Bourbia A, Cruz MA, Rozycki HJ. NF-κB in tracheal lavage fluid from intubated premature infants: association with inflammation, oxygen and outcome. Arch Dis Child Fetal Neonatal Ed 2006; 91(1):F36–F39.

68. Vancurova I, Bellani P, Davidson D. Activation of NF-κB and its suppression by dexamethasone in polymorphonuclear leukocytes: newborn versus adult. Pediatr Res 2001; 49:257–262.

69. Zentay Z, Sharaf M, Qadir M, et al. Mechanism for dexamethasone inhibition of neutrophil migration upon exposure to lipopolysaccharide in vitro: role of neutrophil interleukin-8 release. Pediatr Res 1999; 46:233–242.

70. Harju K, Ojaniemi M, Rounioja S, et al. Expression of Toll-like receptor 4 and endotoxin responsiveness in mice during perinatal period. Pediatr Res 2005; 57:644–648.

71. Levy O, Zarember KA, Roy RM, et al. Selective impairment of TLR-mediated innate immunity in human newborns: neonatal blood plasma reduces monocyte TNF-α induction by bacterial lipopeptides, lipopolysaccharide, and imiquimod, but preserves the response to R-848. J Immunol 2004; 173:4627–4634.

72. Viemann D, Dubbel G, Schleifenbaum S, et al. Expression of Toll-like receptors in neonatal sepsis. Pediatr Res 2005; 58:654–659.

73. Murch SH, Costeloe K, Klein NJ, et al. Mucosal tumor necrosis factor-α production and extensive disruption of sulfated glycosaminglycans begin within hours of birth in neonatal respiratory distress syndrome. Pediatr Res 1996; 40:484–489.

74. Schmidt B, Cao L, Mackensen-Haen S, et al. Chorioamnionitis and inflammation of the fetal lung. Am J Obstet Gynecol 2001; 185(1):173–177.

75. Jones CA, Cayabyab RG, Kwong KY, et al. Undetectable interleukin (IL)-10 and persistent IL-8 expression early in hyaline membrane disease: a possible developmental basis for the predisposition to chronic lung inflammation in preterm newborns. Pediatr Res 1996; 39:966–975.

76. Kakkera DK, Siddiq MM, Parton LA. Interleukin-1 balance in the lungs of preterm infants who develop bronchopulmonary dysplasia. Biol Neonate 2004; 87(2):82–90.

77. Baier RJ, Loggins J, Kruger TE. Interleukin-4 and 13 concentrations in infants at risk to develop bronchopulmonary dysplasia. BMC Pediatr 2003; 3(1):8.

78. Jonsson B, Li YH, Noack G, et al. Down regulatory cytokines in tracheobronchial aspirate fluid from infants with chronic lung disease of prematurity. Acta Paediatr 2000; 89(11):1375–1380.

79. Nakatani-Okuda A, Ueda H, Kashiwamura SI, et al. Protection against bleomycin-induced lung injury by IL-18 in mice. Am J Physiol Lung Cell Mol Physiol 2005; 289(2):L280–L287.

80. Kwong KYC, Jones CA, Cayabyab R, et al. The effects of IL-10 on proinflammatory cytokine expression (IL-1ß and IL-8) in hyaline membrane disease (HMD). Clin Immunol Immunopathol 1998; 88:105–113.

81. Welty SE. CC10 administration to premature infants: in search of the "silver bullet" to prevent lung inflammation. Pediatr Res 2005; 58(1):7–9.

82. Miller TL, Shashikant BN, Pilan AL, et al. Effects of an intratracheally delivered anti-inflammatory protein (rhCC10) on physiological and lung structural indices in a juvenile model of acute lung injury. Biol Neonate 2005; 89(3):159–170.

83. Levine C, Gewolb IH, Allen K, et al. The safety, pharmacokinetics and anti-inflammatory effects of intratracheal recombinant human Clara cell protein in premature infants with respiratory distress syndrome. Pediatr Res 2005; 58(1):15–21.

84. Gahr M, Schulze M, Scheffczyk D, et al. Diminished release of lactoferrin from polymorphonuclear leukocytes of human neonates. Acta Haematol 1987; 77:90–94.

85. Merritt TA, Stuard ID, Puccia J, et al. Newborn tracheal aspirate cytology: classification during respiratory distress syndrome and bronchopulmonary dysplasia. J Pediatr 1981; 98:949–956.

86. Speer CP, Ruess D, Harms K, et al. Neutrophil elastase and acute pulmonary damage in neonates with severe respiratory distress syndrome. Pediatrics 1993; 91:794–799.

87. Bland RD. Neonatal chronic lung disease in the post-surfactant era. Biol Neonate 2005; 88(3):181–191.

88. Pierce RA, Albertine KH, Starcher BC, et al. Chronic lung injury in preterm lambs: disordered pulmonary elastin deposition. Am J Physiol 1997; 272 L452–L460.

89. Alnahhas MH, Karathanasis P, Martich Kriss V, et al. Elevated laminin concentrations in lung secretions of preterm infants supported by mechanical ventilation are correlated with radiographic abnormalities. J Pediatr 1997; 131:555–560.

90. Juul SE, Kinsella MG, Jackson JC, et al. Changes in hyaluronan deposition during early respiratory distress syndrome in premature monkeys. Pediatr Res 1994; 35:238–243.

91. Murch SH, MacDonald TT, Walker-Smith JA, et al. Disruption of sulphated glycosaminoglycans in intestinal inflammation. Lancet 1993; 341:711–714.

92. Altiok O, Ysumatsu R, Bingol-Karakoc G. Imbalance between cysteine proteases and inhibitors in a baboon model of bronchopulmonary dysplasia. Am J Respir Crit Care Med 2006; 173(3):318–326.

93. Schock BC, Sweet DG, Ennis M, et al. Oxidative stress and increased type-IV collagenase levels in bronchoalveolar lavage fluid from newborn babies. Pediatr Res 2001; 50(1):29–33.

94. Cederquist K, Sorsa T, Tervahartiala T, et al. Matrix metalloproteinases-2, -8, and -9 and TIMP-2 in tracheal aspirates from preterm infants with respiratory distress. Pediatrics 2001; 108:686–692.

95. Curley AE, Sweet DG, MacMahon KJ, et al. Chorioamnionitis increases matrix metalloproteinase-8 concentrations in bronchoalveolar lavage fluid from preterm babies. Arch Dis Child Fetal Neonatal Ed 2004; 89:F61–F64.

96. Masumoto K, de Rooij JD, Suita S, et al. Expression of matrix metalloproteinases and tissue inhibitors of metalloproteinases during normal human pulmonary development. Histopathology 2005; 47(4):410–419.

97. Miller TL, Touch SM, Shaffer TH. Matrix metalloproteinase and tissue inhibitor of matrix metalloproteinase expression profiles in tracheal aspirates do not adequately reflect tracheal or lung tissue profiles in neonatal respiratory distress: observations from an animal model. Pediatr Crit Care Med 2006; 7:63–69.

98. Cederqvist K, Haglund CAJ, Heikkilä P, et al. High expression of pulmonary proteinase-activated receptor 2 in acute and chronic lung injury in preterm infants. Pediatr Res 2005; 57:831–836.

99. Speer CP, Ambruso DR, Grimsley JA, Johnston RB. Oxidative metabolism in cord blood monocytes and monocyte-derived macrophages. Infect Immun 1985; 50(3):919–921.

100. Drossou V, Kanakoudi F, Tzimuoli V, et al. Impact of prematurity, stress and sepsis on neutrophil respiratory burst activity on neonates. Biol Neonate 1997; 72:201–209.

101. Yang RB, Mark MR, Gurney AL, Godowski PJ. Signaling events induced by lipopolysaccharide-activated Toll-like receptor 2. J Immunol 1999; 163:639–643.

102. Matsuoka T. A sedative effect of dopamine on the respiratory burst in neonatal polymorphonuclear leukocytes. Pediatr Res 1990; 28:24–27.

103. Henneke P, Osmers I, Bauer K, et al. Impaired CD14-dependent and independent response of polymorphonuclear leukocytes in preterm infants. J Perinatol Med 2003; 31:176–183.

104. Qing G, Howelett S, Bortolussi R. Lipopolysaccharide binding proteins on polymorphonuclear leukocytes: Comparison of adult and neonatal cells. Infect Immun 1996; 64:4638–4642.

105. Pagano A, Barazzone-Argiroffo C. Alveolar cell death in hyperoxia-induced lung injury. Ann N Y Acad Sci 6, 2003; 1010:405–416.

106. Saugstad OD. Bronchopulmonary dysplasia and oxidative stress: are we closer to an understanding of the pathogenesis of BPD? Acta Paediatr 1997; 86:1277–1282.

107. Saugstad OD. Oxidative stress in the newborn – a 30 years perspective. Biol Neonate 2005; 88(3):228–236.

108. Gerber CE, Bruchelt G, Stegmann H, et al. Presence of bleomycin-detectable free iron in the alveolar system of preterm infants. Biochem Biophys Res Commun 1999; 257:218–222.

109. Speer CP, Pabst M, Hedegaard HB, et al. Enhanced release of oxygen metabolites by monocyte-derived macrophages exposed to proteolytic enzymes: activity of neutrophil elastase and cathepsin G. J Immunol 1994; 133:2151–2156.

110. Kramer BW, Kramer S, Ikegami M, et al. Injury inflammation and remodelling in fetal sheep lung after intraamniotic endotoxin. Am J Physiol Lung Cell Mol Physiol 2002; 283:L452–L459.

111. Collard KJ, Godeck S, Holley JE, et al. Pulmonary antioxidant concentrations and oxidative damage in ventilated premature babies. Arch Dis Child Fetal Neonatal Ed 2004; 89:F412–F416.

112. Bancalari E, Claure N, Gonzalez A. Patent ductus arteriosus and respiratory outcome in premature infants. Biol Neonate 2005; 88(3):192–201.

113. Davidson D, Drafta D, Wilkens BA. Elevated urinary leukotriene E4 in chronic lung disease of extreme prematurity. Am J Respir Crit Care Med 1995; 151:841-845.

114. Gaylord MS, Smith ZL, Lorch V, et al. Altered platelet-activating factor levels and acetylhydrolase activities are associated with increasing severity of bronchopulmonary dysplasia. Am J Med Sci 1996; 312:149–154.

115. Kojima T, Hattori K, Hirata Y, et al. Endothelin-1 has a priming effect on production of superoxide anion by alveolar macrophages: its possible correlation with bronchopulmonary dysplasia. Pediatr Res 1996; 39:112–116.

116. Mirro R, Armstead W, Leffler C. Increased airway leukotriene levels in infants with severe bronchopulmonary dysplasia. AJDC 1990; 144:160–161.

117. Niu JO, Munshi UK, Siddiq MM, Parton LA. Early increase in endothelin-1 in tracheal aspirates of preterm infants: correlation with bronchopulmonary dysplasia. J Pediatr 1998; 132:965–970.

118. Adams EW, Harrison MC, Counsell SJ, et al. Increased lung water and tissue damage in bronchopulmonary dysplasia. J Pediatr 2004; 145(4):503–507.

119. Brus F, Oeveren W van, Okken A, et al. Activation of the plasma clotting, fibrinolytic, and kinin-kallikrein system in preterm infants with severe idiopathic respiratory distress syndrome. Pediatr Res 1994; 36:647–653.

120. Brus F, Oeveren W van, Okken A, et al. Activation of circulating polymorphonuclear leukocytes in preterm infants with severe idiopathic respiratory distress syndrome. Pediatr Res 1996; 39:456–463.

121. Saugstad OD, Buo L, Johansen HT, et al. Activation of the plasma kallikrein-kinin system in respiratory distress syndrome. Pediatr Res 1992; 32:431–435.

122. Jaarsma AS, Braaksma MA, Geven WB, et al. Early activation of inflammation and clotting in the preterm lamb with neonatal RDS. Comparison of conventional ventilation and high frequency oscillatory ventilation. Pediatr Res 2001; 50:650–657.

123. Nupponen I, Pesonen E, Andersson S, et al. Neutrophil activation in preterm infants who have respiratory distress syndrome. Pediatrics 2002; 110:36–41.

124. Sitaru AG, Holzhauer S, Speer CP, et al. Neonatal platelets from cord blood and peripheral blood. Platelets 2005; 16(3–4):203–210.

125. Bartram U, Speer CP. The role of transforming growth factor ß in lung development and disease. Chest 2004; 125:754–765.

126. Sime PJ, Marr RA, Gauldie D, et al. Transfer of tumor necrosis factor-α to rat lung induces severe pulmonary inflammation and patchy interstitial fibrogenesis with induction of transforming growth factor-ß1 and myofibroblasts. Am J Pathol 1998; 153:825–832.

127. Adcock KG, Martin J, Loggins J, et al. Elevated platelet derived growth factor-BB concentrations in premature neonates who develop chronic lung disease. BMC Pediatr 2004; 4:10.

128. Kotecha S, Wangoo A, Silverman M, et al. Increase in the concentration of transforming growth factor-ß1 in bronchoalveolar lavage fluid before the development of chronic lung disease of prematurity. J Pediatr 1996; 128:464–469.

129. Lecart C, Cayabyab R, Bockley S, et al. Bioactive transforming growth factor-ß in the lungs of extremely low birthweight neonates predicts the need for home oxygen supplementation. Biol Neonate 2000; 77:217–223.

130. Jónsson B, Li Y-H, Noack G, et al. Downregulatory cytokines in tracheobronchial aspirate fluid from infants with chronic lung disease of prematurity. Acta Paediatr 2000; 89:1375–1380.

131. Kunzmann S, Kramer BW, Jobe AH, et al. Bedeutung von transforming growth factor (TGF-beta) und connective tissue factor (CTGF) in der Pathogenese der bronchopulmonalen Dysplasie (BPD). Z Geburtsh Neonatol 2005; 209:S2.

132. Danan C, Franco ML, Jarreau PH, et al. High concentrations of keratinocyte growth factor in airways of premature infants predicted absence of bronchopulmonary dysplasia. Am J Respir Crit Care Med 2002; 165(10):1384–1387.

133. Lassus P, Heikkila P, Andersson LC, et al. Lower concentration of pulmonary hepatocyte growth factor is associated with more severe lung disease in preterm infants. J Pediatr 2003; 143(2):199–202.

134. Asikainen TM, Ahmad A, Schneider BK, et al. Effect of preterm birth on hypoxia-inducible factors and vascular endothelial growth factor in primate lungs. Pediatr Pulmonol 2005; 40(6):538–546.

135. Tambunting F, Beharry KD, Waltzman J, et al. Impaired lung vascular endothelial growth factor in extremely premature baboons developing bronchopulmonary dysplasia/chronic lung disease. Investig Med 2005; 53(5):253–263.

136. Thebaud B, Ladha F, Michelakis ED, et al. Vascular endothelial growth factor gene therapy increases survival, promotes lung angiogenesis, and prevents alveolar damage in hyperoxia-induced lung injury: evidence that angiogenesis participates in alveolarization. Circulation 2005; 112(16):2477–2486.

137. Tsao PN, Wei SC, Chou HC, et al. Vascular endothelial growth factor in preterm infants with respiratory distress syndrome. Pediatr Pulmonol 2005; 39(5):461–465.

138. Balasubramaniam V, Maxey AM, Fouty BW, et al. Nitric oxide augments fetal pulmonary artery endothelial cell angiogenesis in vitro. Am J Physiol Lung Cell Mol Physiol 2006; 290(6):L1111–L1116.
139. May M, Marx A, Seidenspinner S, Speer CP. Apoptosis and proliferation in lungs of human fetuses exposed to chorioamnionitis. Histopathology 2004; 45:283–290.
140. Yoon BH, Romero R, Jun JK, et al. Amniotic fluid cytokines (interleukin-6, tumor necrosis factor-alpha, interleukin-1 beta, and interleukin-8) and the risk for the development of bronchopulmonary dysplasia. Am J Obstet Gynecol 1997; 177(4):825–830.
141. Gomez R, Romero R, Ghezzi F, et al. The fetal inflammatory response syndrome. Am J Obstet Gynecol 1998; 179:194–202.
142. Van Marter LJ, Dammann O, Allred EN, et al. Chorioamnionitis, mechanical ventilation, and postnatal sepsis as modulators of chronic lung disease in preterm infants. J Pediatr 2002; 140:171–176.
143. Groneck P, Götze-Speer B, Speer CP. Inflammatory bronchopulmonary response of preterm infants with microbial colonisation of the airways at birth. Arch Dis Child Fetal Neonatal Ed 1996; 74:F51–F55.
144. Cordero L, Ayers LW, Davis K. Neonatal airway colonization with Gram-negative bacilli: association with severity of bronchopulmonary dysplasia. Pediatr Infect Dis J 1997; 16:18–23.
145. Rojas MA, Gonzalez A, Bancalari E, et al. Changing trends in the edpidemiology and pathogenesis of neonatal chronic lung disease. J Pediatr 1995; 126:605–610.
146. Gonzales A, Sosenko IRS, Chandar J, et al. Influence of infection on patent ductus arteriosus and chronic lung disease in premature infants weighing 1000 grams or less. J Pediatr 1996; 128:470–478.
147. Wang EE, Matlow AG, Ohlsson A, Nelson SC. Ureaplasma urealyticum infections in the perinatal period. Clin Perinatol 1997; 24:91–105.
148. Yoder BA, Coalson JJ, Winter VT, et al. Effects of antenatal colonization with Ureaplasma urealyticum on pulmonary disease in the immature baboon. Pediatr Res 2003; 54:797–807.
149. Kotecha S, Hodge R, Schaber JA, et al. Pulmonary Ureaplasma urealyticum is associated with the development of acute lung inflammation and chronic lung disease in preterm infants. Pediatr Res 2004; 55:61–68.
150. Schelonka RL, Katz B, Waites KB, et al. Critical appraisal of the role of Ureaplasma in the development of bronchopulmonary dysplasia with metaanalytic techniques. Pediatr Infect Dis J 2005; 12:1033–1039.
151. Fleer A, Krediet TG. Innate immunity: Toll-like receptors and some more. A brief history, basic organization and relevance for the human newborn. Neonatology 2007; 92:145–157.
152. Muscedere JG, Mullen JBM, Gan K, et al. Tidal ventilation at low airway pressures can augment lung injury. Am J Respir Crit Care Med 1994; 149:1327–1334.
153. Dreyfuss D, Saumon G. Ventilator-induced lung injury: lessons from experimental studies. Am J Respir Crit Care Med 1998; 157:294–323.
154. Albertine KH, Jones GP, Starcher BC, et al. Chronic lung injury in preterm lambs. Disordered respiratory tract development. Am J Respir Crit Care Med 1999; 159:945–958.
155. Tremblay L, Valenza F, Ribeiro SP, et al. Injurious ventilatory strategies increase cytokines and c-fos m-RNA expression in an isolated rat lung model. J Clin Invest 1997; 99:944–952.
156. Thome U, Goetze-Speer B, Speer CP, et al. Comparison of pulmonary inflammatory mediators in preterm infants treated with intermittent positive pressure ventilation or high frequency oscillatory ventilation. Pediatr Res 1998; 44:330–337.
157. May M, Ströbel P, Seidenspinner S, et al. Apoptosis and proliferation in lungs of stillborn fetuses and ventilated preterm infants with respiratory distress syndrome. Eur Respir J, 2004; 23:113–121.
158. Copland IB, Martinez F, Kavanagh BP, et al. High tidal volume ventilation causes different inflammatory responses in newborn versus adult lung. Am J Respir Crit Care Med 2004; 169:739–748.
159. Ricard JD, Dreyfuss D, Saumon G. Production of inflammatory cytokines in ventilator-induced lung injury: a reappraisal. Am J Respir Crit Care Med 2001; 163(5):1176–1180.
160. Tsuchida S, Engelberts D, Roth M, et al. Continuous positive airway pressure causes lung injury in a rat model of sepsis. Am J Physiol Lung Cell Mol Physiol 2005; 289(4):L554–L564.
161. Vlahakis NE, Schroeder MA, Limper AH, Hubmayr RD. Stretch induces cytokine release by alveolar epithelial cells in vitro. Am J Physiol 1999; 277(1):L167–L173.
162. Coalson JJ. Experimental models of bronchopulmonary dysplasia. Biol Neonate 1997; 71:35–38.
163. Bonikos DS, Bensch KG, Ludwin SK, et al. Oxygen toxicity in the new born: the effect of prolonged 100% O_2 exposure on the lungs of new born mice. Lab Invest 1975; 32:619–635.
164. Wagenaar GT, ter Horst SA, van Gastelen MA, et al. Gene expression profile and histopathology of experimental bronchopulmonary dysplasia induced by prolonged oxidative stress. Free Radic Biol Med 2004; 36(6):782–801.
165. Warner BB, Stuart LA, Papes RA, et al. Functional and pathological effects of prolonged hyperoxia in neonatal mice. Am J Physiol 1998; 275:L110–L117.
166. Roberts FJ, Weesner KM, Bucher RJ. Oxygen-induced alterations in lung vascular development in the newborn rat. Pediatr Res 1983; 17:368–375.
167. Han RNN, Buch S, Tseu I, et al. Changes in structure, mechanics and insulin-like growth factor-related gene expression in the lungs of newborn rats exposed to air or 60% oxygen. Pediatr Res 1996; 39:921–929.
168. Chen Y, Martinze MA, Frank L. Prenatal dexamethasone administration to premature rats exposed to prolonged hyperoxia: a new rat model of pulmonary fibrosis (bronchopulmonary dysplasia). J Pediatr 1997; 130:409–416.

169. Bustani P, Hodge R, Tellabati A, et al. Differential response of the epithelium and interstitium in developing human fetal lung explants to hyperoxia. Pediatr Res 2006; 59(3):383–388.

170. Rozycki HJ, Comber PG, Huff TF. Cytokines and oxygen radicals after hyperoxia in preterm and term alveolar macrophages. Am J Physiol Lung Cell Mol Physiol 2002; 282(6):L1222–L1228.

171. Maniscalco WM, Watkins RH, Roper JM, et al. Hyperoxic ventilated premature baboons have increased p53, oxidant DNA damage and decreased VEGF expression. Pediatr Res 2005; 58(3):549–556.

172. Vuichard D, Ganter MT, Schimmer RC, et al. Hypoxia aggravates lipopolysaccharide-induced lung injury. Clin Exp Immunol 2005; 141:248–260.

173. Speer CP. Pulmonary inflammation and bronchopulmonary dysplasia. J Perinatol 2006; 26(Suppl 1):S57–S64.

Chapter 9

New Developments in the Presentation, Pathogenesis, Epidemiology and Prevention of Bronchopulmonary Dysplasia

Ilene R.S. Sosenko MD • Eduardo Bancalari MD

Changes in Clinical Presentation

Changes in Pathogenesis

Epidemiology

Prevention

Conclusion

The modern era of neonatology has witnessed the implementation of antenatal steroids, postnatal surfactant therapy and new modalities of respiratory and nutritional intervention. This has resulted in both the resuscitation and support of smaller and more immature infants, but more importantly, an increase in their ultimate survival. However, associated with the improved survival of these "micropremies" is the high risk of developing chronic lung damage, known as bronchopulmonary dysplasia (BPD). BPD continues to be one of the most common long-term complications of premature infants requiring prolonged mechanical ventilation. Its incidence varies among institutions, ranging between 15 and 50% of all infants who weigh less than 1500 g at birth (1). Four decades have elapsed since the original description of BPD by Northway in 1967 (2). During this time, its clinical presentation, evidence about its pathogenesis and epidemiology have changed. As a consequence, basic translational research has increased understanding of this process and has provided new possibilities for BPD prevention.

CHANGES IN CLINICAL PRESENTATION

With the introduction of mechanical ventilation to neonatal intensive care in the 1960s, the natural course of severe RDS in the premature infant was altered. At that time, mechanical ventilation brought about improved survival of premature infants who would have previously died; however, many survivors were left with the sequelae of chronic lung damage, not previously seen. Northway and colleagues described this chronic lung process in a group of surviving premature infants weighing > 1500 g at birth, all of whom had received *prolonged* mechanical ventilation with high airway pressures and high inspired oxygen concentrations.

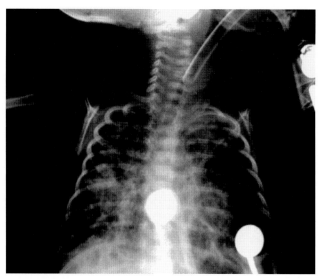

Figure 9-1 X-ray of infant with Stage 4 BPD (Northway classification) with cystic abnormalities, hyperinflation, and interstitial changes.

This process was attributed to multiple injuries to the immature lung, and was characterized by a progression of its clinical and radiological course through four stages, which culminated in severe respiratory failure with hypoxemia and hypercapnea, often with cor pulmonale, and with chest X-ray findings of increased densities due to fibrosis and large areas of emphysema, juxtaposed against areas of collapse (Fig. 9-1). Northway and colleagues, in 1967, gave a name to this chronic lung process: bronchopulmonary dysplasia (2).

Forty years later the severe classic presentation of BPD originally described by Northway is infrequently seen. Instead, the clinical presentation is more often that of a considerably milder form of lung disease, which appears in much smaller and more immature infants than those in the original description. Like their predecessors, essentially all present-day premature infants developing chronic lung disease have required mechanical ventilation early in life. However, one of the most striking differences in clinical presentation is the small size of these infants (400–1000 g). In addition, many of these infants, most of whom have benefited from antenatal steroids and/or postnatal surfactant, now present initially with only minimal or mild respiratory failure, and may require mechanical ventilation with *low inspiratory pressures and low oxygen* concentrations for mild RDS, pneumonia, apnea or poor respiratory effort. Unlike the original infants with BPD who required many days of mechanical ventilation with high oxygen, present-day infants often have weaned to room air within the first day or days of life. In fact, they often experience a "honeymoon period" at that time, where they usually remain on mechanical ventilation, though their need for supplemental oxygen is minimal (1) (Fig. 9-2). It is only after a few days or weeks that these infants begin to show a progressive deterioration in their lung function, characterized by an increase in ventilator and oxygen requirements and signs of ongoing respiratory failure. This deterioration is often triggered by bacterial infection and/or the development of a symptomatic patent ductus arteriosus (3). By this time, these infants have developed a chronic lung process: the "new" BPD. Radiographic manifestations of this present-day BPD differ substantially from the X-ray picture described by Northway. Instead of evidence of significant lung destruction resulting in fibrosis and emphysema (Fig. 9-1), radiographic findings now may range from diffuse haziness to areas of hyperinflation, non-homogeneity of lung tissue and fine or coarse densities extending to the periphery (Fig. 9-3) (4).

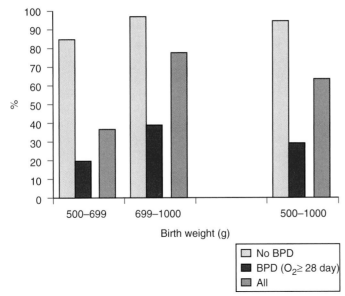

Figure 9-2 Proportion of infants breathing room air for more than one week during the first 28 days of life. (Fig. 4, from Bancalari E, Claure N, et al. BPD: changes in pathogenesis, epidemiology and definition. Seminars in Neonatology 2003; 8:67.)

Once lung damage has occurred, these infants often require mechanical ventilation and supplemental oxygen for several weeks or months. Their clinical progression is a slow one, with steady improvement in both lung function and chest radiographic appearances, gradual weaning from mechanical ventilation, followed by weaning from supplemental oxygen. However, after extubation, these infants

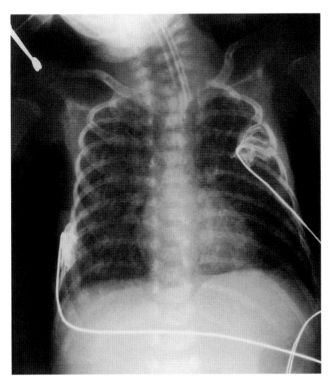

Figure 9-3 Chest X-ray of infant with milder BPD changes (diffuse haziness only). (Fig. 3, from Bancalari E. Bronchopulmonary dysplasia. In: Laurent G, Shapiro S, eds. Encyclopedia of respiratory medicine. Oxford: Elsevier; 2006:301.)

may have persistence of tachypnea and chest retractions and may demonstrate lobar or migratory segmental atelectasis secondary to airway damage and increased secretions, leading to obstruction. Most infants with BPD in the antenatal steroid/surfactant era, with this relatively milder form of lung disease, have resolution of the majority of signs and symptoms by discharge (1).

Nonetheless, a small number of BPD infants demonstrate a more severe process ($\sim< 25\%$ of all infants with BPD at our institution). Their lung picture may evolve into progressive respiratory failure and even death as a result of severe lung damage, pulmonary hypertension and cor pulmonale, signs of right heart failure, including cardiomegaly, hepatomegaly and fluid retention. In addition to developing significant lung parenchymal damage, these more severely affected infants may also develop severe airway damage consisting of bronchomalacia with subsequent airway obstruction, especially during spells of agitation and increased intrathoracic pressure and may have episodes of severe cyanosis with wheezing (5, 6). Infants with this severe form of BPD are at risk for acute pulmonary infection, either bacterial or viral, which may complicate their respiratory course, may increase the degree of lung damage and may even be the precipitating cause of death (7).

CHANGES IN PATHOGENESIS (FIG. 9-4)

Original Concepts of BPD Pathogenesis

The pathogenesis of BPD is clearly multifactorial. Specific pathogenetic factors for BPD were postulated by Northway in his original description, including: (i) respiratory distress or failure; (ii) prematurity; (iii) oxygen supplementation; and (iv) positive pressure mechanical ventilation (2). These same four pathogenetic factors are still felt to play a major role in the evolution of BPD today.

Immaturity of Lung Development

In relation to immaturity, BPD rarely develops, at the present time, in infants greater than 32 weeks of gestation. In fact, the incidence of BPD in premature infants requiring mechanical ventilation is inversely proportional to gestational age and birth weight (1). A possible explanation for the increased vulnerability of the extremely preterm infant relates to the immature state of lung development. For example, at 24 weeks of gestation, the lung is in the canalicular stage of development, progressing to the saccular stage by 30 weeks of gestation. Thus, the extremely immature lungs of an infant born at this time would be easily damaged by therapeutic interventions, such as mechanical ventilation and oxygen, which are required to ensure survival. As important, however, may be the possibility that premature birth plus therapeutic interventions could disrupt the normal progression of lung architecture, in relation to the development of alveoli and lung vasculature. This dysregulation of lung morphologic maturation may produce significant long-term sequelae and may explain some of the pathological changes described with the "new" BPD, including inhibition of acinar development and reduction in numbers of alveoli and capillaries, with a reduction in the gas exchange surface area (8, 9). It is of interest that de Felice and coworkers describe disordered oral mucosal vascularization in infants developing BPD, which they suggest could be an early marker for BPD, and which they contend is consistent with the hypothesis that early vascular abnormalities are important in the pathogenesis of BPD (10).

Other Concepts of BPD Pathogenesis

Two other pathogenetic mechanisms proposed by Northway, specifically, toxicity from oxygen exposure and trauma due to mechanical ventilation, are the focus of

BRONCHOPULMONARY DYSPLASIA PATHOGENESIS

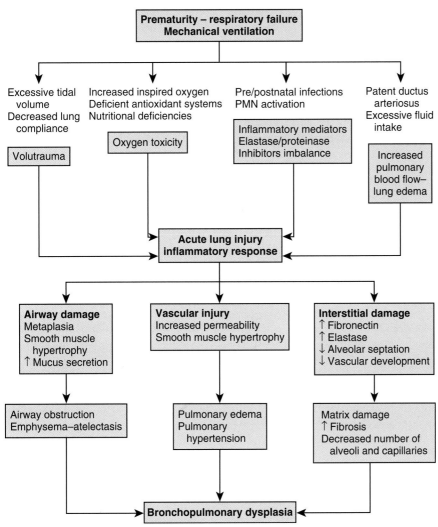

Figure 9-4 Complex interplay of pathogenetic possibilities for BPD. (Fig. 5, from Bancalari E. Bronchopulmonary dysplasia. In: Laurent G, Shapiro S, eds. Encyclopedia of respiratory medicine. Oxford: Elsevier; 2006:303.)

the chapter by Belik in this publication and will not be discussed here. However, other concepts have emerged in relation to BPD pathogenesis, including inflammation (alone or associated with infection) (also the focus of the chapters by Jobe and coworkers and by Speer in this publication), pulmonary edema as the result of PDA or excess fluid administration, nutritional deficiencies, predisposition to airway reactivity, and early adrenal insufficiency (1). The following discussion will further elaborate these concepts.

Inflammation and Infection

There are strong epidemiologic associations between infection/inflammation and preterm birth, including the observation that amniotic fluid samples with elevated IL-6 levels are predictive of preterm delivery (11). In addition, women who deliver extremely preterm infants have been found to have an increased likelihood of having bacterial vaginosis and/or elevated amniotic fluid pro-inflammatory cytokines compared to women who deliver infants later in gestation (12). What is surprising is that premature infants born to mothers with chorioamnionitis have initial evidence of accelerated lung maturation, with reduced incidence of hyaline membrane disease (HMD), but a paradoxical increase in the chronic lung damage of BPD. Watterberg and colleagues reported that only 33% of infants delivered to mothers with histologic chorioamnionitis developed HMD, whereas 67% of these infants subsequently developed BPD (13). In fact, elevations in a number of pro-inflammatory stimuli (including interleukin (IL)-6, TNF-α, IL-1β, and IL-8) in amniotic fluid sampled within 5 days of premature delivery were found to correlate with the development of BPD (as well as with periventricular leukomalacia and cerebral palsy) in these offspring (14, 15).

Though there is now substantial evidence that pulmonary inflammation is a major risk factor for the development of BPD, exactly what factors trigger and sustain the inflammatory response in regard to BPD remain as yet unknown. Although infection is a major trigger of inflammation, it is important to mention that inflammation may be triggered by factors other than those associated with infection, including oxygen free radicals, positive pressure ventilation, particularly with high tidal volume, and increased pulmonary blood flow caused by a PDA (16). These factors, either independently, or through the triggering of the inflammatory response, have all been implicated in the pathogenesis of BPD.

Infection itself, either antenatal or postnatal, is likely to be a major trigger for the lung inflammation that plays a role in the evolution of BPD. One antenatal infectious process that may be responsible for initiating inflammation in utero is the mycoplasma organism *Ureaplasma urealyticum*, which has been isolated from the lungs of infants who develop BPD (17). Kotecha and colleagues utilized reverse transcriptase PCR to determine the presence of *U. urealyticum*, group B streptococci and other organisms in premature infants with lung inflammation but without clinical or laboratory evidence of infection, who went on to develop BPD. They found the majority of these infants to have both evidence of significant lung inflammation and to have *U. urealyticum* in bronchoalveolar lavage fluid at day 10 of age, suggesting that this organism, acquired antenatally, may play a role in the progression of pulmonary inflammation to BPD (18). Coalson and coworkers, using a premature baboon model of BPD, performed intra-amniotic inoculation with *U. urealyticum*, and demonstrated that those colonized with *U. urealyticum* had persistent cytokine elevation in tracheal aspirate fluid and worse lung function than non-colonized controls (19). Nonetheless, a randomized trial of erythromycin failed to reduce the incidence of BPD, though it is not clear whether this intervention actually was able to eradicate the *U. urealyticum* from the trachea (20). Other studies suggesting that antenatal infection might be related to BPD pathogenesis are those that demonstrate increased cord blood IgM levels for viruses such as adenovirus, in infants who later develop BPD (21).

Circumstantial evidence also indicates postnatal infection as a risk factor for the development of BPD. The presence of nosocomial infections during the first month of life increases the risk of BPD in preterm infants requiring prolonged mechanical ventilation (3). In fact, Liljedahl and coworkers reported that the relative risk of BPD was significantly increased in premature infants with sepsis due to a common nosocomial organism, coagulase-negative staphylococcus (22). This risk is increased even further when the nosocomial infection occurs concomitantly with the presence of a PDA (3). Postnatal cytomegalovirus infection has also been associated with an increased risk of BPD (23), whereas respiratory syncytial virus infection is known to cause respiratory deterioration as well as re-hospitalization in infants with evolving or established BPD (24).

Fluid Administration, Pulmonary Edema, and PDA

Premature infants with excess fluid, whether related to excessive fluid administration or to lack of diuresis during the first days of life, are at increased risk of BPD.

Although initially reported almost 30 years ago (25), this has been confirmed in a recent retrospective analysis from the NICHD Neonatal Research Network, examining data of > 1000 very low birth weight (400–1000 g) infants, and reporting that those who either received higher fluid intakes or had less weight loss during the first 10 days of life had increased incidence of PDA and were at increased risk of BPD (26). An explanation for these findings is that excessive fluid intake with retention of extracellular fluid may increase symptomatic PDA, and result in interstitial edema, decreased lung compliance and respiratory compromise, necessitating increased oxygen and ventilatory support, thereby increasing the risk of BPD (27). As mentioned above, increased pulmonary blood flow resulting from excessive fluid intake and/or PDA could also initiate the inflammatory cascade by inducing neutrophil margination and activation in the lung, which could produce lung damage (28). Because of the role that the PDA might play in precipitating respiratory compromise or in inducing lung inflammation, a strong association has been reported between the presence and duration of PDA and the increased risk of BPD (3) (Fig. 9-5, Table 9-1 (29)).

Nutritional Deficiencies

Several studies have indicated that deficiency in vitamin A may play a role in the development of BPD. Reports have demonstrated that infants with lower vitamin A levels in the first weeks of life are at increased risk of BPD compared to those with normal vitamin A levels (30). This hypothesis is further supported by the similarities between airway epithelial changes seen with both BPD and vitamin A deficiency (31) and also by the evidence that administration of vitamin A in the first month of life has a protective effect against development of BPD (32).

Since ~ 80% of the accretion of magnesium occurs during the third trimester and because magnesium deficiency increases the susceptibility of cells to peroxidation and worsens inflammatory reactions, investigators such as Caddell (33) have suggested a possible role for magnesium deficiency in the pathogenesis of BPD. Although others have proposed a role for deficiency of another trace metal, selenium, an essential component of the antioxidant enzyme glutathione peroxidase, in risk for BPD (34), this was not borne out in a recent prospective analysis of selenium levels in preterm infants developing BPD (35).

Increased Airway Resistance

Because infants who develop BPD have been noted to have increased pulmonary resistance as early as the first week of age, it is possible that airway obstruction may be a pathogenetic factor in the development of BPD (36). The airway obstruction

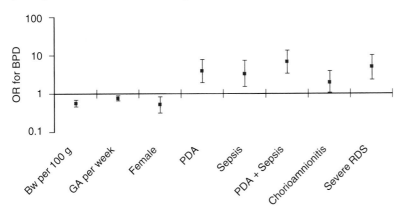

Figure 9-5 Perinatal and postnatal risk factors for BPD. (Fig. 4, from Bancalari E. Bronchopulmonary dysplasia. In: Laurent G, Shapiro S, eds. Encyclopedia of respiratory medicine. Oxford: Elsevier; 2006:303.)

Table 9-1	Odds Ratios for Development of BPD by Multivariate Logistic Regression Analysis (29)	
Factor	Odds ratio for BPD (95% CI)
Symptomatic PDA	6.2 (2.1–18.4)
Sepsis and symptomatic PDA (temporally related)	43.3 (6.3 to >100)
Late symptomatic PDA (after first week of life)	21.1 (5.6–80)
Duration of symptomatic PDA (per week)	3.5 (1.9–6.5)

may be due to bronchiolar epithelial hyperplasia and metaplasia and mucosal edema, and may also be related to pulmonary edema produced by PDA or excessive fluid administration. There may even be some association between increased airway resistance or hyperresponsiveness and vitamin A deficiency, since this finding has been described in experimental animals (37). Inflammation and inflammatory mediators may also be playing a role in the development of increased airway resistance or reactivity and BPD, with findings of increased leukotrienes and platelet activating factor (PAF) in airways of infants with BPD (38).

Finally, as yet unknown genetic factors may be playing a role in abnormal airway reactivity relating to BPD, since infants with BPD have been found to have a stronger family history of asthma compared to those without BPD (39). Because of the report by Manar et al. on an association between BPD and polymorphisms in the glutathione S-transferase P1 gene, it is possible that polymorphisms of this cytoprotective gene could decrease an infant's ability to handle oxidative stress and thus increase susceptibility to developing oxidative lung injury (40). A recent report examined genetic susceptibility to major neonatal morbidities in preterm twins, particularly BPD. When major covariates for BPD such as gender, RDS, birth weight, and treating institution were adjusted for, this study reported that 53% of the variance in liability to BPD is attributable to genetic factors (41).

Early Adrenal Insufficiency

Recent evidence suggests a role for early adrenal insufficiency in the development of BPD. Watterberg and colleagues found that low birth weight infants with lower cortisol values in the first week of life had an increased incidence of PDA, increased lung inflammation and increased risk of BPD (42). Although an initial clinical trial showed that early treatment with low-dose hydrocortisone increased survival without BPD (43), a larger clinical trial demonstrated an advantage of hydrocortisone therapy only in a subgroup of infants exposed to chorioamnionitis, and was stopped early due to excessive complications (spontaneous gastrointestinal perforations) in the early hydrocortisone-treated group, although this may have been related to an interaction between the hydrocortisone and indomethacin therapy (44).

Blood Transfusions

Several studies have linked early packed red blood cell transfusions and the risk of BPD. Silvers and coworkers found, by logistic regression, that the greater the number of packed cell transfusions received during an infant's NICU stay, the greater the risk of developing BPD (45). This clinical observation was studied mechanistically by the recent investigation of whether the lung could be a site of increased oxidative damage following blood transfusions. Malondialdehyde, a biochemical marker of lipid peroxidation, measured in bronchoalveolar lavage fluid from ventilated premature infants, was found to be elevated after transfusion, suggesting that blood transfusions may be a source of pulmonary oxidative stress, thereby increasing the risk of BPD (46). However, an alternate explanation for the findings of these two studies could be that the sickest infants are those who receive the most transfusions and are at the highest risk of BPD as well, and that no causal relationship exists.

In contrast, the administration of erythropoietin to experimental animals exposed to hyperoxia was found to have a protective effect on hyperoxia-induced lung injury, improving alveolar structure, enhancing vascularity and decreasing fibrosis, and in this capacity may be functioning as a growth factor rather than as an antioxidant (47).

Markers of BPD and Possible Clues to Pathogenesis

The literature is replete with various markers for BPD in preterm infants that promise diagnostic and predictive possibilities, and could, in addition, suggest additional pathogenetic mechanisms or confirm previously proposed mechanisms. One marker found to be elevated in plasma of infants with BPD was D-galactosidase (both α and ß), suggesting a possible role for lysosomes in the pathogenesis of BPD (48). Serum soluble E-selectin (an adhesion molecule involved with neutrophil attachment to endothelial cells) levels in the first 3 days were found to be higher in infants developing BPD, another indicator that inflammation is involved with BPD evolution (49). Endothelin-1, with features of both proinflammatory substance and potent vasoconstrictor, was found to be elevated in tracheal aspirate samples during the first week of life in infants progressing to BPD (50). Whereas levels of vascular endothelial growth factor (VEGF) were not found to be elevated in tracheal aspirates of infants developing BPD, levels of basic fibroblast growth factor (bFGF), important in mediating lung development, maturation, injury and repair, were found to correlate with BPD (51). Conversely, increased concentrations of another growth factor, important in enhancing lung repair, keratinocyte growth factor (KGF), were found in tracheal aspirate samples of infants who did not develop BPD (52). Other potential biomarkers for BPD include basement membrane biomarkers, which were lower in early serum samples of infants developing BPD, suggesting a defect in pulmonary basement membrane remodeling (53) and elevations in urine bombesin-like peptide, derived from pulmonary neuroendocrine cells, which may serve merely as a marker for lung injury (54).

Figure 9-4 provides a schematic summary of potential mechanisms for pathogenesis of BPD.

EPIDEMIOLOGY

In order to study the epidemiology of BPD, one must deal with several discrepancies. Most involve the major variations in BPD incidence which appear in the literature. For example, in infants with birth weights between 500 and 1500 g, the incidence of BPD (defined as oxygen dependency at 36 weeks postmenstrual age) in the different centers of the National Institute of Child Health and Human Development Neonatal Research Network ranged between 3 and 43% (55).

The variations in reported incidence of BPD relate to several issues, including differences in patient susceptibility amongst different populations of infants and differences in management from institution to institution, including frequency of antenatal steroid and postnatal surfactant utilization. Antenatal steroids have played an important role in the increased survival of the smallest and sickest infants who are at greatest risk of BPD. Surfactant therapy has resulted in a decrease in mortality from RDS but has not been shown to independently decrease the incidence of BPD. However, when death and BPD as endpoints are combined,

Table 9-2	Incidence of BPD According to Different Diagnostic Criteria among Extremely Premature Infants Born at UM/JMC during the Period 1995–2000 (29)	
Definition of BPD		**Incidence (%)**
On continuous O_2 during the first 28 days of life		5.9
On O_2 at 28 days of life		57.2
On O_2 for $\geq$ 28 days during hospitalization		47.1
On O_2 for $\geq$ 84 days during hospitalization		11.0
On O_2 at 36 weeks corrected age		25.0
On O_2 at 36 weeks corrected age and for $\geq$ 28 days		22.8

surfactant has been found to significantly increase the number of infants surviving without BPD (56–58). Similarly, changing survival rates among populations also influence BPD incidence, because as the survival of very low birth weight infants increases, so does the number of infants at risk for BPD (59).

Differences in gestational age of patient populations also can drastically influence the incidence of BPD. Since BPD incidence is inversely related to birth weight or gestational age, data from our institution indicate a 67% incidence of BPD for infants weighing between 500 and 750 g at birth compared to a < 1% incidence in infants weighing 1251–1500 g (1). As a reflection of the change in epidemiology of BPD, it is noteworthy that BPD today rarely occurs in infants born after 32 weeks, whereas the BPD described by Northway occurred in relatively mature infants (weighing 1500–2000 g at birth) (2). Another important explanation for differences in incidence relates to inconsistencies in the definition of BPD (discussed further in Chapter 11). Table 9-2 illustrates the widely varying incidences of BPD from our institution during the period 1995–2000 based on the application of different BPD definitions (1).

Another explanation for differences in BPD incidence relates to differences in base populations from which BPD incidence is calculated. The incidence will be different if it is determined in relation to *all* premature infants compared to only *surviving* premature infants or compared to only *ventilated* premature infants.

To further explore the epidemiology of BPD, a study of the relationship of perinatal and postnatal risk factors to the incidence of BPD was undertaken from the data of very low birth weight (500–1000 g) premature infants born at the University of Miami/Jackson Memorial Medical Center (UM/JMC) for the years 1995–2000. The results of the logistic regression analysis (with > 28 days of supplemental oxygen requirement during an infant's hospital course used as the definition of BPD) are seen in Figure 9-5. The data revealed the expected inverse relationship between birth weight and gestational age and the incidence of BPD, as well as the very striking association between PDA and sepsis individually plus their powerful combined influence on BPD risk (1).

PREVENTION

As outlined above, the pathogenesis of BPD is both complex and multifactorial. There is not, and probably never will be, a "silver bullet" representing a single modality which will completely prevent the lung damage of BPD. Instead the approach to successful BPD prevention should be one where many of the known risk factors are effectively addressed. Many of these potential protective modalities will be discussed below.

Antenatal Prevention

Preventing Preterm Labor/Acceleration of Lung Maturity

Since prematurity is an overriding risk factor for the development of BPD, the first strategy for BPD prevention actually begins before birth. The avoidance of preterm labor or postponing preterm birth by weeks, or even just days, with interventions that include treatment of urinary tract infection, cervical cerclage, or treatment of bacterial vaginosis, could potentially reduce the severity of RDS and the development of BPD (60). A recent report has demonstrated the efficacy of α-hydroxyprogesterone administered by weekly injection in preventing preterm labor in at-risk women (61). The administration of antenatal glucocorticoid hormones clearly has been shown to reduce the risk and severity of RDS, although the effect on BPD incidence has been less clear (62–64).

Preventing Antenatal Oxidative Stress

Another possible perinatal intervention that could potentially impact on the development of BPD is avoidance of oxidative stress around the time of birth. With intrauterine inflammation, usually due to chorioamnionitis, the infant is exposed to oxidative stress due to activated phagocytes, pro-inflammatory cytokines and accumulation of activated neutrophils in the lungs (65). Although without documented positive effects, potential therapies around the time of birth to reduce oxidant stress could include maternal antibiotic administration, early delivery to avoid ongoing inflammatory exposure, and the use of air rather than 100% oxygen for delivery room resuscitation (66).

Neonatal Interventions

Surfactant Therapy

The addition of exogenous surfactant therapy to the standard therapeutic regimen of premature infants born with lung immaturity was greeted with great promise; yet its effect on reducing the incidence of BPD has not been convincing. Although clearly reducing neonatal mortality, surfactant usage has not clearly reduced the incidence of BPD. Several large controlled clinical trials have not demonstrated a significant decrease in BPD incidence with surfactant administration. This may be due, in part, to its effect on improving survival of extremely ill infants who would have died without surfactant therapy, thus paradoxically increasing the number of surviving infants who go on to develop BPD. However, when the endpoints of BPD and death are combined, infants who had received surfactant were shown to have a significant advantage. It is important to note that very premature infants who are born with minimal lung disease and do not receive surfactant after birth but require prolonged mechanical ventilation for poor respiratory effort or apnea are still at risk for developing BPD (67–69).

Mechanical Ventilation

Once a preterm infant with immature lungs is born, some form of assisted ventilation with supplemental oxygen is usually required to sustain life. The goal in providing ventilatory assistance to a preterm infant at risk of BPD is to deliver these life-saving measures, but with the goal of attempting to avoid high airway pressures, high tidal volumes and high FiO_2, known to be damaging to the lung. One recent approach to this dilemma has been the early initiation of nasal CPAP, even in the delivery room. In fact, Wung and colleagues have used nasal CPAP as a primary ventilatory strategy and have reported a low incidence of BPD relative to comparable neonatal centers (70, 71), although this reduction in BPD from increased or early use of CPAP has yet to be substantiated in large-scale randomized controlled trials.

Another approach to ventilatory support for preterms at risk for BPD is that of "gentle ventilation," specifically the avoidance of high airway pressures and duration of positive pressure ventilation and acceptance of higher values for $PaCO_2$, or "permissive hypercapnea." Again, these potentially protective interventions have not been conclusively proven by rigorous clinical testing (72). Despite its potential to limit volutrauma, high-frequency ventilation has not been shown to be substantially protective in preventing or decreasing BPD in premature infants (73, 74). Other possible protective modalities of mechanical ventilation which require further investigation include proportional assist ventilation (75), volume-targeted ventilation (76, 77), and the addition of pressure support ventilation to SIMV (78). Finally, it is possible that studies may uncover a role for nasal intermittent positive pressure ventilation, either as a primary treatment modality or for use post-extubation, in protection against lung injury (79).

Oxygen Therapy

Although the toxicity of oxygen and free radicals is well known, evidence for BPD protection by reducing oxygen exposure is largely circumstantial. Two major trials have been conducted in preterm infants where randomization to different target oxygen saturation groups occurred. However, both of these studies were conducted when infants were several weeks of age, and BPD was already evolving. In addition, neither study looked specifically at primary pulmonary endpoints, especially BPD. In the STOP-ROP trial (Supplemental Therapeutic Oxygen for Prethreshold Retinopathy of Prematurity), infants with prethreshold ROP (post-menstrual age at enrollment ~35 weeks) were randomly assigned to what was called the "conventional oxygen arm" (target saturations of 89–94%) or a "supplemental arm" (target oxygen saturations of 96–99%). Although the objective was to determine whether high oxygen saturations would reduce progression to threshold ROP, which was not found to be the case, secondary outcome analysis demonstrated that pneumonia and/or exacerbations of BPD (e.g., increased need for oxygen, diuretics, and hospitalization at 3 months corrected age) occurred more in the infants randomized to high oxygen saturations (13.2%) vs. those receiving conventional oxygen therapy (8.5%) (80). The second trial examining different oxygen saturation targets in extremely preterm infants was designed to explore growth and neurodevelopmental outcome at 12 months corrected age. The two target oxygen saturations assigned in this study were what was called "standard" oxygen saturation (91–94%) and "high oxygen saturation" (95–98%). Infants were randomly assigned to one of these target saturation groups at 32 weeks postmenstrual age, 3 weeks sooner than study entry for the STOP-ROP trial, but still advanced enough in age to have established or evolving BPD. Although there were no significant differences in weight, length, head circumference or neurodevelopmental outcome at 12 months corrected age between the groups assigned to the two target saturations, those in the high saturation group had evidence of adverse pulmonary outcome (specifically, six deaths due to pulmonary causes vs. one death in the standard saturation group, longer requirement for supplemental oxygen, 40% increase in number of infants on oxygen at 36 weeks postmenstrual age, and 70% increase in infants needing home oxygen therapy) (81). The definitive question of whether extremely premature infants would have improved pulmonary outcome (decreased incidence or severity of BPD) when randomized to lower vs. higher target oxygen saturations from a very early age (first day or week of life) remains to be answered.

Exogenous Antioxidants

Because of the role oxygen free radicals are felt to play in BPD as well as data indicating immaturity of the pulmonary antioxidant enzyme (AOE) system in animals and infants delivered before term, studies have explored the efficacy of exogenously administered AOE in protecting against BPD. Although numerous animal studies have demonstrated significant efficacy in terms of lung protective effects from exogenously administered AOE, human studies have yielded disappointing results. A large randomized placebo-controlled trial of recombinant human copper/zinc superoxide dismutase (CuZn SOD) studied 302 premature infants (birth weights of 600–1200 g) with RDS and needing exogenous surfactant at birth. These infants were randomized to receive either intra-tracheal CuZn SOD or placebo every 48 hours until either extubation or 1 month of age. Treated infants showed no reduction in incidence of BPD at either 28 days or 36 weeks or death. However, at one year corrected age, follow-up data on 80% of surviving infants demonstrated a 36% reduction in wheezing episodes requiring bronchodilator medications, 55% decrease in emergency room visits and 44% decrease in subsequent hospitalizations (82).

Because of its relationship to glutathione, a major lung antioxidant, N-acetylcysteine (NAC), was administered during the first week of life in a randomized controlled trial of 33 premature infants with birth weights of 500–999 g. The specific endpoint, lung function measurements before discharge, was not improved in infants who had received NAC compared to placebo-treated infants, suggesting lack of protection against lung injury (83). However, glutathione levels may not have been elevated by this intervention.

Another substance with a potential role in protection against oxidative lung injury is allopurinol, an inhibitor of xanthine oxidase, an enzyme which catalyzes reactions in which superoxide radicals are generated. When 400 infants between 24 and 32 weeks of gestation were randomized to receive either enteral allopurinol or placebo for 7 days, no differences were found in incidence of BPD (84).

Because of animal studies showing that induction of cytochrome $P450$ by oxygen exposure may release free radicals that can produce oxidant lung injury, cimetadine, an inhibitor of cytochrome $P450$, was tested in a randomized controlled trial of premature infants to determine whether lung injury might be reduced. However, cimetadine, administered beginning at < 24 h and continuing for 10 days, was found to have no effect on severity of respiratory insufficiency at 10 days of age or on reduction of F_2-isoprostane levels in tracheal aspirates (a marker of oxidant injury); it is possible that cimetadine in this situation was not an adequate inhibitor of cytochrome $P450$ (85).

Other antioxidants have been examined in experimental animals and shown to have a lung protective effect. One substance, the catalytic antioxidant metalloporphyrin AEOL 10113, was tested in the fetal baboon model of BPD and found to produce partial reversal of abnormal alveolar structure and thickness associated with hyperoxia (86). Another antioxidant, deferoxamine, which functions as an iron chelator, decreased markers of oxidative lung damage and enabled partial preservation of lung architecture, in newborn rats exposed to hyperoxia (87). It is unknown whether these or other synthetic antioxidants will be tested for potential future application to the human premature infant with BPD.

Inhaled Nitric Oxide

The potential for inhaled nitric oxide in protection against BPD is a controversial one. Its theoretical role could be one of pulmonary vasodilatation, bronchodilatation and/or inhibition of lung inflammation (88). A single-site randomized placebo-controlled trial studied the effect of inhaled NO in the first week of life in premature infants with RDS. Results from this trial were a significant decrease in combined outcome of death or BPD in infants receiving NO (89). However, a recent multicenter trial was conducted, whereby 420 preterm neonates with respiratory failure despite surfactant therapy, < 34 weeks of gestation, weighing 401–1500 g at birth, were randomized early to receive either NO or placebo. Results showed no reduction in death or BPD in infants randomized to early NO treatment (90). Additional multicenter randomized controlled trials investigating this question have recently been completed but await publication (91, 92).

Fluid Restriction, PDA Closure

As discussed above, major pathogenetic mechanisms for BPD include excessive fluid intake and/or decreased early weight loss and prolonged PDA. Therefore, both fluid restriction and early closure of a symptomatic PDA are standard treatments in the care of the premature infant, with the goal of reducing BPD risk. Despite these therapeutic approaches, prospective studies of these interventions have failed to produce conclusive BPD risk reduction. Bell and coworkers conducted a meta-analysis of four randomized trials on fluid restriction and BPD and found that restricted fluid intake significantly reduced the risks of PDA and death; however, there were merely trends toward reduced risk of BPD (93). Similarly, meta-analysis of 19 controlled trials of 2872 infants receiving prophylactic indomethacin or placebo failed to show reduction in BPD despite increased PDA closure. However, in terms of analysis of indomethacin trials, BPD was not the primary endpoint of these investigations. In addition, many placebo infants received indomethacin later to close a symptomatic PDA (94, 95).

Nutritional Issues

GENERAL UNDERNUTRITION

Because of a number of concerns, including their critically ill state, attempts at fluid restriction, questions of the integrity of their gastrointestinal tract, and frequent glucose intolerance, extremely premature infants are often exposed soon after birth to days, and even weeks, of inadequate nutrition. Though not approached in prospective clinical trials, the influence of undernutrition on tolerance to oxidative lung injury has been inferred from studies on experimental animals. For example, when rat pups were exposed to conditions of undernutrition and then exposed to 7 days of $> 95\%$ O_2 exposure, these undernourished pups demonstrated only 44% survival vs. 73% for normally nourished pups; in addition, there were additive effects of conditions of undernutrition and hyperoxia on inhibition of lung DNA (96). Similar findings were reported for food-restricted preterm guinea pigs, which had decreased lung glutathione associated with decreased 72 h survival in hyperoxia (44% vs. 80%) (97). In addition, protein-deficient rats also showed increased median death time in hyperoxia (49–50 h vs. 58–69 h) associated with decreased lung glutathione (98). Therefore, these data would suggest that premature infants suffering from inadequate nutrition would have increased vulnerability to lung damage, and that attempts at providing adequate nutrition to these at-risk prematures could potentially decrease their chances of developing BPD.

LIPID NUTRITION

Although classical biochemistry teaches that increasing cellular polyunsaturated fatty acids (PUFA) increases cellular vulnerability to oxidative damage, an "alternate hypothesis" proposes that increased intracellular PUFA, if located in noncritical, nonmembrane sites, and if immediately replenished after autoxidation, could serve to scavenge excess oxygen free radicals, prevent their interaction with critical membrane PUFA, and actually protect cells from oxidative damage (99).

Evidence from experimental animals provided with increased PUFA diets and exposed to hyperoxia seems to support this alternate hypothesis. When pregnant rats were fed diets rich in various forms of PUFA, they gave birth to offspring with substantially increased PUFA in lung lipids and with markedly superior tolerance to hyperoxia when compared to rats born of dams fed regular diets and, even more strikingly, to those fed low PUFA diets (100, 101).

As a result of these animal studies demonstrating a positive effect of high PUFA intake on tolerance to hyperoxia, multiple clinical trials were undertaken to determine whether early high PUFA in the form of intravenous lipid (intralipid) could protect premature infants against BPD. At least five randomized, prospective clinical trials failed to demonstrate a protective effect of early intralipid on pulmonary outcome of ventilator and oxygen-dependent premature infants (102–106). One possible explanation for the inability to demonstrate a positive, protective effect against BPD by the administration of early intralipid might have related to the presence of toxic lipid hydroperoxides present in the lipid preparations used at that time, which might have obscured a protective PUFA effect (107). Since then, intralipid has been manufactured by a different process, thereby virtually eliminating lipid hydroperoxides. Therefore, the possibility remains that the present-day intralipid preparations, if administered early, might protect against the development of BPD; however, further investigation is required.

Despite the lack of positive findings from the clinical trials mentioned above, certain clinical observations do support a role for PUFA and BPD protection. One example is the report that initially higher levels of PUFA in tracheal effluent during the first day of mechanical ventilation were found to be associated with a reduced risk of BPD (108).

Inositol

Inositol is incorporated into cell membranes within the lung, serves as a precursor for synthesis of pulmonary surfactant and has been reported to be deficient in premature infants. Hallman and colleagues conducted a double-blind, placebo-controlled randomized trial of inositol supplementation in 221 infants with RDS between the gestational ages of 24 and 32 weeks. They reported improved survival without BPD in inositol-supplemented infants (109). Since that initial report, there have been two additional randomized clinical trials. When the three trials were analyzed together, results continued to demonstrate a significant reduction of death or BPD in infants who had received inositol (110). Despite these findings from meta-analysis, inositol supplementation is not part of the standard care of the very low birth weight infant.

Vitamin A

Vitamin A plays an important role in differentiation and maintenance of the integrity of the epithelial cells in the conducting airways. In addition, retinoic acid is important in alveolar development. The acquisition of vitamin A by the fetus is largely a third-trimester event (111). Thus, the very preterm infant is born without the vitamin A stores of a more mature infant, and studies have demonstrated a positive relationship between decreased plasma vitamin A concentrations during the first month of life and the development of BPD in the preterm infant (112, 113). These findings provided the basis for several double-blind controlled trials of vitamin A supplementation in preterm infants at risk for BPD, including the trial of vitamin A supplementation for the first 28 days of life to more than 400 infants (vs. > 400 placebo-treated infants) conducted by the NICHD Neonatal Research Network (114). This trial revealed a small, but significant reduction (55% vs. 62%) in the primary outcome variable, death or BPD, in vitamin A-supplemented vs. control infants respectively, without increasing mortality or neurodevelopmental impairment at 18–22 months (115).

Meta-analysis of seven trials showed reduction in death or oxygen requirement at 1 month of age and at 36 weeks post-menstrual age with vitamin A supplementation and concluded that despite clear evidence of efficacy from multiple trials, utilization of vitamin A appears dependent on the willingness of clinicians to utilize repeated intramuscular injections and the relative value placed on the modest reduction in BPD outcome (116). In fact, a recent survey of the practice of vitamin A supplementation revealed that most neonatal programs surveyed (69–82%) did not practice routine vitamin A supplementation to premature infants at risk for BPD. The conclusion from this survey was that despite data demonstrating efficacy for vitamin A in BPD prevention, neonatal practice was inconsistent in relation to practicing evidence-based medicine (117).

Reduction of Lung Inflammation

CORTICOSTEROIDS

Several strategies have been explored in an attempt to reduce the risk of BPD by reducing pulmonary inflammation. One extremely controversial anti-inflammatory modality that has received significant attention is postnatal corticosteroids. Reviews of numerous studies of postnatal treatment with corticosteroids have grouped the trials on the basis of age at start of corticosteroid administration, i.e., "early" (< 96 h), "moderately early" (7–14 days) and "delayed" (> 3 weeks). These meta-analyses have demonstrated a significant reduction of BPD, defined as oxygen dependence at 36 weeks post-conceptional age, for all three steroid treatment strategies. In addition, steroid-treated infants were extubated earlier than controls and were less likely to be treated with late postnatal steroids. However, associated with the reduction in BPD in several trials was evidence of abnormal neurodevelopmental outcome (118–120). For example, in the early steroid-treated neonates, the risk of cerebral palsy was approximately double that of infants who did not receive steroids. As described by Grier and Halliday, for every 100 babies receiving early steroids, BPD would be prevented in 10 at the expense of an additional 6 infants with gastrointestinal hemorrhage, 12 infants with cerebral palsy and 14 with abnormal follow-up neurological exam (121). Because of this unfavorable risk:benefit ratio, corticosteroids, administered either *early* or *moderately early*, are not an accepted approach to BPD prevention. However, because of lack of evidence of poor neurodevelopmental outcome when steroids are administered after 2–3 weeks of life, the late use of steroids in BPD prevention still remains a possibility, requiring further focused investigation. A recent follow-up study of children at 7 years of age who had received systemic dexamethasone at > 15 days of age failed to show differences in cognitive function, disability rates or cerebral palsy in those who had received dexamethasone vs. inhaled budesonide. In fact, this study failed to show differences at 7 years even in the infants receiving dexamethasone at < 3 days of age (122).

α_1-PROTEINASE INHIBITOR

Although not technically an anti-inflammatory agent, α_1-proteinase inhibitor functions to prevent proteolysis in the lung by forming a complex with neutrophil elastase. When α_1-proteinase inhibitor was administered in a randomized controlled trial for BPD prevention, no significant reduction in BPD incidence was apparent (123).

RECOMBINANT HUMAN CLARA CELL 10-kDA PROTEIN (CC10)

This secretory protein, produced mainly in pulmonary clara cells, is thought to have anti-inflammatory properties (with in vitro evidence of inhibition of neutrophil, monocyte and fibroblast chemotaxis, and suppression of cytokine release from lymphocytes) as well as the capacity to inhibit secretory phospholipase A_2, an enzyme which degrades surfactant and facilitates prostaglandin synthesis. A small, randomized placebo-controlled trial of CC10 administered by the intra-tracheal route to premature infants at risk for BPD ($n = 22$ infants) demonstrated a favorable safety profile with evidence of reduction in pulmonary inflammation (e.g., decreased cell counts and protein concentration in tracheal aspirates), though the study was small and not powered to determine decrease in BPD. Future studies with optimal dosing of CC10 may prove promising in terms of BPD protection (124).

Methylxanthines

Methylxanthines function as phosphodiesterase inhibitors, which play a key role in regulating intracellular levels of the second messengers cAMP and cGMP, and hence cell function. Caffeine is one of the methylxanthines which is frequently used to reduce apnea in premature infants. A recent randomized placebo-controlled multi-center trial of caffeine was undertaken to determine potential effect on long-term developmental outcome at 18–21 months. In this trial, infants were randomized to receive caffeine or placebo if determined by their clinicians to be candidates for respiratory stimulant therapy (e.g., for apnea or to facilitate removal of the endotracheal tube) during the first 10 days of age. When the short-term outcome of BPD, defined as the need for supplemental oxygen at postmenstrual age of 36 weeks, was analyzed, those who had received caffeine showed a significantly reduced incidence of BPD (OR 0.64 (0.52–0.78)). Because extremely low birth weight infants tend to remain ventilator-dependent during the first 10 days of life, they were not candidates for enrollment in this trial; yet these are the infants at highest risk for BPD (125, 126). Thus, additional studies would be required to determine whether early administration of caffeine to the most immature infants (prior to their ability to be extubated) would provide protection against BPD in this most vulnerable group.

Pentoxifylline is also a methylxanthine and phosphodiesterase inhibitor, which appears to inhibit multiple processes leading to hyperoxic lung injury, including influencing lung antioxidant enzymes, growth factors, inflammation, coagulation, and edema. Recent work in experimental animals has shown that pentoxifylline improves survival in hyperoxia, induces a protective lung antioxidant enzyme response, reduces fibrin deposition, and reverses downregulation of VEGF (127–129). Though these findings in experimental animals appear promising, the potential role that pentoxifylline could play in decreasing BPD risk will require testing in human premature infants.

CONCLUSION

It has been 40 years since the process of BPD was described and the term "bronchopulmonary dysplasia" became part of the vocabulary of those caring for premature infants. During these decades, the clinical process of BPD has evolved and has remained the focus of extensive investigation of pathogenesis and epidemiology. From these investigations have emerged possibilities and promises for therapies that could potentially reduce the risk or severity of BPD, thus having a major impact on the morbidity and mortality as well as long-term outcome of premature infants.

REFERENCES

1. Bancalari E, Claure N, Sosenko IRS. Bronchopulmonary dysplasia: changes in pathogenesis, epidemiology and definition. Semin Neonatol 2003; 8:63–71.
2. Northway WH Jr, Rosan RC, Porter DY. Pulmonary disease following respirator therapy of hyaline membrane disease: bronchopulmonary dysplasia. N Engl J Med 1967; 276:357–368.
3. Gonzalez A, Sosenko IRS, Chandar J, et al. Influence of infection on patent ductus arteriosus and chronic lung disease in premature infants weighing 1000 grams or less. J Pediatr 1996; 128:470–478.

4. Hyde I, English ER, Williams JA. The changing pattern of chronic lung disease of prematurity. Arch Dis Child 1989; 64:448–451.

5. McCubbin M, Frey EE, Wagener JS, et al. Large airway collapse in bronchopulmonary dysplasia. J Pediatr 1989; 114:304–307.

6. Miller RW, Woo P, Kellman RK, Slagle TS. Tracheobronchial abnormalities in infants with broncho-pulmonary dysplasia. J Pediatr 1987; 111:779–782.

7. Groothuis JR, Gutierrez KM, Lauer BA. Respiratory syncytial virus infection in children with bronchopulmonary dysplasia. Pediatrics 1988; 82:199–203.

8. Coalson JJ. Pathology of chronic lung disease of early infancy. In: Bland RJ, Coalson JJ, eds. Chronic lung disease in early infancy. New York: Marcel Dekker; 2003:85–124.

9. Husain AN, Siddiqui NH, Stocker JT. Pathology of arrested acinar development in postsurfactant bronchopulmonary dysplasia. Human Pathol 1998; 29:710–717.

10. De Felice C, Latini G, Parrini S, et al. Oral mucosal microvascular abnormalities: an early marker of bronchopulmonary dysplasia. Pediatr Res. 2004; 56:927–931.

11. Wenstrom KD, Andrews WW, Hauth JC, et al. Elevated second trimester amniotic fluid interleukin-6 levels predict preterm delivery. Am J Obstet Gynecol 1998; 178:546–550.

12. Watts DH, Krohn MA, Hillier SL, Eschenbach DA. The association of occult amniotic fluid infection with gestational age and neonatal outcome among women in preterm labor. Obstet Gynecol 1992; 79:351–357.

13. Watterberg KL, Demers SM, Scott SM, Murphy S. Chorioamnionitis and early lung inflammation in infants in whom bronchopulmonary dysplasia develops. Pediatrics 1996; 97:210–215.

14. Yoon BH, Romero R, Jun JK, et al. Amniotic fluid cytokines (interleukin-6, tumor necrosis factor-a, interleukin-lß, and interleukin-8) and the risk for the development of bronchopulmonary dysplasia. Am J Obstet Gynecol 1997; 177:825–830.

15. Yoon BH, Romero, Kim CJ, et al. High expression of tumor necrosis factor-a and intereukin-6 in periventricular leukomalacia. Am J Obstet Gynecol 1997; 177:406–411.

16. Pierce MR, Bancalari E. The role of inflammation in the pathogenesis of bronchopulmonary dysplasia. Pediatr Pulmonol 1995; 19:371–378.

17. Van Waarde WM, Brus F, Okken A, Kimpen JL. Ureaplasma urealyticum colonization, prematurity and bronchopulmonary dysplasia. Eur Respir J 1997; 10:886–890.

18. Kotecha S, Hodge R, Schraber JA, et al. Pulmonary Ureaplasma urealyticum is associated with the development of acute lung inflammation and chronic lung disease in preterm infants. Pediatr Res 2004; 55:61–68.

19. Yoder BA, Coalson JJ, Winter VT, et al. Effects of antenatal colonization with Ureaplasma urealy-ticum on pulmonary disease in the immature baboon. Pediatr Res 2003; 54:797–807.

20. Lyon AJ, McColm J, Middlemist L, et al. Randomised trial of erythromycin on the development of chronic lung disease in preterm infants. Arch Dis Child Fetal Neonatal Ed 1998; 78:F10–F14.

21. Couroucli XI, Welty SE, Ramsay PL, et al. Detection of microorganisms in the tracheal aspirates of preterm infants by polymerase chain reaction: association of adenovirus infection with broncho-pulmonary dysplasia. Pediatr Res 2000; 47:225–232.

22. Liljedahl M, Bodin L, Schollin J. Coagulase negative staphylococcal sepsis as a predictor of bronchopulmonary dysplasia. Acta Pediatrica 2004; 93:211–215.

23. Sawyer MH, Edwards DK, Spector SA, 1987 Cytomegalovirus infection and bronchopulmonary dysplasia in premature infants. Am J Dis Child 141: 303–305.

24. Smith VC, Zupancic JA, McCormick MC, et al. Rehospitalization in the first year of life among infants with bronchopulmonary dysplasia. J Pediatr 2004; 144:799–803.

25. Brown ER, Stark A, Sosenko I, et al. Bronchopulmonary dysplasia: possible relationship to pulmonary edema. J Pediatr 1978; 92:982–984.

26. Oh W, Poindexter BB, Perritt R, et al. Association between fluid intake and weight loss during the first ten days of life and risk of bronchopulmonary dysplasia in extremely low birth weight infants. J Pediatr 2005; 147:786–790.

27. Gerhardt T, Bancalari E. Lung compliance in newborns with patent ductus arteriosus before and after surgical ligation. Biol Neonate 1980; 38:96–105.

28. Varsila E, Hallman M, Venge P, Andersson S. Closure of patent ductus arteriosus decreases pulmo-nary myeloperoxidase in premature infants with respiratory distress syndrome. Biol Neonate 1995; 67:167–171.

29. Bancalari E, Claure N, Gonzalez A. Patent ductus arteriosus and respiratory outcome in premature infants. Biol Neonate 2005; 88:192–201.

30. Shenai JP, Chytil F, Stahlman MT. Vitamin A status of neonates with bronchopulmonary dysplasia. Pediatr Res 1985; 19:185–189.

31. Takahashi Y, Miura T, Takahashi K. Vitamin A is involved in maintenance of epithelial cells on the bronchioles and cells in the alveoli of rats. J Nutr 1993; 123:634–641.

32. Tyson JE, Wright LL, Oh W, et al. Vitamin A supplementation for extremely low birth weight infants. N Engl J Med 1999; 340:1962–1968.

33. Caddell JL. Evidence for magnesium deficiency in the pathogenesis of bronchopulmonary dysplasia. Magnesium Res 1996; 9:205–216.

34. Falciglia HS, Johnson JR, Sullivan J, et al. Role of antioxidant nutrients and lipid peroxidation in premature infants with respiratory distress syndrome and bronchopulmonary dysplasia. Am J Perinatol 2003; 20:97–107.

35. Merz U, Peschgens T, Dott W, Hornchen H. Selenium status and bronchopulmonary dysplasia in premature infants. Zeit Geburt Neonatol 1998; 202:203–206.

36. Goldman SL, Gerhardt T, Sonni R, et al. Early prediction of chronic lung disease by pulmonary function testing. J Pediatr 1983; 102:613–617.

37. McGowan SE, Holmes AJ, Smith J. Retinoic acid reverses the airway hyperresponsiveness but not the parenchymal defect that is associated with vitamin A deficiency. Am J Physiol Lung Cell Mol Physiol 2004; 286:L437–L444.

38. Groneck P, Gotze-Speer B, Oppermann M et al. Association of pulmonary inflammation and increased microvascular permeability during the development of bronchopulmonary dysplasia: a sequential analysis of inflammatory mediators in respiratory fluids of high-risk preterm neonates. Pediatrics 1994; 93:712–718.

39. Nickerson BG, Taussig LM. Family history of asthma in infants with bronchopulmonary dysplasia. Pediatrics 1980; 65:1140–1144.

40. Manar MH, Brown MR, Gauthier TW, et al. Association of glutathione-S-transferase-P1 poly-morphisms with bronchopulmonary dysplasia. J Perinatol 2004; 24:30–35.

41. Bandari V, Bizzaro MJ, Shetty A, et al. Familial and genetic susceptibility to major neonatal morbidities in preterm twins. Pediatrics 2006; 117:1901–1906.

42. Watterberg KL, Scott SM, Backstrom C, et al. Links between early adrenal function and respiratory outcome in preterm infants: airway inflammation and patent ductus arteriosus. Pediatrics 2000; 105:320–324.

43. Watterberg KL, Gerdes JS, Gifford KL, Lin HM. Prophylaxis against early adrenal insufficiency to prevent chronic lung disease in premature infants. Pediatrics 1999; 104:1258–1263.

44. Watterberg KL, Gerdes JS, Cole CH, et al. Prophylaxis of early adrenal insufficiency to prevent bronchopulmonary dysplasia: a multicenter trial. Pediatrics 2004; 114:1649–1657.

45. Silvers KM, Gibson AT, Russell JM, Powers HJ. Antioxidant activity, packed cell transfusions and outcome in premature infants. Arch Dis Child Fetal Neonat Ed 1998; 78:F214–219.

46. Collard KJ, Godeck S, Holley JE. Blood transfusion and pulmonary lipid peroxidation in ventilated premature babies. Pediatr Pulmonol 2005; 39:257–261.

47. Ozer EA, Kumral A, Ozer E, et al. Effects of erythropoietin on hyperoxic lung injury in neonatal rats. Pediatr Res 2005; 58:38–41.

48. Goi G, Bairati C, Massaccesi L, et al. Lysosomal enzymes in preterm infants with bronchopulmon-ary dysplasia: a potential diagnostic marker. Clin Chim Acta 1998; 278:23–34.

49. Ramsay PL, O'Brian Smith E, Hegemier E, Welty SE. Early clinical markers for the develop-ment of bronchopulmonary dysplasia: soluble E-selectin and ICAM-1. Pediatrics 1998; 102:927–932.

50. Niu JO, Munshi UK, Siddiq MM, Parton LA. Early increase in endothelin-1 in tracheal aspirates of preterm infants: correlation with bronchopulmonary dysplasia. J Pediatr 1998; 132:965–970.

51. Ambalavanan N, Novak ZE. Peptide growth factors in tracheal aspirates of mechanically ventilated preterm neonates. Pediatr Res 2003; 53:240–244.

52. Danan C, Franco ML, Jarreau PH, et al. High concentrations of keratinocyte growth factor in airways of premature infants predicted absence of bronchopulmonary dysplasia. Am J Resp Crit Care Med 2002; 165:1384–1387.

53. Aghai ZH, Areval R, Lumicao L, et al. Basement membrane biomarkers in very low birth weight premature infants: association with length of NICU stay and bronchopulmonary dysplasia. Biol Neonate 2002; 81:16–22.

54. Cullen A, Van Marter LJ, Allred EN et al. Sunday ME. Urine bombesin-like peptide elevation precedes clinical evidence of bronchopulmonary dysplasia. Am J Resp Crit Care Med 2002; 165:1093–1097.

55. Lemons A, Bauer CR, Oh W, et al. Very low birth weight outcomes of the National Institute of Child Health and Human Development Neonatal Research Network, January 1995 through December 1996. Pediatrics 2001; 107:1–8.

56. Kendig W, Notter RH, Cox C, et al. Surfactant replacement therapy at birth: final analysis of a clinical trial and comparisons with similar trials. Pediatrics 1988; 82:756–762.

57. Jobe AH. Pulmonary surfactant therapy. N Engl J Med 1993; 328:861–868.

58. Schwartz RM, Luby AM, Scanlon JW, Kellogg RJ. Effect of surfactant on morbidity, mortality, and resource use in newborn infants weighing 500–1500 g. N Engl J Med 1994; 330:1476–1480.

59. Parker RA, Pagano M, Allred EN. Improved survival accounts for most, but not all, of the increase in bronchopulmonary dysplasia. Pediatrics 1992; 90:663–668.

60. Goldberg RL, Rouse DJ. Prevention of premature birth. N Engl J Med 1998; 339:313–320.

61. Meis PJ, Klebanoff M, Thom E, et al. Prevention of recurrent preterm delivery by 17-a-hydroxy-progesterone caproate. N Engl J Med 2003; 348:2379–2385.

62. Van Marter LJ, Leviton A, Kuban CKC, et al. Maternal glucocorticoid therapy and reduced risk of bronchopulmonary dysplasia. Pediatrics 1990; 86:331–336.

63. Van Marter LJ, et al. Antenatal glucocorticoid treatment does not reduce chronic lung disease among preterm infants. J Pediatr 2001; 138:198–202.

64. Crowley P. Antenatal corticosteroid therapy: a meta-analysis of the randomized trials, 1972–1994. Am J Obstet Gynecol 1995; 173:322–335.

65. Saugstad OD. Bronchopulmonary dysplasia: oxidative stress and oxidants. Semin Neonatol 2003; 8:29–38.

66. Saugstad OD, Rootwelt T, Aalen O. Resuscitation of asphyxiated newborn infants with room air or oxygen: an international controlled trial: the Resair 2 study. Pediatrics 1998; 102:e1–7.

67. Collaborative European Multicenter Study Group. Surfactant replacement therapy for severe neonatal respiratory distress syndrome: an international randomized clinical trial. Pediatrics 1988; 82:683–691.

68. Jobe AH. Pulmonary surfactant therapy. N Engl J Med 1993; 328:861–868.

69. Schwartz RM, et al. Effect of surfactant on morbidity, mortality and resource use in newborn infants weighing 500 to 1500 grams. N Engl J Med 1994; 330:1476–1480.

70. Avery ME, Tooley WJ, Keller JB, et al. Is chronic lung disease in low birth weight infants preventable? A survey of eight centers. Pediatrics 1987; 79:26–30.

71. Van Marter LJ, Allred EN, Pagano M, et al. Do clinical markers of barotraumas and oxygen toxicity explain interhospital variation in rates of chronic lung disease? The neonatology committee for the developmental nework. Pediatrics 2000; 105:1194–1201.

72. Woodgate PG, Davies MW. Permissive hypercapnea for the prevention of morbidity and mortality in mechanically ventilated newborn infants. Cochrane Database Syst Rev 2001; w:CD002061.

73. Courtney SE, Durand DJ, Asselin JM, et al. High frequency oscillatory ventilation versus conventional mechanical ventilation for very low birth weight infants. N Engl J Med 2002; 347:643–652.

74. Johnson AH, Peacock JL, Greenough A, et al. High frequency oscillatory ventilation for the prevention of chronic lung disease of prematurity. N Engl J Med 2002; 347:633–642.

75. Schulze A, Bancalari E. Proportional assist ventilation in infants. Clin Perinatol 2001; 28:561–578.

76. Sinha SK, Donn, SM, Gavey J, et al. Randomised trial of volume controlled versus time cycled, pressure limited ventilation in preterm infants with respiratory distress syndrome. Arch Dis Child Fetal Neonatal Ed 1997; 77:F202–F205.

77. Cheema I, Ahluwalia J. Feasibility of tidal volume-guided ventilation in newborn infants: a randomized crossover trial using the volume guarantee modality. Pediatrics 2001; 107:1323–1328.

78. Reyes ZC, Claure N, Tauscher MK, et al. Randomized, controlled trial comparing synchronized intermittent mandatory ventilation and synchronized intermittent mandatory ventilation plus pressure support in preterm infants. Pediatrics 2006; 118:1409–1417.

79. B Lemyre, PG Davis, De Paoli AG. Nasal intermittent positive pressure ventilation (NIPPV) versus nasal continuous positive airway pressure (NCPAP) for apnea of prematurity. Cochrane Database of Systematic Reviews 2006; 2:CD002272.

80. STOP-ROP Multicenter Study Group. Supplemental therapeutic oxygen for prethreshold retinopathy of prematurity (STOP-ROP), a randomized controlled trial. I: Primary outcomes. Pediatrics 2000; 105:295–310.

81. Askie LM, Henderson-Smart DJ, Irwig L, Simpson JM. Oxygen-saturation targets and outcomes in extremely preterm infants. N Engl J Med 2003; 349:959–967.

82. Davis JM, Parad RB, Michele T, et al. North American Recombinant Human CuZn SOD Study Group. Pediatrics 2003; 111:469–476.

83. Sandberg KI, Fellman V, Stigson L, et al. N-acetylcysteine administration during the first week of life does not improve lung function in extremely low birth weight infants. Biol Neonate 2004; 86:275–279.

84. Russell GA, Cooke RW. Randomised controlled trial of allopurinol prophylaxis in very preterm infants. Arch Dis Child Fetal Neonat Ed 1995; 73:F27–F31.

85. Cotton RB, Hazinski TA, Morrow JD, et al. Cimetidine does not prevent lung injury in newborn premature infants. Pediatr Res 2006; 59:795–800.

86. Chang LY, Subramaniam M, Yoder BA, et al. A catalytic antioxidant attenuates alveolar structural remodeling in bronchopulmonary dysplasia. Am J Resp Crit Care Med 2003; 167:57–64.

87. Frank L. 1991. Hyperoxic inhibition of newborn rat lung development: protection by deferoxamine. Free Rad Biol Med 11:341–348.

88. Potter CF, Dreshaj IA, Haxhie MA, et al. Effects of exogenous and endogenous nitric oxide on the airway and tissue components of lung resistance in the newborn piglet. Pediatr Res 1997; 41:886–891.

89. Screiber MD, Gat-Mestan K, Marks JD, et al. Inhaled nitric oxide in premature infants with respiratory distress syndrome. N Engl J Med 2003; 349:2099–2107.

90. Van Meurs KP, Wright LL, Ehrenkranz RA, et al. Inhaled nitric oxide for premature infants with severe respiratory failure. N Engl J Med 2005; 353:82–84.

91. Kinsella JP, Cutter GR, Walsh WF, et al. Early inhaled nitric oxide in premature newborns with respiratory failure. PAS Late-breaker abstract: 2006; 1.

92. Ballard RA, Truog WE, Martin RJ, et al. Improved outcome with inhaled nitric oxide in preterm infants mechanically ventilated at 7–21 days of age. PAS Late-breaker abstract: 2006; 2.

93. Bell EF, Acarregui MJ. Restricted versus liberal water intake for preventing morbidity and mortality in preterm infants. Cochrane Review. In: Cochrane Library 2001; 3:CD000503.

94. Blakely ML, Kennedy KA, Lally KP, Tyson JE. Intravenous indomethacin for symptomatic patent ductus arteriosus in preterm infants. The Cochrane Database of Systematic Reviews 2002; 1:CD003479.

95. Schmidt B, Roberts RS, Fanaroff A, et al. and the TIPP investigators. Indomethacin prophylaxis, patent ductus arteriosus and the risk of bronchopulmonary dysplasia: further analyses from the trial of indomethacin prophylaxis in preterms (TIPP). J Pediatr 2006; 148:730–734.

96. Frank L, Groseclose EE. Oxygen toxicity in newborns: the adverse effects of undernutrition. J Appl Physiol 1982; 53:1248–1255.

97. Langley SC, Kelly FJ. Effect of food restriction on hyperoxia-induced lung injury in preterm guinea pig. Am J Physiol Lung 1992; 263:L357–362.

98. Deneke SM, Gershoff SN, Fanberg BL. Potentiation of oxygen toxicity in rats by dietary protein or amino acid deficiency. J Appl Physiol 1983; 54:147–151.

99. Dormandy TL. Biological rancidification. Lancet 1969; 2:684–686.

100. Sosenko IRS, Innis SM, Frank. Polyunsaturated fatty acids and protection of newborn rats from oxygen toxicity. J Pediatr 1988; 112:630–637.
101. Sosenko IRS, Innis SM, Frank L. Intralipid increases lung polyunsaturated fatty acids and protects newborn rats from oxygen toxicity. Pediatr Res 1991; 30:413–417.
102. Hammerman C, Aramburo MJ. Decreased lipid intake reduces morbidity in sick, premature neonates. J Pediatr 1988; 113:1083–1088.
103. Gilbertson N, Kovar IZ, Cox DJ, et al. Introduction of intravenous loipi administration on the first day of life in the very low birth weight neonate. J Pediatr 1991; 119:615–623.
104. Sosenko IRS, Rodriguez-Pierce M, Bancalari E. Effect of early initiation of intravenous lipid administration on the incidence and severity of chronic lung disease. J Pediatr 1993; 123:975–982.
105. Brownlee KG, Kelly E, Ng PC, et al. Early or late parenteral nutrition for the sick preterm infant? Arch Dis Child 1993; 69:281–283.
106. Alwaidh MH, Bowden L, Shaw B, Ryan SW. Randomised trial of effect of delayed intravenous lipid administration on chronic lung disease in preterm neonates. J Pediatr Gastro Nutr 1996; 22:303–306.
107. Pitkanen O, Hallman M, Anderson S. Generation of free radicals in lipid emulsion used in parenteral nutrition. Pediatr Res 1991; 29:56–59.
108. Rudiger M, von Baehr A, Haupt R, et al. Preterm infants with high polyunsaturated fatty acid and plasmalogen content in tracheal aspirates develop bronchopulmonary dysplasia less often. Crit Care Med 2000; 28:1572–1577.
109. Hallman M, Bry K, Hoppu K, et al. Inositol supplementation in premature infants with respiratory distress. N Engl J Med 1992; 326:1233–1239.
110. Howlett A, Ohlsson A. Inositol for respiratory distress syndrome in preterm infants. Cochrane Database Syst Rev 2000; 4:CD000366.
111. Widdowson EM. Chemical composition and nutritional needs of the fetus at different stages of gestation. In: Aebi H, Whitehead R, eds. Maternal nutrition during pregnancy and lactation. Berne: H Huber; 1980: 39–48.
112. Husted VA, Gutcher GR, Anderson SA, et al. Relationships of vitamin A (retinol) status and lung disease in the preterm infant. J Pediatr 1984; 105:610–615.
113. Shenai JP, Chytil F, Jhaveri A, et al. Plasma vitamin A and retinol-binding protein in premature and term infants. J Pediatr 1981; 99:302–305.
114. Tyson JE, Wright LL, Oh W, et al. Vitamin A supplementation for extremely low birth weight infants: National Institute of Child Health and Human Development Neonatal Research Network. N Engl J Med 1999; 340:1962–1968.
115. Ambalavanan N, Tyson JE, Kennedy KA, et al. National Institute of Child Health and Human Development Neonatal Research Network. Vitamin A supplementation for extremely low birth weight infants: outcome at 18 to 22 months. Pediatrics 2005; 115:e249–254.
116. Darlow BA, Graham PJ. Vitamin A supplementation for preventing morbidity and mortality in very low birth weight infants. Cochrane Database Syst Rev 2002; 4:CD000501.
117. Ambalavanan N, Kennedy KA, Tyson JE, Carlo WA. Survey of vitamin A supplementation for extremely low birth weight infants: is clinical practice consistent with evidence? J Pediatr 2004; 145:304–307.
118. Halliday HL, Ehrenkranz RA. Early postnatal (< 96 hours) corticosteroids for preventing chronic lung disease in preterm infants. Oxford: The Cochrane Library; 2001; Update Software: 3.
119. Halliday HL, Ehrenkranz RA. Moderately early postnatal (7–14 days) corticosteroids for preventing chronic lung disease in preterm infants. Oxford: The Cochrane Library; 2001; Update Software: 3.
120. Halliday HL, Ehrenkranz RA. Delayed (> 3 weeks) postnatal corticosteroids for preventing chronic lung disease in preterm infants. Oxford: The Cochrane Library; 2001; Update Software: 3.
121. Grier DG, Halliday HL. Corticosteroids in the prevention and management of bronchopulmonary dysplasia. Semin Neonatol 2003; 8:83–91.
122. Wilson TT, Waters L, Patterson CC, et al. Neurodevelopmental and respiratory follow-up results at 7 years for children from the United Kingdom and Ireland enrolled in a randomized trial of early and late postnatal corticosteroid treatment, systemic and inhaled (the Open Study of Early Corticosteroid Treatment). Pediatrics 2006; 117:2196–2205.
123. Stiskal JA, Dunn MS, Shennan AT, et al. α$_1$-Proteinase inhibitor therapy for the prevention of chronic lung disease of prematurity: a randomized controlled trial. Pediatrics 1998; 1011:89–94.
124. Levine CR, Gewolb IH, Allen K, et al. Safety, pharmacokinetics, and anti-inflammatory effects of intratracheal recombinant human clara cell protein in premature infants with respiratory distress syndrome. Pediatr Res 2005; 58:15–21.
125. Schmidt B, Roberts RS, Davis P, et al. Caffeine therapy for apnea of prematurity. N Engl J Med 2006; 354:2112–2121.
126. Bancalari E. Caffeine for apnea of prematurity. N Engl J Med 2006; 354:2179–2181.
127. ter Horst SA, Wagenaar GT, de Boer E, et al. Pentoxifylline reduces fibrin deposition and prolongs survival in neonatal hyperoxic lung injury. J Appl Physiol 2004; 97:2014–2019.
128. Almario B, Sosenko IRS. Pentoxifylline improves survival, decreases lung injury and augments catalase and glutathione peroxidase activity during prolonged exposure to hyperoxia in newborn rats. PAS Abstract 2006; 5168:10.
129. Almario B, Wu S, Peng J, Sosenko IRS. Pentoxifylline up-regulates lung vascular endothelial growth factor (VEGF) gene expression and prolongs survival in hyperoxia-exposed newborn rats. PAS Abstract 2006; 4132:8.

Chapter 10

What is the Evidence for Drug Therapy in the Prevention and Management of Bronchopulmonary Dysplasia?

Henry L. Halliday MD FRCPE FRCP FRCPCH
• Conor P. O'Neill MB BCh BAO MRCPCH

Diagnosis

Prevention

Treatment of BPD

Conclusions

DIAGNOSIS

Bronchopulmonary dysplasia (BPD) is a chronic disease of the lung primarily affecting about 20% of the preterm infants who need respiratory support with mechanical ventilation. In the post-surfactant era BPD has become more of a problem because of increased survival of very preterm infants. Furthermore, the spectrum of patients affected by BPD has changed since Northway et al. (1) published their classic description in 1967. BPD is the result of abnormal repair processes following inflammatory lung injury leading to remodeling of the lung (2). Inflammation may be initiated by a variety of stimuli including mechanical ventilation, oxidative stress and infection. The resultant neutrophil chemotaxis and degranulation lead to release of enzymes that cause proteolysis of lung extracellular matrix (ECM). Abnormal healing with remodeling leads to poorly compliant lungs with reduced capacity for gas exchange.

The modern milder clinical form of BPD, termed "new" BPD, is found in very preterm infants who survive following a gentler form of assisted ventilation. These infants have usually not been exposed to high mechanical ventilation pressures or volumes and high ambient oxygen concentrations, the major factors in the pathogenesis of "classic" BPD (1). In the search for a drug therapy to prevent or manage BPD it is important to consider the pathogenesis of this "new" form of BPD.

We will discuss current knowledge of the pathophysiology of BPD before addressing its management in three stages: (i) antenatal drug and management strategies aimed at preventing development of BPD, (ii) postnatal drug and management strategies aimed at preventing BPD, including those aimed at reducing lung injury or influencing airway remodeling, and (iii) those strategies aimed at improving clinical outcomes in babies with established BPD.

Pathology

The principal risk factors in the pathogenesis of BPD are lung immaturity, barotrauma and volutrauma, associated with mechanical ventilation, oxidative stress, prenatal and nosocomial infections as well as increased pulmonary blood flow secondary to a patent ductus arteriosus (3). However, the exact pathogenetic mechanisms of lung injury and repair are incompletely understood and are the subject of ongoing research. Coalson has recently reviewed the pathology of BPD (4). In "classic" BPD there are alternating areas of atelectasis and over-inflation, severe airway epithelial lesions, airway and vascular smooth muscle hyperplasia, extensive fibroproliferation and decreased internal surface area and number of alveoli. In contrast, in "new" BPD there are fewer and larger simplified alveoli, negligible airway lesions and variable airway smooth muscle hyperplasia, variable interstitial fibroproliferation, fewer and dysmorphic capillaries and less-severe arterial lesions. This is accompanied by a change in patient population to a smaller more preterm group who have been managed with more gentle mechanical ventilation and conservative use of inspired oxygen. It has been hypothesized that the "new" BPD represents an arrest of lung development at the time the fetus becomes an infant (5).

Normal Lung Development

Normal lung development occurs in four phases. The airways begin to develop from rudimentary lung buds during the pseudoglandular phase up to about 17 weeks gestation. Airways branching is completed and type II pneumocytes begin to appear during the canalicular phase, which finishes about the 26th week of gestation. The saccular phase of lung development begins about 22 weeks gestation when the walls of the air sacs begin to thin out and septate in preparation for the final stage of alveolarization. Secondary septae grow out from the primary septae beginning around 30–32 weeks gestation for the final alveolar stage of lung development, which continues well into the first decade of life. In neonatal intensive care units babies of gestational ages as low as 23–24 weeks gestation are cared for with a reasonable chance of survival despite the absence of alveoli. However, the stage of lung development is a major factor influencing outcome.

Prenatal lung growth is under the influence of many genetic, hormonal and physical factors. Glucocorticoid receptors are present in the lungs from as early as 8 weeks gestation during the pseudoglandular phase of lung development (6) and without endogenous glucocorticoids alveolar air spaces fail to develop (7). Thyroid hormones are also essential for normal lung growth and maturation (8).

The canalicular phase of lung development is marked by growth of capillaries and differentiation of type I and type II pneumocytes from undifferentiated epithelial cells. Vascular endothelial growth factor (VEGF) is a powerful inducer of endothelial cell proliferation and it promotes growth of blood vessels (9). Vascular development in the lung is closely linked to alveolar development and inhibition of vascular growth directly impairs vascularization (10). During early lung development the airways act as a template for the vasculogenesis of capillaries, defined as the organization of undifferentiated endothelial cells into vascular structures in the mesenchyme. During the canalicular phase capillaries form by angiogenesis. In this process endothelial cells proliferate and sprout from the previously formed vessels giving rise to new vascular structures. The dividing cells are in the existing capillaries and not in the existing mesenchyme. VEGF, which is involved in the vasculogenesis and angiogenesis, is expressed in bronchial epithelial cells early in the course of lung development but later expression is more localized in alveolar epithelial cells (11). It is strongly expressed at the tip of branching airways where it stimulates vascular growth. Impairment of VEGF signaling is thought to have a role in the pathogenesis of BPD (12). Other factors that may modulate fetal lung vascular development include nitric oxide (13).

This normal process of lung growth, differentiation and alveolarization may be influenced by preterm birth and its management. Many of the common therapies used for management of preterm babies can result in abnormal lung growth and remodeling, ultimately resulting in chronic respiratory insufficiency characterized by BPD.

Lung Injury

Airways remodeling can occur as a consequence of lung injury (2). A variety of factors may precipitate lung injury and the pathway that leads to remodeling is through initiation of an uncontrolled inflammatory response. The link between early lung inflammation and lung injury is clearly established, since levels of many pro-inflammatory cytokines are increased in bronchoalveolar lavage (BAL) fluid of babies who subsequently develop BPD (14, 15). Lung inflammation may begin either before birth in the setting of infection such as chorioamnionitis or after birth as a result of mechanical ventilation, oxidative stress or nosocomial infection.

Oxidative Stress and Lung Inflammation

Preterm babies are at risk of oxidative stress for a number of reasons. They are often exposed to high concentrations of inspired oxygen for resuscitation and to maintain normal arterial oxygen tensions after birth. High oxygen exposure leads to generation of oxygen free radicals, which are highly reactive molecules that can cause oxidative damage to tissues and trigger an inflammatory response. Preterm babies have low levels of antioxidant protection and an inability to increase antioxidant production in response to oxidative stress. This has been extensively studied in animal models by Frank and Sosenko (16) and, although data from human newborns are more scanty, they support the role of oxidative stress in the development of pulmonary inflammation and subsequent BPD.

Newborn baboons exposed to high levels of inspired oxygen have reduced alveolarization and airways remodeling similar to that seen in BPD (17). The mechanism is not fully understood but it may be by inhibition of DNA synthesis (18) or indirectly by initiation of inflammation from oxidation of lung structures at the interface with the atmosphere. Oxidative stress may also upregulate collagenolytic enzymes such as the matrix metalloproteinases. Antioxidants have therefore been considered as a potential preventive treatment strategy for BPD.

Neutrophil degranulation and subsequent respiratory (or oxidative) burst with the release of reactive oxygen species (ROS) may contribute to oxidative stress and this is the subject of ongoing research. Neutrophils appear rapidly in the BAL fluid of preterm infants with RDS peaking at day 4 and declining rapidly in infants who do not later develop BPD, whereas in those who do this decrease is delayed (19, 20). In animal models, neutrophil depletion can limit the effect of hyperoxia-induced lung injury, suggesting a role for the neutrophil in lung damage.

The proinflammatory cytokines that attract cells into the lung have also been extensively studied (15). TNF-α, IL-1ß, IL-6 and IL-8 are just some proinflammatory cytokines that are increased in BAL fluid of preterm infants. With influx of neutrophils their degranulation and release of ROS and proteases will result in cell injury. In babies developing BPD the balance between proteases and anti-proteases appears to be tilted in favor of proteolysis. Elastase levels are increased in babies with RDS but those who subsequently develop BPD have even higher levels (20). This, accompanied with a decreased level of α-1-proteinase inhibitor levels compared with babies who recover from RDS without BPD, as well as higher levels of urinary elastin degradation products suggest ongoing proteolysis (21). Therefore drugs which modify the oxidative burst response such as superoxide dismutase (22) and proteolysis such as α-1-proteinase inhibitor (23) are potential candidates to prevent or treat BPD.

Prenatal Infection and Lung Inflammation

The association between chorioamnionitis and preterm labor is well established (24). This, often subclinical, infection is not only responsible for many preterm births but can also cause serious neonatal multi-organ morbidity as a result of a systemic fetal inflammatory response (25). The inflammation, however, may be limited to the fetal lung and predispose the affected fetus to develop BPD (26, 27). How chorioamnionitis-induced lung inflammation affects alveolarization and pulmonary angiogenesis in preterm babies is unknown; however, it has been hypothesized that destruction of the lung ECM by inflammatory collagenases may be important (28, 29).

The pathophysiology of BPD may be thought of as separate processes of inflammation, architectural disruption, fibrosis and disordered or delayed development. "Classic" BPD is heavily influenced by inflammation and fibrosis, while "new" BPD is primarily an arrest of development. This should be viewed as a spectrum, with "classic" BPD being more influenced by lung injury and "new" BPD being more influenced by disordered and delayed pulmonary development (also termed modeling and remodeling).

Once BPD has developed it is difficult to treat and emphasis should therefore be directed at prevention. Drugs that may influence lung modeling and remodeling can broadly be divided into three groups: (i) those administered prenatally to induce lung maturation thereby reducing the need for mechanical ventilation and oxygen exposure, (ii) drugs administered postnatally to prevent or minimize initiation of and effects of inflammatory stimuli and (iii) drugs that may influence the inflammatory response in order to limit airways remodeling. Ventilator strategies to minimize ventilatory barotrauma and volutrauma include use of CPAP, high-frequency oscillation and synchronized mechanical ventilation but randomized clinical trials have shown only modest reductions in BPD. This is not surprising in view of evidence that airways remodeling may begin before birth. The last group of therapies that we will discuss are those that aim to maximize pulmonary function of babies who have BPD.

PREVENTION

The ideal treatment strategy for BPD would be to prevent it altogether as it is so difficult to treat once it has developed. Prevention may be attempted using a spectrum of interventions ranging from the ideal of prevention of preterm birth to the, at present, more realistic minimization of lung injury.

Prenatal Interventions (See Table 10-1)

Prevention of Preterm Birth

This ideal aspiration is unlikely to be achieved as there is such a diverse range of causes of preterm birth. Most studies have targeted at-risk women such as those who have had a previous preterm birth. Overall advances in reducing preterm birth have been modest. The prevalence remains high in many countries, including the USA (11%) (30), Canada (7%) (31) and France (7%) (32). Furthermore, the incidence of preterm birth in these countries has increased by 10–20% in the last

Table 10-1   Prenatal Interventions

	Outcome	No. of patients	No. of studies	RR	95% CI	NNT	95%CI
Progesterone (36)	Preterm birth	988	6	0.65	0.54–0.79	8	5–14
Antibiotic treatment in cases of asymptomatic bacteriuria (37)	Preterm birth	1923	10	0.64	0.50–0.82	20	13–50
Treatment for bacterial vaginosis (38)	Preterm birth	622	5	0.89	0.71–1.11	–	
Antibiotics for preterm, prelabor rupture of membranes (39)	Preterm birth	4931	3	1.0	0.97–1.03	–	
	BPD 28 days	5597	4	0.75	0.53–1.06	–	
	BPD 36 weeks	4809	1	0.91	0.70–1.17	–	
Prenatal corticosteroid (44)	RDS	3735	18	0.64	0.56–0.72	11	9–15
	BPD 28 days	411	3	1.38	0.90–2.11	–	
Prenatal thyrotrophin releasing hormone (200)	BPD 28 days	2511	5	1.01	0.85–1.19	–	
	Death/BPD 28 days	3694	6	1.08	0.94–1.25	–	

few years (31, 32). Various intervention programs to prevent preterm labor based on identification of women at risk have been tried but they have no effect on the frequency of preterm birth (33, 34).

Progesterone has also been used to try to prevent preterm birth in at-risk women. A systematic review and meta-analysis of progesterone supplementation for preventing preterm birth identified seven randomized controlled trials (35) (Table 10-1). Women who received progesterone were statistically significantly less likely to give birth before 37 weeks (seven studies, 1020 women, RR = 0.58, 95%CI = 0.48–0.70), to have an infant with birth weight of ≤ 2.5 kg (six studies, 872 infants, RR = 0.62, 95%CI = 0.49–0.78), or to have an infant diagnosed with intraventricular hemorrhage (one study, 458 infants, RR = 0.25, 95%CI = 0.08–0.82). Progesterone treatment was associated with a 50% decrease in the risk of preterm birth but had no effect on neonatal outcomes. However, there is currently insufficient information to allow recommendations regarding the optimal dose, route and timing of administration of progesterone supplementation (36).

One other type of drug treatment is effective in reducing the risks of preterm birth. Antibiotic treatment in cases of asymptomatic bacteriuria reduces the frequency of preterm birth in women at risk (RR = 0.64, 95%CI = 0.5 to 0.82; NNT = 20, 95%CI = 13–50) (37). However, in a recent systematic review (38) in women with a previous preterm birth, treatment for bacterial vaginosis did not affect the risk of subsequent preterm birth (RR = 0.89, 95%CI = 0.71–1.11). It may, however, decrease the risk of preterm prelabor rupture of membranes (RR = 0.14, 95%CI = 0.05–0.38) and low birthweight (RR = 0.31, 95%CI = 0.13–0.75). This review provides little evidence that screening and treating all pregnant women with asymptomatic bacterial vaginosis will prevent preterm birth and its consequences (38). Another approach is based on antibiotic treatment after the onset of labor or after membrane rupture. Antibiotic treatment does not reduce preterm labor (RR = 1.00, 95%CI = 0.97–1.03), whereas it has been found to decrease the risk of chorioamnionitis (RR = 0.57, 95%CI = 0.37–0.86), neonatal sepsis (RR = 0.68, 95%CI = 0.53–0.87) and cerebral abnormalities (RR = 0.82, 95%CI = 0.68–0.98) following preterm rupture of the membranes (39). This treatment did not affect the need for oxygen at 28 days (RR = 0.75, 95%CI = 0.53–1.06) or at 36 weeks corrected age (RR = 0.91, 95%CI = 0.70–1.17), nor did it decrease the need for assisted ventilation (RR = 0.90, 95%CI = 0.8–1.02) despite reducing the need for surfactant (RR = 0.83, 95%CI = 0.72–0.96) (39).

Prevention of RDS – Prenatal Glucocorticoids

Glucocorticoids given prenatally promote maturation of the surfactant system (40), increase antioxidant capacity (41), increase activity of lung endothelial nitric oxide synthase (42) and histologic lung maturation with increased size of the air spaces and thinner more mature epithelium (43). The net result is a decreased risk of RDS (RR = 0.64, 95%CI = 0.56–0.72) (44). Ideally glucocorticoids should be given between 1 and 7 days before birth. However, although the effect on RDS is well established there is no clear evidence that glucocorticoids reduce the risk of BPD (44), indeed there is a trend towards an increased risk (RR = 1.38, 95%CI = 0.90–2.11). Furthermore, it has been shown that with multiple courses of glucocorticoids there is a significantly increased incidence of BPD (45) (RR = 3.01, 95%CI = 1.54–5.88) (44). This is supported by animal data suggesting that while some glucocorticoids are necessary for normal lung development an excess inhibits normal lung maturation (43, 46). Knockout mice bred to be deficient in corticotrophin-releasing hormone show early failure of development of the air spaces and the newborn pups all die of respiratory failure. Conversely, animals exposed repeatedly to glucocorticoids during the period of lung development have a reduced number of alveoli which are larger and more mature-looking than those of controls due to reduction in thickness of septal mesenchyme (43). There is improved lung compliance but changes in lung elastin and collagen content during this abnormal modeling may increase the tendency for mechanical ventilation-induced alveolar disruption (47). A further concern is the observation in rats that although the lungs are more mature following prenatal glucocorticoid treatment there is a reduction in lung weight and lung weight to body ratio (48). In a systematic review of repeat doses of prenatal corticosteroids for women at risk of preterm birth when multiple courses were compared to a single course there was no increase in BPD for all women (RR = 1.01, 95%CI = 0.63–1.65) or for those with preterm prelabor rupture of the membranes (RR = 0.77, 95%CI = 0.42–1.41). Currently available evidence suggests that repeat courses of prenatal corticosteroids reduce the severity of acute neonatal lung disease. However, there is insufficient evidence on benefits and risks to recommend repeat courses of prenatal corticosteroids for women at risk of preterm birth for prevention of neonatal respiratory disease (49). The National Institutes of Health recently recommended that no more than one course of glucocorticoids be used routinely outside clinical trials (50).

There is increased expression of VEGF following dexamethasone administration during the period of postnatal alveolarization (9). Glucocorticoids may therefore inhibit alveolarization by increasing the expression of VEGF which alters normal alveolar septal vascular maturation. Tropoelastin expression is also upregulated, leading to increased elastin production and this may contribute to improved lung compliance (51). Prenatal glucocorticoid treatment may have beneficial effects in terms of outcome but this is mediated through a process of early lung maturation and abnormal airways modeling which may predispose to subsequent ventilation-induced lung injury and BPD.

Many cases of preterm labor are associated with a concomitant chorioamnionitis and fetal lung inflammation and this also results in lung maturation. Glucocorticoids and inflammation appear to work synergistically to induce lung maturation. Therefore the apparent benefit of prenatal glucocorticoids in the presence of inflammation may lead to preterm babies with more functionally mature lungs enabling them to survive but be offset in part by an increased susceptibility to ventilation-induced lung injury (2).

Recent studies in animal models suggest that prenatal glucocorticoids in the presence of inflammation have short-term anti-inflammatory effects with a later rebound of inflammation to higher levels than before glucocorticoids were

Table 10–2   Postnatal Intervention – Surfactant Therapy

	Outcome	No. of patients	No. of studies	RR	95% CI	NNT	95%CI
Early surfactant and short ventilation vs ongoing ventilation (60)	BPD 28 days	68	1	0.94	0.20–4.35	–	
	Death before 28 days	68	1	0.38	0.08–1.81	–	
Early vs. delayed selective surfactant (201)	BPD 28 days	3039	3	0.97	0.88–1.06	33	20–100
	BPD 36 weeks	3007	2	0.70	0.55–0.88	–	
	Mortality	3039	3	0.90	0.79–1.01	–	
Multiple vs. single dose of surfactant (62)	BPD 28 days	343	1	1.10	0.63–1.93	–	
	Mortality	394	2	0.63	0.39–1.02	–	
Natural vs. synthetic surfactant (61)	BPD 28 days	3515	8	1.02	0.93–1.11	–	
	BPD 36 weeks	3179	5	1.01	0.90–1.12	–	
	Mortality	4588	10	0.86	0.76–0.98	–	
Prophylactic natural surfactant (63)	BPD 28 days	932	7	0.93	0.80–1.07	–	
	Mortality	932	7	0.60	0.44–0.83	14	8–33
Prophylactic synthetic surfactant(64)	BPD 28 days	1086	4	1.06	0.83–1.36	–	
	Mortality	1500	7	0.70	0.58–0.85	–	
Prophylactic surfactant vs. selective surfactant (65)	BPD 28 days	2816	8	0.96	0.82–1.12	–	
	Mortality	2613	7	0.61	0.48–0.77	14	9–33
Synthetic surfactant for RDS(66)	BPD 28 days	2248	5	0.75	0.61–0.92	25	16–100
	Mortality	2352	6	0.73	0.61–0.88	20	14–50

administered (52). This may help explain why improved early pulmonary outcome is not associated with a reduction in BPD (44).

Prevention of RDS – Prenatal Thyrotrophin-Releasing Hormone

Thyroid hormones are involved in fetal lung growth and maturation (53, 54) and in fetal sheep they act synergistically with glucocorticoids to improve surfactant synthesis (55). Thyrotrophin-releasing hormone (TRH) has been studied as a means of maturing the fetal lung and early small clinical trials were promising but showed conflicting results (55, 56). In the Australian ACTOBAT study (186) and later in a large North American clinical trial involving 996 women prenatal TRH given with glucocorticoids was no more effective in preventing RDS or death than glucocorticoids alone (55). Furthermore, in the ACTOBAT study those treated with TRH had an increased risk of motor and sensory impairment at 12-month follow-up (57). For these reasons further research into antenatal TRH has been suspended and its administration to women expected to deliver prematurely cannot be recommended.

Postnatal Interventions (See Tables 10-2 and 10-3)

Surfactant Therapy

Since surfactant therapy was introduced into routine clinical practice in the early 1990s there has been improved survival particularly of the smallest preterm infants who are at greatest risk of developing BPD. Surfactant has also allowed more gentle forms of ventilation as evidenced by fewer pneumothoraces and as a result there are now increasing numbers of neonates surviving with mainly "new" BPD (4, 187). This has skewed the population of infants with BPD to the more premature end of the scale. The early trials of surfactant found an increase in survival without BPD but these were in bigger more mature babies. Recent estimates of the prevalence of BPD at 28 days of age are about 40% in infants with birthweights between 500 and 1000 g who require ventilation (59). Several randomized controlled trials (RCTs) have confirmed the safety and efficacy of surfactant therapy. Several meta-analyses (60–66) of various approaches to the use of surfactant replacement have been performed (Table 10-2). The results indicate that surfactant treatment significantly reduces mortality, but without a statistically significant effect on the incidence of BPD.

Table 10–3   Postnatal Interventions Other Than Surfactant

	Outcome	No. of patients	No. of studies	RR	95% CI	NNT	95%CI
Inositol (70)	BPD 28 days	336	3	0.68	0.45–1.02	12	6–1000
	Death/BPD 28 days	295	2	0.56	0.42–0.77	5	3–9
Early steroids (79)	BPD 28 days	2621	16	0.85	0.79–0.92	14	9–25
	BPD 36 weeks	2415	15	0.69	0.60–0.80	11	8–20
Inhaled steroids (173)	BPD 28 days	292	1	1.06	0.88–1.26	–	
Bronchodilators (76)	BPD 28 days	173	1	1.03	0.78–1.37	–	
Prophylactic ibuprofen (94)	BPD 28 days	41	1	0.88	0.32–2.42	–	
	BPD 36 weeks	626	3	1.10	0.91–1.33	–	
Prophylactic indomethacin (202)	BPD 28 days	1022	9	1.08	0.92–1.22	–	
	BPD 36 weeks	999	1	1.06	0.92–1.22	–	
Caffeine (97)	BPD	2006	1	0.78	0.69–0.86	10	7–17
Retinol (114)	BPD 36 weeks	793	2	0.87	0.77–0.99	–	
Superoxide dismutase (203)	BPD 28 days	33	1	3.65	0.10–9.86	–	
	BPD 36 weeks	33	1	1.00	0.21–65.05	–	
α-1-Antitrypsin (204)	BPD 28 days	151	2	0.81	0.64–1.01	–	
	BPD 36 weeks	151	2	1.56	0.58–4.17	–	
Nitric oxide (127)	BPD 36 weeks	748	7	0.89	0.78–1.02	–	
	Death/BPD 36 weeks	460	5	0.96	0.77–1.18	–	

As with prenatal glucocorticoids the effects of surfactant replacement may have been concealed because of the increased survival of extremely immature infants.

Inositol

Inositol is an essential nutrient required by human cells in culture for growth and survival. It is a six-carbon sugar alcohol found widely throughout mammalian tissues in its free form as the phospholipid phosphatidylinositol, and in cell membranes as a phosphoinositide. Inositol promotes maturation of several components of surfactant and may play a critical role in fetal and early neonatal life. Three RCTs of inositol supplementation after birth, the first using oral inositol supplementation for 10 days (67), the second intravenous inositol supplementation in the first 5 days of life (68) and the third a supplemented formula high in inositol (69), have been reported. A recent meta-analysis of these trials showed a strong trend favoring a reduction in BPD at 28 days (RR = 0.68, 95%CI 0.45–1.02; NNT = 12, 95%CI 6–1000) (70). Other effects of inositol supplementation include important reductions in the rates of death, death or BPD, intraventricular hemorrhage of grades III or IV, and retinopathy of prematurity of stage 4 or needing treatment. However, these conclusions are based on a limited number of patients. They require confirmation in large multicenter trials before inositol supplementation can be recommended as a routine part of the nutritional management of preterm infants with RDS (70).

Early Systemic Postnatal Glucocorticoids

The story of postnatal glucocorticoids has evolved from one of potential short-term benefit to one of long-term harm and it is a warning against using treatments in the newborn without long-term follow-up studies to establish risk-benefit ratio. In the early 1980s high-dose dexamethasone was used to successfully wean babies with BPD from ventilation (71, 72). In 1989 Cummings et al. treated 36 infants with a high risk of BPD who remained on ventilation at 14 days with either an 18-day or a prolonged 42-day tapering course of dexamethasone and these also resulted in faster weaning from the ventilator and reductions in need for supplemental oxygen (73). This study suggested that the prolonged course was associated with a reduced risk of long-term neurodevelopmental sequelae and high-dose dexamethasone became almost standard practice during the 1990s. At that time it was known that there were some acute adverse effects such as hypertension, hyperglycemia, gastrointestinal bleeding, infection, cardiac hypertrophy and poor growth but these were felt to be manageable and reversible once treatment was discontinued. The general feeling of many neonatologists was that the benefit of improved lung function, earlier extubation and less BPD outweighed the known adverse effects.

This all changed after 1998 with the publication of three follow-up studies suggesting increases in adverse neurodevelopmental sequelae, including cerebral palsy in infants who had been treated with dexamethasone (74–76). In 2001 and 2002 the European Association of Perinatal Medicine (77) and the American Academy of Pediatrics (78) recommended that glucocorticoids should not be used for treatment of preterm infant unless as a last resort or as part of a well-designed randomized trial with long-term follow-up.

Glucocorticoids had been used early in the course of RDS to try to prevent BPD (79) or later when BPD was developing (58) or had developed (80). Later use of glucocorticoids is discussed under Treatment of BPD (see below). The rationale for early postnatal glucocorticoid use was based upon the belief that the course of RDS could be altered, although an earlier study published in 1972 suggested that this was not the case (81). Indeed in addition to finding no apparent benefits from early hydrocortisone in babies with RDS these researchers found adverse neurological effects, including severe intraventricular hemorrhage (82) and abnormal EEG (83) in the treated group of infants in two follow-up studies. More recent studies have shown that infants with RDS have higher levels of endogenous glucocorticoids, probably due to a stress response, but the levels in babies who subsequently develop BPD are reduced (83). This finding provided another rationale for early glucocorticoid treatment.

A third rationale for early treatment was the knowledge that inflammation begins early in RDS and early glucocorticoid treatment may help prevent the progression to BPD. Early glucocorticoid treatment reduces levels of proinflammatory cytokines in BAL from ventilated preterm infants (84). In the 1980s and 1990s there were about 20 RCTs of early glucocorticoids to prevent BPD in preterm babies with RDS and these have been summarized in a meta-analysis (79). Dexamethasone, starting at 0.5 mg/kg/day halving every 3 days for a total of 12 days, was the most usual drug regimen but hydrocortisone has also been used as well as other dosing regimens. The systematic review confirmed the acute adverse effects of raised blood pressure and blood glucose and in addition the increased risk of cerebral palsy (RR = 1.69, 95%CI = 1.20–2.38). Early glucocorticoids did lead to earlier extubation (risk of extubation failure before day 28) (RR = 0.84, 95%CI = 0.72–0.98) and reduced risk of BPD at 28 days (RR = 0.85, 95%CI = 0.79–0.92) and 36 weeks corrected age (RR = 0.69, 95%CI = 0.60–0.80) but had no effect on neonatal mortality (RR = 1.05, 95%CI = 0.90–1.22).

Early Inhaled Postnatal Glucocorticoids

These offer an attractive option of trying to get the beneficial pulmonary effects of glucocorticoids while hoping to avoid the adverse systemic side-effects. There have been several studies looking at inhaled glucocorticoids in neonates at risk of developing BPD. In these beclamethasone, budesonide, flunisolide and fluticasone have all been compared with placebo (85–88, 75). Some studies showed a trend towards reduced time on mechanical ventilation and need for oxygen at 36 weeks but they were insufficiently powered to detect significant differences. A systematic review of inhaled glucocorticoids given in the first 2 weeks of life showed a trend towards reduced mortality, earlier extubation and reduced BPD without significant side-effects, but the results were not statistically significant (174).

More research is needed to determine whether there is a role for inhaled glucocorticoids, and studies assessing the effects of lower systemic doses of other glucocorticoids in physiological rather than pharmacological doses are also warranted (78, 89).

Other Anti-inflammatory Agents

Since glucocorticoids are effective in prevention of BPD other anti-inflammatory drugs have also been studied. Sodium cromoglycate with a nebulized dose of 20 mg 6 hourly lowered levels of proinflammatory cytokines in bronchoalveolar lavage fluid but had no effect on the incidence of BPD at 28 days in a study of 26 infants at high risk of developing BPD (90).

Bronchodilators

One RCT used metered-dose inhalers to administer salbutamol 200 μg every 4 h or a placebo to 173 preterm infants at risk of developing BPD. Treatment was given on the 10th or 11th postnatal day and was given for 28 days with the dose tapering over a period of 8 days (91). This trial was the subject of a recent systematic review which showed that there was no statistically significant difference in duration of ventilatory support or age of weaning from respiratory support with salbutamol treatment (76). There were insufficient data to reliably assess the use of salbutamol for the prevention of BPD (76, 91).

Prostaglandin Synthetase Inhibitors

The effectiveness of indomethacin-induced closure of PDA in preventing the development of BPD has been confirmed in a systematic review (92, 93). This review also suggests that earlier therapy, when symptoms of PDA first appear, may be more effective in preventing pulmonary morbidity than therapy commencing after signs of congestive heart failure are present (92). However, prophylactic therapy with indomethacin did not appear to decrease the incidence of oxygen need at 36 weeks corrected age in a study of 1202 infants of 500–999 g birthweight despite reducing the incidence of symptomatic PDA (93). With the easy availability and high efficacy of indomethacin for PDA closure, prompt medical or surgical closure of symptomatic PDA is a reasonable method of BPD prevention.

Two recent systematic reviews have looked at ibuprofen for the prevention (94) and treatment (95) of PDA in preterm and/or low birth weight infants. Ibuprofen did not prevent BPD at 28 days (RR = 0.88, 95%CI = 0.32–2.42), or BPD at 36 weeks (RR = 1.10, 95%CI = 0.91–1.33) (94). However, in the meta-analysis, there was a statistically significant increase in the incidence of BPD at 28 days in the ibuprofen group compared to the indomethacin group (RR = 1.37, 95%CI = 1.01–1.86). The incidence of BPD at 36 weeks was not significantly different (RR = 1.28, 95%CI = 0.77–2.10) (95).

Fluid restriction as a preventive measure for BPD has also been studied and was the subject of a meta-analysis. The risk of BPD was not significantly affected by fluid intake in any of the three trials in which this was analyzed nor in the overall analysis (RR = 0.80, 95%CI = 0.56–1.14) (96).

Caffeine

Caffeine and other similar drugs known as the methylxanthines have been used for more than 25 years to treat apnea of prematurity. The caffeine for apnea of prematurity (CAP) study enrolled 2006 premature infants between 1999 and 2004. This was an RCT comparing 1000 control infants receiving placebo to 1006 infants treated with 20 mg/kg of caffeine citrate. At 36 weeks corrected age there was a significant reduction in BPD in the caffeine-treated group (RR = 0.78, 95%CI = 0.69–0.86; NNT = 10, 95%CI = 7–17) (97). The authors speculated that the reduction in BPD may have been due to the placebo group having longer exposure to positive pressure ventilation. However, caffeine may improve lung mechanics in the immature injured lung in ventilator-dependent preterm infants and it has also been shown to reduce pulmonary resistance and increase lung compliance (98). Reducing ventilator-induced lung damage may be an important factor in preventing BPD but caffeine also has a diuretic effect that could reduce lung fluid and improve lung mechanics and gas exchange. Caffeine may also have anti-inflammatory effects in the immature lung and others have hypothesized that methylxanthines act as antioxidants (99). Animal models have also demonstrated improvement in airway resistance and compliance with the administration of caffeine (100).

Antibiotic Treatment

The association between chorioamnionitis and preterm labor is well established (24). Chorioamnionitis appears to decrease the risk of RDS but increase the risk of BPD in intubated preterm infants (59, 101). Infection with *Ureaplasma urealyticum* appears to be specifically related to a subsequent increased risk of BPD (102). This appears to be more pronounced in infants weighing less than 1000 g (103). In a recent meta-analysis colonization with *Ureaplasma* was associated with an increased risk of later BPD (RR = 1.72, 95%CI = 1.5–1.96) compared to uncolonized neonates. However, RCTs of erythromycin treatment do not show any reduction in BPD (104). This may be because erythromycin fails to eliminate airway colonization with *U. urealyticum* in very low birthweight infants (105).

Antioxidant Therapy

Since the immature infant is deficient in endogenous pulmonary antioxidants (106, 107) and is exposed to multiple sources of oxidative stress (108) a number of antioxidant therapies have been used to try to prevent BPD. Antioxidants such as vitamin A (124) vitamin E (109), and superoxide dismutase (110) as well as the free radical scavenger *N*-acetylcysteine (111) and allopurinol (112), an inhibitor of xanthine oxidase (an enzyme capable of generating superoxide radicals following hypoxia ischemia), have been administered to preterm babies at risk of BPD in an attempt to reduce oxygen free radical-induced lung damage. To date only vitamin A has shown any encouraging results, with a statistically significant if modest reduction in BPD (RR = 0.89, 95%CI = 0.80–0.99) in babies treated with intramuscular vitamin A (113, 114). Vitamin A is a retinoid and its benefits may not be due entirely to antioxidant effects. It is known that retinoic acid promotes alveolar septation (115). Rats treated with trans-retinoic acid during the postnatal period of alveolarization show increased lung septation per unit volume of lung by 50% (116). The beneficial effect of vitamin A may be due to a reduction in prenatal glucocorticoid-induced alveolar hypoplasia.

Recombinant human superoxide dismutase (rh SOD) given intratracheally to piglets reduces lung damage caused by hyperoxia and hyperventilation (117). However, studies in preterm babies have produced disappointing results. In a multi-center RCT of intratracheal human copper zinc SOD (CuZnSOD) administered every 48 h for up to 1 month in mechanically ventilated extremely preterm infants Davis et al. found no difference in mortality or oxygen-dependence at 36 weeks between the two study groups at 1 year of age (118). The treated infants had lower rates of hospitalization, emergency room visits and treatment with asthma medications, suggesting a potential CuZnSOD-mediated pulmonary benefit that was not evident on the early assessments. Clearly further trials will be needed before this drug can be recommended for prevention of BPD.

Although the antioxidant and free radical scavenger *N*-acetylcysteine recently has been shown to reduce markers of injury in a rat model of endotoxin-mediated acute lung injury (111) a Nordic randomized placebo-controlled clinical trial of 6 days of intravenous treatment with *N*-acetylcysteine in mechanically ventilated infants of 500–999 g birthweight showed no significant improvement in lung function (119) or reduction in mortality or requirement for supplemental oxygen at 28 days or 36 weeks corrected age (120).

In an RCT of allopurinol in 400 very preterm infants of between 24 and 32 weeks gestation randomly allocated to receive either enteral allopurinol (20 mg/ml) or an equivalent dose of placebo for 7 daily doses the rate of BPD was not reduced despite plasma hypoxanthine concentrations at birth being significantly higher in infants who subsequently developed BPD (112).

More effective antioxidant therapies now being tested in animals might offer greater short-term benefits. In the moderately preterm baboon model of BPD induced by oxygen toxicity Chang et al. (121) found that an intravenous infusion of a catalytic antioxidant metalloporphyrin, AEOL 10113, partially reversed the morphological changes induced by 100% oxygen exposure and inhibited hyperoxia-induced increases in pulmonary neuroendocrine cells and urine bombesin-like peptide. This compound has yet to be evaluated in clinical trials. It should also be noted that oxygen free radicals play a role in cell signaling during tissue growth and differentiation and for this reason others have cautioned against using antioxidant therapy in newborn (122).

Proteinase Inhibitors

Lung injury by proteolytic enzymes accompanies unopposed antioxidant stress and pulmonary inflammation, and disruption of the pulmonary proteinase:antiproteinase balance has been associated with the occurrence of BPD (123). A recent approach for prevention of BPD has been administration of α-1-proteinase inhibitor in an attempt to reduce the destructive effects of elastase on lung extracellular matrix (ECM). Neutrophil elastase is released in the lungs as part of the inflammatory process. α-1-Proteinase inhibitor forms a complex with neutrophil elastase preventing destruction of the ECM. In a RCT intravenous α-1-proteinase inhibitor (60 mg/kg) or placebo was infused on four occasions during the first 2 weeks of life (23). There was a reduction of BPD at 36 weeks (RR = 0.48, 95%CI = 0.23–1.00) in the treated group which just failed to reach statistical significance but there was a significant reduction in pulmonary hemorrhage (RR = 0.22, 95%CI = 0.05–0.98). A number of investigators have suggested that neutrophil elastase excess and proteinase:antiproteinase imbalance might be of less importance in the pathogenesis of "new" BPD (125, 126). However, the benefits of antiproteinase therapy are biologically plausible, the number of infants studied to date is small, and no adverse effects of α-1-proteinase inhibitor treatment have been observed, making this a preventive therapy for BPD worthy of larger-scale clinical trials.

Inhaled Nitric Oxide

Nitric oxide (NO) is a potent vasodilator and inhaled NO (iNO) is a selective pulmonary vasodilator, reversing pulmonary hypertension and improving oxygenation without affecting the systemic circulation. NO therapy is of proven benefit in term and near-term infants with persistent pulmonary hypertension, reducing the need for ECMO (127). In preterm babies with early lung disease iNO may reduce pulmonary vascular resistance and selectively increase blood flow to areas of lung that are being adequately ventilated, thereby improving oxygenation and reducing ventilatory requirements and the risk of oxygen toxicity. Moreover, in animal studies NO reduces pulmonary inflammation directly (128) and decreases pulmonary artery remodeling in rat pups (129). The capacity of NO to improve ventilation:perfusion (V:Q) (130, 131) matching as well as its anti-inflammatory (130) and antioxidant (132) effects offer potential benefit to the preterm infant at risk of developing BPD. Early studies of iNO by Kinsella et al. (133), Mercier et al. (134) and Subhedar and colleagues (135) showed no benefit of iNO for prevention of BPD, either independently or in a meta-analysis (RR = 0.93, 95%CI = 0.79–1.09) (136).

However, in a recent RCT low-dose (10 ppm) iNo in preterm infants with mild or moderate RDS reduced risk of death or BPD from 64% to 49% (137). The magnitude of this effect was greater among infants whose respiratory illness was less severe (oxygenation index< 6.94). Any benefits need to be weighed against potential adverse effects of NO, which include prolonged bleeding time (138), surfactant dysfunction (139) and increased pulmonary inflammation (140), all more likely at higher doses. In this study, however, no adverse effects of iNO were detected with respect to rates of severe intraventricular hemorrhage or periventricular leukomalacia, although the study protocol did not provide standardized assessment of these outcomes. At 24-month follow-up of 138 (82%) of 168 survivors, Mestan and colleagues (141) found improved outcomes among the iNO-treated group (24% abnormal neurodevelopment vs. 46% among placebo-treated subjects).

Van Meurs and colleagues (142) reported the results of a multicenter RCT of iNO treatment of extremely preterm infants at 15 NICHD Neonatal Network centers. This study enrolled 420 newborns with gestations below 34 weeks and birthweights of 401–1500 g who had signs of ongoing respiratory failure more than 4 h after receiving surfactant. They found no difference in the primary outcome, death or BPD at 36 weeks corrected age, between study groups (80% of the iNO treatment group and 82% of the placebo group; RR = 0.97, 95%CI = 0.86–1.08). There were no apparent effects of iNO treatment on rates of intraventricular hemorrhage or white matter damage. Post hoc analyses suggested that iNO effects differed by birthweight. Among infants above 1000 g iNO was associated with improved primary outcome (death or BPD); however, infants born at or below 1000 g who were treated with iNO had higher rates of mortality and intraventricular hemorrhage than controls and the study was eventually terminated due to this increase (143).

The most recent meta-analysis published in 2006 (144) of five published RCTs involving a total of 808 infants below 34 weeks gestation showed a reduction in BPD with iNO (RR = 0.83, 95%CI = 0.72–0.95). The results of two further reasonably large RCTs have recently been published. The first, involving 798 infants, 398 treated with iNO (5 ppm) and 395 with placebo gas (controls), found overall no difference in the incidence of death or BPD between groups (145). However, iNO therapy reduced the incidence of BPD in infants with birthweight > 1000 g by 50% ($p = 0.001$) in a post hoc analysis and this result needs to be treated with caution. The second RCT enrolled infants < 1250 g birthweight who required ventilatory support at 7–21 days of age (146). Treated infants received decreasing concentrations of iNO, beginning at 20 ppm, for a minimum exposure of 24 days. Severity of lung disease, based on hospitalization and requirement for ventilatory support, was less at 36 ($p = 0.012$), 40 ($p = 0.014$) and 44 ($p = 0.033$) weeks. There were no differences between groups with regard to co-morbidities occurring after entry. In post hoc analyses, iNO improved survival without CLD for infants enrolled at 7–14 days (49.1% vs. 27.8%, $p = 0.001$), but not for infants enrolled at 15–21 days (40.7% vs. 42.8%), and benefit was restricted to infants with less severe lung disease at entry.

NO may not be the magic bullet it was hoped to be and its role, if any, is likely to be early, in low dose, for babies with mild or moderate lung disease. Its use in babies of less than 1000 g birthweight remains uncertain. Further studies with appropriate neurodevelopmental and respiratory follow-up need to be undertaken before iNO can be recommended as a routine therapy to prevent BPD in very low birthweight infants.

Cytokines and Anticytokines

Future preventive therapies for BPD are likely to include targeted cytokine or anti-cytokine therapies aimed at upregulating beneficial and blocking harmful humoral factors. Lung maturation is potentially induced by the administration of low-dose pro-inflammatory cytokines. Endotoxin is a potent inducer of synthesis of pro-inflammatory cytokines. Prenatal endotoxin exposure in a preterm sheep model causes lung maturational effects similar to those following prenatal gluco-corticoids (147). This effect is not mediated by upregulation of endogenous cortisol (148), acts synergistically with the glucocorticoid effect and requires direct contact of lung epithelium with endotoxin (149). However, inflammation also leads to remodeling and alveolar hypoplasia, so that concerns about longer-term adverse effects may limit the usefulness of endotoxin as a therapeutic agent.

Another potential therapy is antimacrophage chemokine (anti-MCP-1). In a report of anti-MCP-1 treatment in a newborn rat model of lung injury at 1 week (150), anti-MCP-1-treated rats showed reduced pulmonary macrophages and neu-trophils in BAL fluid, suggesting suppression of harmful inflammatory factors. Other candidates for future therapies include: anti-inflammatory agents (such as interleukin-10), surfactant proteins (151), clara cell secretory protein (152), and bombesin blocking molecules (153, 154).

TREATMENT OF BPD

The major postnatal risk factors for BPD include over-ventilation, nosocomial infection, oxidative stress and PDA. Avoiding fluid overload and maintaining good nutrition are important factors in reducing lung damage and aiding repair. However, when prevention is not possible early intervention is desirable.

The use of mechanical ventilation is associated with an increased risk of BPD and there is now compelling evidence that ventilation is harmful because of over-distension of the lung. Babies with the lowest arterial carbon dioxide tensions at 48 h of age appear to be at greatest risk of developing BPD, implying that over-ventilation may be a key causative factor (155). Lung injury may occur when lungs are inflated to volumes exceeding total lung capacity, a situation that has been described as volutrauma (156). Over-inflation of the lung by ventilating at the higher end of the pressure-volume curve can disrupt developing alveolar structures and initiate the release of chemokines (157). The inflammatory response appears to amplify the initial lung injury. Conversely, suboptimal ventilation at volumes below functional residual capacity can also initiate inflammation (158). The ideal tidal volume for an individual baby is very difficult to determine and the margin between the low-volume lung injury zone and the high-volume lung injury zone is small.

Preterm babies are at risk of oxidative stress for a number of reasons. They are often exposed to high concentrations of inspired oxygen for resuscitation and to maintain normal arterial oxygen tensions after birth. High oxygen exposure leads to generation of oxygen free radicals, which are highly reactive molecules that can cause oxidative damage to tissues and trigger an inflammatory response. The presence of lipid peroxidation products in lung lavage has been linked to the later development of BPD (159). Preterm babies have low levels of antioxidant protection and an inability to increase antioxidant production in response to oxidative stress. The aim of management of preterm infants has traditionally been to maintain arterial oxygen saturations in the range that is normal for a term baby (94–97%), believing that this is optimal for growth and brain development and for promoting closure of the ductus arteriosus. These saturations are much higher than those needed for maintenance of well-being in utero. An acceptance of lower oxygen saturations might reduce the risk of BPD. The STOP-ROP trial was designed to see if maintaining preterm babies with pre-threshold retinopathy of prematurity at higher oxygen saturations (96–99% vs. 89–94%) would reduce progression to retinopathy of prematurity (160). There were no significant differences in ophthalmologic outcomes but the group maintained at lower oxygen saturations had less respiratory morbidity, suggesting that further studies are warranted to define safe oxygen saturation targets for the very preterm baby (161).

As previously discussed, prenatal infections increase the risk of BPD; however, postnatal infections also increase the risk (162, 163). Several investigators have found an association between respiratory colonization of premature infants with organisms such as *U. urealyticum* and later development of BPD (104, 164–166).

Interstitial edema is a pathological feature of infants with BPD. PDA and excessive fluid administration may contribute to development of interstitial edema and worsening of respiratory status (167). Symptomatic PDA has also been associated with development of BPD (59, 168). Both PDA and systemic infection increase serum levels of proinflammatory cytokines and this may be the mechanism of action (168).

Preterm infants are born before they can maximally accumulate nutrients. Their limited stores, inadequate postnatal nutrient intake, the simultaneous use of other medications such as glucocorticoids and diuretics, oxidative stress, and infections may result in a prolonged hypercatabolic state which may further impair the process of healing (169). Thus, the interactions of several factors, such as proinflammatory cytokines, mechanical ventilation, oxygen, the relative lack of antioxidant defenses, and the release of cytotoxic enzymes such as elastases and proteinases, interfere with normal developmental signals and result in BPD. In the previous section we looked at drugs used to prevent BPD and in this section we will consider drug management of established BPD.

Late Systemic Postnatal Glucocorticoids (Table 10-4)

Systematic reviews of the numerous RCTs examining benefits and risks of systemic glucocorticoids for babies with or developing BPD are divided into two groups, depending on the timing of treatment after birth: moderately early treatment (7–14 days) (58) and late treatment (>3 weeks) (80). With moderately early glucocorticoids there is a reduction in neonatal mortality before 28 days and a clear trend towards reduction in mortality before discharge in treated babies. Treatment started between 7 and 14 days also facilitates earlier extubation and significantly reduces the risk of BPD at 36 weeks. However, side-effects include hypertension and cardiac hypertrophy. Late systemic glucocorticoids also lead to more rapid weaning from mechanical ventilation but mortality is not affected and there is also an increased risk of side-effects. Overall glucocorticoid treatment exerts short-term beneficial effects on the neonatal lung, with improved lung mechanics and gas exchange that facilitate early extubation, perhaps through a reduction of pulmonary inflammation. The additional benefit of a reduction in supplemental oxygen requirement only occurs when treatment is given within the first 14 days of life. Side-effects occur regardless of timing of treatment. However, as with prenatal glucocorticoids there is evidence from rat studies that postnatal treatment also inhibits alveolarization and reduces lung growth (170). There is conflicting evidence regarding persistence of this effect, with one study showing persistence into

Table 10–4 Treatment of BPD

	Outcome	No. of patients	No. of studies	RR	95% CI	NNT	95%CI
Moderately early steroids(58)	BPD 28 days	623	6	0.87	0.81–0.94	9	6–20
	BPD 36 weeks	247	5	0.62	0.47–0.82	5	3–11
Late steroids(80)	BPD 36 weeks	118	1	0.76	0.58–1.00	6	3–100
	Death or BPD 36 weeks	118	1	0.73	0.58–0.93	5	3–14

adulthood (170) but another using doses more equivalent to those used in neonates showing resolution (171).

Late Inhaled Glucocorticoids

Inhaled glucocorticoids are an alternative method for delivering anti-inflammatory activity locally without the risks associated with systemic administration. When given to intubated infants with BPD for periods of 1–4 weeks, inhaled glucocorticoids significantly improve the rate of successful extubation during treatment (RR = 0.12, 95%CI = 0.03–0.43) (172). Inhaled steroids are as good as systemic steroids at weaning babies from the ventilator (173, 174). Although the studies that measured adverse effects such as adrenal function, infection, retinopathy of prematurity and/or intraventricular hemorrhage generally did not find an increase in adverse effects in glucocorticoid-treated infants, they were small and lacked the power to detect clinically significant rises. A recent study of adrenal function in premature infants being treated with inhaled glucocorticoids showed decreases in basal cortisol levels, but normal responses to stimulation (175). Further RCTs are needed which address the risk/benefit ratio of different delivery techniques, dosing schedules and long-term effects of inhaled steroids, with particular attention to neurodevelopmental outcome.

Diuretics

Diuretics are drugs that could also potentially improve pulmonary compliance and airway resistance by reducing lung edema. Two Cochrane reviews have assessed the effects of enteral loop diuretics (such as furosemide) (176) and those acting on the distal renal tubule (such as thiazides and spironolactone) (177) in either preventing or treating BPD in preterm infants. Chronic administration of furosemide improves oxygenation and lung compliance in infants with established BPD (176). A small study of 17 infants with BPD suggested that furosemide (1 mg/kg 12 hourly intravenously or 2 mg/kg 12 hourly orally) may also hasten ventilator weaning when compared with placebo (178). However, in light of the paucity of controlled trials in this area, a recent systematic review concluded that routine use of furosemide could not be recommended in BPD (176). Although a single dose of aerosolized furosemide improves lung mechanics, lack of data regarding important clinical outcomes means that routine or sustained use of this therapy cannot be recommended based on current evidence (179). Furosemide also has significant metabolic side-effects, ranging from displacing bilirubin from albumin at high doses to decreased weight gain, ototoxicity, hypercalciuria, and electrolyte abnormalities (180, 181). Distal tubular diuretics (thiazides and spironolactone) to treat BPD have also been assessed in a systematic review (176). A 1-week course of these diuretics improves pulmonary function in some studies, but not in others (182, 183). A 4-week course improved pulmonary function and decreased the need for concomitant furosemide in a study of 43 infants with BPD (184). In addition, in a study of 19 intubated infants, oxygen requirement and survival improved in those receiving a 4-week course of a thiazide diuretic and spironolactone (185). Although distal tubular diuretics may also cause significant electrolyte abnormalities, the incidence of nephrocalcinosis and hearing loss do not appear to be increased by these drugs (180, 184).

The beneficial effects of diuretic drugs on lung function in infants with BPD cannot be solely explained by an increased diuresis. It has been hypothesized that diuretics exert a direct effect on lung fluid balance by altering ion water transport or pulmonary vascular tone (187). Whilst both types of diuretic resulted in short-term improvements of lung compliance, there is little evidence of benefit of diuretic therapy on the need for ventilatory support, length of hospital stay, or other important long-term infant outcomes. Their use remains empirical in established BPD, although they may be effective in improving lung compliance and airway resistance as a short-term measure during acute decompensations.

Bronchodilators

Infants with severe BPD frequently have airway smooth muscle hypertrophy and airway hyperreactivity, and both systemic and inhaled bronchodilators have been used to treat BPD. However, most of the literature on these drugs deals with their short-term effects on pulmonary function, and little new research has been done (185). Up-to-date evidence for a long-term benefit of bronchodilators both in prevention and treatment of BPD does not exist (188). Inhaled bronchodilators that have been used in infants with BPD include ß-agonists and anticholinergic agents alone or in combination. Some acute improvement of lung function in both ventilated preterm infants early in life and in non-ventilator-dependent infants with overt BPD have been reported but response rates are variable (188). The inhaled ß-agonists, salbutamol, isoprenaline, orciprenaline and isoetarine, all lead to acute improvement in airflow (188). Terbutaline, another ß-agonist, improved short-term pulmonary mechanics when given subcutaneously to eight preterm infants with severe BPD (190). The inhaled anticholinergic agents, atropine and ipratropium bromide, also cause bronchodilatation and improve pulmonary function in infants with BPD in the short term (191) but long-term efficacy has not been studied for any of these drugs (76, 185). The inhaled anti-inflammatory agent sodium cromoglycate has been studied to a limited extent in intubated infants with BPD. Although it decreased leukocyte concentrations in BAL fluid and improved pulmonary function, there have been no long-term studies of its use in BPD (90).

Other Anti-inflammatory Drugs

Methylxanthines (aminophylline and caffeine) reduce airway resistance in infants with BPD and they have other potential beneficial effects, such as respiratory stimulation and a mild diuretic effect. Aminophylline may also improve respiratory muscle contractility. Like other drugs that inhibit phosphodiesterases, they may also have anti-inflammatory effects. The improvement in pulmonary function in infants with BPD is additive to the effects of diuretics (98, 192). Although there have been case reports attributing improved weaning of infants from mechanical ventilation to the use of theophylline, long-term studies of methylxanthine effectiveness in BPD have not been performed (193). Methylxanthines also have significant side-effects, such as gastroesophageal reflux, which is undesirable in preterm infants with BPD.

Mucolytics

Recombinant human deoxyribonuclease I (rhDNase, dornase alpha), administered by inhalation, is currently used as a mucolytic agent in the treatment of cystic fibrosis. There have been several case reports of the use of DNase (dornase alpha), administered intratracheally or by nebulization, to relieve the mucus plugging that occurs in BPD. Dornase alpha appears to improve radiographic evidence of plugging and to decrease oxygen requirements (194) but no RCTs have been performed (189).

Antibiotics for Postnatal Infection

Prevention of nosocomial infection is important in preventing long-term pulmonary consequences. To date, the impact of strategies to prevent nosocomial infection on the incidence of BPD has not been established. In a study of 28 infants born at < 30 weeks gestation colonized with *U. urealyticum*, although erythromycin treatment was effective in reducing colonization, there was no evidence that treatment altered the severity of lung disease (166). However, as we have already said, other studies showed that some antibiotics such as erythromycin fail to eliminate airway colonization with this organism in very low birthweight infants (105).

Immunization and Monoclonal Antibodies

Infants with BPD are at increased risk of recurrent respiratory tract infections and frequent hospitalizations. The most significant respiratory tract infection is that due to respiratory syncytial virus (RSV). A meta-analysis of RCTs found that RSV immunoglobulin or RSV monoclonal antibody was effective in preventing read-mission to the hospital and to the pediatric intensive care unit (195). A large multicenter study of palivizumab, a humanized monoclonal antibody against RSV, found that monthly injections of 15 mg/kg for 5 months reduced the hospi-talization rate for RSV infection by 4.9% (from 12.8% to 7.9%) in infants with BPD (195). This means that 20 infants with BPD need to receive a course of palivizumab to prevent one patient with RSV being hospitalized. Many centers now routinely administer palivizumab either to all preterm infants or to all those with established BPD who are likely to be discharged home prior to or during their first annual encounter with the peak RSV season. The AAP recommendations are that palivizumab or RSV-IGIV prophylaxis should be considered for infants and children younger than 2 years of age with BPD who have required medical therapy for their lung disease within 6 months before the anticipated RSV season. Patients with more severe BPD may benefit from prophylaxis for two RSV seasons (196).

New Treatments

SILDENAFIL

Sildenafil is a cGMP-specific phosphodiesterase inhibitor. In rat studies sildenafil improves alveolar growth and reduces pulmonary hypertension in hyperoxia-induced lung injury. Rat pups were randomly exposed from birth to normoxia, hyperoxia (95% FiO_2; BPD model), and hyperoxia plus sildenafil (100 mg/kg/day subcutaneously). Rat pups exposed to hyperoxia showed fewer and enlarged air spaces as well as decreased capillary density, mimicking pathologic features seen in human BPD. Sildenafil preserved alveolar growth and lung angiogenesis, and decreased pulmonary vascular resistance, right ventricular hypertrophy and medial wall thickness (197).

PENTOXIFYLLINE

Pentoxifylline is a methylxanthine with anti-inflammatory and anticytokine effects. Its anti-inflammatory effects include inhibition of neutrophils, macrophages, and monocytes. In a small, uncontrolled trial of five infants with BPD, 7 days of therapy with nebulized pentoxifylline was associated with a tendency to reduction in oxygen requirement and improvement in pulmonary mechanics. This intervention has not been studied in RCTs (198). Interim analysis of a prophylactic trial (199) suggests pentoxifylline may reduce treatment requirements after the neonatal period and that, in established BPD, pentoxifylline and dexamethasone may be of similar efficacy.

CONCLUSIONS

It is almost 40 years since Northway et al. (1) published the classic description of BPD in 1967. BPD continues to be a major complication of preterm birth as well as a major therapeutic challenge. Future developments will depend on a combination of understanding the interplay between lung injury and lung development, and the development of novel treatments to interrupt the pathogenesis of BPD and deal with its sequelae. It is likely that treatments for BPD may involve a combination (cocktail) of anti-inflammatory, antioxidant and anti-apoptotic agents. Further basic science research combined with appropriate clinical trials will we hope lead to prevention or amelioration of the effects of BPD in the near future.

REFERENCES

1. Northway WH, Jr, Rosan RC, Porter DY. Pulmonary disease following respirator therapy of hyaline-membrane disease. Bronchopulmonary dysplasia. N Engl J Med 1967; 276:357–368.
2. Sweet DG, Halliday HL. Modeling and remodeling of the lung in neonatal chronic lung disease: implications for therapy. Treat Respir Med 2005; 4:347–359.
3. Van Marter LJ, Allred EN, Pagano M. Do clinical markers of barotrauma and oxygen toxicity explain interhospital variation in rates of chronic lung disease? The Neonatology Committee for the Developmental Network. Pediatrics 2000; 105:1194–1201.
4. Coalson JJ. Pathology of new bronchopulmonary dysplasia. Semin Neonatol 2003; 8:73–81.
5. Jobe AH. The new BPD: an arrest of lung development. Pediatr Res 1999; 46:641–643.
6. Condon J, Gosden C, Gardener D. Expression of type 2 11beta-hydroxysteroid dehydrogenase and corticosteroid hormone receptors in early human fetal life. J Clin Endocrinol Metab 1998; 83:4490–4497.
7. Muglia LJ, Bae DS, Brown TT. Proliferation and differentiation defects during lung development in corticotropin-releasing hormone-deficient mice. Am J Respir Cell Mol Biol 1999; 20:181–188.
8. Ballard PL. Hormones and lung maturation. Monogr Endocrinol 1986; 28:1–354.
9. Bhatt AJ, Amin SB, Chess PR. Expression of vascular endothelial growth factor and Flk-1 in developing and glucocorticoid-treated mouse lung. Pediatr Res 2000; 47:606–613.
10. Ambalavanan N, Carlo WA. Bronchopulmonary dysplasia: new insights. Clin Perinatol 2004; 31:613–628.
11. Lassus P, Turanlahti M, Heikkila P. Pulmonary vascular endothelial growth factor and Flt-1 in fetuses, in acute and chronic lung disease, and in persistent pulmonary hypertension of the newborn. Am J Respir Crit Care Med 2001; 164:1981–1987.
12. Zeng X, Wert SE, Federici R. VEGF enhances pulmonary vasculogenesis and disrupts lung morphogenesis in vivo. Dev Dyn 1998; 211:215–227.
13. Shaul PW, Afshar S, Gibson LL. Developmental changes in nitric oxide synthase isoform expression and nitric oxide production in fetal baboon lung. Am J Physiol Lung Cell Mol Physiol 2002; 283:1192–1199.
14. Kotecha S, Wilson L, Wangoo A. Increase in interleukin (IL)-1 beta and IL-6 in bronchoalveolar lavage fluid obtained from infants with chronic lung disease of prematurity. Pediatr Res 1996; 40:250–256.
15. Groneck P, Speer CP. Inflammatory mediators and bronchopulmonary dysplasia. Arch Dis Child Fetal Neonatal Ed 1995; 73:F1–3.
16. Frank L, Sosenko IR. Development of lung antioxidant enzyme system in late gestation: possible implications for the prematurely born infant. J Pediatr 1987; 110:9–14.
17. Coalson JJ, Winter V, deLemos RA. Decreased alveolarization in baboon survivors with broncho-pulmonary dysplasia. Am J Respir Crit Care Med 1995; 152:640–646.
18. Han RN, Buch S, Tseu I. Changes in structure, mechanics, and insulin-like growth factor-related gene expression in the lungs of newborn rats exposed to air or 60% oxygen. Pediatr Res 1996; 39:921–929.
19. D'Angio CT, Basavegowda K, Avissar NE. Comparison of tracheal aspirate and bronchoalveolar lavage specimens from premature infants. Biol Neonate 2002; 82:145–149.
20. Ogden BE, Murphy SA, Saunders GC. Neonatal lung neutrophils and elastase/proteinase inhibitor imbalance. Am Rev Respir Dis 1984; 130:817–821.
21. Bruce MC, Wedig KE, Jentoft N. Altered urinary excretion of elastin cross-links in premature infants who develop bronchopulmonary dysplasia. Am Rev Respir Dis 1985; 131:568–572.
22. Narayanan PK, Carter WO, Ganey PE. Impairment of human neutrophil oxidative burst by polychlorinated biphenyls: inhibition of superoxide dismutase activity. J Leukoc Biol 1998; 63:216–224.
23. Stiskal JA, Dunn MS, Shennan AT. alpha1-Proteinase inhibitor therapy for the prevention of chronic lung disease of prematurity: a randomized, controlled trial. Pediatrics 1998; 101:89–94.
24. Goldenberg RL, Hauth JC, Andrews WW. Intrauterine infection and preterm delivery. N Engl J Med 2000; 342:1500–1507.
25. Yoon BH, Jun JK, Romero R. Amniotic fluid inflammatory cytokines (interleukin-6, interleukin-1 beta, and tumor necrosis factor-alpha), neonatal brain white matter lesions, and cerebral palsy. Am J Obstet Gynecol 1997; 177:19–26.
26. Yoon BH, Romero R, Jun JK. Amniotic fluid cytokines (interleukin-6, tumor necrosis factor-alpha, interleukin-1 beta, and interleukin-8) and the risk for the development of bronchopulmonary dysplasia. Am J Obstet Gynecol 1997; 177:825–830.
27. Schmidt B, Cao L, Mackensen-Haen S. Chorioamnionitis and inflammation of the fetal lung. Am J Obstet Gynecol 2001; 185:173–177.
28. Curley AE, Sweet DG, Thornton CM. Chorioamnionitis and increased neonatal lung lavage fluid matrix metalloproteinase-9 levels: implications for antenatal origins of chronic lung disease. Am J Obstet Gynecol 2003; 188:871–875.

29. Curley AE, Sweet DG, MacMahon KJ. Chorioamnionitis increases matrix metalloproteinase-8 concentrations in bronchoalveolar lavage fluid from preterm babies. Arch Dis Child Fetal Neonatal Ed 2004; 89:F61–64.

30. Goldenberg RL. The management of preterm labor. Obstet Gynecol 2002; 100:1020–1037.

31. Heaman MI, Sprague AE, Stewart PJ. Reducing the preterm birth rate: a population health strategy. J Obstet Gynecol Neonatal Nurs 2001; 30:20–29.

32. Blondel B, Norton J, du Mazaubrun C. Development of the main indicators of perinatal health in metropolitan France between 1995 and 1998. Results of the national perinatal survey. J Gynecol Obstet Biol Reprod 2001; 30:552–564.

33. Alexander GR, Weiss J, Hulsey TC. Preterm birth prevention: an evaluation of programs in the United States. Birth 1991; 18:160–169.

34. Goldenberg RL, Rouse DJ. Prevention of premature birth. N Engl J Med 1998; 339:313–320.

35. Dodd JM, Crowther CA, Cincotta R. Progesterone supplementation for preventing preterm birth: a systematic review and meta-analysis. Acta Obstet Gynecol Scand 2005; 84:526–533.

36. Dodd JM, Flenady V, Cincotta R. Prenatal administration of progesterone for preventing preterm birth. Cochrane Database Syst Rev 2006; 004947.

37. Smaill F. Antibiotics for asymptomatic bacteriuria in pregnancy. Cochrane Database Syst Rev 2001; 000490.

38. McDonald H, Brocklehurst P, Parsons J. Antibiotics for treating bacterial vaginosis in pregnancy. Cochrane Database Syst Rev 2005; 000262.

39. Kenyon S, Boulvain M, Neilson J. Antibiotics for preterm rupture of membranes. Cochrane Database Syst Rev 2003; 001058.

40. Ballard PL, Ning Y, Polk D. Glucocorticoid regulation of surfactant components in immature lambs. Am J Physiol 1997; 273:1048–1057.

41. Keeney SE, Mathews MJ, Rassin DK. Antioxidant enzyme responses to hyperoxia in preterm and term rats after prenatal dexamethasone administration. Pediatr Res 1993; 33:177–180.

42. Asoh K, Kumai T, Murano K. Effect of antenatal dexamethasone treatment on Ca2+-dependent nitric oxide synthase activity in rat lung. Pediatr Res 2000; 48:91–95.

43. Willet KE, Jobe AH, Ikegami M. Lung morphometry after repetitive antenatal glucocorticoid treatment in preterm sheep. Am J Respir Crit Care Med 2001; 163:1437–1443.

44. Crowley P. Prophylactic corticosteroids for preterm birth. Cochrane Database Syst Rev 2000; 000065.

45. Banks BA, Macones G, Cnaan A. Multiple courses of antenatal corticosteroids are associated with early severe lung disease in preterm neonates. J Perinatol 2002; 22:101–107.

46. Kutzler MA, Ruane EK, Coksaygan T. Effects of three courses of maternally administered dexamethasone at 0.7, 0.75, and 0.8 of gestation on prenatal and postnatal growth in sheep. Pediatrics 2004; 113:313–319.

47. Willet KE, Jobe AH, Ikegami M. Pulmonary interstitial emphysema 24 hours after antenatal betamethasone treatment in preterm sheep. Am J Respir Crit Care Med 2000; 162:1087–1094.

48. Adamson IY, King GM. Postnatal development of rat lung following retarded fetal lung growth. Pediatr Pulmonol 1988; 4:230–236.

49. Crowther CA, Harding J. Repeat doses of prenatal corticosteroids for women at risk of preterm birth for preventing neonatal respiratory disease. Cochrane Database Syst Rev 2003; 003935.

50. National Institutes of Health Consensus Development, Panel. Antenatal corticosteroids revisited: repeat courses – National Institutes of Health Consensus Development Conference Statement, August 17–18, 2000. Obstet Gynecol 2001; 98:144–150.

51. Pierce RA, Mariencheck WI, Sandefur S. Glucocorticoids upregulate tropoelastin expression during late stages of fetal lung development. Am J Physiol 1995; 268:491–500.

52. Kallapur SG, Kramer BW, Moss TJ. Maternal glucocorticoids increase endotoxin-induced lung inflammation in preterm lambs. Am J Physiol Lung Cell Mol Physiol 2003; 284:633–642.

53. Schellenberg JC, Liggins GC, Manzai M. Synergistic hormonal effects on lung maturation in fetal sheep. J Appl Physiol 1988; 65:94–100.

54. Ballard PL. Hormones and lung maturation. Monogr Endocrinol 1986; 28:1–354.

55. Ballard PL, Ballard RA, Ning Y. Plasma thyroid hormones in premature infants: effect of gestational age and antenatal thyrotropin-releasing hormone treatment. TRH Collaborative Trial Participants. Pediatr Res 1998; 44:642–649.

56. Knight DB, Liggins GC, Wealthall SR. A randomized, controlled trial of antepartum thyrotropin-releasing hormone and betamethasone in the prevention of respiratory disease in preterm infants. Am J Obstet Gynecol 1994; 171:11–16.

57. Crowther CA, Hiller JE, Haslam RR. Australian Collaborative Trial of Antenatal Thyrotropin-Releasing Hormone: adverse effects at 12-month follow-up. ACTOBAT Study Group. Pediatrics 1997; 99:311–317.

58. Halliday HL, Ehrenkranz RA, Doyle LW. Moderately early (7–14 days) postnatal corticosteroids for preventing chronic lung disease in preterm infants. Cochrane Database Syst Rev 2003; 001144.

59. Rojas MA, Gonzalez A, Bancalari E. Changing trends in the epidemiology and pathogenesis of neonatal chronic lung disease. J Pediatr 1995; 126:605–610.

60. Stevens TP, Blennow M, Soll RF. Early surfactant administration with brief ventilation vs selective surfactant and continued mechanical ventilation for preterm infants with or at risk for respiratory distress syndrome. Cochrane Database Syst Rev 2004; 003063.

61. Soll RF, Blanco F. Natural surfactant extract versus synthetic surfactant for neonatal respiratory distress syndrome. Cochrane Database Syst Rev 2001; 000144.

62. Soll RF. Multiple versus single dose natural surfactant extract for severe neonatal respiratory distress syndrome. Cochrane Database Syst Rev 2000; 000141.

63. Soll RF. Prophylactic natural surfactant extract for preventing morbidity and mortality in preterm infants. Cochrane Database Syst Rev 2000; 000511.

64. Soll RF. Prophylactic synthetic surfactant for preventing morbidity and mortality in preterm infants. Cochrane Database Syst Rev 2000; 001079.

65. Soll RF, Morley CJ. Prophylactic versus selective use of surfactant in preventing morbidity and mortality in preterm infants. Cochrane Database Syst Rev 2001; 000510.

66. Soll RF. Synthetic surfactant for respiratory distress syndrome in preterm infants. Cochrane Database Syst Rev 2000; 001149.

67. Hallman M, Jarvenpaa AL, Pohjavuori M. Respiratory distress syndrome and inositol supplementation in preterm infants. Arch Dis Child 1986; 61:1076–1083.

68. Hallman M, Bry K, Hoppu K. Inositol supplementation in premature infants with respiratory distress syndrome. N Engl J Med 1992; 326:1233–1239.

69. Friedman CA, McVey J, Borne MJ. Relationship between serum inositol concentration and development of retinopathy of prematurity: a prospective study. J Pediatr Ophthalmol Strabismus 2000; 37:79–86.

70. Howlett A, Ohlsson A. Inositol for respiratory distress syndrome in preterm infants. Cochrane Database Syst Rev 2003; 000366.

71. Mammel MC, Green TP, Johnson DE. Controlled trial of dexamethasone therapy in infants with bronchopulmonary dysplasia. Lancet 1983; 1:1356–1358.

72. Avery GB, Fletcher AB, Kaplan M. Controlled trial of dexamethasone in respirator-dependent infants with bronchopulmonary dysplasia. Pediatrics 1985; 75:106–111.

73. Cummings JJ, D'Eugenio DB, Gross SJ. A controlled trial of dexamethasone in preterm infants at high risk for bronchopulmonary dysplasia. N Engl J Med 1989; 320:1505–1510.

74. Yeh TF, Lin YJ, Huang CC. Early dexamethasone therapy in preterm infants: a follow-up study. Pediatrics 1998; 101:E7.

75. O'Shea TM, Kothadia JM, Klinepeter KL. Randomised placebo controlled trial of a 42-day tapering course of dexamethasone to reduce the duration of ventilator dependency in very low birthweight infants: outcome of study participants at 1-year adjusted age. Pediatrics 1995; 104:15–21.

76. Shinwell ES, Karplus M, Reich D, Early postnatal dexamethasone treatment and increased incidence of cerebral palsy. Arch Dis Child Fetal Neonatal Ed 2000; 83:F177–181.

77. Halliday HL. Guidelines on neonatal steroids. Prenat Neonat Med 2001; 6:371–373.

78. Committee on Fetus and,Newborn. Postnatal corticosteroids to treat or prevent chronic lung disease in preterm infants. Pediatrics 2002; 109:330–338.

79. Halliday HL, Ehrenkranz RA, Doyle LW. Early postnatal (< 96 hours) corticosteroids for preventing chronic lung disease in preterm infants. Cochrane Database Syst Rev 2003; 001146.

80. Halliday HL, Ehrenkranz RA, Doyle LW. Delayed (> 3 weeks) postnatal corticosteroids for chronic lung disease in preterm infants. Cochrane Database Syst Rev 2003; 001145.

81. Baden M, Bauer CR, Colle E. A controlled trial of hydrocortisone therapy in infants with respiratory distress syndrome. Pediatrics 1972; 50:526–534.

82. Taeusch HW, Jr, Wang NS, Baden N. A controlled trial of hydrocortisone therapy in infants with respiratory distress syndrome: II. Pathology. Pediatrics 1973; 52:850–854.

83. Fitzhardinge PM, Eisen A, Lejtenyi C. Sequelae of early steroid administration to the newborn infant. Pediatrics 1974; 53:877–883.

84. Groneck P, Reuss D, Gotze-Speer B. Effects of dexamethasone on chemotactic activity and inflammatory mediators in tracheobronchial aspirates of preterm infants at risk for chronic lung disease. J Pediatr 1993; 122:938–944.

85. Zimmerman JJ, Gabbert D, Shivpuri C. Meter-dosed, inhaled beclomethasone attenuates bronchoalveolar oxyradical inflammation in premature infants at risk for bronchopulmonary dysplasia. Am J Perinatol 1998; 15:567–576.

86. Merz U, Kusenbach G, Hausler M. Inhaled budesonide in ventilator-dependent preterm infants: a randomized, double-blind pilot study. Biol Neonate 1999; 75:46–53.

87. Konig P, Shatley M, Levine C. Clinical observations of nebulized flunisolide in infants and young children with asthma and bronchopulmonary dysplasia. Pediatr Pulmonol 1992; 13:209–214.

88. Dugas MA, Nguyen D, Frenette L. Fluticasone inhalation in moderate cases of bronchopulmonary dysplasia. Pediatrics 2005; 115:e566–572.

89. Grier DG, Halliday HL. Management of bronchopulmonary dysplasia in infants: guidelines for corticosteroid use. Drugs 2005; 65:15–29.

90. Viscardi RM, Hasday JD, Gumpper KF. Cromolyn sodium prophylaxis inhibits pulmonary proinflammatory cytokines in infants at high risk for bronchopulmonary dysplasia. Am J Respir Crit Care Med 1997; 156:1523–1529.

91. Denjean A, Paris-Llado J, Zupan V. Inhaled salbutamol and beclomethasone for preventing broncho-pulmonary dysplasia: a randomised double-blind study. Eur J Pediatr 1998; 157:926–931.

92. Clyman RI. Recommendations for the postnatal use of indomethacin: an analysis of four separate treatment strategies. J Pediatr 1996; 128:601–607.

93. Cooke L, Steer P, Woodgate P. Indomethacin for asymptomatic patent ductus arteriosus in preterm infants. Cochrane Database Syst Rev 2003; 003745.

94. Shah SS, Ohlsson A. Ibuprofen for the prevention of patent ductus arteriosus in preterm and/or low birth weight infants. Cochrane Database Syst Rev 2006; 004213.

95. Ohlsson A, Walia R, Shah S. Ibuprofen for the treatment of patent ductus arteriosus in preterm and/or low birth weight infants. Cochrane Database Syst Rev 2005; 003481.

96. Bell EF, Acarregui MJ. Restricted versus liberal water intake for preventing morbidity and mortality in preterm infants. Cochrane Database Syst Rev 2001; 000503.

97. Schmidt B, Roberts RS, Davis P. Caffeine therapy for apnea of prematurity. N Engl J Med 2006; 354:2112–2121.

98. Davis JM, Bhutani VK, Stefano JL. Changes in pulmonary mechanics following caffeine administration in infants with bronchopulmonary dysplasia. Pediatr Pulmonol 1989; 6:49–52.

99. Lapenna D, De Gioia S, Mezzetti A. Aminophylline: could it act as an antioxidant in vivo? Eur J Clin Invest 1995; 25:464–470.

100. Yoder B, Thomson M, Coalson J. Lung function in immature baboons with respiratory distress syndrome receiving early caffeine therapy: a pilot study. Acta Paediatr 2005; 94:92–98.

101. Watterberg KL, Demers LM, Scott SM. Chorioamnionitis and early lung inflammation in infants in whom bronchopulmonary dysplasia develops. Pediatrics 1996; 97:210–215.

102. Lyon A. Chronic lung disease of prematurity. The role of intra-uterine infection. Eur J Pediatr 2000; 159:798–802.

103. Wang EE, Ohlsson A, Kellner JD. Association of Ureaplasma urealyticum colonization with chronic lung disease of prematurity: results of a metaanalysis. J Pediatr 1995; 127:640–644.

104. Iles R, Lyon A, Ross P. Infection with Ureaplasma urealyticum and Mycoplasma hominis and the development of chronic lung disease in preterm infants. Acta Paediatr 1996; 85:482–484.

105. Baier RJ, Loggins J, Kruger TE. Failure of erythromycin to eliminate airway colonization with Ureaplasma urealyticum in very low birth weight infants. BMC Pediatrics 2003; 3:10.

106. Collard KJ, Godeck S, Holley JE. Pulmonary antioxidant concentrations and oxidative damage in ventilated premature babies. Arch Dis Child Fetal Neonatal Ed 2004; 89:F412–416.

107. Kaarteenaho-Wiik R, Kinnula VL. Distribution of antioxidant enzymes in developing human lung, respiratory distress syndrome, and bronchopulmonary dysplasia. J Histochem Cytochem 2004; 52:1231–1240.

108. Zoban P, Cerny M. Immature lung and acute lung injury. Physiol Res 2003; 52:507–516.

109. Watts JL, Milner R, Zipursky A. Failure of supplementation with vitamin E to prevent bronchopulmonary dysplasia in infants less than 1,500 g birth weight. Eur Respir 1991; 4:188–190.

110. Davis JM. Superoxide dismutase: a role in the prevention of chronic lung disease. Biol Neonate 1998; 74:29–34.

111. Kao SJ, Wang D, Lin HI. N-acetylcysteine abrogates acute lung injury induced by endotoxin. Clin Exp Pharmacol Physiol 2006; 33:33–40.

112. Russell GA, Cooke RW. Randomised controlled trial of allopurinol prophylaxis in very preterm infants. Arch Dis Child Fetal Neonatal Ed 1995; 73:F27–31.

113. Tyson JE, Wright LL, Oh W. Vitamin A supplementation for extremely-low-birth-weight infants. National Institute of Child Health and Human Development Neonatal Research Network. N Engl J Med 1999; 340:1962–1968.

114. Darlow BA, Graham PJ. Vitamin A supplementation for preventing morbidity and mortality in very low birthweight infants. Cochrane Database Syst Rev 2002; 000501.

115. Ross SA, McCaffery PJ, Drager UC. Retinoids in embryonal development. Physiol Rev 2000; 80:1021–1054.

116. Massaro GD, Massaro D. Postnatal treatment with retinoic acid increases the number of pulmonary alveoli in rats. Am J Physiol 1996; 270:305–310.

117. Nakamura T, Ogawa Y. Prophylactic effects of recombinant human superoxide dismutase in neonatal lung injury induced by the intratracheal instillation of endotoxin in piglets. Biol Neonate 2001; 80:163–168.

118. Davis JM, Rosenfeld WN, Sanders RJ. Prophylactic effects of recombinant human superoxide dismutase in neonatal lung injury. J Appl Physiol 1993; 74:2234–2241.

119. Sandberg K, Fellman V, Stigson L. N-acetylcysteine administration during the first week of life does not improve lung function in extremely low birth weight infants. Biol Neonate 2004; 86:275–279.

120. Ahola T, Lapatto R, Raivio KO. N-acetylcysteine does not prevent bronchopulmonary dysplasia in immature infants: a randomized controlled trial. J Pediatr 2003; 143:713–719.

121. Chang LY, Subramaniam M, Yoder BA. A catalytic antioxidant attenuates alveolar structural remodeling in bronchopulmonary dysplasia. Am J Respir Crit Care Med 2003; 167:57–64.

122. Jankov RP, Negus A, Tanswell AK. Antioxidants as therapy in the newborn: some words of caution. Pediatr Res 2001; 50:681–687.

123. Merritt TA, Cochrane CG, Holcomb K. Elastase and alpha 1-proteinase inhibitor activity in tracheal aspirates during respiratory distress syndrome. Role of inflammation in the pathogenesis of bronchopulmonary dysplasia. J Clin Invest 1983; 72:656–666.

124. Ambalavanan N, Tyson JE, Kennedy KA. Vitamin A supplementation for extremely low birth weight infants: outcome at 18 to 22 months. Pediatrics 2005; 115:e249–e254.

125. Sluis KB, Darlow BA, Vissers MC. Proteinase-antiproteinase balance in tracheal aspirates from neonates. Eur Respir J 1994; 7:251–259.

126. Sveger T, Ohlsson K, Polberger S. Tracheobronchial aspirate fluid neutrophil lipocalin, elastase- and neutrophil protease-4-alpha1-antitrypsin complexes, protease inhibitors and free proteolytic activity in respiratory distress syndrome. Acta Paediatr 2002; 91:934–937.

127. Barrington KJ, Finer NN. Inhaled nitric oxide for respiratory failure in preterm infants. Cochrane Database Syst Rev 2006; 000509.

128. Kinsella JP, Parker TA, Galan H. Effects of inhaled nitric oxide on pulmonary edema and lung neutrophil accumulation in severe experimental hyaline membrane disease. Pediatr Res 1997; 41:457–463.

129. Roberts JD, Jr, Chiche JD, Weimann J. Nitric oxide inhalation decreases pulmonary artery remodeling in the injured lungs of rat pups. Circ Res 2000; 87:140–145.

130. El Kebir D, Hubert B, Taha R. Effects of inhaled nitric oxide on inflammation and apoptosis after cardiopulmonary bypass. Chest 2005; 128:2910–2917.

131. Wang T, El Kebir D, Blaise G. Inhaled nitric oxide in 2003: a review of its mechanisms of action. Can J Anaesth 2003; 50:839–846.

132. Hamon I, Fresson J, Nicolas MB. Early inhaled nitric oxide improves oxidative balance in very preterm infants. Pediatr Res 2005; 57:637–643.

133. Kinsella JP, Walsh WF, Bose CL. Inhaled nitric oxide in premature neonates with severe hypoxaemic respiratory failure: a randomised controlled trial. Lancet 1999; 354:1061–1065.

134. Anonymous. Early compared with delayed inhaled nitric oxide in moderately hypoxaemic neonates with respiratory failure: a randomised controlled trial. The Franco-Belgium Collaborative NO Trial Group. Lancet 1999; 354:1066–1071.

135. Subhedar NV, Ryan SW, Shaw NJ. Open randomised controlled trial of inhaled nitric oxide and early dexamethasone in high risk preterm infants. Arch Dis Child Fetal Neonatal Ed 1997; 77:F185–190.

136. Barrington KJ, Finer NN. Inhaled nitric oxide for respiratory failure in preterm infants. Cochrane Database Syst Rev 2006; 000509.

137. Schreiber MD, Gin-Mestan K, Marks JD. Inhaled nitric oxide in premature infants with the respiratory distress syndrome. N Engl J Med 2003; 349:2099–2107.

138. Hogman M, Frostell C, Arnberg H. Bleeding time prolongation and NO inhalation. Lancet 1993; 341:1664–1665.

139. Hallman M, Waffarn F, Bry K. Surfactant dysfunction after inhalation of nitric oxide. J Appl Physiol 1996; 80:2026–2034.

140. Robbins CG, Davis JM, Merritt TA. Combined effects of nitric oxide and hyperoxia on surfactant function and pulmonary inflammation. Am J Physiol 1995; 269:545–550.

141. Mestan KK, Marks JD, Hecox K. Neurodevelopmental outcomes of premature infants treated with inhaled nitric oxide. N Engl J Med 2005; 353:23–32.

142. Van Meurs KP, Wright LL, Ehrenkranz RA. Inhaled nitric oxide for premature infants with severe respiratory failure. N Engl J Med 2005; 353:13–22.

143. Field D, Elbourne D, Truesdale A. Neonatal ventilation with inhaled nitric oxide versus ventilatory support without inhaled nitric oxide for preterm infants with severe respiratory failure: the INNOVO multicentre randomised controlled trial (ISRCTN 17821339). Pediatrics 2005; 115:926–936.

144. Hoehn T, Krause MF, Buhrer C. Meta-analysis of inhaled nitric oxide in premature infants: an update. Klin Padiatr 2006; 218:57–61.

145. Kinsella J, Cutter G, Walsh W. Early inhaled nitric oxide therapy in premature newborns with respiratory failure. N Engl J Med 2006; 355:354–364.

146. Ballard RA, Truog WE, Cnaan A. Inhaled nitric oxide in preterm infants undergoing mechanical ventilation. N Engl J Med 2006; 355:343–353.

147. Jobe AH, Newnham JP, Willet KE. Effects of antenatal endotoxin and glucocorticoids on the lungs of preterm lambs. Am J Obstet Gynecol 2000; 182:401–408.

148. Jobe AH, Newnham JP, Willet KE. Endotoxin-induced lung maturation in preterm lambs is not mediated by cortisol. Am J Respir Crit Care Med 2000; 162:1656–1661.

149. Moss TJ, Nitsos I, Kramer BW. Intra-amniotic endotoxin induces lung maturation by direct effects on the developing respiratory tract in preterm sheep. Am J Obstet Gynecol 2002; 187:1059–1065.

150. Vozzelli MA, Mason SN, Whorton MH. Antimacrophage chemokine treatment prevents neutrophil and macrophage influx in hyperoxia-exposed newborn rat lung. Am J Physiol Lung Cell Mol Physiol 2004; 286:488–493.

151. Chiba H, Piboonpocanun S, Mitsuzawa H. Pulmonary surfactant proteins and lipids as modulators of inflammation and innate immunity. Respirology 2006; 11:S2–6.

152. Levine CR, Gewolb IH, Allen K. The safety, pharmacokinetics, and anti-inflammatory effects of intratracheal recombinant human Clara cell protein in premature infants with respiratory distress syndrome. Pediatr Res 2005; 58:15–21.

153. Chang LY, Subramaniam M, Yoder BA. A catalytic antioxidant attenuates alveolar structural remodeling in bronchopulmonary dysplasia. Am J Respir Crit Care Med 2003; 167:57–64.

154. Sunday ME, Shan L, Subramaniam M. Immunomodulatory functions of the diffuse neuroendocrine system: implications for bronchopulmonary dysplasia. Endocr Pathol 2004; 15:91–106.

155. Kraybill EN, Runyan DK, Bose CL. Risk factors for chronic lung disease in infants with birth weights of 751–1000 grams. J Pediatr 1989; 115:115–120.

156. Auten RL, Vozzelli M, Clark RH. Volutrauma. What is it, and how do we avoid it?. Clin Perinatol 2001; 28:505–515.

157. Dreyfuss D, Saumon G. Ventilator-induced lung injury: lessons from experimental studies. Am J Respir Crit Care Med 1998; 157:294–323.

158. Muscedere JG, Mullen JB, Gan K. Tidal ventilation at low airway pressures can augment lung injury. Am J Respir Crit Care Med 1994; 149:1327–1334.

159. Buss IH, Darlow BA, Winterbourn CC. Elevated protein carbonyls and lipid peroxidation products correlating with myeloperoxidase in tracheal aspirates from premature infants. Pediatr Res 2000; 47:640–645.

160. Anonymous supplemental therapeutic oxygen for prethreshold retinopathy of prematurity (STOP-ROP), a randomized, controlled trial. I: primary outcomes. Pediatrics 2000; 105:295–310.

161. Cole CH, Wright KW, Tarnow-Mordi W. Resolving our uncertainty about oxygen therapy. Pediatrics 2003; 112:1415–1419.

162. Gonzalez A, Sosenko IR, Chandar J. Influence of infection on patent ductus arteriosus and chronic lung disease in premature infants weighing 1000 grams or less. J Pediatr 1996; 128:470–478.

163. Bancalari E. Changes in the pathogenesis and prevention of chronic lung disease of prematurity. Am J Perinatol 2001; 18:1–9.

164. Ruf B, Klauwer D, Reiss I. Colonisation of the airways with Ureaplasma urealyticum as a risk factor for bronchopulmonary dysplasia in VLBW infants? Z Geburtshilfe Neonatol 2002; 206:187–192.

165. Viscardi RM, Manimtim WM, Sun CC. Lung pathology in premature infants with Ureaplasma urealyticum infection. Pediatr Dev Pathol 2002; 5:141–150.

166. Jonsson B, Rylander M, Faxelius G. Ureaplasma urealyticum, erythromycin and respiratory morbidity in high-risk preterm neonates. Acta Paediatrica 1998; 87:1079–1084.

167. Van Marter LJ, Leviton A, Allred EN. Hydration during the first days of life and the risk of bronchopulmonary dysplasia in low birth weight infants. J Pediatr 1990; 116:942–949.

168. Gonzalez A, Sosenko IR, Chandar J. Influence of infection on patent ductus arteriosus and chronic lung disease in premature infants weighing 1000 grams or less. J Pediatr 1996; 128:470–478.

169. Frank L. Antioxidants, nutrition, and bronchopulmonary dysplasia. Clin Perinatol 1992; 19:541–562.

170. Blanco LN, Frank L. The formation of alveoli in rat lung during the third and fourth postnatal weeks: effect of hyperoxia, dexamethasone, and deferoxamine. Pediatr Res 1993; 34:334–340.

171. Schwyter M, Burri PH, Tschanz SA. Geometric properties of the lung parenchyma after postnatal glucocorticoid treatment in rats [erratum appears in Biol Neonate. 2003;84(2):141]. Biol Neonate 2003; 83:57–64.

172. Lister P, Iles R, Shaw B. Inhaled steroids for neonatal chronic lung disease. Cochrane Database Syst Rev 2000; 002311.

173. Shah SS, Ohlsson A, Halliday H. Inhaled versus systemic corticosteroids for the treatment of chronic lung disease in ventilated very low birth weight preterm infants. Cochrane Database Syst Rev 2003; 002057.

174. Halliday HL, Patterson CC, Halahakoon CW. A multicenter, randomized open study of early corticosteroid treatment (OSECT) in preterm infants with respiratory illness: comparison of early and late treatment and of dexamethasone and inhaled budesonide. Pediatrics 2001; l07:232–240.

175. Cole CH. Inhaled glucocorticoid therapy in infants at risk for neonatal chronic lung disease. J Asthma 2000; 37:533–543.

176. Brion LP, Primhak RA. Intravenous or enteral loop diuretics for preterm infants with (or developing) chronic lung disease. Cochrane Database Syst Rev 2002; 001453.

177. Brion LP, Primhak RA, Ambrosio-Perez I. Diuretics acting on the distal renal tubule for preterm infants with (or developing) chronic lung disease. Cochrane Database Syst Rev 2002; 001817.

178. McCann EM, Lewis K, Deming DD. Controlled trial of furosemide therapy in infants with chronic lung disease. J Pediatr 1985; 106:957–962.

179. Brion LP, Primhak RA, Yong W. Aerosolized diuretics for preterm infants with (or developing) chronic lung disease. Cochrane Database Syst Rev 2001; 001694.

180. Farrell PA, Fiascone JM. Bronchopulmonary dysplasia in the 1990s: a review for the pediatrician. Curr Probl Pediatr 1997; 27:129–163.

181. Cashore WJ, Oh W, Brodersen R. Bilirubin-displacing effect of furosemide and sulfisoxazole. An in vitro and in vivo study in neonatal serum. Dev Pharmacol Ther 1983; 6:230–238.

182. Engelhardt B, Blalock WA, DonLevy S. Effect of spironolactone-hydrochlorothiazide on lung function in infants with chronic bronchopulmonary dysplasia. J Pediatr 1989; 114:619–624.

183. Kao LC, Warburton D, Cheng MH. Effect of oral diuretics on pulmonary mechanics in infants with chronic bronchopulmonary dysplasia: results of a double-blind crossover sequential trial. Pediatrics 1984; 74:37–44.

184. Kao LC, Durand DJ, McCrea RC. Randomized trial of long-term diuretic therapy for infants with oxygen-dependent bronchopulmonary dysplasia. J Pediatr 1994; 124:772–781.

185. Davis JM, Sinkin RA, Aranda JV. Drug therapy for bronchopulmonary dysplasia. Pediatr Pulmonol 1990; 8:117–125.

186. Australian collaborative trial of antenatal thyrotropin-releasing; hormone (ACTOBAT) for prevention of neonatal respiratory disease. Lancet 1995; 8:345:877–882.

187. Thomas W, Speer CP. Management of infants with bronchopulmonary dysplasia in Germany. Early Hum Dev 2005; 81:155–163.

188. Allen J, Zwerdling R, Ehrenkranz R. Statement on the care of the child with chronic lung disease of infancy and childhood. Am J Respir Crit Care Med 2003; 168:356–396.

189. D'Angio CT, Maniscalco WM. Bronchopulmonary dysplasia in preterm infants: pathophysiology and management strategies. Paediatr Drugs 2004; 6:303–330.

190. Sosulski R, Abbasi S, Bhutani VK. Physiologic effects of terbutaline on pulmonary function of infants with bronchopulmonary dysplasia. Pediatr Pulmonol 1986; 2:269–273.

191. Wilkie RA, Bryan MH. Effect of bronchodilators on airway resistance in ventilator-dependent neonates with chronic lung disease. J Pediatr 1987; 111:278–282.
192. Kao LC, Durand DJ, Phillips BL. Oral theophylline and diuretics improve pulmonary mechanics in infants with bronchopulmonary dysplasia. J Pediatr 1987; 111:439–444.
193. Costalos C, Houlsby WT, Manchett P. Weaning very low birthweight infants from mechanical ventilation using intermittent mandatory ventilation and theophylline. Arch Dis Child 1979; 54:404–405.
194. Reiter PD, Townsend SF, Velasquez R. Dornase alfa in premature infants with severe respiratory distress and early bronchopulmonary dysplasia. J Perinatol 2000; 20:530–534.
195. Wang EE, Tang NK. Immunoglobulin for preventing respiratory syncytial virus infection. Cochrane Database Syst Rev 2000; 001725.
196. Meissner HC, Long SS and American Academy of Pediatrics. Committee on Infectious Diseases and Committee on Fetus and, Newborn. Revised indications for the use of palivizumab and respiratory syncytial virus immune globulin intravenous for the prevention of respiratory syncytial virus infections. Pediatrics 2003; 112:1447–1452.
197. Ladha F, Bonnet S, Eaton F. Sildenafil improves alveolar growth and pulmonary hypertension in hyperoxia-induced lung injury. Am J Respir Crit Care Med 2005; 172:750–756.
198. Lauterbach R, Szymura-Oleksiak J. Nebulized pentoxifylline in successful treatment of five premature neonates with bronchopulmonary dysplasia. Eur J Pediatr 1999; 158:607.
199. Lauterbach R, Pawlik D, Zembala M. Pentoxifylline in and prevention and treatment of chronic lung disease. Acta Paediatrica Supplement 2004; 93:20–22.
200. Crowther CA, Alfirevic Z, Haslam RR. Thyrotropin-releasing hormone added to corticosteroids for women at risk of preterm birth for preventing neonatal respiratory disease. Cochrane Database Syst Rev 2004; 000019.
201. Yost CC, Soll RF. Early versus delayed selective surfactant treatment for neonatal respiratory distress syndrome. Cochrane Database Syst Rev 2000; 001456.
202. Fowlie PW, Davis PG. Prophylactic intravenous indomethacin for preventing mortality and morbidity in preterm infants. Cochrane Database Syst Rev 2002; 000174.
203. Suresh GK, Davis JM, Soll RF. Superoxide dismutase for preventing chronic lung disease in mechanically ventilated preterm infants. Cochrane Database Syst Rev 2001; 001968.
204. Shah P, Ohlsson A. Alpha-1 proteinase inhibitor (a1PI) for preventing chronic lung disease in preterm infants. Cochrane Database Syst Rev 2001; 002775.

Chapter 11

Definitions and Predictors of Bronchopulmonary Dysplasia

Michele C. Walsh MD MS

Northway's Original Description

Clinical Definitions

NIH Consensus Definition

Physiologic Definition

The New BPD

Predictors of BPD

Future Directions

The development of mechanical ventilation in the 1960s changed the natural history of respiratory distress syndrome (RDS) and resulted in the survival of smaller and sicker infants. Soon thereafter the pulmonary sequelae of mechanical ventilation were described by Northway and colleagues, who introduced the term bronchopulmonary dysplasia (BPD) (1). Both the terms bronchopulmonary dysplasia (BPD) and chronic lung disease (CLD) have been used interchangeably to describe the pulmonary sequelae. At a National Institutes of Health sponsored workshop held in 2001 participants recommended that the term BPD be used to describe the pulmonary sequelae of RDS and prematurity because BPD emphasized the involvement of all of the tissues of the lung, and was a term reserved solely to survivors of preterm birth (2). Since the original description by Northway the natural history of BPD has evolved and newer definitions have been proposed. These definitions serve to clarify the diagnosis of BPD as an outcome measure of clinical care and research trials. In this chapter, we will discuss definitions of BPD and early predictors of the risk of BPD.

NORTHWAY'S ORIGINAL DESCRIPTION

All infants originally described by Northway and colleagues had severe RDS, received prolonged mechanical ventilation, and were exposed to high concentrations of inspired oxygen (1). Northway described a progression of disease through four stages that ended with severe chronic changes characterized by persistent respiratory failure, hypoxemia, and hypercapnia. Radiographs of infants with stage IV disease showed areas of increased density due to fibrosis alternating with areas of hyperinflation. Late follow-up of these infants at age 14–23 years demonstrated persistent and significant pulmonary morbidity (3). By the late 1970s there was increasing recognition that damage from large tidal volume ventilation strategies contributed to BPD. Modifications of these strategies decreased the incidence of the classic stages described by Northway. Therefore, investigators proposed definitions based on clinical and radiographic characteristics.

CLINICAL DEFINITIONS

Bancalari and colleagues were the first to propose a definition based on clinical characteristics, including the need for oxygen on 28 of the first 28 days, together with a compatible chest radiograph (4). Subsequently, Tooley and O'Brodovich provided additional support for this definition (5, 6). Palta explored the utility and predictive validity of various definitions of BPD in the Newborn Lung Project in the late 1980s (7). Her group found that clinical characteristics combined with chest radiograph were predictive of later pulmonary morbidity. These early definitions focused on outcomes at the first month of life. However, as smaller and more immature neonates were resuscitated, treated for RDS and survived, the significance of a continued oxygen requirement during the first 28 days was questioned. By the late 1970s authors noted that the radiographic abnormalities in ELBW differed from those described by Northway (8). Fletcher and colleagues compared different definitions of BPD and found that radiographic findings did not improve either the sensitivity or specificity of the diagnosis (9).

In 1988 Shennan and co-workers compared the ability of continued treatment with oxygen at 28 days of age or at 36 weeks post-menstrual age to predict outcome in neonates < 1500 g birth weight (10). The authors defined abnormal pulmonary outcomes as one or more of the following in the first 2 years of life: death in the first 2 years of life, oxygen at 40 weeks postmenstrual age, surgical procedure involving respiratory tract, two or more hospitalizations for respiratory cause, wheezing requiring drug treatment, and persistent radiographic changes at 1 year of age. The study cohort had a mean birth weight of 1132 g in those with a normal outcome ($n = 486$) and 992 g in those with an abnormal outcome ($n = 119$). Seventy-four of the 119 (62%) with abnormal outcome were ventilated. The 28 day definition did correctly identify neonates less than 30 weeks gestation who went on to have an abnormal pulmonary outcome; however, it performed less well for older infants. A requirement for oxygen at 28 days had a positive predictive value of only 38% for later abnormal pulmonary function. In contrast, oxygen requirement at 36 weeks PMA increased the positive predictive value to 63% and the sensitivity from 79% to 83%.

Since the original work by Shennan, many studies have validated the utility of this definition. The diagnosis of clinical BPD at 36 weeks post-menstrual age has been firmly established as a significant risk factor for future pulmonary and neurodevelopmental impairment (11–16) (Table 11-1). Even after adjustment for gestational age and initial severity of illness, BPD is among the most significant predictors of future neurodevelopmental impairment in infancy, early childhood and adolescence. In a longitudinal study by Short and coworkers evaluating survivors at 8 years of age neonates with BPD (54%) were more likely to be enrolled in special education classes (54%) compared to a

Table 11-1	Early Childhood Neurodevelopmental Outcomes Associated with the Diagnosis of Bronchopulmonary Dysplasia			
Study	Year published	Years included in cohort	MDI < 70	PDI < 70	Cerebral palsy
Hack	2000	1992–1995	2.18 (1.20–3.94)	NA	3.09 (1.51–6.35)
Vohr	2000	1993–1994	1.84 (1.28–2.61)	1.47 (1.1–2.2)	2.20 (1.6–3.74)
Vohr	2005	1993–1998	2.15 (1.38–2.31)	2.00 (1.50–2.60)	2.00 (1.25–2.75)

Adapted from references 11–13.

matched VLBW cohort (37%) or to term children (25%) (16). In addition, more BPD children (20%) had full-scale IQ scores < 70, in the mental retardation range, compared with either VLBW (11%) or term (3%) children. Only recently have the pulmonary outcomes of these infants been studied (17). The findings are sobering, with higher rates of asthma and diminished pulmonary function into adolescence. The longer-term impact on the development of chronic obstructive pulmonary disease in the presence and absence of tobacco exposure is not known, nor is the impact on longevity.

NIH CONSENSUS DEFINITION

While moving the definition of BPD to a time point at 36 weeks post-menstrual age improved the specificity and positive predictive value of the BPD definition, many remained concerned that neonates who might have suffered significant pulmonary injury were not included in the 36 week definition. In addition, neonates >32 weeks were not well classified by the 36 week definition, as it was possible for a 2 week old 34 week GA neonate who remained in oxygen to be classified as BPD at 36 weeks PMA but to have resolved lung injury and weaned to room air shortly after 36 weeks PMA.

The NIH Consensus definition addressed these competing needs (2). In addition, the definition increased the information contained in the definition to include a range of severity of outcomes from no BPD, to mild, moderate or severe BPD (Table 11-2). Neonates are assessed for the outcome BPD at different time points to account for different gestational trajectories. Those < 32 weeks gestation are assessed at 36 weeks PMA or discharge home, whichever comes first. Those = 32 weeks gestational age are assessed at > 28 days, but less than 56 days, or discharge home, whichever comes first. The severity of the lung injury is assessed

Table 11-2 NIH Consensus Definition of Bronchopulmonary Dysplasia

Gestational age	< 32 weeks	≥ 32 weeks
Time point of assessment	36 weeks PMA or discharge to home, whichever comes first	> 28 day, but < 56 day postnatal age or discharge to home, whichever comes first
Mild BPD	Treatment with oxygen > 21% for at least 28 days **plus** Breathing room air at 36 weeks PMA or discharge, whichever comes first	Breathing room air by 56 days postnatal age or discharge, whichever comes first
Moderate BPD	Need for < 30% oxygen at 36 weeks PMA or discharge, whichever comes first	Need for < 30% oxygen at 56 days postnatal age or discharge, whichever comes first
Severe BPD	Need for ≥ 30% oxygen and/or positive pressure (PPV or NCPAP) at 36 weeks PMA or discharge, whichever comes first	Need for ≥ 30% oxygen and/or positive pressure (PPV or NCPAP) at 56 days postnatal age or discharge, whichever comes first

Definition of abbreviations: BPD = bronchopulmonary dysplasia; NCPAP = nasal continuous positive airway pressure; PMA = post-menstrual age; PPV = positive-pressure ventilation

A physiologic test confirming that the oxygen requirement at the assessment time point remains to be defined. This assessment may include a pulse oximetry saturation range. BPD usually develops in neonates being treated with oxygen and positive-pressure ventilation for respiratory failure, most commonly respiratory distress syndrome. Persistence of clinical features of respiratory disease (tachypnea, retractions, rales) is considered common to the broad description of BPD and has not been included in the diagnostic criteria describing the severity of BPD. Infants treated with oxygen > 21% and/or positive pressure for non-respiratory disease (e.g., central apnea or diaphragmatic paralysis) do not have BPD unless they also develop parenchymal lung disease and exhibit clinical features of respiratory distress. A day of treatment with oxygen > 21% means that the infant received oxygen > 21% for more than 12 h on that day. Treatment with oxygen > 21% and/or positive pressure at 36 week PMA, or at 56 days postnatal age or discharge, should not reflect an "acute" event, but should rather reflect the infant's usual daily therapy for several days preceding and following 36 weeks PMA, 56 days postnatal age, or discharge.

Adapted from reference 2.

Table 11-3   **BPD Definitions and Selected Pulmonary Outcomes at 18 to 22 Months' Corrected Age**

BPD definition (consensus)	NICU infants, n (%; n = 4866)	Follow-up infants, n (%; n = 3848)	Pulmonary medications (% of follow-up[†])	Rehospitalized pulmonary cause (% of follow-up[†])	RSV Prophylaxis (% of follow-up[‡])
None	1124 (23.1)	876 (22.8)	27.2	23.9	12.5
Mild	1473 (30.3)	1186 (30.8)	29.7	26.7	16.6
Moderate	1471 (30.2)	1143 (29.7)	40.8	33.5	19.2
Severe	798 (16.4)	643 (16.7)	46.6[‡]	39.4[‡]	28.4[‡]

Missing data: 28 days – CXR, 17 infants (13 for follow-up cohort); 36 weeks – CXR, 12 (8 for follow-up cohort); pulmonary medications, 17; rehospitalizations for pulmonary causes, 35; RSV prophylaxis, 17.
    †Cohort of infants who were seen at 18 to 22 months' corrected age.
    ‡$P < .0001$, Mantel-Haenszel χ^2 for linear association across the categories of the consensus definition (none to severe), Mantel-Haenszel χ^2.
    Data from reference 18.

by a combination of early support and degree of support needed at the assessment endpoint. In every case, the definition requires the need for supplemental oxygen for a minimum of 28 days plus continued support at the assessment endpoint (Table 11-2). The definition was constructed by consensus from a panel of neonatal experts. While the definition had high face validity with neonatologists and pediatric pulmonologists it was not derived from a body of evidence.

Ehrenkranz, Walsh and coauthors explored the validity of the NIH Consensus definition in the large NICHD Neonatal Research Network database (18). Use of the consensus definition increases the number of infants diagnosed with BPD by adding the group who were on oxygen at 28 days of age but in room air at 36 weeks to those defined as having BPD. The overall rate of BPD was increased from 46% to 77%. The assessment of severity of BPD adds richness to the outcome measure and identifies a spectrum of adverse pulmonary and neurodevelopmental outcomes. As the severity of BPD increases the incidence of adverse events also increases (Table 11-3).

PHYSIOLOGIC DEFINITION

All of the previous definitions are based on the use of oxygen at varying time points. The need for oxygen is determined by individual physicians, rather than on the basis of a physiologic assessment. Implicit in the definition is the assumption that the criteria on which the decision to administer oxygen are uniform and applied similarly across institutions. However, such an assumption is erroneous. Because there is no consensus in the literature, neonatologists have widely divergent practices regarding oxygen saturation targets (19). Indeed, published literature cites acceptable saturation ranges from 84 to 98%. Thus, we developed a definition of BPD at 36 weeks postmenstrual age based on a timed challenge in room air in selected infants receiving < 30% effective oxygen (20, 21). Infants in room air were assumed to have no BPD. Infants receiving > 30% effective oxygen, support on a ventilator or continuous positive airway pressure were defined as BPD without a challenge. The physiologic definition identified infants treated with oxygen who were able to maintain saturations exceeding 90% in room air. Overall, the physiologic definition resulted in a 6% reduction in the number of infants diagnosed as having BPD compared to the clinical definition of BPD by oxygen use alone, from 31% to 25% (Fig. 11-1). One hundred and one of 227 infants challenged with a reduction of oxygen to room air passed the challenge. The magnitude of the impact did differ by center, with the largest impact

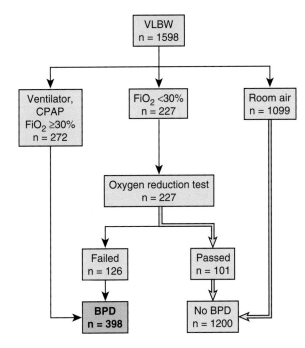

Figure 11-1 Impact of the physiologic definition on the diagnosis of BPD. From Walsh M, Yao Q, Gettner P, et al. Impact of a physiologic definition on bronchopulmonary dysplasia rates. Pediatrics 2004; 114:1305–1311.

being a reduction in the BPD rate from 60% to 16% (Fig. 11-2). It became apparent through this study that large numbers of infants were receiving oxygen for reasons other than compromised pulmonary function. Such reasons included treatment of retinopathy of prematurity and apnea of prematurity. The main utility of this definition will be in the context of clinical trials; however, the room air challenge may also be useful clinically in identifying infants who are candidates for trials of room air. Many of these infants are receiving oxygen by nasal cannulae, which may make it difficult to determine the true amounts of oxygen delivered, and may lead to additional days of treatment with low amounts of oxygen that are not needed (22).

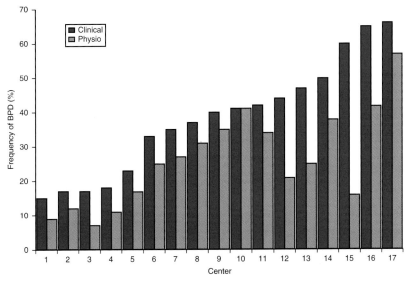

Figure 11-2 Variation in the impact of the physiologic definition by center. From Walsh M, Yao Q, Gettner P, et al. Impact of a physiologic definition on bronchopulmonary dysplasia rates. Pediatrics 2004; 114:1305–1311.

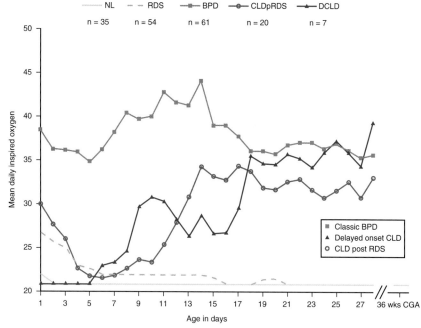

Figure 11-3 Oxygen patterns of neonates with typical and atypical BPD. From Charafeddine L, D'Angio CT, Phelps DL. Atypical chronic lung disease patterns in neonates. Pediatrics 1999; 103:759–765.

THE NEW BPD

Charafeddine and colleagues studied a cohort of neonates born at < 1250 g birthweight and classified their outcomes as no BPD, typical BPD or atypical BPD based on their initial duration of mechanical ventilation (23). They identified 31% as having atypical disease. These infants with atypical BPD were drawn from two groups: (i) infants who developed symptoms after the first week of life and following a well interval in room air; and (ii) infants with resolved respiratory distress syndrome with a symptom-free period of at least 72 h before the onset of chronic respiratory illness (Fig. 11-3). Most infants had onset of symptoms between 7 and 9 days. Jobe described these infants as the "new" BPD and attributed the disease to the arrest of alveolar development associated with preterm birth (24). Hodgeman has argued that the "new" BPD is actually not new, but instead was described as Wilson-Mikity syndrome in prior eras (25, 26). Whatever the name used to describe the respiratory insufficiency, all agree that this disease appears to be different from typical BPD that follows severe RDS. It is unknown if the outcome of these infants will be different from those with typical BPD.

PREDICTORS OF BPD

It is clear from all these definitions that the endpoint BPD occurs late in the neonatal course. However, increasing evidence from studies and meta-analyses suggests that markers of inflammation can be identified in the first days of life that differentiate those neonates who will resolve their RDS from those who will progress to BPD. In addition, data suggest that the optimal time to intervene and potentially modify the illness is early in the course between 7 and 21 days (27–29). In the clinical arena biochemical markers of airway inflammation are generally not available. Thus, there has been increasing interest in developing scores that identify

Table 11-4	Scores to Predict Risk of BPD					
Study	Assessment time point	Outcome time point	Sensitivity	Specificity	ROC
Toce, 84	21 days	30 days	correlation	na	na
Palta, 90 (*n* = 42)	first days of life	—	correlation	na	na
Sinkin, 90 (validation *n* = 160)	12 h, day 10	28 days	57	96	na
Corcoran, 93	not stated	28 days	65	88	na
Ryan, 96 (*n* = 204, <32 weeks)	4 days	36 weeks	88	90	0.85
Romagnoli, 98 (*n* = 228, <1250g)	3 days, 5 days	28 days	93	97	0.96

Data from references 30–34.

infants at high predicted risk of BPD. A number of different risk scores have been proposed (30, 31–34) (Table 11-4). The score developed by Ryan appears to have a desirable combination of both sensitivity and specificity with a high value for the Receiver Operating Curve. The elements included in the Ryan risk score include birth weight, peak inspiratory pressure and the need for ventilation on day 4 of life (33). Using a cut point of 0.4 for the score leads to sensitivity and specificity, as shown in the table. The Romagnoli score requires similar information and includes clinical data up to and including day 5 of life: birth weight, gestational age, concentration of inspired oxygen, and peak inspiratory pressure (34). Both of these scores are also attractive as they do not require knowledge of the partial pressure of oxygen for their calculation. An alternative score, the oxygenation index, has been validated as a predictor of mortality in preterm infants with respiratory failure. It has not been validated as a predictor of BPD (35). It has the disadvantage of requiring knowledge of the arterial partial pressure of oxygen, which may not be available in every patient. None of these scores has been validated in an independent cohort.

FUTURE DIRECTIONS

The ideal definition of BPD would be both sensitive and specific. Definitions have evolved to meet this goal. The next step will be to combine the specificity of a diagnosis based on a room air challenge with the severity assessment inherent in the NIH Consensus Definition.

REFERENCES

1. Northway WH Jr, Rosan RC, Porter DY. Pulmonary disease following respirator therapy of hyaline-membrane disease: bronchopulmonary dysplasia. N Engl J Med 1967; 276:357–368.
2. Jobe A, Bancalari E. NICHD/NHLBI/ORD Workshop Summary – Bronchopulmonary Dysplasia. Am J Respir Crit Care Med 2001; 163:1723–1729.
3. Northway WM, Moss RB, Carlisle KB, et al. Late pulmonary sequelae of bronchopulmonary dysplasia. N Engl J Med 1990; 323:1793–1799.
4. Bancalari E, Abdenour GE, Feller R, Gannon J. Bronchopulmonary dysplasia: clinical presentation. J Pediatr 1979; 85:819–823.
5. Tooley WH. Epidemiology of bronchopulmonary dysplasia. J Pediatr 1979; 85:851–855.
6. O'Brodovich HM, Mellins RB. Bronchopulmonary dysplasia: unresolved neonatal acute lung injury. Am Rev Respir Dis 1985; 132:694–709.
7. Palta MG, Gabbart D, Weinstein MR, et al. Multivariate assessment of traditional risk factors for chronic lung disease in VLBW neonates. J Pediatr 1991; 119:285–292.

8. Heneghan MA, Sosulski R, Baquero JM. Persistent pulmonary abnormalities in newborns: the changing picture of bronchopulmonary dysplasia. Pediatr Radiol 1986; 16:180–184.
9. Fletcher BD, Wright LL, Oh W, et al. Evaluation of radiographic (CXR) scoring system for predicting outcomes of very low birthweight (VLBW) infants with BPD. Pediatr Res 1993; 33:326A.
10. Shennan A, Dunn MS, Ohlsson A, et al. Abnormal pulmonary outcomes in premature infants: prediction from oxygen requirements in the neonatal period. Pediatrics 1988; 82:527–532.
11. Hack M, Taylor HG, Klein N, Mercuri-Minich N. Functional limitations and special health care needs of 10- to 14-year-old children weighing < 750 grams at birth. Pediatrics 2000; 106:554–600.
12. Hack M, Wilson-Costello D, Friedman H, et al. Neurodevelopment and predictors of outcomes of children with birthweights of less than 1000 g: 1992–1995. Arch Pediatr Adolesc Med 2000; 154:725–731.
13. Vohr BR, Wright LL, Dusick AM, et al. Neurodevelopmental and functional outcomes of extremely low birth weight infants in the National Institute of Child Health and Human Development Neonatal Research Network, 1993–1994. Pediatrics 2000; 105:1216–1226.
14. Vohr BR, Wright LL, Poole WK, McDonald SA. Neurodevelopmental outcomes of extremely low birth weight infants < 32 weeks gestation between 1993–1998. Pediatrics 2005; 116:635–643.
15. Singer L, Yamashita T, Lilien L, et al. A longitudinal study of developmental outcome of infants with bronchopulmonary dysplasia and very low birth weight. Pediatrics 1997; 100(6):987–993.
16. Short EJ, Klein NK, Lewis BA, et al. Cognitive and academic consequences of bronchopulmonary dysplasia and very low birth weight: 8-year-old outcomes. Pediatrics 2003; 112(5):e359.
17. Baraldi E, Bonetto G, Zacchello F, Filippone M. Low exhaled nitric oxide in school-age children with bronchopulmonary dysplasia and airflow limitation. Am J Resp Crit Care Med 2005; 171:68–72.
18. Ehrenkranz RA, Walsh MC, Vohr BR, et al. Validation of the National Institutes of Health Consensus Definition of bronchopulmonary dysplasia. Pediatrics 2005; 116:1353–1360.
19. Ellsbury DL, Acarregui M, McGuinness G, Klein J. Variability in the use of supplemental oxygen for bronchopulmonary dysplasia. J Pediatr 2002; 140:247–249.
20. Walsh M, Wilson-Costello D, Zadell A, et al. Safety, reliability, and validity of a physiologic definition of bronchopulmonary dysplasia. J Perinatol 2003; 23:451–456.
21. Walsh M, Yao Q, Gettner P, et al. Impact of a physiologic definition on bronchopulmonary dysplasia rates. Pediatrics 2004; 114:1305–1311.
22. Walsh M, Engle W, Laptook A, et al. Oxygen delivery through nasal cannulae to preterm infants: can practice be improved? Pediatrics 2005; 116:857–861.
23. Charafeddine L, D'Angio CT, Phelps DL. Atypical chronic lung disease patterns in neonates. Pediatrics 1999; 103:759–765.
24. Jobe AH. The new BPD: an arrest of lung development. Pediatr Res 1999; 66:641–643.
25. Wilson MG, Mikity VG. A new form of respiratory disease in premature infants. J Dis Child 1960; 99:489–499.
26. Hodgman JE. Relationship between Wilson-Mikity syndrome and the new bronchopulmonary dysplasia. Pediatrics 2003; 112:1414–1415.
27. Halliday HL, Ehrenkranz RA, Doyle LW. Early postnatal (< 96 hours) corticosteroids for preventing chronic lung disease in preterm infants. The Cochrane Database Syst Rev 2003.
28. Halliday HL, Ehrenkrantz RA, Doyle LW. Moderately early (7–14 days) postnatal corticosteroids for chronic lung disease in preterm infants. Cochrane Database Syst Rev 2003; 1(CD001144).
29. Halliday HL, Ehrenkrantz RA, Doyle LW. Delayed (> 3 weeks) postnatal corticosteroids for chronic lung disease in preterm infants. Cochrane Database Syst Rev 2003; 1(CD001145).
30. Toce SS, Farrell PM, Leavitt LA, et al. Clinical and roentgenographic scoring systems for assessing bronchopulmonary dysplasia. Am J Dis Child 1984; 138:581–585.
31. Palta M, Gabbert D, Fryback D, et al. Development and validation of an index for scoring baseline respiratory disease in the very low birth weight neonate. Severity Index Development and Validation Panels and Newborn Lung Project. Pediatrics 1990; 86:714–721.
32. Sinkin RA, Cox C, Phelps DL. Predicting risk for bronchopulmonary dysplasia: selection criteria for clinical trials. Pediatrics 1990; 86:728–736.
33. Ryan SW, Nycyk J, Shaw BNJ. Prediction of chronic neonatal lung disease on day 4 of life. Eur J Pediatr 1996; 155:668–671.
34. Romagnoli C, Zecca E, Tortorolo L, et al. A scoring system to predict the evolution of respiratory distress syndrome into chronic lung disease in preterm infants. Intensive Care Med 1998; 24:476–480.
35. Subhedar NV, Tan AT, Sweeney EM, Shah NJ. A comparison of indices of respiratory failure in ventilated preterm infants. Arch Dis Child Fetal Neonatal Ed 2000; 83:F97–F100.

Chapter 12

New Developments in the Pathogenesis and Management of Neonatal Pulmonary Hypertension

Judy L. Aschner MD • Candice D. Fike MD

Transitional Physiology

Presentation and Clinical Management of PPHN

Clinical Management and Therapeutic Interventions

Novel and Experimental Therapies

An Unmet Challenge

Conclusions

Pulmonary hypertension in infants, regardless of the etiology or age at onset, represents a clinical, diagnostic and therapeutic challenge. Infants with persistent pulmonary hypertension of the newborn (PPHN), a syndrome of failed circulatory adaptation at birth, have benefited from advances in basic, clinical and translational research. Yet some infants with PPHN and most infants with later-onset pulmonary hypertension associated with lung and heart disease are refractory to currently approved therapies. Advancements in this field will require a better understanding of normal and abnormal pulmonary vascular development and the processes involved in vascular remodeling. The first part of this chapter will review fetal-to-neonatal transitional physiology, including (a) fetal circulatory anatomy, (b) events critical to postnatal circulatory adaptation, (c) determinants of fetal pulmonary vascular tone, (d) biochemical modulators of fetal pulmonary vasoconstriction and vasodilatation, and (e) the factors involved in successful and failed circulatory adaptation. Part two of this chapter addresses the clinical presentation and management of PPHN, including (a) etiology, (b) diagnosis, and (c) treatment. Both proven therapeutic interventions and novel therapies under investigation in the clinical arena and in the laboratory will be discussed.

TRANSITIONAL PHYSIOLOGY

Transitional physiology refers to the process of postnatal circulatory adjustments made by the newborn in the minutes to hours after birth. It is conceivably the most dramatic event in human physiology. This process converts the high pulmonary vascular resistance (PVR) of the fetal lung to the low PVR of the postnatal lung. It is accompanied by an 8–10-fold increase in pulmonary blood flow which is essential for the neonatal lung to assume its gas exchange function and for postnatal survival.

To appreciate successful and failed transitional circulatory physiology it is necessary to understand the unique fetal circulatory anatomy and the determinants of fetal pulmonary vascular tone.

Fetal Circulatory Anatomy

To understand the physiological changes that must occur at the time of birth, it is important to understand the anatomy and performance of the cardiovascular system prior to birth. The fetal circulation is characterized by three unique structures: the ductus arteriosus, which connects the pulmonary artery to the aorta, the foramen ovale, which connects the right and left atria, and the ductus venosus, which joins the umbilical vein to the inferior vena cava (Fig. 12-1). The fetal right and left ventricles basically perform the same tasks prenatally as they do postnatally: the right ventricle delivers the majority of its output to the organ of gas exchange, i.e. the placenta prenatally and the lungs postnatally, and the left ventricle delivers the majority of its output to the heart, brain and upper body.

Knowledge of the human fetal circulation is derived primarily from studies in the fetal lamb. Oxygenated blood leaves the placenta via the umbilical vein with a partial pressure of oxygen (PaO$_2$) of 30–40 mmHg and an oxygen saturation of approximately 80% (1). The umbilical venous blood splits in the liver, with slightly more than

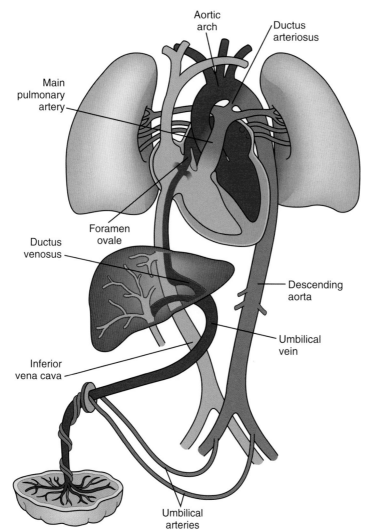

Figure 12-1 Schematic illustration of the fetal circulation. Oxygenated blood leaves the placenta via the umbilical vein and deoxygenated blood returns to the placenta via the umbilical arteries. There are three important fetal shunts: the ductus venosus, which connects the umbilical vein to the inferior vena cava; the foramen ovale, which connects the right and left atria; and the ductus arteriosus, which connects the pulmonary artery to the aorta. Relative oxygen saturations in specific vascular segments are indicted by a red-pink color scale.

half passing through the ductus venosus into the inferior vena cava (IVC), which is carrying blood from the lower part of the body. The remainder perfuses the liver and returns to the IVC via the portal vein. The oxygenated blood passing through the ductus venosus tends to follow a different path from the deoxygenated blood, entering the IVC from the lower body by hugging the medial aspect of the IVC near its junction with the right atrium (Fig. 12-1). At the right atrial junction, the septum primum and the eustachian valve (also known as the crista dividens) split the IVC stream so that 2/3 of the IVC flow is directed toward the left atrium, across the foramen ovale. The remaining 1/3 of the IVC flow mixes with desaturated blood from the superior vena cava and is pumped into the right ventricle. It is believed that the magnitude of the right atrial to left atrial shunt is critical to the proper development of the left atrium and ventricle (2). It has been postulated that a premature decrease of this right to left shunt may contribute to the development of left heart hypoplasia (3).

Blood from the left atrium enters the left ventricle to be pumped predominantly to the head and upper extremities. Thus, the left ventricular output has higher oxygen content than does the right ventricular output, resulting in enhanced oxygen delivery to the brain (Fig. 12-1). Blood from the right ventricle is pumped into the pulmonary artery. Approximately 90% of the right ventricular output is directed to the systematic circulation via the ductus arteriosus. The remaining 10% supplies the lungs via the pulmonary artery (4). This ratio of blood flow is supported by both the high resistance of the fetal pulmonary circulation and by low systemic resistance, attributable to the presence of the low-impedance placenta. Blood from the aorta returns to the placenta via the umbilical artery, where the PaO_2 is 15–25 torr, or 50–60% saturated. The placenta receives approximately 40% of the total cardiac output (1).

A typical umbilical arterial blood gas in a healthy human fetus is: pH 7.33, pCO_2 42 mmHg and PaO_2 34 mmHg. These values were obtained by cordocentesis at fetoscopy in the second trimester (5). Mean blood gas values in the umbilical vein have a slightly higher pH (7.35), lower pCO_2 (37 mmHg) and much higher PaO_2 (55 mmHg) (5). The low PaO_2 and slightly lower pH are physiologically acceptable to the fetus as they help maintain a high PVR and patency of the ductus arteriosus, thus contributing to the unique configuration of the fetal circulation. Despite relative hypoxemia, the fetus is not hypoxic, meaning that there is adequate oxygen delivery to the tissues for the fetus to thrive and grow in this environment.

Events Critical to Postnatal Circulatory Adaptation

Many of the changes in cardiovascular hemodynamics at birth result directly from gaseous lung inflation (Box 12-1). With the first breaths of life, the majority of fetal lung fluid is cleared and a functional residual capacity is established. Ventilation alone causes an increase in pulmonary blood flow and is also a stimulus for surfactant secretion (6–8). Ventilation creates a gas-liquid interface and stimulates pulmonary stretch receptors producing reflex dilatation of the peripheral pulmonary vascular beds (9). In experimental animals, ventilation of fetal lungs with a non-oxygen-containing gas mixture increases pulmonary blood flow from 8% to 31% of the combined cardiac output (6). Pulmonary venous return likewise increases, thereby increasing left ventricular output. These alterations in cardiac output exert a large influence on blood flow across the foramen ovale and ductus arteriosus, with ductal blood flow reduced to 24% of combined ventricular output (6). The direction of blood flow, however, remains predominantly right to left.

In experimental animals, when expanded lungs are ventilated with 100% oxygen rather than an inert gas, further changes in blood flow patterns occur (6, 10) (Box 12-1). Pulmonary blood flow and pulmonary venous return increase slightly, further increasing left atrial pressure and functionally closing the

Box 12-1 *Events Critical to Postnatal Circulatory Adaptation*

Ventilation
- clears fetal lung fluid
- establishes a functional residual capacity
- creates a gas-fluid interface within the alveolus
- reduces pressure on the pulmonary capillary vessels
- stimulates surfactant secretion
- increases pulmonary blood flow
- increases pulmonary venous return
- increases left ventricular output
- increases oxygen tension
- stimulates pulmonary stretch receptors
- produces reflex vasodilatation of the peripheral vascular beds

Oxygenation
- increases oxygen tension
- further reduces pulmonary vascular resistance
- further increases pulmonary blood flow and pulmonary venous return
- increases left atrial pressure
- functionally closes the foramen ovale
- decreases ductal level shunting

Cord Clamping
- removes low resistance placenta
- increases systemic vascular resistance

foramen ovale. Some of the increased pulmonary blood flow is derived from the reversal of ductal flow so that the net flow is from the aorta to the pulmonary artery producing a left to right shunt. The left-to-right blood flow across the ductus arteriosus steals blood from the lower body. This ductal "steal" from the lower body continues until complete ductal closure occurs.

The removal of the low-impedance placenta is another major mechanical event that takes place at birth (Box 12-1). Although this is an important event which significantly increases systemic resistance, its effect on central blood flow patterns is limited (10, 11). With cord clamping, blood flow to the lower body increases because of the elimination of blood flow to the placenta.

Despite marked alterations in blood flow patterns with oxygenation and ventilation, mean blood pressures do not change significantly. However, vascular resistance changes dramatically.

Using the fetal lamb as a model, Teital et al. estimated that left atrial pressure rises with ventilation from approximately 3 mmHg to 7 mmHg, mean systemic arterial pressure initially falls, then rises slightly with cord clamping, and pulmonary artery pressure falls minimally from 53 mmHg to 47 mmHg following ventilation and oxygenation (10). Pulmonary blood flow increases dramatically at birth, reflecting a marked fall in PVR relative to the fetal condition. Yet, pulmonary artery pressure remains elevated compared with the adult, taking weeks to months to decline toward adult norms.

Determinants of Fetal Pulmonary Vascular Tone

To understand the factors involved in the dramatic circulatory changes necessary for successful transition at birth, it is helpful to understand the factors that determine pulmonary vascular resistance in the fetus. Two physical laws are important to this understanding: Poiseulle's law, which states that resistance is proportional to the fourth power of the radius: $R = ((8 \times \text{viscosity})(\text{length})/\pi(\text{Number of vessels})(\text{vessel radius})^4)$, and Ohm's law, which states that resistance to flow between two points along a tube equals the decrease in pressure between the two points divided by flow: pulmonary vascular resistance (PVR) = pulmonary arterial pressure − pulmonary venous pressure/pulmonary blood flow.

Most of the knowledge of transitional circulatory physiology is derived from the application of Poiseulle's and Ohm's laws in studies in fetal sheep. Early in gestation, a paucity of small arteries contributes to the extremely high PVR of the fetus (12). During the last half of gestation, new arteries develop, leading to a 40-fold increase in pulmonary vascular cross-sectional area (12). At the same time, the mass of the lung increases 4-fold such that the increase in pulmonary vessels is only 10-fold when normalized to the lung mass. Pulmonary blood flow also increases progressively with gestational age (13). If not corrected for changes in lung weight, calculated total PVR decreases in the last half of gestation (14). However, when corrected for the increase in lung or body weight, total pulmonary vascular resistance remains elevated and in fact increases late in gestation (15, 16).

Identifying the factors responsible for the maintenance of high PVR despite the dramatic increase in vessel surface area during the last half of gestation has been the subject of decades of research. Early studies suggested that vessel wall thickness increases with gestational age, progressively reducing vascular lumen diameter, thereby maintaining high PVR (17). This idea was refuted by later findings showing no change in the thickness of the medial muscular layers in the small pulmonary arteries in human or lamb during the last half of gestation (12, 18). An alternative theory is that smooth muscle contractile properties mature with advancing gestational age. Although gestational age-related changes in the intrinsic properties of vascular smooth muscle cells (VSMC) have not been well studied, the available data indicate that fetal pulmonary VSMC have a lower actin-myosin ratio and a reduced potential for vasoconstriction compared to the newborn and adult (19, 20). The limitations of these studies, including the use of larger, conduit level pulmonary arteries studied at only a few points during fetal development, make it difficult to ascertain the contribution of changing muscle VSMC contractile properties in the maintenance of high fetal pulmonary vascular resistance.

More conclusive evidence excludes sympathetic tone as the reason for increased fetal pulmonary vascular tone. Vagotomy or atropine infusion does not change basal fetal PVR (14). Bilateral thoracic sympathectomy causes only slight decreases in PVR (21). Although not important to basal PVR, the ability to respond to adrenergic and cholinergic stimuli is present in the fetal pulmonary circulation and may help modulate fetal PVR during stress (14, 22).

It seems certain that mechanical factors contribute to maintenance of high fetal PVR. An infusion of saline increases and withdrawal of fetal lung fluid decreases fetal PVR (23). Expanding fetal lungs with air, oxygen, or nitrogen, but not with saline, decreases PVR (24). Taken together, these studies indicate that lack of an air-liquid interface and compressions of the pulmonary vasculature when fetal lungs are progressively distended with fetal lung fluid are factors that help maintain elevated fetal PVR.

The ability to autoregulate blood flow with a myogenic response may also contribute to the maintenance of high fetal PVR (25–28). It is well accepted that the myogenic response, whereby increases in intravascular pressure cause constriction and decreases in intravascular pressure cause dilatation, helps regulate blood flow to the brain, kidneys, and other systemic vascular beds (29). The existence of a myogenic response in the pulmonary circulation is controversial (30–32). In vivo studies with fetal sheep show that the fetal pulmonary circulation responds to ductal constriction and increased intravascular pressure or certain dilator stimuli with a transient increase in pulmonary blood flow followed by return to basal levels of pulmonary blood flow despite persistence of the dilator stimulus (26, 27, 33). This myogenic response in the pulmonary circulation may be unique to the fetus. The presence of this response provides the fetus with a physiologically important vasoconstrictor mechanism to oppose pulmonary vasodilatation and may help the fetus maintain a high PVR and low pulmonary blood flow in the face of prolonged exposure to a dilator stimulus.

Oxygen is an important determinant of pulmonary vascular tone at all ages. Strong evidence suggests that fetal pulmonary vascular responses to low systemic oxygen tension contribute to elevated PVR in the last half of gestation. As early as 0.7 term gestation, fetal sheep increase PVR in response to lowered oxygen tension; the magnitude of this response increases with gestational age (22). Conversely, increasing systemic oxygen tension causes marked decreases in PVR in fetal sheep close to term, but does not decrease PVR in fetal sheep before 0.7 term gestation. Even a 5 torr increase in PaO_2 can markedly decrease PVR in the near term ovine fetus (26, 34). It seems certain that a potent constrictor response to low oxygen tension and not the inability to dilate to oxygen helps maintain high fetal PVR.

Biochemical Mediators of Fetal Pulmonary Vasoconstriction

It is generally accepted that production of vasoconstrictors helps maintain elevated fetal PVR. Yet, to date, the responsible vasoconstrictors have not been conclusively identified. Candidates for this role include vasoconstrictor products of arachidonic acid metabolism.

Cyclooxygenase Products of Arachidonic Acid Metabolism

It was shown in the 1970s and 1980s that arachidonic acid infusions cause elevation of PVR in fetal goats and lambs (35–37). The arachidonate-induced constriction was abolished or diminished by either a cyclooxygenase (COX) inhibitor or a thromboxane synthetase inhibitor, providing evidence that the responsible arachidonic acid metabolite is the COX-dependent constrictor, thromboxane (36–38). However, studies by other investigators failed to substantiate a role for thromboxane in maintaining elevated fetal PVR (39).

Leukotrienes

Leukotrienes, products of the 5′-lipoxygenase pathway of arachidonic acid metabolism, are also possible mediators of elevated fetal PVR. The strongest evidence comes from studies showing that leukotriene synthesis inhibitors and receptor blockers decrease fetal PVR (40, 41). This evidence is weakened by the knowledge that the agents used are not selective against leukotrienes and that the vasoconstrictor effect of leukotrienes is mediated, at least in part, by thromboxane production (42). Furthermore, if leukotrienes contribute significantly to elevated fetal PVR, one would expect high lung concentrations of these metabolites. Instead, leukotriene concentrations are low in fetal lung fluid and the leukotriene content in fetal lung is lower than that in maternal lung (43). Thus, the role of leukotrienes in maintaining fetal PVR is uncertain.

Cytochrome P450 Metabolites of Arachidonic Acid

Another arachidonate pathway that might produce constrictors capable of contributing to elevated fetal PVR is the cytochrome *P*450 (CYP450) pathway. The CYP450 metabolism of arachidonic acid results in the formation of four regioisomers of epoxyeicosatrienoic acids (EETs), their corresponding

vic-dihdroxyeicosatetraenoic acids (DHETs), and 19- and 20-hydroxyeicosatetrae-
noic acids (HETEs). The CYP450 enzymes that convert arachidonic acid to EETs
are known as epoxygenases and the enzymes that produce 19- and 20-HETE are
referred to as ω-1 and ω-hydroxylases, respectively. There is growing evidence that
the EETs and HETEs are important modulators of tone in a number of vascular
beds (44). EETs are generally potent dilators so would not be good candidates to
maintain high fetal PVR (44, 45). HETEs have been shown to be constrictors in
a number of vascular beds (44), including the neonatal pulmonary circulation (46).
Enthusiasm for a role of HETEs in maintaining elevated fetal PVR is dampened by
the finding that infusion of a specific 20-HETE inhibitor had no effect on basal PVR
in fetal lambs (28). Of interest, 20-HETE inhibition did attenuate the pulmonary
myogenic response (28). The currently available data, albeit limited, point to a
possible role for HETEs in the fetal pulmonary vascular response to hemodynamic
stress, but do not implicate an important role for HETEs in maintaining high basal
fetal PVR.

Isoprostanes

Isoprostanes are a complex family of compounds produced nonenzymatically from
arachidonic acid via a free radical-catalyzed mechanism (47). Isoprostanes elicit
vasoconstrictor responses in the neonatal pulmonary circulation (48, 49) but their
vasoactive effects in the fetal pulmonary circulation have not been reported. Since
these compounds are generated at sites of free radical production and are considered markers of oxidant stress (47), they may contribute to the modulation of PVR
during the transition period when the lung is exposed to higher oxygen concentrations. Their role in maintaining elevated basal fetal PVR is unknown.

Endothelins

Endothelins (ETs) have garnered much attention as possible mediators of increased
fetal PVR. The ETs are a family of vasoactive peptides with at least three distinct
isoforms, ET-1, ET-2, and ET-3 (50). Each ET is derived from post-translational
processing of a preprohormone. For example, ET-1 is synthesized stepwise by
proteolytic cleavage of preproET-1 to form big ET-1, which in turn is cleaved
to form ET-1. The hemodynamic effects of the ETs are mediated by at least two
distinct receptors, ET_A and ET_B.

Of the ETs, ET-1 is the best characterized and its actions in the fetal pulmonary
circulation are the best studied. In vitro preparations have clearly shown that ET-1
constricts pulmonary arteries from fetal lambs and rabbits (51–53). In contrast,
intrapulmonary infusion of ET-1 dilates the vascular bed of the intact fetal lamb
(54, 55). This vasodilatory effect is transient since there is a return to baseline tone
when the infusion is prolonged (55). The biphasic response to ET-1 has been
described in other vascular beds and is likely to be due to initial activation of
the ET_B receptor, which stimulates release of the vasodilator nitric oxide (NO)
(56–58), followed by activation of the ET_A receptor, which mediates vasoconstriction (50, 57, 59). Notably, infusion of big ET-1, the precursor to ET-1, causes
sustained pulmonary vasoconstriction in the intact fetal lamb (60). Thus, stimulating endogenous ET-1 may have different effects than exogenous infusions of ET-1.
Indeed, selective ET_A receptor blockade causes fetal pulmonary vasodilatation,
supporting the contention that intrinsic lung ET-1 activity, as compared to
exogenous infusion, causes vasoconstriction (57, 61). Of note, ET_A receptor blockade has no effect on PVR in 120 day (approx. 0.8 gestation) fetal lambs but
decreases PVR in fetal lambs later in gestation (62). This latter finding would
support a role for ET in maintaining high PVR as pulmonary vascular surface
area increases. However, it is curious that whole lung ET_A receptor expression
decreases, rather than increases, as the fetal lamb approaches term gestation (62).

Moreover, the magnitude of decrease in PVR in response to ET_A receptor blockade was found to be minimal in studies by some investigators (61). Therefore, the role for basal ET-1 in maintaining high fetal PVR is complex and may be minor.

Rho/Rho Kinase

Although the responsible fetal pulmonary vasoconstrictor remains uncertain, evidence points to RhoA/Rho kinase as the signal transduction pathway responsible for maintaining an elevated fetal PVR (63). Rho kinase stabilizes myosin light chain by phosphorylating and inactivating myosin light chain phosphatase, thereby increasing the calcium sensitivity of VSMC, leading to sustained contraction. Brief infusion of pharmacologic inhibitors of Rho kinase cause sustained reductions in pulmonary vascular resistance in late-gestation fetal lambs (63). Rho kinase can be activated by hypoxia and by a variety of biochemical mediators, including ET-1, thromboxane, reactive oxygen species (ROS) and serotonin (64), and might serve a central role in sustaining an elevated fetal PVR.

Biochemical Mediators of Fetal Pulmonary Vasodilatation

An alternative theory for the maintenance of elevated PVR is an inability of the fetal pulmonary circulation to synthesize or respond to circulating and locally produced vasodilators.

Cyclooxygenase-dependent Vasodilators

The fetal lung produces a number of COX-dependent metabolites, including PGI_2, PGE_1, PGE_2, and PGD_2 (65, 66), that have been clearly demonstrated to function as dilators in the pulmonary circulation of fetal lambs and goats (42, 67–70). The lack of pharmacologic agents that selectively inhibit production of these specific COX metabolites has made it difficult to ascertain their individual contribution to maintenance of fetal pulmonary vascular tone. Indomethacin, an agent that inhibits all COX-dependent products, i.e. dilators and constrictors, increases PVR in the intact ovine fetus (36). Although this finding suggests a greater contribution from COX-dependent dilators than constrictors to basal fetal pulmonary vascular tone, the degree of pulmonary constriction to indomethacin is negligible in preparations not influenced by concurrent changes in ductal patency, e.g. the excised fetal goat lung (71). Hence, the production of COX-dependent dilators and constrictors may be fairly balanced in the late gestation fetal pulmonary circulation.

Nitric Oxide

NO, another pulmonary vasodilator, is synthesized from L-arginine by one of three nitric oxide synthase (NOS) isoforms, NOS I (neuronal or nNOS), NOS II (inducible or iNOS) and NOS III (endothelial or eNOS). One or more NOS isoforms have been identified in the lungs of fetal rats (72), lambs (73), pigs (74), baboons (75), and humans (76). Immunostaining with a specific monoclonal antibody against type III NOS demonstrates that the endothelial isoform of NOS is present in the fetal lungs very early in gestation (72, 73, 77). The presence of type I NOS and type II NOS has also been demonstrated in the fetal lung and may contribute to pulmonary NO production (75, 78).

Despite high PVR, there is strong evidence that NO modulates baseline fetal PVR from early in gestation. The infusion of a NOS antagonist increases PVR in the ovine fetus (15, 79). Moreover, both the 0.95 and 0.86 gestation ovine fetuses respond to inhaled NO with pulmonary vasodilatation (15, 80). NO-mediated vasodilatation may occur via direct activation of ion channels or via the second messenger, cyclic GMP (cGMP). Infusions of type V cGMP-specific phosphodiesterase antagonists, such as sildenafil (81, 82), dipyridamole (83, 84), and zaprinast

(85–88), which increase the half-life and intracellular concentrations of cGMP, cause marked pulmonary vasodilatation in the fetus and newborn. Thus, although the responsible constrictor(s) continue to evade definitive identification, combined evidence strongly suggests that a preponderance of constrictors, and not the absence of or inability to respond to dilators, underlies the elevated fetal PVR that persists into late gestation and up to the time of birth.

Factors Involved in Successful Circulatory Adaptation

For successful pulmonary circulatory transition to occur, the mechanical, physiological and biochemical factors that maintain the high PVR of the fetus must be eliminated or reversed.

Mechanical Events

An important event in successful circulatory transition is the replacement of the fluid-filled fetal lung with an air-filled postnatal lung. Even in the absence of changes in oxygen tension, lung inflation with a gaseous mixture lowers PVR (89–91). With establishment of an air-liquid interface, mechanical distension of the lungs physically increases vessel lumen diameter and changes the conformation and arrangement of smooth muscle and endothelial cells in the vascular wall (92, 93). Based on Poiseulle's law, the resulting increase in arterial lumen diameter with lung inflation will dramatically lower PVR at the time of birth. It is important to understand that the increase in vessel lumen diameter is not due to a decrease in smooth muscle cell mass but rather is due to a structural reorganization of the vessel wall which includes a flattening of the endothelial lining (92–94). Nor is there evidence for diminished contractile ability of smooth muscle cells in the initial rapid change in vessel diameter (19, 95).

Another sentinel event in the normal transition of the pulmonary circulation is an increase in oxygen tension. By approximately 0.7 gestation, the fetal pulmonary circulation is capable of responding to increases in oxygen tension by lowering PVR. Even small changes in oxygen tension above fetal levels lower PVR (26, 34).

Independent of gaseous lung inflation and increases in oxygen tension, the birth-related increase in pulmonary blood flow (shear stress) independently lowers pulmonary vascular resistance. Lung inflation, increased oxygen tension, and flow-induced elevations in shear stress interact to release biochemical mediators at the time of birth. These mediators serve as transducers to lower pulmonary smooth muscle tone. Thus, while the pulmonary circulation of both the fetus and the newborn are capable of vasoconstrictor and vasodilator responses, there is a shift from the fetal state where a preponderance of constrictors help sustain the elevated fetal PVR to the postnatal state where production of dilators predominates and contributes to the dramatic decrease in PVR at the time of birth.

Biochemical Events

Changes in the synthesis and release of biochemical modulators of vascular tone occur at the time of birth. Prime candidates for the biochemical mediators of pulmonary vasodilatation at birth are prostacyclin (PGI_2) and NO. Inhibition of the COX pathway of arachidonic acid metabolism with meclofenamate or indomethacin attenuates the decrease in pulmonary vascular resistance that occurs with the first inflation of newborn rabbit lungs (96). There is strong evidence that the COX-dependent dilator, PGI_2, is one of the prostanoids involved. COX inhibition blocks the decrease in PVR and the concomitant increase in PGI_2 production that occur over the first 2 h after birth in the spontaneously breathing term lamb (97). Ventilation, not oxygenation, is the primary stimulus for increased PGI_2 production (98–100). Molecular events that take place at birth to optimize production of COX metabolites, such as PGI_2, include an increase in COX mRNA and protein between late gestation and the first days of life (101). The amount of PGI_2 produced by lamb pulmonary arteries also increases progressively between an early fetal period and the first few weeks of life (101). Taken together, evidence strongly supports a role for increased production of COX metabolites, and particularly that of the COX-dependent dilator, PGI_2, in transitional circulatory adaptation.

Despite the above evidence, a functioning COX pathway may not be essential for successful fetal to neonatal circulatory adaptations to occur, providing other dilator pathways are intact. In term lambs, acute COX inhibition attenuated, but did not abolish, the decline in PVR at birth. Other physiologic adjustments, including the rise in arterial oxygenation, were not adversely affected by COX inhibition (97). Studies in the 1970s found that chronic in utero COX inhibition could result in pulmonary hypertension (102), presumably caused by in utero ductal constriction. Nonetheless, human use of COX inhibitors as tocolytics or chronic ingestion of COX inhibitors during pregnancy has been associated with pulmonary hypertension in only a very small proportion of infants (103). As long as other vasodilator pathways are functioning, COX-dependent metabolites may not be critical to normal fetal pulmonary vascular function or to successful transition at the time of birth.

There is strong evidence that NO is an important vasodilator involved in the normal decrease in PVR at birth. Treatment with the NO antagonist nitro-L-arginine attenuates the decline in PVR that occurs during caesarean-section delivery of near-term fetal lambs by almost 50% (79). Ventilation, oxygenation, and shear stress are independent stimuli capable of increasing NO production in the pulmonary circulation of the near-term fetal lamb (98). In some species, molecular events take place to optimize production of NO at the time of birth. For example, amounts of two of the NOS proteins increase during fetal life in the rat, reach maximal expression near term, and then fall after birth (72, 104, 105). The developmental pattern of NOS expression is somewhat different in fetal sheep, peaking at 0.8 gestation, and then declining before birth (77). One study performed with human lungs found that expression of endothelial NOS fell markedly after mid-gestation and remained low postnatally (76), while another found no change with advancing fetal gestation from 22 to 42 weeks (106). It is important to realize that molecular events do not always correlate with enzyme function and physiology. For example, despite a decline in NOS protein amounts (77), studies with ovine lungs show that there are developmental increases in NO-mediated relaxation between the late fetal and the early postnatal period (107). Furthermore, pulmonary arteries from fetal and newborn lambs show a maturational rise in amounts of the NO downstream messenger, cyclic GMP (108). The discordance between changes in NOS amounts and NO function are not surprising as the regulation of pulmonary vascular NO production, which unfortunately cannot be directly measured, is complex and determined by much more than NOS protein amount, as will be discussed in more detail below.

Despite strong experimental evidence that NO contributes to the normal decline in PVR at birth, it is not clear that pulmonary vascular NO production is essential for successful adaptation to extrauterine life. Chronic in utero NO inhibition caused persistently elevated pulmonary arterial pressures in fetal lambs but did not attenuate the immediate decrease in PVR in the first few minutes after birth (109). Transgenic fetal and newborn mice deficient in eNOS have structural evidence of pulmonary hypertension with increased arterial muscularization but they survive into adulthood (110). Interestingly, the pulmonary hypertension in eNOS knockout mice persists into adult life only in male mice (110). Whereas eNOS expression is diminished in lungs of lambs with PPHN induced by in utero ductal ligation (105, 111), an increase in eNOS expression is found in lungs from lambs that develop PPHN due to in utero exposure to high pulmonary blood flow (112).

Clearly, to better understand the role of NO in the perinatal pulmonary circulation information beyond the amount of NOS enzyme expressed is needed. Regardless of the amount of NOS, other alterations in NO biochemistry and metabolism might change NO bioavailability and modulate the normal decline in PVR at birth. This could result from alterations in (a) NOS activity, (b) substrate and cofactor availability, (c) amounts of the endogenous NO inhibitor, asymmetric dimethyl arginine (ADMA), (d) amounts of soluble guanylate cyclase, the downstream target of NO that produces the second messenger, cGMP, (e) cGMP metabolism by the type V phosphodiesterase or (e) concentrations of the oxygen free radical, superoxide. Superoxide radicals have high affinity for and will combine with NO radicals to form peroxynitrite, a cellular toxin, thus limiting NO bioavailability. Combinations of these biochemical alterations may occur simultaneously to modulate NO action in the perinatal pulmonary circulation. Which elements of NOS signaling are involved with normal pulmonary vascular transition is far from resolved. However, clearly there is more to the story than is reflected by changes in NOS protein amounts.

Reduced production of vasoconstrictors, such as endothelin, could also contribute to the successful decline in PVR at birth. In support of this theory, it has been shown that whole lung ET protein content and ET_A receptor mRNA decline as term approaches in fetal sheep (62). Moreover, the converse situation appears to be true in the context of failed circulatory adaptation at birth. That is, lung ET-1 content is increased, ET_A-mediated constriction is increased, and ET_B-mediated dilatation is decreased in lambs with pulmonary hypertension caused by in utero ductal ligation (59, 113). Similar alterations in the ET-1 cascade are found in lambs with pulmonary hypertension due to in utero elevations in pulmonary blood flow (114). Furthermore, some human infants with PPHN have elevated ET-1 levels (115, 116). Unfortunately, it is not clear whether the altered ET-1 cascade is the cause or the consequence of pulmonary hypertension. Recall that at least in some situations, the ET-1 cascade mediates dilatation, not constriction (55, 61), so that changes in ET-1 could reflect an attempt to counteract pulmonary hypertension. Furthermore, endogenous ET-1 activity does not appear to play a role in the vasodilatory response to ventilation with oxygen in utero (117). Studies with fetal sheep show that dual ET receptor blockade has no effect on the pulmonary or hemodynamic changes during ventilation with oxygen at birth (117). Thus, although evidence is strong that the ET-1 cascade is altered in pathological states where pulmonary arterial pressure is elevated, there is no clear evidence that ET-1 is involved with the normal transitional circulation.

Decreased production of other vasoconstrictors, such as those downstream of arachidonic acid metabolism including thromboxane and leukotrienes, has been postulated to contribute to the successful reduction in PVR at birth. However, no changes in either total leukotriene or thromboxane content were found in lungs of late-gestation lambs obtained before and after caesarean-section delivery (43). Similar to the case for the ET-1 cascade, elevations in the arachidonate pathway constrictors may be found in situations where neonates maintain an elevated PVR at birth. Levels of thromboxane, but not leukotrienes, were elevated in lungs of lambs with pulmonary hypertension induced by in utero ductal ligation (43). Elevated thromboxane and leukotriene levels have been measured in human infants with persistent pulmonary hypertension (118–120). Yet, there is no evidence that a reduction in any of these constrictors is necessary for the successful transition from the higher fetal PVR to lower postnatal PVR to occur.

The evidence strongly suggests that lung inflation shifts the balance of biochemical mediators towards production of dilators and thereby facilitates the reduction in PVR that occurs at birth. There is good evidence that PGI_2 and NO facilitate, but at least individually may not be required, for successful transition. Additional potential dilators include other arachidonate dilators, such as the EETS, and the elusive endothelial-derived hyperpolarizing factor (EDHF). In fact, it is logical that there would be sufficient redundancy of dilators available to compensate for failure or inadequacy of any single pathway, given that this process is essential for postnatal survival.

Factors Involved in Failed Circulatory Adaptation

Hypoxia

Failure to adapt normally to extrauterine life causes PPHN. The failure of PVR to decline at birth is often associated with inappropriate perinatal hypoxia. Remember that elevated oxygen tension is a potent stimulus for the decrease in PVR that normally occurs with onset of ventilation at birth. It is not surprising that when fetal oxygen levels persist or are resumed shortly after birth, the pulmonary circulation responds with hypoxic pulmonary vasoconstriction (HPV) and persistence of the fetal pattern of circulation. Fortunately, the neonate appears to have some defenses against HPV. In particular, the magnitude of HPV is less in younger than in older newborns (121–124). The explanation for attenuated HPV in newborns in the first few days of life is not completely understood but it could be due to immature contractile ability of the pulmonary VSMC (19). In addition, hypoxia acutely increases PGI_2 synthesis in pulmonary arteries from newborn lambs, whereas in fetal lamb pulmonary arteries acute hypoxia reduces PGI_2 production (108). Despite these defense mechanisms, the HPV response of the neonatal pulmonary circulation may be sufficient to lead to resumption of right-to-left shunting across the fetal cardiovascular channels.

pH

Elevated hydrogen ions ($[H^+]$) in the pulmonary capillaries may contribute to failed pulmonary circulatory transition. In newborn calves, resting pulmonary artery pressure was shown to be dependent on age and blood pH, being higher in the younger (< 24 h of age) and more acidotic animals (125). PVR was dramatically increased by hypoxia when the pH was below 7.3, whereas only minor changes were noted when blood pH was above 7.3. The lower the pH, the greater was the pulmonary vasoconstrictor response to hypoxia.

Conversely, alkalosis has been shown to reverse vasoconstriction induced by hypoxia in multiple species, developmental stages and laboratory preparations (126–130). Alkalosis is also effective in reversing pulmonary vasoconstriction caused by infusion of the prostaglandin vasoconstrictor, thromboxane, and group B streptococcus (131, 132). Although the pulmonary vascular bed responds to both respiratory and metabolic alkalosis with dilatation, increased arterial pH, not decreased $PaCO_2$, is thought to mediate the decrease in PVR (133).

Hypothermia and Polycythemia

Other factors affecting successful perinatal reduction in PVR include temperature and hematocrit. Hypothermia causes pulmonary venous constriction, an effect that can be abolished by adrenergic blockade (134). Polycythemia or hyperviscosity also elevates PVR with a sharp increase when the hematocrit level is above 40% (134). This knowledge suggests that babies with PPHN should be transfused judiciously based on their degree of anemia and that partial exchange transfusion for infants with PPHN and polycythemia may be beneficial.

Atelectasis

A number of local pulmonary factors can influence pulmonary vascular tone. The degree of lung inflation is one such factor. When lung volumes are low, alveolar recruitment reduces PVR; when lung volumes are high, further inflation increases PVR (135). Atelectasis causes regional elevations in PVR. Local hypoxia and acidosis may also contribute to elevations in PVR in areas of atelectasis, which serves as an important mechanism for ventilation/perfusion matching. Lung inflation also causes release of surfactant; pulmonary surfactant itself reduces PVR (7). Positive pressure mechanical ventilation impedes pulmonary blood flow as does overdistension with PEEP. However, PEEP in the range of 5–8 in premature lambs had no effect on PVR (136).

Pulmonary Hypoplasia and Structural Changes

Structural changes in the pulmonary vasculature in utero can also contribute to failed circulatory adaptation at birth. Some infants dying from PPHN exhibit distal extension of smooth muscle, thickening of the media and adventitia, and excessive accumulation of matrix protein in the pulmonary vessel walls (137, 138). Many of these same pathological features are found in fetal lambs with PPHN induced by in utero ligation of the ductus arteriosus (139–141), by in utero placement of aortopulmonary shunts (142), and by in utero placement of systemic arteriovenous fistulas (143).

Lung hypoplasia is another class of pulmonary structural abnormality that often results in persistent elevation of PRV after birth. Pulmonary hypoplasia is associated not only with a reduction in the number of alveoli but also with a decrease in total cross-sectional area of the pulmonary vasculature (144). Increased smooth muscle in the pulmonary resistance arteries may also contribute to pulmonary hypertension in some infants with lung hypoplasia, particularly those with congenital diaphragmatic hernia (CDH) (145). It is important to recognize that the increased vascular wall thickness exhibited in the pulmonary circulation of human infants and newborn animals with PPHN does not necessarily imply a hypercontractile phenotype of the pulmonary vessels. Compared with control lambs, the pulmonary vascular smooth muscle of lambs with PPHN induced by in utero ductal ligation developed less force (146). Increased wall thickness found in newborn piglets with chronic hypoxia-induced pulmonary hypertension is not invariably associated with increased contractile responsiveness (147).

Rather than enhanced contractility, there is convincing evidence that pulmonary vascular structural abnormalities are associated with impaired dilatation in animal models of PPHN. The reduced potential for dilatation is due in part to changes in pulmonary VSMC relaxant properties. Pulmonary vascular content of myosin light chain phosphatase, a key enzyme responsible for muscle relaxation in the pulmonary vasculature, is diminished in the ductal ligation model of PPHN in fetal sheep (148). Abnormalities in endothelial cell function have also been shown to contribute to impaired dilatation and maintenance of an elevated PVR in animal models of PPHN (149–151). Endothelial cells synthesize and metabolize many vasoactive mediators. A dysfunctional endothelium can contribute to impaired dilatation at birth by failure to produce dilators, by overproduction of constrictors, or failure to metabolize and remove constrictors.

Impact of Postnatal Age

Some infants initially adapt successfully with a drop in PVR at the time of birth but subsequently develop pulmonary hypertension. Resumption of an elevated PVR may happen within hours after birth, as is often the case in sepsis, or may develop over days to months, such as occurs with chronic lung disease and some forms of congenital heart disease. It is important to realize that the pathogenesis of and treatments for postnatally acquired pulmonary hypertension may be quite different than for infants with PPHN. Factors that regulate PVR change with postnatal age. For example, the COX metabolites PGE_1, PGE_2, and PGD_2 dilate the fetal and immediate postnatal pulmonary circulation. Yet, these specific COX products cause pulmonary vasoconstriction in older animals of some species (42). The relative contribution of COX vs. NOS pathways to appropriate dilator responses changes with postnatal age 9 (152). The degree of vascular contractility to various agonists, including hypoxia, also changes with postnatal age and the presence of structural changes. The timing and degree of pulmonary vascular structural changes varies with the underlying etiology and length of exposure to the stimuli responsible for the development of pulmonary hypertension (147, 153, 154). Thus, as will be discussed in the next section, responses to various therapies may vary with the stage and type of pulmonary hypertension (155, 156).

PRESENTATION AND CLINICAL MANAGEMENT OF PPHN

Successful postnatal circulatory adaptation depends upon a fall in PVR and a rapid increase in pulmonary blood flow. Failure of the pulmonary circulation to achieve or sustain the normal decline in PVR at birth results in the clinical syndrome of PPHN. This condition is characterized by altered pulmonary vascular tone, reactivity and/or structure. Infants with PPHN display severe hypoxemia as a result of continued right-to-left shunting of blood across the ductus arteriosus and foramen ovale. Intractable hypoxemia, inadequate tissue oxygenation, acidosis, and eventual cardiac failure may ensue, resulting in death. Although advances in neonatology have led to improved survival rates for many neonatal conditions, the morbidity and mortality of infants with PPHN remain high (157). In the following sections, the pathogenesis and management of PPHN will be addressed, including (a) epidemiology, (b) presentation and diagnosis, (c) etiology and (d) evidenced-based therapies. We will also discuss (e) novel, but as yet unproven, therapies for PPHN based on current understanding of the pathobiology of this condition and promising results in neonatal animal models of PPHN and clinical trials in older patients with other forms of pulmonary hypertension.

Epidemiology of Neonatal Respiratory Failure and PPHN

Neonatal respiratory failure is a common reason for admission to the NICU, accounting for 30–50% of neonatal mortality in the United States (158). Respiratory failure severe enough to require mechanical ventilator support occurs in about 2% of all newborns. While the majority of these infants are premature, more than 30% are born at or near full-term gestation (158). PPHN often accompanies respiratory failure not only in term and near-term infants but also in premature infants. Among infants of 34 weeks gestational age with respiratory failure requiring mechanical ventilation, approximately 50% will display echocardiographic evidence of abnormally elevated pulmonary artery pressure (159). PPHN with or without associated parenchymal lung disease has been estimated to occur in 2–6 per 1000 live births, accounting for up to 10% of NICU admissions (160). The diagnosis of PPHN carries a mortality rate of 11%, resulting in the death of more than 900 newborns in the United States each year (160).

Presentation and Diagnosis of PPHN

A diagnosis of PPHN should be considered in any infant manifesting hypoxemia that is disproportional to the degree of parenchymal lung disease. On physical examination, a single, loud second heart sound may be appreciated, reflecting systemic or suprasystemic pulmonary artery pressure. Evaluation should include assessment of simultaneous pre- and post-ductal oxygen saturations. A difference of 5% or more with pre-ductal saturations (measured in the right hand) higher than post-ductal saturations (measured on a lower extremity) is presumptive evidence of PPHN with right-to-left shunting of blood at the ductal level. However, similar pre- and post-ductal saturations do not preclude PPHN. It simply implies the absence of a ductal level shunt. An atrial level shunt alone will fail to produce a differential in pre- and post-ductal oxygen saturations, but nevertheless result in venous admixture and hypoxemia; alternatively pulmonary hypertension may manifest in right-sided heart failure, particularly in the absence of a right-to-left shunt. Additional clinical assessment tools include the "hyperoxia test," conducted by placing the infant in 100% FiO_2 for 5–10 min. Longer periods of exposure to 100% FiO_2 are not necessary and may be contraindicated, as this assessment is used to differentiate between PPHN and cyanotic congenital heart disease, where a fall in PVR may be contraindicated. A post-ductal arterial $PaO_2 > 150$ mmHg excludes most forms of cyanotic congenital heart disease. However, an arterial $PaO_2 < 150$ mmHg does not differentiate between congenital heart disease and PPHN. The gold standard for diagnosis of PPHN is 2-D echocardiography with color flow Doppler demonstrating a right-to-left shunt at the ductal and/or atrial level or other evidence of elevated pulmonary artery pressures with bowing of the atrial septum or tricuspid regurgitation.

Optimal management of infants with PPHN must address both the alveolar and vascular components of the lung disease. Assessments of airway patency, the extent of alveolar recruitment and the underlying parenchymal lung pathology are as important as determinations of the degree of pulmonary vascular disease and the level of shunt. Evaluation of myocardial function is also an essential aspect of the clinical management of infants with PPHN. This should include assessment of filling volumes, myocardial contractility and diagnosis of structural cardiac abnormalities. Ventilation-perfusion matching is critical to the successful medical management of infants with PPHN. Failure of an infant with PPHN to respond to vasodilator therapy, such as inhaled nitric oxide (iNO), should trigger careful reassessment of underlying airway or parenchymal pathology and institution of appropriate targeted therapies (surfactant, antibiotics and/or volume recruitment strategies as indicated), as well as attention to myocardial function and judicious use of volume replacement and inotropic support. Poor cardiac function and ventilation-perfusion mismatch are common reasons for failed medical management and referral for extracorporeal membrane oxygenation (ECMO).

Etiologies of PPHN

PPHN is not a single entity; rather it is a clinical syndrome associated with diverse diseases. Some infants with PPHN have an underlying anatomic etiology. Infants with pulmonary hypoplasia and inadequate development of the pulmonary vascular bed often present with PPHN, as do infants with cardiovascular malformations. However, most infants who suffer from PPHN have structurally normal cardiopulmonary development. Most often, PPHN is triggered by a perinatal insult such as perinatal asphyxia, meconium aspiration, shock or sepsis that impairs the functional response of the neonatal pulmonary vasculature to extrauterine life. Other cases of PPHN appear to be idiopathic and are characterized by clear, hypovascular lung fields on chest radiograph and no identifiable risk factors. Whether PPHN is considered a primary vascular disease or is secondary to associated parenchymal lung disease, its occurrence imposes a significant toll in morbidity and mortality.

Nearly any form of parenchymal lung disease, including meconium aspiration syndrome, aspiration of blood, amniotic fluid or gastric contents, pneumonia and respiratory distress syndrome, can be associated with PPHN (161, 162). Infants with some forms of congenital heart disease are also at increased risk of PPHN. Congenital heart disease associated with increased pulmonary blood flow, such as atrial and ventricular septal defects, and pulmonary venous hypertension associated with disorders of left heart filling, such as mitral stenosis, obstructed pulmonary veins and left ventricular failure, may result in pulmonary hypertension. Pulmonary vascular disease related to congenital heart disease (Eisenmenger's syndrome) is thought to develop after a period of normal pulmonary vascular resistance but increased pulmonary blood flow. Approximately one-third of patients with uncorrected congenital heart disease will die from their pulmonary vascular disease. Severe pulmonary hypertension occurs in approximately 2% of infants following cardiothoracic surgery (163, 164).

PPHN is also seen in infants with lung diseases associated with arrest of alveolar and/or vascular development. This includes infants with congenital pulmonary anomalies such as congenital diaphragmatic hernia, congenital cystic adenomatoid malformation of the lung and Scimitar syndrome, an association of congenital cardiopulmonary anomalies consisting of a partial anomalous pulmonary venous connection of the right lung to the inferior vena cava, right lung hypoplasia, dextroposition of the heart and anomalous systemic arterial supply to the right lung. Infants with other forms of pulmonary hypoplasia, including Potter's syndrome caused by renal agenesis, polycystic kidney disease or prolonged oligohydramnios of any etiology also have associated maldevelopment of their pulmonary vasculature and PPHN. Other conditions associated with pulmonary hypertension and abnormal prenatal or postnatal vascular development include alveolar capillary dysplasia and severe bronchopulmonary dysplasia with coordinated arrest of alveolar and vascular development.

Drug-induced PPHN has been described following in utero exposure to non-steroidal anti-inflammatory drugs, such as indomethacin and ibuprofen (165), and the serotonin reuptake inhibitor class of antidepressant drugs (166). PPHN has also been reported in preterm infants given prophylactic postnatal ibuprofen for prevention of a patent ductus arteriosus (167).

PPHN has been described as "reactive" versus "fixed" depending on the reversibility of the vasoconstriction and the presence or extent of vascular remodeling. The terms "maladaptative" and "nonreactive" PPHN have also been used to distinguish between forms of the syndrome that are responsive to supportive care and vasodilator therapies versus those that ultimately prove fatal. These classifications, however, are somewhat capricious as abnormal vasoreactivity and structural remodeling most likely represent a continuum in which vasoconstriction induces progressive hypertensive structural changes, further altering vascular responsiveness, creating a vicious cycle. Environmental factors, such as hypoxia and acidosis, endothelial dysfunction and structural alterations in the smooth muscle and the adventitia, lead to the inability to sustain dilator release and/or to enhanced vasoconstrictor production, further elevating PVR.

CLINICAL MANAGEMENT AND THERAPEUTIC INTERVENTIONS

The clinical approach to the management of infants with PPHN has evolved over decades, paralleling the dissemination of available technologies, such as ECMO and high-frequency ventilation, and advances in our fundamental understanding of the biochemical and molecular signals that regulate vascular tone. A transition from "experienced-based" to "evidence-based" interventions for PPHN has been facilitated by the conduct of appropriately powered randomized controlled trials (RCTs). The development, investigation and implementation of iNO for PPHN are excellent examples of translational research that have resulted in a fundamental change in clinical practice. Yet, we must be mindful of a long history of adopting new therapies into wide-spread practice before efficacy and safety have been rigorously evaluated and validated. The following section will review evidenced-based as well as non-evidenced-based therapies in common use currently to treat PPHN and other forms of pulmonary hypertension in the neonatal intensive care unit.

Commonly Employed but Unproven Therapies for PPHN

Before the development of iNO therapy, medical treatment options for infants with PPHN were limited by the lack of a pharmacologic vasodilator specific for the pulmonary vascular bed. Aggressive medical therapies, such as hyperoxia, hyperventilation, alkaline infusions, paralysis, sedation and high-frequency ventilation, were commonly employed but have never been validated by RCTs (160).

Oxygen Therapy

Oxygen is an important determinant of pulmonary vascular tone and supplemental oxygen is the mainstay of therapy for hypoxemic respiratory failure and PPHN. Alveolar hypoxia and a low systemic arterial PaO_2 are known to cause pulmonary vasoconstriction and are thought to contribute to the physiology of PPHN (26, 34). Recall that babies with uncorrected transposition of the great arteries develop pulmonary hypertension, despite normal alveolar PaO_2, high svO_2 but low systemic arterial PaO_2.

The data in human infants and animal models of PPHN strongly support the avoidance of hypoxia in the management of infants with PPHN. However, the optimal target range for PaO_2 or oxygen saturations is unknown. It was common practice in the era before approval of iNO to target supraphysiological PaO_2 levels in infants with PPHN. Infants were traditionally managed on an FiO_2 of 1.0 throughout the acute phase of their pulmonary vascular disease, despite PaO_2 levels which, in some cases, were in the 200–300 mmHg range. A preference for weaning ventilator settings over weaning FiO_2, a complacent attitude about the tolerance of neonates to hyperoxia, and a fear of labile PVR and acute, life-threatening hypoxic pulmonary vasoconstriction perpetuated this non-evidence-based approach to oxygen therapy for many years.

Recently, there has been a growing appreciation for the potential injurious effects of hyperoxia and oxygen free radicals in the newborn lung (168, 169). In the newborn lamb, exposure to 100% oxygen for even a brief period after birth increased the contractile responses of small pulmonary arteries, presumably due to production of ROS (168). A longer duration of exposure to 100% oxygen resulted in even more exaggerated vasoconstriction compared to lambs ventilated with room air. Human studies have shown that brief exposure to oxygen during resuscitation results in prolonged biochemical changes lasting up to a month or more (170).

Contemporary strategies for the management of infants with PPHN now include avoidance of hyperoxia as well as avoidance of hypoxia. Data from a cardiac catheterization study in older infants with pulmonary hypertension associated with severe BPD support the avoidance of hypoxia through the use of supplemental oxygen, but do not suggest that hyperoxia is likely to cause further improvement in pulmonary hypertension (171). In this study there was little further decrease in pulmonary artery pressure with oxygen supplementation that achieved a PaO_2 greater than 70 mmHg. Dr. Jen Wung and colleagues at Columbia have advocated the avoidance of hyperoxia and hyperventilation in the management of infants with PPHN since the 1980s (172). Unfortunately, no randomized trials comparing ventilator strategies or oxygenation targets for infants with PPHN have been conducted. That being said, at this time there is no evidence to support a PaO_2 target that exceeds 70–80 mmHg in infants with PPHN. Neither the safety nor the efficacy of a higher oxygen target has been demonstrated.

Hyperventilation and Alkaline Infusion

It has been known since the 1960s that alkalosis selectively dilates the pulmonary circulation of newborn animals (125). In the 1970s, this animal model observation was recapitulated in human infants with PPHN treated with hyperventilation and monitored with an indwelling pulmonary artery catheter (173). Because treatment options for infants with PPHN were limited by the absence of pulmonary-specific vasodilators other than oxygen, respiratory alkalosis produced by mechanically induced hyperventilation became the mainstay of treatment for infants with PPHN in the 1980s and early 1990s (160, 174, 175). However, to achieve adequate pulmonary vasodilatation, hyperventilation to a pH greater than 7.6 and a $PaCO_2$ less than 25 were often necessary (174). Buffer infusions were also frequently used to achieve and maintain an alkalotic pH (160). Hypocarbic alkalosis and infusion of sodium bicarbonate were soon advocated to treat other conditions associated with pulmonary hypertension, including post-operative congenital heart disease (176) without good evidence of safety or efficacy. Although both hypocapnic and metabolic alkalosis *acutely* reduce pulmonary vasoconstriction, the long- or short-term consequences of prolonged intentional hyperventilation or alkali therapy were not addressed in the early clinical reports and remain unknown. Alternative strategies advocating avoidance of hypocapnic alkalosis and demonstrating good outcomes appeared in the literature (172, 177). Unfortunately, neither approach had the support of RCTs. A lack of equipoise in both camps and the difficulty and expense of conducting a large RCT in this population hampered a head-to-head comparison trial of these divergent ventilator approaches.

In the absence of strong evidence to guide management, wide variations in clinical practice evolved. Walsh-Sukys et al. (160) reported the outcomes of 385 infants with PPHN cared for in 12 NICHD network centers in the years 1993–1994, prior to approval of iNO for clinical use. Hyperventilation was used in 65% and continuous alkali infusion was used in 75% of infants in the cohort, with marked center-to-center differences in practice. The mean pH achieved was 7.63 ± 0.09 with a remarkable range of 7.58–7.85. Hyperventilation and alkali infusions were often used together (53% of the cohort) but interestingly did not appear to produce the same safety and efficacy profile. In this retrospective study hyperventilation alone (13% of the cohort) was shown to reduce the risk of ECMO without increasing the use of oxygen at 28 days. Continuous alkali infusion alone (21% of the cohort) was associated with increased use of ECMO and increased use of oxygen at 28 days. Only 13% of the infants with PPHN in this cohort were managed without hyperventilation or alkali therapy. Mortality was 11% overall and was not significantly influenced by the choice of management. However, most neonates who failed medical management were offered ECMO, which probably explains the relatively low mortality rate. Nonetheless, the four centers that used the least hyperventilation and alkali infusion had the highest survival rates (160).

Unfortunately, RCTs comparing long-term pulmonary and neurodevelopmental outcomes of infants with PPHN treated with alkalosis vs. "gentle ventilation" have not been conducted. Yet, there is growing awareness of the potential side-effects of hyperventilation and hypocapnia. Hypocapnia is often achieved at the expense of lung injury and frequently cannot be sustained. Furthermore, hypocarbia and hypertonic alkali infusions may cause cerebral hypoperfusion and are associated with poor neurodevelopmental outcomes (178) and hearing loss (179).

Deliberate induction of hypocapnia for short periods while definitive treatment measures are being instituted remains a common therapeutic strategy in the clinical context of severe PPHN. However, evidence to support the therapeutic or prophylactic use of induced hypocapnia is lacking, even in this life-threatening situation. Gradually, hyperventilation has been abandoned as newer therapies for PPHN have been introduced. Because of the accumulating data that this therapeutic approach is associated with lung injury, cerebral hypoperfusion and worse clinical outcomes, therapeutic alkalosis cannot be recommended as a strategy for the management of infants with PPHN.

Sedation and Paralysis

Data to support or refute the use of sedation or paralysis in infants with PPHN are limited and anecdotal. Walsh-Sukys et al. (2000) reported that use of sedation was common in the mid 1990s but there was wide variability among centers (160). Importantly, the authors noted that use of paralysis was associated with increased mortality. The odds ratio of death associated with paralysis was 2.84, exceeding that associated with ECMO (odds ratio of 2.1). Notably, the centers with the lowest mortality also had the lowest use of muscle relaxants (160). Avoidance of paralysis has also been advocated by Dr. Wung in the Columbia approach to management of PPHN (172). Unfortunately, there are no RCTs examining the safety or efficacy of paralysis in the management of PPHN. In light of the potential for increased risk of death, this common practice cannot be recommended for the routine management of PPHN patients.

Tolazoline

Tolazoline is a nonselective vasodilator that has been used for several decades to treat pulmonary hypertension in neonates. Its primary action appears to be as a competitive α-adrenergic antagonist. Although tolazoline can lower mean pulmonary artery pressure and increase cardiac index (180), it produces unpredictable responses in individual patients (174). Furthermore, systemic hypotension and thrombocytopenia are common adverse effects associated with its intravenous use in neonates. Stevenson et al. (1979) treated 39 infants with severe hypoxemic respiratory failure with slow bolus infusions of tolazoline (180). Improved oxygenation was observed in 67% of the infants, but the response was not correlated with survival. Side-effects were common, including significant systemic hypotension in 67%, thrombocytopenia in 31%, and either pulmonary or gastrointestinal hemorrhages in 20% of infants so treated.

Endotracheal tolazoline may produce more selective pulmonary vasodilatation. Parida et al. (1997) reported the use of endotracheal tolazoline in 12 neonates with PPHN with gestational ages ranging from 25 to 42 weeks (181). In this small case series, the treated infants demonstrated significant increases in arterial oxygen saturation and PaO_2, and significant decreases in oxygenation index, without systemic hypotension. However, this drug is now off the market so further trials with this route of administration are unlikely.

Magnesium Sulfate

Mg^{2+} antagonizes calcium ion entry into smooth muscle cells, thus promoting nonselective vasodilatation. Potentially desirable effects of Mg^{2+} include antithrombosis, sedation, muscle relaxation, and the alleviation of oxidant-mediated tissue injury (182). Mg^{2+} may also affect prostaglandin metabolism, activate adenylate cyclase, and reduce the responsiveness of smooth muscles to vasopressors (182, 183). Accordingly, there has been interest in the use of this readily available and inexpensive therapy for the treatment of infants with PPHN. Although prospective RCTs have not been performed, several groups have reported beneficial effects of $MgSO_4$ in nonrandomized series of patients (182, 184). However, beneficial effects on the pulmonary circulation may be complicated by decreases in systemic blood pressure, as has been demonstrated in neonatal models of hypoxic or septic pulmonary hypertension (185). The possibility of adverse effects on the systemic circulation combined with the success of iNO therapy has reduced the enthusiasm for $MgSO_4$ as a primary treatment for infants with PPHN.

Evidenced-based Therapies for PPHN

Inhaled Nitric Oxide

In late 1999, the US Food and Drug Administration (FDA) approved iNO for treatment of pulmonary hypertension in newborns 35 weeks gestation and older. This inhalation therapy represented the first evidence-based medical therapy for the treatment of infants with PPHN associated with hypoxemic respiratory failure.

The US FDA approval of iNO was based on the results of two large, multicenter RCTs of term and near-term neonates with hypoxic respiratory failure demonstrating improved outcome with iNO therapy compared with placebo. The Neonatal Inhaled Nitric Oxide Study Group (NINOS) trial showed that iNO reduced the need for ECMO (186), without increasing neurodevelopmental, behavioral or medical morbidities at 2 years of age (187). The Clinical Inhaled Nitric Oxide Research Group (CINRGI) trial demonstrated that iNO reduced both the need for ECMO and the incidence of chronic lung disease (188). Numerous subsequent clinical trials in the US and in Europe have supported the safety and efficacy of iNO in term and near-term infants with hypoxic respiratory failure and PPHN (189–194). Individual clinical trials and several systematic reviews have shown that iNO improves outcomes by reducing the need for ECMO without influencing length of hospital stay or ventilator days in neonates with PPHN (188, 195). In centers where ECMO is available, iNO has not been shown to reduce mortality. In the short term, iNO improves oxygenation with a lowering of the oxygenation index (OI = mean airway pressure in cm of $H_2O \times FiO_2 \times 100/PaO_2$ in mmHg) in about 50–60% of treated infants (195). Long-term neurodevelopmental outcome does not appear to be affected by treatment with iNO (196).

The neonatology community now has considerable experience with the use of iNO in the treatment of PPHN in term and near-term infants. A review of the evidence-based indications for its use and gaps in our knowledge regarding the optimal dosing, administration and patient selection should help optimize the efficacious and cost-effective use of this agent and expose opportunities for the study of novel therapies for infants unresponsive to iNO therapy.

WHICH INFANTS SHOULD BE TREATED WITH iNO THERAPY?

Gestational Age Limitations. Inhaled NO is indicated for the treatment of term and near-term infants with hypoxic respiratory failure and clinical or echocardiographic evidence of pulmonary hypertension. The initial RCT of iNO for PPHN restricted enrollment to infants of 34 weeks (186, 188); currently this drug is not approved by the FDA for infants below 35 weeks gestation. RCTs of iNO in preterm infants (197–200) have generated new interest in this drug for the extremely low birth weight infant to prevent BPD. However, until the results of the neurodevelopmental assessments at 2 years are known, use of iNO in this population should be considered experimental and restricted to randomized clinical trials with informed parental consent.

Postnatal Age Limitations. Inhaled NO is specifically approved for use in the neonatal population; currently this drug does not have an FDA-approved indication in older children or adults. Several trials enrolled infants up to age 14 days although the majority of patients were enrolled in the first few days of life. For example, the average age at enrollment in the NINOS study was 1.7 days (186). There is great uncertainty about whether there is a postnatal age beyond which iNO should not be initiated, except as part of an IRB-approved investigation. In many centers clinical use of iNO has been extended well beyond the first 2 weeks of life. However, the efficacy of iNO in older infants and children with pulmonary hypertension attributable to conditions other than PPHN has not been as clearly demonstrated. Initiation or resumption of iNO after ECMO in infants with persistence of pulmonary hypertension, and prolonged therapy for refractory pulmonary hypertension beyond 2 weeks of age are well described (201), although not well supported in the literature. Despite limited evidence from RCTs for the efficacy and safety of iNO beyond the neonatal period, this therapy has been widely adopted in pediatric and neonatal intensive care units for older infants and children with pulmonary hypertension caused by a wide range of pulmonary, cardiac and systemic diseases (171, 201–208). Lack of equipoise has hampered the conduct of well-powered trials for patients with congenital heart disease and pulmonary hypertension following cardiopulmonary bypass surgery.

Another controversial area that has not been well studied is the use of iNO in very preterm infants who are several months old with a corrected age greater than 34 weeks who have severe BPD, pulmonary hypertension and cor pulmonale. These infants are often refractory to medical management, including short-term therapy with iNO, and die of cardiorespiratory failure. The management of pulmonary hypertension and cor pulmonale in infants with severe BPD will be discussed in greater detail later in this chapter.

Severity of Hypoxemia. Infants enrolled in the original trials had severe hypoxemic respiratory failure; the mean OI of the infants in both the NINOS and CINRGI trials was greater than 40 (186, 188), although the criteria for eligibility was an OI = 25. An OI of 25 is associated with a 50% risk of requiring ECMO or dying. An OI of 40 is often used as a criterion to initiate ECMO therapy. Even in the absence of echocardiographic confirmation of right-to-left shunt, iNO demonstrated efficacy in the population of critically ill infants with OI > 40. Two trials that enrolled less severely ill infants or infants at an earlier stage of their disease failed to demonstrate an effect on the primary outcome of death or ECMO; however, this may have been related to slow enrollment and inadequate power, as both trials were stopped before the targeted enrollments had been reached (194, 209). The question of whether waiting to initiate iNO until an infant with lung disease and pulmonary hypertension has an OI greater than 25 will delay timely transfer to an ECMO center or the institution of other appropriate therapies has not been addressed in any of the published studies. With the wide dissemination of this inhalation therapy to non-ECMO centers, it seems unlikely there will be an answer to this question.

iNO appears to reduce the likelihood of progression to ECMO in those infants with an OI between 25 and 40 and documented extrapulmonary right-to-left shunt. Thus, acceptable indications for treatment with iNO include (a) an OI > 25 or $PaO_2 < 100$ with $FiO_2 = 1$ with echocardiographic evidence of extrapulmonary right-to-left shunting and (b) severe hypoxic respiratory failure with an OI > 40 with or without echocardiographic evidence of pulmonary hypertension. It is important to note that several trials demonstrating efficacy did not require the presence of clinical or echocardiographic evidence of pulmonary hypertension (186, 194, 210, 211). Infants without documented extrapulmonary right-to-left shunt may respond with improved oxygenation based on iNO-mediated reductions in ventilation/perfusion mismatching. There does not appear to be a strong indication to use iNO in less severely ill infants at this time. As shown by Konduri et al. (209), iNO improves oxygenation but does not reduce the incidence of death or need for ECMO in infants with an OI between 15 and 25 when compared to infants in whom iNO therapy was initiated at an OI of 25 or greater.

Underlying Pulmonary Pathology. The underlying pulmonary pathology clearly influences the likelihood of a positive response to iNO. Among infants with meconium aspiration syndrome, pneumonia, idiopathic PPHN and respiratory distress syndrome more than 65% will respond to iNO with improved oxygenation and survival without the need for ECMO. In contrast, less than 35% of infants with congenital diaphragmatic hernia (CDH) respond favorably to iNO or survive without ECMO (188). The poor response to iNO in infants with CDH has been shown in numerous clinical trials with more deaths or ECMO in the iNO group than in the control group (188, 212, 213). In a trial that exclusively studied infants with CDH, there was a suggestion that outcomes of infants with CDH were worse when treated with iNO (186).

Despite lack of efficacy, it is not uncommon for a trial of iNO to be used in infants with CDH and other forms of pulmonary hypoplasia prior to ECMO cannulation and after decannulation in those with persistently elevated pulmonary artery pressures (214). Until more effective therapies for this group of infants are developed, this non-evidence-based practice is unlikely to change.

Congenital Heart Disease. Another controversial area is use of iNO for infants with congenital heart disease, an indication for which there is no FDA approval. Yet, iNO is used widely for postoperative hypertensive crisis. Extensive anecdotal data exist and several case series have been published suggesting that iNO decreases pulmonary artery pressure and improves oxygenation in infants and children after open heart surgery (204, 207). Unfortunately, there have been few RCTs. In a small (20 in each group) RCT of iNO after cardiothoracic surgery iNO did not substantially improve pulmonary hemodynamics and gas exchange in the immediate post-operative period or decrease the incidence of pulmonary hypertensive crisis (204). In contrast, a larger ($n = 124$) randomized masked study in children (median age 3 months) undergoing surgical correction of congenital heart disease showed that routine prophylactic use of 10 parts per million (ppm) iNO after surgery lessens the risk of pulmonary hypertensive crisis by 30% and shortens post-operative course with no obvious toxicity (207). Mortality was not affected, nor was pulmonary hypertensive crisis abolished. It is not clear whether higher doses would have been more efficacious although it has been shown that doses as low as 2 ppm are sufficient to reverse acute pulmonary hypertensive crises. This RCT (207) supports the anecdotal reports of acute improvement in postoperative pulmonary hypertension with iNO therapy.

iNO DOSING RECOMMENDATIONS

Starting Dose. The recommended starting dose of iNO is 20 ppm. This was the starting dose in both the NINOS (212) and CINRGI (188) trials. The NINOS trial allowed escalation of dosing to 80 ppm in infants who failed to respond to lower concentrations. Increasing the dose to 40 or 80 ppm has not been shown to improve oxygenation in infants who fail to respond to a dose of 20 ppm (194, 212, 215). In fact, only 6% of infants in the NINOS trial had an improvement in oxygenation following an increase in iNO dose to 80 ppm. It is not possible to determine from the study design whether the improvement in oxygenation was caused by the increase in dose or by chance.

Davidson et al. evaluated the effects of different doses of iNO in a randomized, controlled, dose-response trial (194). Doses of 5, 20 and 80 ppm NO were compared to placebo. All doses of iNO improved oxygenation relative to placebo and efficacy were similar among all iNO dosing groups. However, evidence of toxicity was seen at the highest dose of 80 ppm. Methemoglobinemia occurred in 35% and elevated levels of inspired nitrogen dioxide (NO_2) in 19% of infants treated with 80 ppm. NO_2, the product of NO plus O_2, can cause epithelial damage, airway reactivity and pulmonary edema (216, 217). Methemoglobin, which is formed when NO combines with hemoglobin, causes tissue hypoxia when present at high levels in the circulation (212).

Guthrie et al. reviewed registry data on 476 patients from 36 centers that voluntarily reported outcomes of infants treated with iNO (218). The patients were divided into three groups based on the starting dose of iNO: a low-dose group with starting doses less than 18 ppm, a mid-dose group with starting doses of 18–22 ppm, and a high-dose group with starting doses above 22 ppm. Treatment failure and ECMO referral were lowest in the low-dose group and highest in the high-dose group. Survival without need for supplemental oxygen at 28 days or at discharge was 93% in the low-dose group and 76% in the high-dose group, with no differences in mortality or length of hospital stay between the groups. Higher levels of methemoglobin were seen in the high-dose group (218). This study has a number of limitations. It was retrospective and the groups were not randomized. It is certainly possible that infants deemed to be sicker were started on higher doses of iNO and therefore differences in the populations might explain the worse outcomes of infants in the high-dose group. However, to date there are no data to suggest that doses higher than 20 ppm are more efficacious than lower doses and extensive data to suggest that toxicity is more likely at doses of 80 ppm or higher. Thus, it is reasonable to consider 20 ppm both an appropriate starting dose and maximal dose of iNO.

Controversy remains about the lowest effective dose of iNO. One human trial that evaluated a starting dose of 2 ppm suggested that this initial low starting dose impaired responses to subsequent higher doses (98). The limitations of this study include a small sample size of 38 infants and an unblinded trial design. Current recommendations for dosing, therefore, include starting therapy at 20 ppm and weaning rapidly to 5 ppm within 4–24 h. The approach to weaning from iNO therapy is discussed in greater detail below.

Timing of Response and Duration of Therapy. Among infants with a positive response to iNO therapy, the response time is rapid. A reduction in OI and increase in PaO_2 are typically seen within 30–60 min after commencing therapy.

According to the package insert for INOmax®, therapy should continue for up to 14 days or "until the underlying oxygen desaturation has resolved." The maximum duration of therapy in several early RCTs was 14 days (189, 191, 194, 212). The exception was the CINRGI trial, which allowed a maximum duration of therapy of 4 days (188). Most infants in the reported trials were treated for 5 days or less with the exception of infants with CDH, who, despite lack of efficacy, have typically been exposed to the drug for extended periods (206, 219). Unfortunately, there are no data to indicate the maximal safe duration of iNO therapy.

The need for iNO therapy beyond 5 days should trigger evaluation of causes of pulmonary hypertension that are less likely to respond to vasodilator therapy. This should include consideration of conditions such as alveolar capillary dysplasia, congenital anomalies of the lung leading to pulmonary hypoplasia, cardiovascular anomalies such as anomalous pulmonary venous drainage and cyanotic congenital heart disease and genetic defects of surfactant biosynthesis.

Use of Adjunctive Therapies with iNO

When PPHN is associated with parenchymal lung disease, the combination of iNO plus a ventilation strategy that optimizes alveolar recruitment is more efficacious than iNO alone. High-frequency oscillatory ventilation (HFOV) has been shown to recruit lung volume and improve the response to iNO among infants with parenchymal lung disease and PPHN (190). Infants with parenchymal lung disease were less likely to be referred for ECMO when treated with HFOV combined with iNO than when treated with either therapy alone. This was not true for infants with idiopathic pulmonary hypertension, where iNO was highly effective and the addition of HFOV was not synergetic with iNO therapy. Likewise, surfactant decreased the use of ECMO in infants with RDS, meconium aspiration syndrome and sepsis, but not in infants with idiopathic PPHN (220).

Thus, effective vasodilator therapy with iNO requires adequate lung inflation to optimize drug delivery to resistance-level pulmonary arteries. Conversely, suboptimal lung inflation may compromise the efficacy of iNO therapy for infants with PPHN. It has been suggested that poor lung inflation with inadequate alveolar recruitment is the most common cause of treatment failure (190). An infant who fails to respond to iNO therapy should be evaluated by chest radiograph for airway obstruction and atelectasis and by echocardiogram for cardiac performance. Lung volume recruitment strategies with therapies such as HFOV, optimal positive end expiratory pressure or surfactant therapy should be used to address the underlying parenchymal lung disease. Lung volume optimization, in combination with iNO to treat the pulmonary vascular disease, and blood pressure and blood volume support to maximize cardiac output and systemic hemodynamics are interrelated components of the optimal medical management of infants with PPHN.

Strategies for weaning iNO

RCTs have provided clinicians with useful information to help select patients who may benefit from initiating iNO therapy. Information about appropriate weaning of patients off iNO therapy is scarce. Even before FDA approval of iNO, it was known that with or without an obvious clinical response, sudden discontinuation of iNO can be associated with "rebound" pulmonary hypertension (212, 221–225). In part because the rebound can be severe, infants who are candidates for ECMO therapy should be started on iNO only in centers where ECMO is available or transport while receiving iNO can be performed. All infants should be carefully monitored during weaning from iNO. The mechanism for this rebound phenomenon is not certain but has been attributed to downregulation of endogenous NO and elevations in free radicals and endothelin-1 levels caused by iNO therapy (226–229).

It is imperative that clinicians adopt a strategy to safely wean iNO at the time the therapy is initiated and a means to monitor compliance with this weaning protocol. This is important for both patient safety and for cost-containment purposes. The cost of iNO therapy is high and reimbursement is quite variable, putting iNO usage under close scrutiny in many hospitals. Surprisingly, there are few published protocols that provide parameters to guide clinicians in weaning, dosing escalation or reinitiation of iNO therapy.

When Should iNO Weaning be Started? The weaning protocol for the CINRGI trial included a rapid wean at the end of 4 h of treatment at 20 ppm to 5 ppm in those patients whose oxygenation improved with 20 ppm (188). The NINOS trial (212) incorporated an iNO weaning attempt when the patient had an arterial PaO_2 greater than 50 torr (230). Davidson et al. addressed the safety of withdrawing iNO in infants with PPHN (223). iNO weaning was initiated when the patient achieved an oxygenation index less than 10. These published studies support the safety of attempting to wean iNO within a few hours of initiating therapy if the infant is clinically stable with an improvement in respiratory status after treatment with 20 ppm.

FiO$_2$ Versus iNO: Which Drug Should be Weaned First? The relative timing of weaning FiO$_2$ versus iNO has not been studied. There is some evidence that iNO, particularly at doses less than 80 ppm, has beneficial effects other than those attributed to lowering PVR (231). For example, animal studies have shown that iNO reduces the accumulation of neutrophils in the lung and diminishes the inflammatory cascade associated with lung injury (232, 233). The CINRGI trial showed an association between use of iNO and a decrease in the occurrence of chronic lung disease (188). Therefore, a logical argument can be made to start weaning FiO$_2$ prior to weaning iNO. Supportive of this approach, clinical success has been reported using algorithms for weaning FiO$_2$ to approximately 50–60% prior to reducing iNO (221, 223, 234). Regardless of whether FiO$_2$ or iNO is reduced first, it should be noted that the neonatal pulmonary vasculature is fully dilated when arterial oxygenation tension exceeds approximately 70–80 torr (121, 171, 235). There is no need or justification to maintain oxygen saturations of 100% or an arterial PO$_2$ greater than 100 torr. Instead, attempts to wean FiO$_2$ should be made once the infant is stable with an arterial PaO$_2$ greater than 50–80 torr and within the first few hours of initiating iNO therapy.

Dose-Reduction Strategies. A variety of dose-reduction paradigms have been used to wean iNO. In the CINRGI trial, infants were weaned from 20 ppm to 5 ppm with no intermediate reductions in iNO (188). In the NINOS trial, the iNO concentration was weaned by 50% until a dose of 5 ppm was achieved (212). Attempts were made to discontinue iNO from 5 ppm, but if this strategy failed, iNO was reduced by 1 ppm decrements from 5 ppm to 0 (230). Other published weaning strategies have incorporated either 5 ppm or 20% step-wise reductions in iNO (221, 223, 234). Unfortunately, there is no evidence to support any particular step-wise weaning decrement in iNO as superior to another. On the other hand, a number of studies have demonstrated a much greater success rate when discontinuing iNO from 1 ppm than from 5 ppm or higher doses of iNO (221, 223, 230). Thus, it seems clear that discontinuation of therapy should be avoided until iNO is weaned to 1 ppm. Some decline in arterial oxygenation should be anticipated and an increase in FiO$_2$ of 10–20% considered reasonable when discontinuing iNO. In other words, iNO therapy should not be reinstated simply because of a need to modestly increase FiO$_2$.

Should an Echocardiogram be Used to Guide iNO Weaning and Discontinuation? An initial echocardiogram is important to rule out structural heart disease and can sometimes provide helpful information to explain failure to respond to therapy. An example of the latter case is when left or right ventricular dysfunction is so severe that pulmonary vasodilatation by itself is not sufficient to improve systemic oxygenation. It is important to remember that the NINOS trial did not use echocardiographic evidence of pulmonary hypertension as entry criteria since it was recognized that iNO can improve oxygenation by enhancing ventilation-perfusion matching. Nor have any clinical trials used resolution of echocardiographic evidence of pulmonary hypertension as criteria to initiate weaning from or to discontinue iNO therapy. There is no evidence that an echocardiogram should be obtained prior to discontinuing iNO. An echocardiogram may be useful when an infant fails to wean from iNO within the typical duration of therapy, which is less than 5 days (221, 223, 230), or demonstrates progressive clinical deterioration at any time during iNO therapy.

A Suggested iNO Weaning Strategy. Based on the currently available evidence, the following is a suggested strategy for weaning iNO.

- Administer 20 ppm of iNO until FiO_2 has been weaned to < 0.6 or for 4 hours, whichever comes first.
- If a patient responds to iNO, weaning of oxygen can begin immediately by small decrements of 2–5%; attempts to wean FiO_2 or iNO should occur within 4 hours of initiation of iNO therapy.
- Weaning of FiO_2 or iNO should be attempted in clinically stable patients when the following conditions are met:
  1. Preductal $SPO_2 > 92\%$
  2. $PaO_2 > 60$ torr
  3. Pre-post ductal SPO_2 difference $< 5\%$
- iNO weaning attempts should be made at least as often as every 24 h.
- iNO can be weaned in decrements of 5 ppm as frequently as every 15 min until a dose of 5 ppm is achieved.
- iNO should be weaned from 5 ppm to 1 ppm using decrements of 1 ppm.
- FiO_2 may be increased by 15% to a maximum of 0.75 to allow iNO to be discontinued.
- Once iNO is discontinued, the patient should be reevaluated after 60 min and placed back on iNO if any of the following conditions exist:
  1. $FiO_2 > 0.75$ to maintain $PaO_2 > 60$ torr or $SPO_2 > 92$
  2. Evidence of hemodynamic deterioration.

OVERALL SAFETY PROFILE OF iNO

When used in accordance with FDA guidelines, iNO appears to have a good overall safety profile. Its lack of effect on systemic hemodynamics has been well established. It is the only selective pulmonary vasodilator with established efficacy in RCTs. Efficacy has generally been defined as a reduced need for ECMO, with the number needed to treat (NNT) of 5.3 (195). This deserves some discussion as ECMO is itself a therapy of proven benefit in infants with hypoxic respiratory failure. Initial concerns that a delay in the referral for ECMO or a decrease in ECMO usage would result in increased lung injury has not been borne out by clinical trials. In fact, iNO has been associated with a decrease in the incidence of chronic lung disease (188). ECMO is a technologically sophisticated therapy with restricted availability in many parts of the world. A large number of infants who would benefit from ECMO are not born in centers where this technology is available, necessitating an infant transport, often under less than ideal circumstances. ECMO is invasive and expensive and is associated with important complications. Thus, a drug with a satisfactory safety profile that reduces the need for ECMO is a valuable addition to our therapeutic repertoire.

Administration of iNO must be accompanied by careful monitoring for toxicities, including methemoglobinemia and NO_2 levels, and of course accurate monitoring of the delivered concentration of iNO itself. Safety concerns surrounding the phenomenon of rebound pulmonary hypertension upon withdrawal of iNO were discussed under weaning strategies. It cannot be overemphasized that rebound pulmonary hypertension can occur even in infants who fail to respond to initiation of iNO. Deterioration of oxygenation upon discontinuation of iNO in these infants has implications for the use of this drug in non-ECMO centers and for transport of infants between centers (236).

Several studies have provided reassuring information regarding longer-term neurodevelopmental outcome (187, 237–239). Among survivors who were available for follow-up, infants treated with iNO were similar to those who received placebo with regard to their mental, motor and audiological examinations and post-discharge pulmonary complications. Unfortunately, longer-term outcomes for these children at school age and beyond are not available. In 2000, the American Academy of Pediatrics (AAP) issued practice guidelines regarding the use of iNO and made several recommendations that remain valid today (236).

- Generally, iNO should be initiated in centers with ECMO capability. If the center does not have ECMO capability, criteria and procedure for transfer to an ECMO facility should be established between the two centers prospectively. Transfer must occur without interruption of iNO therapy.
- Center-specific criteria for treatment failure should be developed to facilitate timely consideration of alternative therapies.
- Centers that provide iNO should provide comprehensive long-term medical and neurodevelopment follow-up.
- Centers that provide iNO therapy should establish prospective data collection for treatment time course, toxic effects, treatment failure, and use of alternative therapies and outcomes.

Surfactant Therapy

Exogenous surfactant therapy as adjunctive treatment for near-term and term neonates with severe hypoxemic respiratory failure has been studied in RCT and has shown promise. There is evidence for surfactant deficiency in some patients with PPHN (240, 241). Studies have shown that surfactant therapy is associated with sustained clinical improvement in term infants with pneumonia and meconium aspiration syndrome (242), and can reduce the duration of ECMO (243). A multi-center, randomized, double-blind, placebo-controlled trial studied the role of surfactant treatment in term neonates with severe respiratory failure (220). Infants of 36 weeks or greater were randomly assigned to receive four doses of surfactant (beractant) or air placebo before ECMO treatment, if required. They found that the need for ECMO therapy was significantly less in the surfactant group than in the placebo group; this effect was greatest for infants within the lowest OI stratum – 15–22 (220).

NOVEL AND EXPERIMENTAL THERAPIES

Despite a favorable efficacy and safety profile, outcomes for infants treated with iNO are not universally positive and iNO is not consistently efficacious in all infants with PPHN. Only 50–60% of infants receiving iNO respond with an improvement in oxygenation. The response rate for infants with CDH is lower and there is some evidence that iNO is contra-indicated in infants with CDH (186, 195). In light of the multiple etiologies of neonatal pulmonary hypertension, it is not surprising that no single therapy is effective in all cases. The reasons why some infants fail to respond or to maintain a response to iNO are not well understood, but are likely to be related to (a) dysfunctional signaling downstream of nitric oxide release or delivery, (b) abnormalities in other vasoactive pathways and/or (c) vascular remodeling or maldevelopment. Endothelial dysfunction leading to increased expression of endothelin-1 and reduced synthesis or activity of the vasodilators, nitric oxide and prostacyclin, are thought to play an important role in vasoconstriction and progressive vascular remodeling. Novel therapies focusing on the manipulation of these three pathways have formed the backbone of therapeutic advances in the treatment

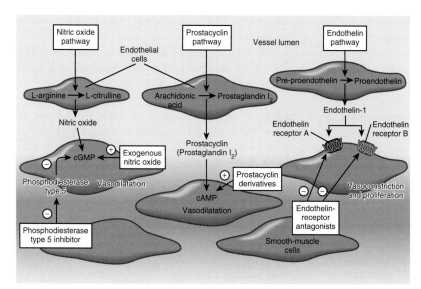

Figure 12-2 Schematic illustration of the nitric oxide, prostacyclin and endothelin pathways. These three biochemical pathways are important in the regulation of pulmonary vascular tone and form the backbone of several novel therapies for patients with pulmonary hypertension.

of pulmonary hypertension in older children and adults (Fig. 12-2). Success in older patients coupled with a 40% non-response rate to iNO has fueled interest in novel therapies for infants with pulmonary hypertension.

Novel and Experimental Therapies Directed at the NO-cGMP Pathway

Alternative Means of Delivering Nitric Oxide

Discussion of novel therapies for PPHN should include alternative means of delivering NO. One such therapy is O-nitrosoethanol gas (ENO) which is designed to replete S-nitrosothiols (SNOs) (244). Most NO is bound in SNO complexes which, unlike nitric oxide gas, do not react with oxygen or superoxide to produce toxic metabolites. SNOs are thought to be involved in ventilation/perfusion matching in the lung. In a small case series published in the Lancet in 2002, inhaled ENO was administered to seven neonates with PPHN (244). ENO administration for 4 h improved oxygenation and systemic hemodynamics. However, even with such short-term therapy, mean methemoglobin concentrations doubled from 1.6% to 3.2%. Thus, it is unclear whether improved oxygenation could be sustained during longer-term therapy without progressive, toxic, increases in methemoglobinemia. Randomized trials with larger patient populations and careful attention to potential toxicity must be performed before conclusions regarding safety and efficacy of this therapy can be made.

Phosphodiesterase Inhibitors

NO mediates vasodilatation by activation of soluble guanylate cyclase, which in turn increases intracellular levels of cGMP. The cGMP-degrading phosphodiesterase, PDE5, is abundantly expressed in lung tissue (245, 246). Inhibitors of PDE5 will prolong the half-life of cGMP and should enhance the biological actions of endogenous or exogenous nitric oxide (Fig. 12-2). PDE5 is therefore an ideal target for the pharmacological treatment of pulmonary hypertension. Development of potent and selective PDE5 inhibitors, such as sildenafil

(Viagra), has heightened interest in this approach for treatment of pulmonary hypertension.

In fetal ovine models of PPHN, lung PDE5 activity and expression were elevated relative to controls (85, 247). The PDE5 inhibitors, zaprinast and dipyridamole, were found to lower PVR in several animal models of PPHN and augment the response to inhaled NO (83, 85, 247). However, the vasodilator effects of systemic dipyridamole were not selective to the pulmonary circulation. Nonetheless, dipyridamole has been used in neonates with CDH and PPHN to enhance the response to iNO or prevent rebound pulmonary hypertension on weaning of iNO (84, 248, 249). Ivy et al. (1998) reported that 7 of 23 patients treated with iNO following surgery for congenital heart disease exhibited significant rebound pulmonary hypertension and that treatment with dipyridamole attenuated this rebound effect (224). Systemic hypotension was not reported to be a significant clinical problem in these case reports.

Recent clinical trials of PDE5 inhibition for pulmonary hypertension have focused mainly on sildenafil, a potent and relatively selective PDE5 inhibitor originally approved for erectile dysfunction. Sildenafil has been shown to selectively reduce PVR in both neonatal animal models (81, 250), and adult humans with pulmonary hypertension (251–255). Uncontrolled human studies of sildenafil in patients with pulmonary hypertension indicate that this drug acutely reduces pulmonary artery pressure and is synergistic with iNO (252). No effects on systemic blood pressure were noted with short-term therapy. In a RCT of 278 adult patients with symptomatic pulmonary arterial hypertension (PAH), oral sildenafil three times daily for 12 weeks significantly improved functional class and hemodynamics (255). Based on the favorable effects of this oral therapy, sildenafil (Revatio), in a dose of 20 mg TID was approved by the FDA in 2005 for the treatment of adult patients with PAH.

The pediatric pulmonary hypertension research community also took note of the potential utility of an orally active drug that could selectively reduce PVR and improve ventilation-perfusion matching and oxygenation. Interest was first stimulated by a case report of the use of sildenafil to attenuate rebound pulmonary hypertension following withdrawal of iNO therapy in patients with congenital heart disease (256). Sildenafil attenuated rebound pulmonary hypertension and increased circulating cGMP (256). Interest in this drug was further stimulated by anecdotal reports of the successful use of oral sildenafil in neonates with PPHN (257). However, the published literature is limited to a single RCT of sildenafil for infants with PPHN. This small, proof-of-concept, placebo-controlled, masked study took place in Colombia, South America, where iNO and ECMO are not available (258). Infants with severe PPHN and OI > 25 were treated with oral sildenafil (1 mg/kg) or placebo by orogastric tube every 6 h. In the treatment group, the OI improved in all infants within 6 to 30 h, without effect on systemic blood pressure. Survival was 6 of 7 in the sildenafil group versus 1 of 6 infants in the placebo group. The authors concluded that oral sildenafil may be effective in the treatment of PPHN and underscored the need for a large, controlled trial (258).

The obvious advantages of this oral agent in countries without access to iNO or ECMO certainly justify larger trials for the primary treatment of PPHN with a focus on long-term safety (259). Only a few small case reports have been published on the long-term effects of oral sildenafil treatment. Concern has been raised about the use of this drug in premature infants at risk for retinopathy of prematurity (260), although this association has been questioned in subsequent reports (261). Moreover, sildenafil inhibits other PDE isoforms, including PDEs found in the brain (262). Thus, attention must be paid to potential adverse or beneficial effects of sildenafil on other vascular beds of the developing newborn, including the cerebral and retinal circulations (263).

In the USA, where iNO is generally available, sildenafil has crept into clinical practice, not as primary therapy for PPHN, but as an adjunct to iNO in infants with inadequate responses and as a therapy to facilitate weaning from iNO in infants requiring both short-term and long-term vasodilator therapy (264). Ease of administration makes it an attractive choice for more chronic forms of postnatal pulmonary hypertension associated with pulmonary maldevelopment or vascular remodeling. Long-term efficacy and safety studies of sildenafil in infants and young children should be a high priority (259). Studies of longer-acting PDE5 inhibitors, such as Tadalafil, are also needed.

L-Arginine Therapy

Arginine is a basic amino acid generated endogenously by the urea cycle. Besides its role as a urea cycle intermediate, L-arginine is the substrate for NO production by nitric oxide synthase (NOS) (Fig. 12-2). On the surface, arginine deficiency seems an improbable cause of NO deficiency. L-Arginine concentrations in the blood are normally about 100 µM, well above the K_m of approximately 3–5 µM for NOS (265). Intracellular concentrations are reported to be much higher. These facts argue against substrate limitation as a likely cause of inadequate endogenous NO production. Yet, numerous studies have demonstrated beneficial effects of L-arginine on vascular responses in vivo in both experimental animals (266, 267) and in humans (268–271). Several mechanisms have been proposed for this "arginine paradox," including overcoming endogenous antagonists of NOS, such as asymmetric dimethyl arginine (ADMA), rapid metabolism of arginine by arginase, or limited bioavailability in cell microdomains, such as in caveolae where NO is synthesized (265). It has been proposed that the rate of transport of L-arginine into caveolae may be more critical than the absolute cellular concentration.

Investigations in animal models and humans with vascular diseases have lent credibility to a possible therapeutic role for arginine supplementation, despite the "arginine paradox." The activity of arginase, which hydrolyzes arginine to ornithine and urea, is elevated in patients with PH (272), and levels of ADMA, the endogenous NOS inhibitor, are elevated in patients with congenital heart disease and pulmonary hypertension (273). The lung is not only a major source of NO, but has recently also been shown to be a major source of ADMA (274). By competitively inhibiting NO synthesis from L-arginine, ADMA can mimic the effects of NO deficiency. ADMA has been implicated in the pathogenesis of systemic and pulmonary hypertension, stroke, diabetes, hyperlipidemia, hyperhomocysteinemia and atherosclerosis (275). High circulating levels of ADMA in patients with vascular disease may explain why exogenous arginine stimulates vascular NO production in a dose-dependent manner (275). Small, uncontrolled studies in pulmonary hypertension patients with heart failure (268), sickle cell disease (272) and congenital heart disease following bypass surgery (270) suggest that L-arginine therapy significantly reduces pulmonary artery pressure and pulmonary vascular resistance, without obvious side-effects. In contrast, little response was observed in patients with scleroderma (268), primary pulmonary hypertension (268) and pre-operative congenital heart disease (270).

Developmental factors add to the rationale for arginine therapy in neonates with pulmonary hypertension. The availability of arginine in the circulation is dependent on the production of new citrulline by the urea cycle in the liver and gut. At 36 weeks gestation, the enzymes in the urea cycle function at only 40–90% of the levels found in adults (276–278). The average plasma arginine level in ill newborns was reported to be only 38 µmol/L, while in adults the average plasma arginine level was 90 µmol/L (159, 279, 280). Furthermore, arginine levels were lower in term and preterm neonates with respiratory failure complicated by pulmonary hypertension compared with infants with lung disease in the absence of pulmonary hypertension. Furthermore, there was an inverse relationship between arginine levels and the severity of lung disease as measured by OI (159). The synthesis of arginine is influenced by a functional polymorphism in carbamoyl-phosphate synthetase (CPS-I), the rate-limiting enzyme of the urea cycle (159). It is possible that a genetically determined limitation in the capacity of CPS-I to produce precursors for NO synthesis predisposes some infants to the development of pulmonary hypertension.

The same functional polymorphism in CPS-I was found to be a significant risk factor for the development of pulmonary hypertension after cardiopulmonary bypass surgery. Infants and children undergoing cardiopulmonary bypass surgery had significantly lower arginine and citrulline plasma levels and lower levels of NO metabolites in the immediate postoperative period (164). The ratio of ornithine to citrulline was elevated postoperatively, indicating decreased urea cycle function. It was speculated that decreased availability of NO precursors may contribute to the risk of postoperative pulmonary hypertension (164).

Despite the biological plausibility and encouraging investigations of arginine administration in animal models of pulmonary hypertension, clinical trials of arginine therapy for neonatal pulmonary hypertension have been few and non-randomized. L-Arginine (500 mg/kg over 30 min) was infused in five consecutive infants with PPHN. After 90 min, there was a rise in PaO_2 from 37 to 84 and a 33–50% reduction in OI in 4/5 babies (271). Unfortunately, RCTs are lacking. Arginine therapy is inexpensive and clinically available. It is tempting to speculate that this may be one reason for a dearth of large randomized human trials. There is little financial incentive for pharmaceutical companies to fund such a trial.

L-Citrulline Therapy

The rapid degradation of oral arginine by hepatic arginase potentially limits its clinical use. Notably, oral citrulline (an arginase-resistant precursor of arginine) was shown to be more effective than oral arginine in increasing circulating levels of L-arginine in healthy subjects (281). Oral citrulline caused a 227% increase in peak arginine concentrations while oral arginine led to only a 90% increase. Addition of citrulline to the diet of arginine-deficient rats supports a normal level of arginine in the blood (282). There is extensive clinical experience using both citrulline and arginine in patients with inborn errors of metabolism (159, 283, 284). It has been hypothesized that oral citrulline therapy may prove more effective than arginine in raising NO levels in patients with pulmonary hypertension.

In a pediatric trial of 40 post-cardiac surgery patients, oral citrulline supplementation in the perioperative period was protective against the development of pulmonary hypertension (285). Median citrulline and arginine concentrations were significantly higher in the citrulline group versus the placebo group 12 h postoperatively. Postoperative pulmonary hypertension only developed in patients with plasma citrulline concentrations less than age-specific norms. Six of these patients were in the placebo group and three were in the citrulline group. The authors speculated that oral citrulline supplementation may be effective in reducing postoperative pulmonary hypertension (285). A large RCT of intravenous citrulline supplementation in infants and children undergoing cardiopulmonary bypass surgery is currently under way.

Antioxidant Therapy

There is accumulating evidence that oxidative stress is increased in patients with pulmonary hypertension and that reactive oxygen species (ROS), including superoxide, are involved in the pathogenesis of pulmonary hypertension (286). Patients with pulmonary hypertension have increased urinary isoprostanes, a marker of oxidative stress (286). Superoxide anions are increased and the amount of superoxide dismutase (SOD), an enzyme responsible for removing superoxide, is reduced in the smooth muscle and adventitia of small pulmonary arteries in the ovine ductal ligation model of PPHN (287).

There are numerous sources of ROS production in cells, including mitochondrial respiration, NADH/NADPH oxidase, xanthine/xanthine oxidase, cyclooxygenase and lipoxygenase. In addition, all NOS isoforms can generate superoxide in a calcium-CaM-dependent manner, especially in the absence of sufficient substrate, L-arginine, or co-factor, tetrahydrobiopterin (BH_4). The availability of arginine or depletion of BH_4 uncouples NOS, leading to the production of superoxide, instead of nitric oxide (288). In the ductal ligation model of PPHN in lambs, there was evidence of eNOS uncoupling as a result of altered binding of NOS to the chaperone protein, Hsp90 (289). eNOS uncoupling was associated with impaired vasodilatation in this model of PPHN (290). Thus, conditions that culminate in PPHN may be associated with post-translational modifications of eNOS that result in an uncoupled enzyme and enhanced eNOS-derived superoxide generation.

The frequent use of hyperoxic ventilation in the management of infants with PPHN may augment the production of ROS. Exaggerated pulmonary vasoconstrictor responses have been described following hyperoxic exposure and ROS formation (168, 169). Excess ROS production may mediate vasoconstriction by a number of mechanisms. For example, superoxide binds avidly to NO, reducing NO bioavailability, and producing peroxynitrite, a potent oxidant that can react with DNA, proteins and lipids to cause cellular damage (291). Peroxynitrite has been shown to be a potent vasoconstrictor of newborn, but not adult, pulmonary arteries from rats (292).

Other mechanisms for ROS-mediated vasoconstriction include the conversion of superoxide by SOD to hydrogen peroxide (H_2O_2) which, in turn, has been reported to elicit pulmonary vasoconstriction (293). In addition, ROS can interact with arachidonic acid to produce isoprostanes. There is evidence that isoprostanes not only serve as reliable markers of in vivo oxidative stress but can have important biological effects. In particular, isoprostanes have been shown to be potent pulmonary vasoconstrictors in newborn piglets and rats (49, 294, 295). Interestingly, when pulmonary arteries are exposed to peroxynitrite, there is a 10-fold rise in the levels of isoprostanes (296). Elevated isoprostane levels have been measured in the tracheal aspirates of babies ventilated with high levels of oxygen compared with those ventilated with room air (297). In addition, ROS may contribute to pulmonary vascular wall injury and thus initiate vascular proliferation and structural remodeling (298).

The local concentration of SOD is thought to be a key determinant of the biological half-life of NO (291). Steinhorn et al. (2001) have shown that SOD enhances the vascular relaxation induced by NO in isolated vessels from lambs with PPHN induced by in utero ductal ligation (299). In contrast, Villamor et al. (2000) reported that SOD had no effect on NO-mediated relaxation in pulmonary arteries from normal piglets (300, 301). These discordant results led Steinhorn and colleagues to speculate that SOD has a more profound effect in remodeled pulmonary vessels than in normal vessels, perhaps because excess superoxide production is a part of the pathophysiology of pulmonary hypertension (299). In ventilated lambs with PPHN, a single intratracheal dose of recombinant human SOD (rhSOD) reduced pulmonary artery pressure and enhanced the pulmonary vasodilator effects of iNO. Intratracheal rhSOD also improved oxygenation and pulmonary hypertension in lambs with severe RDS (302).

A number of animal studies point to the therapeutic potential of SOD for infants with PPHN. In ventilated lambs with PPHN, a single intratracheal dose of rhSOD reduced pulmonary artery pressure and enhanced the pulmonary vasodilator effects of iNO. Intratracheal rhSOD also improved oxygenation and pulmonary hypertension in lambs with severe RDS (302). The effects of intratracheal rhSOD were compared to the effects of inhaled NO in neonatal lambs with PPHN who were ventilated for 24 h with various oxygen concentrations (169). A single dose of intratracheal rhSOD administered at birth caused a sustained improvement in systemic oxygenation lasting 24 h. Oxygenation improved more rapidly with the combination of rhSOD and iNO compared to either intervention alone. Lung isoprostane levels and 3-nitrotyrosine levels (a marker of peroxynitrite formation) were increased by ventilation for 24 h with 100% oxygen, effects that were reversed by rhSOD (169).

The safety profile of intratracheal SOD is well established in human neonates (303). In human preterm infants, rhSOD did not lower the incidence of BPD but reduced late respiratory sequelae, such as use of asthma medications, emergency room visits and rehospitalizations for respiratory illness (304). Clearly, additional studies are needed to clarify the role of superoxide generation in the abnormal pulmonary vascular reactivity of neonates with pulmonary hypertension and to explore the therapeutic potential of exogenous administration of cell-permeable SOD mimetics. In so doing, it must be kept in mind that SODs are present in all vascular tissues. Thus, particularly if modes of delivery other than intratracheal administration are used, careful monitoring for potential adverse effects in other vascular beds must be performed.

Novel and Experimental Therapies Directed at the COX-Prostaglandin Pathway

Prostacyclin Analogues

Prostacyclin (PGI$_2$) is a potent, short-acting, cyclic adenosine monophosphate (cAMP)-dependent vasodilator of the pulmonary and systemic circulations with anti-proliferative and anti-thrombotic effects (Fig. 12-2). There is evidence of decreased expression of prostacyclin synthase and an altered balance of vasoconstrictor and vasodilator prostanoids in neonatal animal models (305) and in patients with various forms of pulmonary hypertension (306). The potential benefits of its use in pulmonary hypertension include its ability to acutely relax vascular smooth muscle, inhibit platelet aggregation, ameliorate endothelial injury, inhibit VSMC migration and proliferation, reverse vascular remodeling, reduce synthesis and improve clearance of ET-1, positive inotropic effects and improved skeletal muscle oxygen use (306). PGI$_2$ is now the mainstay of therapy for adults and older children with pulmonary hypertension (307, 308). However, use in neonates with PPHN or other forms of pulmonary hypertension is largely anecdotal.

PGI$_2$ can be delivered in various forms, although the greatest experience is with continuous i.v. infusions of epoprostenol (Flolan^{TM}). RCTs in adults and older children have demonstrated sustained improvement in symptoms and mortality, even in patients without an immediate hemodynamic response. About 70% of lung-transplant candidates with primary pulmonary hypertension were removed from the transplant list after clinical improvement on epoprostenol therapy (306). Its efficacy has been demonstrated in PAH patients of all ages, and in patients with pulmonary hypertension associated with congenital heart disease. However, epoprostenol therapy has significant drawbacks. It is costly and difficult to administer. A half-life of only 3–5 min necessitates continuous i.v. infusion. It must be reconstituted in alkaline buffer daily and stored in refrigerated reservoirs. Side-effects in adults include jaw pain, hypotension, headache, nausea and anorexia. Escalation of dosing is frequently required to maintain a therapeutic response and acute withdrawal can lead to fatal pulmonary hypertension. Sepsis related to the i.v.

delivery system is another potentially fatal complication (307). Intravenous prostacyclin may lower systemic vascular resistance, worsening ductal or atrial level right-to-left shunting in neonates with PPHN. It may also worsen intrapulmonary shunts by vasodilating non-ventilated areas of the lung, worsening ventilation-perfusion matching and oxygenation (308).

More stable analogues of PGI_2 and alternative routes of administration hold particular attraction for neonates with PPHN and right-to-left extrapulmonary shunts. Aerosolized PGI_2 results in selective pulmonary vasodilatation without decreasing systemic blood pressure and can improve ventilation-perfusion matching and gas exchange in infants with parenchymal lung disease and PPHN by redistributing pulmonary blood flow from nonventilated to ventilated lung regions (308). Its short half-life necessitates continuous inhalation, similar to iNO.

The use of inhaled PGI_2 was reported in four neonates with PPHN refractory to iNO (309). All four infants responded with rapid improvement in oxygenation. One infant later deteriorated and was subsequently found to have alveolar capillary dysplasia at autopsy (309). No systemic vascular effects were observed. The infants were all treated with milrinone, which inhibits cAMP hydrolysis by type 3 phosphodiesterase, which may have increased cAMP availability, further augmenting the response to inhaled PGI_2 (309). This encouraging case series should lay the groundwork for a large RCT of inhaled PGI_2 in infants with an insufficient clinical response to iNO.

Thromboxane Synthase and Receptor Antagonists

Concurrent with reduced PGI_2 production, there is evidence in both animal models and patients with pulmonary hypertension that production of the potent pulmonary vasoconstrictor, thromboxane, is elevated (310). In a neonatal animal model of chronic-hypoxia induced pulmonary hypertension in piglets, terbogrel, an orally active, combined thromboxane synthetase inhibitor and thromboxane receptor antagonist, ameliorated the development of pulmonary hypertension (311). Unfortunately, a multi-center RCT of terbogrel in adult patients with primary pulmonary hypertension was halted early because of the unforeseen side-effect of leg pain which confounded the primary end-point, a 6 min walk test (312). Terbogrel was effective in reducing thromboxane metabolites and was also associated with a modest rise in prostacyclin. Although side-effects preclude the use of terbogrel in humans, other thromboxane inhibitors should be considered. Moreover, use of a novel long-acting prostacyclin agonist with thromboxane synthase inhibitory activity has been shown to attenuate monocrotaline-induced pulmonary hypertension in rats (313). Trials of such combined therapies for pulmonary hypertension should be further pursued in animal models and in the clinical setting.

Novel and Experimental Therapies Directed at the Endothelin Pathway

Non-Selective Endothelin Receptor Antagonists

ET-1 is a potent vasoconstrictor and vascular smooth muscle cell (VSMC[P1]) mitogen whose concentrations in plasma and lung tissue are elevated in patients with pulmonary hypertension (307). Several groups have shown that serum immunoreactive ET-1 is increased in human newborns with established PPHN (115, 116). Bosentan (Tracleer^{TM}) is an orally active, dual endothelin receptor antagonist that can improve exercise capacity, quality of life and hemodynamics in adult patients with pulmonary hypertension (314–316) (Fig. 12-2). It was the first oral drug approved for the treatment of pulmonary arterial hypertension in adults; FDA approval occurred in November 2001. There is some concern that the long-term use of this vasodilator might be limited by liver toxicity, which affects up to 10% of patients treated.

The pharmacokinetics, safety, and efficacy of bosentan were evaluated in an open-label study of 19 pediatric patients with pulmonary arterial hypertension (317). Bosentan produced hemodynamic improvement and was well tolerated. Unfortunately, no neonates were included in this open-label study; the youngest patient enrolled was 2 years of age. In a non-randomized study, Ivy et al. (2004) reported that concomitant use of bosentan allowed a reduction of epoprostenol and decreased its associated side-effects in seven of eight children with idiopathic pulmonary arterial hypertension (318). In young children with congenital heart disease and pulmonary hypertension, bosentan was used as compassionate treatment in seven children when pulmonary hypertension represented a contraindication to corrective surgery or caused right heart failure after surgery (319). After a mean treatment time of 8.6 ± 5 months, the clinical status remained stable or improved in all patients with a mean reduction of the right ventricular systolic pressure.

There are almost no published data on the use of ET receptor antagonists in neonates with pulmonary hypertension. There is a single case report describing the use of bosentan plus epoprostenol in an infant with severe BPD and pulmonary hypertension in which combined treatment decreased systolic right ventricular pressure from 68% to 40% of the systemic level over a 4-month period (320). Despite the lack of published data in infants, bosentan is being prescribed for refractory pulmonary hypertension associated with CDH, BPD and congenital heart disease. There is an urgent need for published data on the efficacy and safety of endothelin antagonists in this population and ultimately for a randomized clinical trial as monotherapy or as an adjunctive therapy for long-term management of neonatal and pediatric pulmonary hypertension.

Selective Endothelin-A Receptor Antagonists

Bosentan is a nonselective inhibitor of both ET_A and ET_B, which is a potential drawback of this drug. ET_B is thought to release NO and mediate vasodilatation. For this reason, there has been interest in the development of drugs such as sitaxsentan, a selective ET_A receptor antagonist. In a double-blind RCT in 245 adult PAH patients, sitaxsentan was associated with functional improvement without evidence of the hepatic toxicity seen with bosentan therapy. Larger studies in adults are sure to follow (321).

Combination Therapies

Combination therapies are of considerable interest for patients who fail to respond adequately to monotherapy. This approach has worked well in other fields such as oncology, and for other cardiovascular diseases such as systemic hypertension and congestive heart failure. Combination therapies may be employed to augment a single pathway. An example of this paradigm is the synergistic affects of a phosphodiesterase inhibitor, such as sildenafil, with inhalation NO therapy. Agents that attack different signaling pathways (Fig. 12-2) hold particular interest as combination therapy for pulmonary hypertension. The first report of the successful long-term use of a combination therapy in patients with severe pulmonary hypertension evaluated the use of oral sildenafil as an adjunct to inhaled iloprost therapy (322). Efficacy of combination therapy in adults with pulmonary hypertension has been shown for epoprostenol and bosentan (323), bosentan and sildenafil (324), and bosentan and inhaled iloprost (325). Hoeper et al. described an algorithm-based approach to combination therapy in 123 consecutive adults with PAH (326). The first-line therapy was bosentan. If functional goals were not met, sildenafil was added, followed by the further addition of inhaled iloprost. Survival at 1, 2 and 3 years was 93.0, 83.1 and 79.9%, respectively, which was significantly better than expected survival. Combination therapy also reduced the need for intravenous prostaglandin treatment and lung transplantation, compared to historical controls (326). However, caution is appropriate as the currently available therapies are relatively expensive, have potential toxicities and may have unanticipated drug-drug interactions. As with all therapies designed and tested in adults, there are limitations and risks when attempting to extrapolate efficacy and safety to infants and children.

Targeting Vascular Remodeling

The clinical introduction of potent vasodilator therapies, such as iNO and PGI_2, has changed the outlook for many patients with pulmonary hypertension, including neonates with PPHN. Yet, a cure for many forms of pulmonary hypertension will require more than acute vasodilator therapy. Reversal of structural remodeling is the next therapeutic frontier for adult patients with PAH and is likely to be the key to treating newborns and older infants who have advanced stages of pulmonary hypertension and who are poorly or insufficiently responsive to acute vasodilator therapy. A recent shift in focus from agents that target vasodilatation to antiproliferative agents reflects the advancement in our understanding of the mechanisms mediating many forms of pulmonary hypertension (327).

Apoptosis, or programmed cell death, is a fundamental biological process that constantly deletes cells to maintain homeostasis. Apoptosis of VSMCs occurs in vivo under both physiological and pathological settings. The delicate balance between VSMC apoptosis and proliferation plays a critical role in maintaining the normal structural and functional integrity of the pulmonary vasculature and the low pulmonary arterial pressure in normal subjects. Remodeling, as occurs during development, is an adaptive process in response to long-term changes in hemodynamics; however, remodeling can also contribute to vascular diseases. Increased pulmonary VSMC proliferation and decreased apoptosis will reduce the inner-lumen diameter of pulmonary arteries, increasing pulmonary vascular resistance (328–331).

The cellular processes underlying remodeling include altered VSMC growth, migration, differentiation and increased extracellular matrix (ECM) abundance leading to neointimal proliferation, intimal fibrosis, medial and adventitial hyperplasia and hypertrophy and neomuscularization of non-muscular arteries (328, 329, 332, 333). Remodeling of the ECM involves increased expression and deposition of elastin, collagen, fibronectin, and the matrix glycoprotein tenascin-C (334–337). Prominent features of many postnatally acquired pulmonary hypertensive diseases include increased elastase activity and deposition of tenascin-C. In the media, impaired apoptosis and excessive proliferation of pulmonary VSMC result from reduced expression of voltage-gated potassium channels (338, 339), de novo expression of the apoptosis inhibitor survivin (340) and increased expression of the serotonin transporter (341). In the adventitia, disordered matrix remodeling (342) and transition of fibroblasts into myofibroblasts (343) may contribute to pathological remodeling (344). Studies have shown that apoptosis plays a key role in resolution of vascular remodeling (330) and that pulmonary arteries have capacity to return to normal architecture (345).

Apoptosis modulators in the vasculature may include NO (346), endothelin (347) and ROS (348). It has been suggested that superoxide induces proliferation and H_2O_2 induces apoptosis. Whether the source of these ROS is the mitochondria, NADPH oxidase or another source is currently controversial. A number of therapeutic targets that exploit the imbalance between VSMC proliferation and apoptosis are under investigation in laboratory models of pulmonary hypertension and hold promise for future clinical trials. Successful therapies are likely to involve strategies that promote endothelial survival while simultaneously promoting VSMC apoptosis, thus remodeling the maldeveloped pulmonary vasculature.

Inhibitors of Serine Elastase Activity

Pulmonary hypertension is associated with an increase in elastase activity (334). Serine elastase activity degrades the extracellular matrix and releases growth factors. The subsequent activation of matrix metalloproteinases (MMPs), clustering of $\alpha_v\beta_3$-integrins, and transcription of the glycoprotein tenascin-C, activates epidermal growth factor receptors (EGFRs), stimulating pulmonary VSMC proliferation (349). The ultimate result is neomuscularization, medial thickening, and reduced number of pulmonary arteries (350–352). Elastase and matrix metalloproteinase inhibitors and tenascin-C antisense suppress VSMC tenascin-C expression and cause apoptosis of cultured VSMCs, presumably by inhibiting EGFR signaling (349, 353).

Monocrotaline is an endothelial toxin that selectively injures the pulmonary endothelium, producing a well-established animal model of rapidly fatal pulmonary hypertension. Administration of a serine elastase inhibitor, Elafin, induces VSMC apoptosis and completely reverses fatal monocrotaline-induced pulmonary hypertension in adult rats (345). Unfortunately, side-effects limit the utility of this agent in human pulmonary hypertension. However, strategies that block downstream effectors, such as MMP inhibitors, $\alpha_v\beta_3$-integrin blockers, or EGFR tyrosine kinase inhibitors are attractive pharmacological strategies for the reversal of vascular remodeling in pulmonary hypertension, as studies with a MMP inhibitor (SC-080), an $\alpha_v\beta_3$-integrin blocker (cilengitide), and an EGFR tyrosine kinase inhibitor, PKI166, have demonstrated (354). These agents are in clinical or preclinical use in cancer patients and might offer a novel approach to the treatment of vascular remodeling in human pulmonary hypertension.

Voltage-Gated Potassium Channels (K_v Channels)

The classical function of K^+ channels is the regulation of membrane potential and thereby the regulation of vascular tone. VSMC from the pulmonary, but not the systemic, circulation possess a delayed rectifier K^+ current that is inhibited by hypoxia (355, 356). Hypoxic pulmonary vasoconstriction (HPV) is initiated by inhibition of these oxygen-sensitive K_v channels (357, 358) and alterations in K_v channel expression and function have been implicated in chronic hypoxia-induced pulmonary hypertension. K^+ channels also participate in vascular remodeling by controlling cell proliferation and apoptosis (357). Decreased K_v expression enhances cell proliferation and inhibits apoptosis (339, 340, 359, 360).

The *redox theory* underlying HPV proposes the existence of an oxygen sensor as an intrinsic property of the VSMC of pulmonary resistance arteries. One candidate for this oxygen sensor is the mitochondria. According to the redox theory, hypoxia decreases the basal, normoxic production of ROS from pulmonary artery VSMC which inhibits K_v channel activity (361). K_v channel inhibition depolarizes the VSMC, activates Ca^{++} channels and increases intracellular Ca^{++}, thereby inducing HPV (358). A number of findings support the redox theory and the important role of K^+ channels in some forms of pulmonary hypertension. For example, the K_v-channel blocker, 4-aminopyridine, causes pulmonary vasoconstriction (362). Oxidants, such as H_2O_2, increase K^+ currents in pulmonary VSMCs and relax resistance-level pulmonary arteries, mimicking the effects of oxygen. Conversely, antioxidants mimic hypoxia, decreasing K^+ currents and causing vasoconstriction (361). Redox signaling appears to involve an interaction between ROS and cysteine and methionine residues in K_v channels, resulting in structural modifications of the channel (357). Despite this supporting evidence, the redox theory remains a topic of scientific debate. The role of the endothelium versus the VSMC in HPV remains controversial (363). Hypoxia has been reported to both decrease (360, 364–366) and increase (367, 368) ROS production. There is disagreement about whether the mitochondria (360, 368, 369) or NADPH oxidase (370–373) is the redox sensor.

In addition to a sensor, the redox theory requires the existence of an effector molecule. The $K_v1.5$ protein is an attractive candidate for this role. $K_v1.5$ expression is increased in pulmonary resistance arteries (374), the site of HPV, compared with expression of this channel in conduit pulmonary arteries or systemic resistance arteries. $K_v1.5$ expression is decreased by chronic hypoxia (375). Conversely, loss of $K_v1.5$ in a knockout mouse attenuates HPV (376, 377). Anorexigens, a pharmacological inducer of human PAH, block $K_v1.5$ (378). Rats with chronic hypoxia-induced pulmonary hypertension have a blunted constrictor response to acute hypoxia. Restoration of expression of this single channel by adenoviral gene transfer restores the normal HPV response in chronically hypoxic rats (375). Chronic K_v downregulation causes VSM hypertrophy and hyperplasia by reducing apoptosis (332), leading to vascular remodeling. Thus, at least some forms of pulmonary hypertension may be considered a K^+ channelopathy (379).

Novel strategies to prevent and reverse chronic hypoxia-induced pulmonary hypertension might therefore include gene therapy with pulmonary VSMC-targeted repletion of K_v channels. Another approach is the use of the metabolic modulator dichloroacetate, which has been shown to restore expression and function of K_v channels in adult rats with chronic hypoxia-induced pulmonary hypertension as described in more detail below (380).

Dichloroacetate (DCA)

Dichloroacetate (DCA) is a metabolic modulator that inhibits mitochondrial pyruvate dehydrogenase kinase and increases mitochondrial oxidative phosphorylation. DCA also depolarizes the mitochondria, causing release of H_2O_2 and cytochrome c. This cascade of events induces a 10-fold increase in apoptosis within the pulmonary artery vascular wall (380, 381). By returning hypertensive pulmonary arteries to an oxidized state, DCA might reverse K_v channel downregulation and restore normal vascular function.

In the monocrotaline rat model of pulmonary hypertension, DCA has been shown to both prevent and reverse pulmonary hypertension and significantly improve mortality. Similar effects of DCA have been shown in a model of chronic hypoxia-induced pulmonary hypertension (380). DCA caused mitochondrial depolarization and restored both the function and expression of K_v channels. DCA also increased apoptosis and reduced proliferation in the media of remodeled pulmonary arteries, without affecting healthy tissues or systemic vessels (381). Thus, at least in some experimental models, DCA seems to be selective for the pulmonary circulation.

A particularly intriguing model of pulmonary hypertension is the faun-hooded rat. This rat strain spontaneously develops pulmonary hypertension in a normoxic environment. In mild hypoxia, the faun-hooded rat develops rapidly progressive pulmonary hypertension and alveolar simplification (344, 382, 383). It is believed that the faun-hooded rat has an inherited mitochondrial defect that reduces ROS production and disrupts oxygen sensing (344). Thus, even in normoxia, the mitochondrial milieu in the faun-hooded rat resembles hypoxia. This activates hypoxia-inducible factor (HIF-1α) and results in $K_v1.5$ downregulation (344, 384). The normoxic activation of HIF-1α and reduced $K_v1.5$ expression could be prevented by exogenous H_2O_2 or by normalization of mitochondrial function with DCA. Both of these treatments improved survival in the faun-hood rat.

DCA has an excellent safety profile; this oral therapy has been used in human infants with mitochondrial diseases (385). Therapeutic benefit in pulmonary hypertension patients may be derived by exploiting DCA's ability to initiate mitochondria-dependent apoptosis, activate K^+ currents, restore dysfunctional or downregulated K_v channels and reverse vascular remodeling. This clinically available oral therapy is worthy of further laboratory and human investigation.

Platelet-Derived Growth Factor (PDGF) Receptor Antagonists

Studies in animal models of pulmonary hypertension and case reports in humans have stimulated interest in the PDGF receptor antagonist imatinib as a novel therapy for pulmonary hypertension refractory to standard vasodilator therapy. PDGF is a potent VSM mitogen that has been associated with vascular proliferation and remodeling in pulmonary hypertension. The PDGF receptors (PDGFR), which belong to a family of transmembrane receptor tyrosine kinases, have been found to be significantly increased in lung tissue from pulmonary hypertension patients compared with healthy donor lung tissue (386). Likewise, in lambs with chronic intrauterine pulmonary hypertension, there is upregulation of both PDGFRα and PDGFRß (387). In several animal models of pulmonary hypertension, daily therapy with the PDGFR antagonist STI571 (imatinib or Gleevec) reversed right ventricular pressures and right ventricular hypertrophy to near normal levels, reversed vascular remodeling and improved survival. This correlated with prevention of PDGFR phosphorylation and initiation of downstream signaling pathways. This drug was effective even in established pulmonary hypertension caused by chronic hypoxia (386).

Imatinib was designed to target the ATP-binding site of tyrosine kinases and is currently approved for the treatment of chronic myelogenous leukemia (CML) and some gastrointestinal tumors (386). In 2005, a case report in the New England Journal of Medicine drew attention to this drug as rescue therapy for human patients with severe pulmonary hypertension (388). An adult male with rapidly progressive familial pulmonary arterial hypertension and right-sided heart failure despite combination therapy with bosentan, inhaled iloprost and oral sildenafil was given compassionate treatment with daily oral imatinib mesylate (Gleevec) in addition to his routine medications while awaiting lung transplantation. He demonstrated impressive improvement after 3 months of imatinib treatment, without obvious side-effects, and was removed from the transplant list. Reports of similar dramatic clinical improvement following the addition of imatinib to a failing regimen of pulmonary vasodilators have since appeared in the literature (389, 390). The limitations of case reports not withstanding, antagonists to the platelet-derived growth factor receptor may be a promising targeted therapy for pulmonary hypertension with the potential to reverse lung vascular remodeling.

Bone Morphogenic Protein (BMP) Signaling and the Survivin Gene

Pulmonary vascular remodeling in pulmonary hypertension is correlated with downregulation of the bone morphogenetic protein axis. Activation of bone morphogenetic protein receptor 2 (BMPR2) suppresses proliferation and initiates apoptosis in normal PASMCs (391) but not in PASMCs from patients with PAH (392). Germ-line and loss-of-function mutations in BMPR2, encoding a TGF-beta receptor, cause familial primary pulmonary hypertension (393). One anti-apoptotic signaling molecule downstream of BMP that has attracted recent attention is survivin.

Survivin (*Birc5*) is a member of the "inhibitor of apoptosis" gene family that plays a role in promoting cell proliferation and antagonizing mitochondria-dependent apoptosis in malignant cells (394). Molecular antagonists of survivin, including antisense and dominant-negative mutants, induce apoptosis and inhibit tumor growth in vivo, without affecting normal cells (394). Interestingly, survivin mutants also prevent vascular remodeling in arterial injury models by inducing apoptosis within the vascular wall (395). Survivin can be induced by exposure of VSMCs to the serum growth factor PDGF, and by vascular injury but is absent in quiescent VSMCs (395). Because survivin is absent from most healthy tissues, it is an attractive target for therapy.

Survivin is expressed in established human and experimental pulmonary hypertension, but not in normal pulmonary arteries (340). In experimental pulmonary hypertension, its expression parallels the rise of PA pressure, although it is not known whether this is true in human pulmonary vascular disease. Adenovirus-mediated overexpression of survivin causes pulmonary hypertension in rats, whereas inhalation of an adenovirus vector encoding a mutant survivin gene with dominant-negative properties reverses established monocrotaline-induced pulmonary hypertension (340). The reversal of vascular remodeling by survivin antagonism is associated with induction of apoptosis, suppression of proliferation, and activation of K_v channels in PASMCs (340). Unfortunately, there is virtually nothing known about the expression and role of survivin in developing human infants or its role, if any, in neonatal forms of pulmonary hypertension. Nonetheless, the use of survivin antagonists to increase cell death and to prevent pathological vascular remodeling might hold therapeutic potential in some patients with pulmonary hypertension associated with vascular remodeling (394).

3-Hydroxy-3-Methylglutaryl-Coenzyme A (HMG-CoA) Reductase Inhibitors

Statins, in addition to their cholesterol-lowering effects, confer potent antiproliferative effects on endothelial cells and VSMCs and have anti-inflammatory properties (396). Statins have been shown to prevent the development of experimental pulmonary hypertension in several different animal models (397, 398). Simvastatin attenuates monocrotaline-induced pulmonary vascular remodeling by increasing apoptosis of VSMCs and improved survival from 0% to 100% (399). Similar results were reported in a rat model of hypoxic pulmonary hypertension (400).

Among the mechanisms of action of statins is inhibition of the rho and ras family of GTPases that couple growth factor receptors to the intracellular MAP/ERK kinase signaling pathways (396). Statins also augment endothelium-dependent NO production and vasodilatation by stabilizing endothelial NO synthase mRNA (401). Additionally, statins may contribute to vascular remodeling by activating the survival factor Akt kinase, which increases circulating endothelial progenitor cells (402). A number of transcriptional changes are associated with statin administration, including downregulation of the inflammatory genes fos, jun, and tumor necrosis factor-alpha and upregulation of endothelial nitric oxide synthase, bone morphogenetic protein receptor typ. 1α and the cell cycle inhibitor p27Kip1. Given the widespread clinical use of these agents, trials of statin therapy for the prevention or treatment of pulmonary hypertension have merit.

Rho/Rho-Associated Kinase Inhibitors

The small GTPase rhoA and its effector protein, rho-kinase, are important regulators of vascular tone. Activation of rho-kinase promotes actin-myosin interaction in VSMCs and reduces expression of eNOS (403). The Rho/rho-kinase system has also been implicated in VSMC migration, proliferation, and apoptosis (404). Activation of the rho-kinase signal transduction pathway is increased in the pulmonary circulation of adult animals with experimental pulmonary hypertension (405–407). Long-term treatment with the rho-kinase inhibitor fasudil reduced pulmonary hypertension and vascular remodeling and improved survival in monocrotaline and hypoxia-induced models of pulmonary hypertension (363, 405–407). Furthermore, as discussed earlier, there is evidence that the rho-kinase signal transduction pathway is an important regulator of the high PVR of the normal fetal lung (63). Thus, rho-kinase inhibitors may be an effective and novel therapy for neonatal pulmonary hypertension (63).

Endothelial Progenitor Cell (EPC) and Stem Cell Therapy

Other novel therapies under investigation in the laboratory include the therapeutic use of mesenchymal stem cells (MSCs) and endothelial progenitor cells (EPCs). Circulating EPCs migrate to the site of injured vascular endothelium, where they differentiate into mature endothelial cells. In a study using the monocrotaline model of pulmonary hypertension in rats, infusion of human EPCs alone modestly attenuated pulmonary hypertension. Transplantation of EPCs carrying the DNA for adrenomedullin, a potent vasodilator, markedly ameliorated pulmonary hypertension and resulted in enhanced survival (408). EPCs migrate to sites of injured endothelium where they differentiate into mature endothelial cells in situ. EPC may be a viable tool for tissue engineering to reconstruct the pulmonary vasculature and also as a vehicle for gene delivery to injured pulmonary endothelium. Given that cord blood is a rich source of EPCs, development of this approach to gene therapy may hold particular promise for neonates, who theoretically could use their own EPCs isolated from cord blood as the vehicle for gene therapy.

MSCs have also been proposed for the treatment of pulmonary hypertension. Intratracheal administration of rat MSCs 2 weeks after administration of mono-crotaline attenuated the rise in pulmonary arterial pressure and pulmonary vascular resistance, decreased the right ventricular hypertrophy and restored pulmonary dilator responses to acetylcholine (409). Immunohistochemistry revealed wide-spread distribution of the MSCs in lung parenchyma surrounding airways in mono-crotaline-treated rats but not in the wall of pulmonary vessels, suggesting a paracrine effect of the transplanted MSCs (409). Likewise, MSCs overexpressing eNOS reduced right ventricular systolic pressure and increased survival time in rats with monocrotaline-induced pulmonary hypertension (410). It is not clear at this time whether stem cell therapy will one day be a viable clinical modality for the treatment of neonatal pulmonary vascular disease or maldevelopment.

Targeted Therapies for Specific Developmental Pulmonary Structural Abnormalities Associated with Pulmonary Hypertension

For neonatal patients with pulmonary hypertension caused by pulmonary hypo-plasia or severe BPD, the therapeutic Holy Grail is reprogramming of arrested vascular development. In both of these conditions innovative therapies are needed to prevent and reverse the progressive pulmonary vascular disease and disturbances in cardiac performance while stimulating new lung growth. Examples of promising therapies for extreme forms of CDH and BPD are discussed next.

Therapies for Congenital Diaphragmatic Hernia (CDH)

Pulmonary hypertension complicates the course of many newborns with CDH. The anatomic pulmonary vascular changes in patients with PPHN and CDH include intra-acinar extension of smooth muscle cells and increased medial hyper-trophy (411) with extensive collagen deposition in the media and adventitia of pulmonary arteries (412). Infants with CDH and PPHN respond poorly to acute vasodilator therapies, including iNO. Downstream signaling abnormalities in the NO-cyclic GMP pathway have been identified in experimental CDH. Thebaud et al.

(2002) found evidence of decreased soluble guanylate cyclase activity in lamb fetuses with surgically created CDH (86). Sakai et al. (2004) reported markedly reduced K_v channel expression in the pulmonary artery VSMC of animals with nitrofen-induced CDH (413). In this animal model, antenatal dexamethasone treatment increased K_v channel protein and mRNA levels in the CDH lung.

Abnormalities in retinoid signaling early in gestation may contribute to the etiology of CDH. Diaphragmatic hernias occur in 25–49% of the offspring of rats with diets deficient in vitamin A (414–416). The incidence of CDH was reduced when vitamin A supplementation was provided during gestation. CDH was also produced in double null-mutant mice that lack both retinoic acid receptors, RARα and RARß (417, 418). Nitrofen (2,4-dichlorophenyl-p-nitrophenyl ether) is a teratogen that induces CDH in rodents (419–422). The developmental pulmonary abnormalities resemble those in human infants with CDH and include lung hypoplasia with a reduction in the number of terminal bronchioles and alveoli, a hypoplastic pulmonary vascular bed, and increased thickness of the pulmonary arterial smooth muscle (423). Nitrofen inhibits retinal dehydrogenase (424) and causes suppression of retinoid response element activation, which can be antagonized in vitro by supplemental retinoic acid. The co-administration of vitamin A and nitrofen can reduce the incidence of CDH by 15% to 30% and attenuate lung hypoplasia (423, 425). In a small clinical study of human infants with CDH, retinol and retinol-binding-protein plasma levels were reduced in cord blood (426). These findings justify a search for candidate genes related to retinoid signaling as a genetic cause of CDH (427).

Abnormal or delayed surfactant synthesis may also contribute to the pathophysiology of CDH. Both the ipsilateral and contralateral lungs exhibit surfactant deficiencies in the lamb model of CDH (428) and surfactant protein A deficiency has been demonstrated in a rat model of CDH (429). The bronchoalveolar lavage fluid of human infants with fatal CDH is deficient in phospholipids; the lungs of these infants demonstrate reduced immunohistochemical staining for surfactant protein A (430). Lotze et al. (1994) reported that infants treated with ECMO for CDH had reduced tracheal aspirate surfactant protein A, relative to infants on ECMO for other diagnoses (431). Prophylactic surfactant therapy, administered to fetal lambs with surgically induced CDH just before birth, dramatically increased pulmonary blood flow and reduced extrapulmonary shunting (432). Unfortunately, the clinical response of human infants with CDH to surfactant treatment postnatally has been disappointing. Administration of surfactant did not improve lung compliance or reduce time to extubation in infants with CDH (431). Effective therapeutic approaches to PPHN associated with CDH or other conditions associated with abnormal lung development must prevent or reverse the vascular structural abnormalities that frequently accompany this condition.

Therapies for Bronchopulmonary Dysplasia (BPD)

Therapies that stimulate lung growth are needed for infants with severe BPD. Reductions in lung surface area and abnormalities of vascular and alveolar structure in severe BPD result in pulmonary hypertension (433–436). A number of animal models of arrested lung growth have been developed to recapitulate the pathobiology of BPD and to study therapies to restore lung growth. One such model is the chronically ventilated preterm lamb, which exhibits elevated postnatal PVR, reduced abundance of eNOS and structural abnormalities of the pulmonary circulation (155). Likewise, reduced alveolar and vascular growth and decreased pulmonary NO production are features of the preterm baboon model of BPD (437). Long-term exposure to iNO has been reported to ameliorate the lung structural abnormalities in chronically ventilated preterm lambs (438) and baboons (437). In the preterm baboon, iNO (5 ppm over 14 days) normalized elastin deposition, stimulated secondary crest formation and achieved rates of lung growth comparable to that in utero (437).

Inhaled NO has also proven protective in several neonatal rat models of BPD (439–441). Exposure of rats to hyperoxia or to a vascular endothelial growth factor (VEGF) inhibitor in the immediate postnatal period impairs alveolar and vascular growth (439, 441). Similar structural abnormalities are seen in rats exposed to mild hypoxia who are genetically deficient in eNOS (440). In all of these rat models of impaired lung growth, iNO treatment was able restore lung structure.

Vascular endothelial growth factor (VEGF) is an endothelial cell-specific survival factor that stimulates angiogenesis and protects endothelial cells against injury (442). NO is a downstream mediator of VEGF-dependent angiogenesis (443). VEGF receptor (VEGFR) activation increases the expression of eNOS mRNA and protein, and stimulates NO release (444). Hyperoxia reduces protein expression of lung eNOS, VEGF and VEGFR-2 (439). Inhibition of the VEGFR reduces alveolarization and vascular growth, resulting in histological changes in lung structure that mimic BPD (445). Bhatt et al. have shown decreased lung VEGF mRNA and protein expression, as well as a reduction of the VEGFR-1 in the lungs of infants with fatal BPD (446). Decreased lung VEGF and VEGFR expression has also been found in the primate model of BPD (447). Studies in eNOS knockout mice suggest that a deficiency of eNOS leads to a failure of lung vascular and alveolar growth and that prolonged iNO treatment can restore lung growth in this animal model (440). Similarly, iNO treatment after hyperoxia or exposure to the VEGFR inhibitor SU-5416 prevents pulmonary hypertension and improves distal lung growth in rats. These results shed light on possible mechanisms by which prolonged iNO treatment improves pulmonary outcomes in some preterm infants at risk for BPD (197, 200).

AN UNMET CHALLENGE

In the 1970s and 1980s persistent echocardiographic evidence of pulmonary hypertension beyond the first few months of life in an infant with BPD or CDH was associated with up to 40% mortality (448, 449). Unfortunately, in the intervening 2–3 decades, no effective therapies have been developed for these infants. Effective approaches to treatment must block progression of the vascular remodeling process and promote regression of established vascular changes. There are many potential targets for pharmacological intervention, as discussed earlier in this chapter. These include extracellular matrix components, vasoregulatory and anti-proliferative proteins, angiogenic proteins, and intracellular signal transduction cascades.

However, much work must be done before the neonatology community can hope to translate any pharmacologic intervention into evidenced-based therapy. This goal will require not just additional basic laboratory research but a focused effort from the clinical community. Unfortunately, the prevalence of pulmonary hypertension beyond the first months of life is unknown; anecdotal data suggest that the condition is under-appreciated and under-diagnosed. There are no standardized definitions of pulmonary hypertension in infants of varying postnatal ages and underlying conditions. Nor do we have recommendations for how to screen for this problem or how to prospectively follow infants at risk or suspected of having mild, moderate or severe pulmonary hypertension. These issues must be addressed before progress can be made on the therapeutic front.

A delay in diagnosis is associated with progressive pulmonary vascular disease. The diagnosis of cor pulmonale is associated with a very high mortality; reversal of pulmonary and cardiovascular disease at this advanced stage is unlikely to meet with success, outside of heart and lung transplantation. An unproven tenet is that identification of infants at earlier stages of pulmonary hypertension will result in more effective interventions and improved outcomes. For this to occur, we must develop guidelines for prospective identification of infants at risk and algorithms for ongoing surveillance and management.

Despite the limitations of echocardiography for serial quantitative assessments of pulmonary hypertension and myocardial dysfunction, Doppler echocardiography is currently the most readily available tool for non-invasive screening. We propose that infants who remain ventilated or who have a fractional inspired oxygen requirement greater than 0.3 be prospectively screened at 30 days of life and monthly thereafter for echocardiographic evidence of pulmonary hypertension. We urge the pediatric cardiology community to define echocardiographic end-points for age-based classifications of mild, moderate and severe pulmonary hypertension that will facilitate prospective monitoring of disease progression and response to therapy. We also applaud efforts to develop new imaging modalities for pulmonary hypertension, including MRI assessment of lung volume, lung vascular area and right heart geometry. Attention should be given to developing therapies for right ventricular dysfunction. The validity and predictive power of biomarkers, such as plasma brain natriuretic peptide (BNP) or troponin, for infants and children with pulmonary hypertension and myocardial dysfunction must be determined. A noninvasive marker for disease progression and efficacy of therapy holds great attraction for the pediatric population. In adults with primary pulmonary hypertension a high level of plasma BNP and, in particular, increasing plasma BNP levels over time have been shown to correlate with increased mortality (450). Also needed are criteria for referral of infants with progressive pulmonary hypertension to an interventional pediatric cardiologist for cardiac catheterization and vasodilator testing.

There are no well-publicized guidelines for the appropriate medical work-up of an infant newly diagnosed with later-onset pulmonary hypertension. We suggest that this work-up should include an assessment of gastroesophageal reflux and chronic aspiration, adequacy of nutrition and the adequacy of ventilation and oxygenation. While the ideal oxygen saturation target for this population is unknown, it is clearly important to avoid recurrent hypoxemic events. For infants with a diagnosis of pulmonary hypertension, it may be necessary to adjust upward the oxygen saturation targets currently thought to be beneficial in the first weeks of life to avoid the development of BPD. Consideration should be given to a metabolic work-up for inborn errors of metabolism, storage diseases and thyroid dysfunction, hematologic diseases such as sickle cell disease, coagulation defects including genetic thrombophilias, such as Factor V Leiden and methyl tetrahydrofolate reductase (MTHFR) mutations and infectious diseases including HIV.

More data are needed on the characteristics of high-risk neonates and the natural history and outcomes of infants who develop pulmonary hypertension beyond the first weeks of life. A wide range of treatment regimens including combination therapies are being used clinically, despite lack of RCTs or efficacy and safety data. We need a mechanism for recording the responses to these therapies and the outcomes of these patients, beyond the occasional case report or case series. We propose the establishment of a database registry of infants with pulmonary hypertension that persists or develops beyond the first weeks of life. Although such registries are, by definition, observational and descriptive, the systematic accrual of data could help clarify patient demographics, risk factors and practice patterns. A registry could provide much-needed information about the timing and antecedents of diagnosis, the types of therapies implemented and whether there is truly a benefit to early detection and treatment. Although hypotheses cannot be tested with registry data, hypotheses can be generated for future testing by comparing outcomes of various treatment regimens reported in the registry. The reality is that there are huge obstacles to the conduct of RCTs in this patient population, including limited patient volumes, disease heterogeneity, lack of standardized definitions for disease onset, severity and progression, multiple treatment paradigms, limited funding and ethical considerations. A database registry will ultimately enable the conduct of RCTs by better defining prevalence and assembling random treatment strategies into a comprehensible pattern.

CONCLUSIONS

Much progress has been made in our understanding and management of infants with reactive pulmonary vascular disease and PPHN. Much work remains to achieve similar success for neonates with pulmonary hypertension-associated structural changes in the lungs. Effective treatment for these infants will most likely require long-term administration of a combination of vasodilator and antiproliferative therapies. Laboratory and clinical studies are needed to define the roles of inflammation and free radical generation, vasodilator/vasoconstrictor imbalance, ion channel dysfunction, angiogenesis and differentiation, thrombosis and hemodynamics in the pathogenesis of neonatal pulmonary hypertensive diseases. A better understanding of normal lung vascular development and the complex regulation of proliferative and apoptotic processes in the maldeveloped, hypertensive neonatal pulmonary circulation is a prerequisite for progress. The challenge lies in developing therapies that induce apoptotic death of abnormal VSMCs without interfering with normal postnatal vascular development. On the clinical front a more systematic approach to the diagnosis, assessment of disease severity and progression, pathophysiology, and clinical and genetic risk factors are necessary first steps to the development of appropriate therapies for persistent forms of neonatal pulmonary hypertension.

REFERENCES

1. Rudolph AM. Distribution and regulation of blood flow in the fetal and neonatal lamb. Circ Res 1985; 57:811.
2. Rudolph AM, Heymann MA. Circulatory changes during growth in the fetal lamb. Circ Res 1970; 26:289.
3. Fishman NH, Hof RB, Rudolph AM, et al. Models of congenital heart disease in fetal lambs. Circulation 1978; 58:354.
4. Rudolph AM. Fetal and neonatal pulmonary circulation. Am Rev Respir Dis 1977; 115:11.
5. Soothill PW, Nicolaides KH, Rodeck CH, et al. Blood gases and acid-base status of the human second-trimester fetus. Obstet Gynecol 1986; 68:173.
6. Teitel DF, Iwamoto HS, Rudolph AM. Changes in the pulmonary circulation during birth-related events. Pediatr Res 1990; 27:372.
7. Lawson EE, Birdwell RL, Huang PS, et al. Augmentation of pulmonary surfactant secretion by lung expansion at birth. Pediatr Res 1979; 13:611.
8. Truog WE. Surface active material: influence of lung distension and mechanical ventilation on secretion. Semin Perinatol 1984; 8:300.
9. Haddad Grellins RB. The role of airway receptors in the control of respiration in infants: a review. J Pediatr 1977; 91:281.
10. Teitel DF, Iwamoto HS, Rudolph AM. Effects of birth-related events on central blood flow patterns. Pediatr Res 1987; 22:557.
11. Iwamoto HS, Teitel D, Rudolph AM. Effects of birth-related events on blood flow distribution. Pediatr Res 1987; 22:634.
12. Levin DL, Rudolph AM, Heymann MA, et al. Morphological development of the pulmonary vascular bed in fetal lambs. Circulation 1976; 53:144.
13. Rudolph AM. The changes in the circulation after birth. Their importance in congenital heart disease. Circulation 1970; 41:343.
14. Rudolph AM. Fetal and neonatal pulmonary circulation. Annu Rev Physiol 1979; 41:383.
15. Kinsella JP, Ivy DD, Abman SH. Ontogeny of NO activity and response to inhaled NO in the developing ovine pulmonary circulation. Am J Physiol 1994; 267:H1955.
16. Morin FC, III, Egan EA. Pulmonary hemodynamics in fetal lambs during development at normal and increased oxygen tension. J Appl Physiol 1992; 73:213.
17. Naeye RL. Arterial changes during the perinatal period. Arch Pathol 1961; 71:121.
18. Hislop A, Reid L. Intra-pulmonary arterial development during fetal life-branching pattern and structure. J Anat 1972; 113:35.

19. Belik J, Halayko A, Rao K, et al. Pulmonary vascular smooth muscle: biochemical and mechanical developmental changes. J Appl Physiol 1991; 71:1129.

20. Ariel Gomez R, Sturgill BC, Chevalier RL, et al. Fetal expression of muscle-specific isoactins in multiple organs of the Wistar-Kyoto rat. Cell Tissue Res 1987; 250:7.

21. Colebatch HJ, Dawes GS, Goodwin JW, et al. The nervous control of the circulation in the foetal and newly expanded lungs of the lamb. J Physiol 1965; 178:544.

22. Lewis AB, Heymann MA, Rudolph AM. Gestational changes in pulmonary vascular responses in fetal lambs in utero. Circ Res 1976; 39:536.

23. Walker AM, Ritchie BC, Adamson TM, et al. Effect of changing lung liquid volume on the pulmonary circulation of fetal lambs. J Appl Physiol 1988; 64:61.

24. Dawes GS, Mott JC, Widdicombe JG, et al. Changes in the lungs of the new-born lamb. J Physiol 1953; 121:141.

25. Abman SH, Accurso FJ. Acute effects of partial compression of ductus arteriosus on fetal pulmonary circulation. Am J Physiol 1989; 257:H626.

26. Accurso FJ, Alpert B, Wilkening RB, et al. Time-dependent response of fetal pulmonary blood flow to an increase in fetal oxygen tension. Respir Physiol 1986; 63:43.

27. Storme L, Rairigh RL, Parker TA, et al. In vivo evidence for a myogenic response in the fetal pulmonary circulation. Pediatr Res 1999; 45:425.

28. Parker TA, Grover TR, Kinsella JP, et al. Inhibition of 20-HETE abolishes the myogenic response during NOS antagonism in the ovine fetal pulmonary circulation. Am J Physiol Lung Cell Mol Physiol 2005; 289:L261.

29. Davis MJ, Hill MA. Signaling mechanisms underlying the vascular myogenic response. Physiol Rev 1999; 79:387.

30. Belik J. Myogenic response in large pulmonary arteries and its ontogenesis. Pediatr Res 1994; 36:34.

31. Kulik TJ, Evans JN, Gamble WJ. Stretch-induced contraction in pulmonary arteries. Am J Physiol 1988; 255:H1391.

32. Lloyd TC, Jr. Pulmonary arterial distension does not cause pulmonary vasoconstriction. J Appl Physiol 1986; 61:741.

33. Accurso FJ, Wilkening RB. Temporal response of the fetal pulmonary circulation to pharmacologic vasodilators. Proc Soc Exp Biol Med 1988; 187:89.

34. Morin FC, III, Egan EA, Ferguson W, et al. Development of pulmonary vascular response to oxygen. Am J Physiol 1988; 254:H542.

35. Tod ML, Cassin S. Perinatal pulmonary responses to arachidonic acid during normoxia and hypoxia. J Appl Physiol 1984; 57:977.

36. Tyler T, Wallis R, Leffler C, et al. The effects of indomethacin on the pulmonary vascular response to hypoxia in the premature and mature newborn goat. Proc Soc Exp Biol Med 1975; 150:695.

37. Tyler TL, Leffler CW, Cassin S. Circulatory responses of perinatal goats to prostaglandin precursors. Prostaglandins Med 1978; 1:213.

38. Tod ML, Cassin S. Thromboxane synthase inhibition and perinatal pulmonary response to arachidonic acid. J Appl Physiol 1985; 58:710.

39. Clozel M, Clyman RI, Soifer SJ, et al. Thromboxane is not responsible for the high pulmonary vascular resistance in fetal lambs. Pediatr Res 1985; 19:1254.

40. Lebidois J, Soifer SJ, Clyman RI, et al. Piriprost: a putative leukotriene synthesis inhibitor increases pulmonary blood flow in fetal lambs. Pediatr Res 1987; 22:350.

41. Soifer SJ, Loitz RD, Roman C, et al. Leukotriene end organ antagonists increase pulmonary blood flow in fetal lambs. Am J Physiol 1985; 249:H570.

42. Cassin S. Role of prostaglandins, thromboxanes, and leukotrienes in the control of the pulmonary circulation in the fetus and newborn. Semin Perinatol 1987; 11:53.

43. Abman SH, Stenmark KR. Changes in lung eicosanoid content during normal and abnormal transition in perinatal lambs. Am J Physiol 1992; 262:L214.

44. Harder DR, Campbell WB, Roman RJ. Role of cytochrome P-450 enzymes and metabolites of arachidonic acid in the control of vascular tone. J Vasc Res 1995; 32:79.

45. Fuloria M, Smith TK, Aschner JL. Role of 5,6-epoxyeicosatrienoic acid in the regulation of newborn piglet pulmonary vascular tone. Am J Physiol Lung Cell Mol Physiol 2002; 283:L383.

46. Fuloria M, Eckman DM, Leach DA, et al. 20-hydroxyeicosatetraenoic acid is a vasoconstrictor in the newborn piglet pulmonary microcirculation. Am J Physiol Lung Cell Mol Physiol 2004; 287:L360.

47. Morrow JD, Roberts LJ. The isoprostanes: their role as an index of oxidant stress status in human pulmonary disease. Am J Respir Crit Care Med 2002; 166:S25.

48. Belik J, Jankov RP, Pan J, et al. Effect of 8-isoprostaglandin F2alpha on the newborn rat pulmonary arterial muscle and endothelium. J Appl Physiol 2003; 95:1979.

49. Gonzalez-Luis G, Perez-Vizcaino F, Garcia-Munoz F, et al. Age-related differences in vasoconstrictor responses to isoprostanes in piglet pulmonary and mesenteric vascular smooth muscle. Pediatr Res 2005; 57:845.

50. Michael JR, Markewitz BA. Endothelins and the lung. Am J Respir Crit Care Med 1996; 154:555.

51. Docherty C, MacLean MR. Development of endothelin receptors in perinatal rabbit pulmonary resistance arteries. Br J Pharmacol 1998; 124:1165.

52. Toga H, Ibe BO, Raj JU. In vitro responses of ovine intrapulmonary arteries and veins to endothelin-1. Am J Physiol 1992; 263:L15.

53. Wang Y, Coceani F. Isolated pulmonary resistance vessels from fetal lambs. Contractile behavior and responses to indomethacin and endothelin-1. Circ Res 1992; 71:320.

54. Cassin S, Kristova V, Davis T, et al. Tone-dependent responses to endothelin in the isolated perfused fetal sheep pulmonary circulation in situ. J Appl Physiol 1991; 70:1228.

55. Chatfield BA, McMurtry IF, Hall SL, et al. Hemodynamic effects of endothelin-1 on ovine fetal pulmonary circulation. Am J Physiol 1991; 261:R182.

56. D'Orleans-Juste P, Labonte J, Bkaily G, et al. Function of the endothelin(B) receptor in cardiovascular physiology and pathophysiology. Pharmacol Ther 2002; 95:221.

57. Ivy DD, Kinsella JP, Abman SH. Physiologic characterization of endothelin A and B receptor activity in the ovine fetal pulmonary circulation. J Clin Invest 1994; 93:2141.

58. Tod ML, Cassin S. Endothelin-1-induced pulmonary arterial dilatation is reduced by N omega-nitro-L-arginine in fetal lambs. J Appl Physiol 1992; 72:1730.

59. Ivy DD, Kinsella JP, Abman SH. Endothelin blockade augments pulmonary vasodilatation in the ovine fetus. J Appl Physiol 1996; 81:2481.

60. Jones OW, III, Abman SH. Systemic and pulmonary hemodynamic effects of big endothelin-1 and phosphoramidon in the ovine fetus. Am J Physiol 1994; 266:R929.

61. Wong J, Fineman JR, Heymann MA. The role of endothelin and endothelin receptor subtypes in regulation of fetal pulmonary vascular tone. Pediatr Res 1994; 35:664.

62. Ivy DD, Le Cras TD, Parker TA, et al. Developmental changes in endothelin expression and activity in the ovine fetal lung. Am J Physiol Lung Cell Mol Physiol 2000; 278:L785.

63. Parker TA, Roe G, Grover TR, et al. Rho kinase activation maintains high pulmonary vascular resistance in the ovine fetal lung. Am J Physiol Lung Cell Mol Physiol 2006; 291:L976.

64. McMurtry IF, Bauer NR, Fagan KA, et al. Hypoxia and Rho/Rho-kinase signaling. Lung development versus hypoxic pulmonary hypertension. Adv Exp Med Biol 2003; 543:127.

65. Printz MP, Skidgel RA, Friedman WF. Studies of pulmonary prostaglandin biosynthetic and catabolic enzymes as factors in ductus arteriosus patency and closure. Evidence for a shift in products with gestational age. Pediatr Res 1984; 18:19.

66. Pace-Asciak CR. Prostaglandin biosynthesis and catabolism in the developing fetal sheep lung. Prostaglandins 1977; 13:649.

67. Cassin S. Role of prostaglandins and thromboxanes in the control of the pulmonary circulation in the fetus and newborn. Semin Perinatol 1980; 4:101.

68. Cassin S, Winikor I, Tod M, et al. Effects of prostacyclin on the fetal pulmonary circulation. Pediatr Pharmacol (New York) 1981; 1:197.

69. Leffler CW, Hessler JR. Pulmonary and systemic vascular effects of exogenous prostaglandin I2 in fetal lambs. Eur J Pharmacol 1979; 54:37.

70. Leffler CW, Hessler JR. Perinatal pulmonary prostaglandin production. Am J Physiol 1981; 241:H756.

71. Leffler CW, Tyler TL, Cassin S. Effect of indomethacin on pulmonary vascular response to ventilation of fetal goats. Am J Physiol 1978; 234:H346.

72. North AJ, Star RA, Brannon TS, et al. Nitric oxide synthase type I and type III gene expression are developmentally regulated in rat lung. Am J Physiol 1994; 266:L635.

73. Halbower AC, Tuder RM, Franklin WA, et al. Maturation-related changes in endothelial nitric oxide synthase immunolocalization in developing ovine lung. Am J Physiol 1994; 267:L585.

74. Arrigoni FI, Hislop AA, Pollock JS, et al. Birth upregulates nitric oxide synthase activity in the porcine lung. Life Sci 2002; 70:1609.

75. Shaul PW, Afshar S, Gibson LL, et al. Developmental changes in nitric oxide synthase isoform expression and nitric oxide production in fetal baboon lung. Am J Physiol Lung Cell Mol Physiol 2002; 283:L1192.

76. Levy M, Maurey C, Chailley-Heu B, et al. Developmental changes in endothelial vasoactive and angiogenic growth factors in the human perinatal lung. Pediatr Res 2005; 57:248.

77. Parker TA, Le Cras TD, Kinsella JP, et al. Developmental changes in endothelial nitric oxide synthase expression and activity in ovine fetal lung. Am J Physiol Lung Cell Mol Physiol 2000; 278:L202.

78. Rairigh RL, Storme L, Parker TA, et al. Role of neuronal nitric oxide synthase in regulation of vascular and ductus arteriosus tone in the ovine fetus. Am J Physiol Lung Cell Mol Physiol 2000; 278:L105.

79. Abman SH, Chatfield BA, Hall SL, et al. Role of endothelium-derived relaxing factor during transition of pulmonary circulation at birth. Am J Physiol 1990; 259:H1921.

80. Skimming JW, DeMarco VG, Cassin S. The effects of nitric oxide inhalation on the pulmonary circulation of preterm lambs. Pediatr Res 1995; 37:35.

81. Shekerdemian LS, Ravn HB, Penny DJ. Intravenous sildenafil lowers pulmonary vascular resistance in a model of neonatal pulmonary hypertension. Am J Respir Crit Care Med 2002; 165:1098.

82. Weimann J, Ullrich R, Hromi J, et al. Sildenafil is a pulmonary vasodilator in awake lambs with acute pulmonary hypertension. Anesthesiology 2000; 92:1702.

83. Dukarm RC, Morin FC, III, Russell JA, et al. Pulmonary and systemic effects of the phosphodiesterase inhibitor dipyridamole in newborn lambs with persistent pulmonary hypertension. Pediatr Res 1998; 44:831.

84. Thebaud B, Saizou C, Farnoux C, et al. Dypyridamole, a cGMP phosphodiesterase inhibitor, transiently improves the response to inhaled nitric oxide in two newborns with congenital diaphragmatic hernia. Intensive Care Med 1999; 25:300.

85. Hanson KA, Ziegler JW, Rybalkin SD, et al. Chronic pulmonary hypertension increases fetal lung cGMP phosphodiesterase activity. Am J Physiol 1998; 275:L931.

86. Thebaud B, Petit T, De Lagausie P, et al. Altered guanylyl-cyclase activity in vitro of pulmonary arteries from fetal lambs with congenital diaphragmatic hernia. Am J Respir Cell Mol Biol 2002; 27:42.

87. Steinhorn RH, Gordon JB, Tod ML. Site-specific effect of guanosine 3',5'-cyclic monophosphate phosphodiesterase inhibition in isolated lamb lungs. Crit Care Med 2000; 28:490.

88. Thusu KG, Morin FC, III, Russell JA, et al. The cGMP phosphodiesterase inhibitor zaprinast enhances the effect of nitric oxide. Am J Respir Crit Care Med 1995; 152:1605.

89. Cassin S, Dawes GS, Mott JC, et al. The vascular resistance of the foetal and newly ventilated lung of the lamb. J Physiol 1964; 171:61.

90. Iwamoto HS, Teitel DF, Rudolph AM. Effects of lung distension and spontaneous fetal breathing on hemodynamics in sheep. Pediatr Res 1993; 33:639.

91. Reid DL, Thornburg KL. Pulmonary pressure-flow relationships in the fetal lamb during in utero ventilation. J Appl Physiol 1990; 69:1630.

92. Allen K, Haworth SG. Human postnatal pulmonary arterial remodeling. Ultrastructural studies of smooth muscle cell and connective tissue maturation. Lab Invest 1988; 59:702.

93. Haworth SG, Hall SM, Chew M, et al. Thinning of fetal pulmonary arterial wall and postnatal remodelling: ultrastructural studies on the respiratory unit arteries of the pig. Virchows Arch A Pathol Anat Histopathol 1987; 411:161.

94. Abman SH. Abnormal vasoreactivity in the pathophysiology of persistent pulmonary hypertension of the newborn. Pediatr Rev 1999; 20:e103.

95. Kelly DA, Hislop AA, Hall SM, et al. Correlation of pulmonary arterial smooth muscle structure and reactivity during adaptation to extrauterine life. J Vasc Res 2002; 39:30.

96. Hammerman C, Scarpelli EM. Indomethacin and the cardiopulmonary adaptations of transition. Pediatr Res 1984; 18:842.

97. Davidson D. Pulmonary hemodynamics at birth: effect of acute cyclooxygenase inhibition in lambs. J Appl Physiol 1988; 64:1676.

98. Cornfield DN, Chatfield BA, McQueston JA, et al. Effects of birth-related stimuli on L-arginine-dependent pulmonary vasodilation in ovine fetus. Am J Physiol 1992; 262:H1474.

99. Velvis H, Moore P, Heymann MA. Prostaglandin inhibition prevents the fall in pulmonary vascular resistance as a result of rhythmic distension of the lungs in fetal lambs. Pediatr Res 1991; 30:62.

100. Leffler CW, Hessler JR, Green RS. Mechanism of stimulation of pulmonary prostacyclin synthesis at birth. Prostaglandins 1984; 28:877.

101. Brannon TS, North AJ, Wells LB, et al. Prostacyclin synthesis in ovine pulmonary artery is developmentally regulated by changes in cyclooxygenase-1 gene expression. J Clin Invest 1994; 93:2230.

102. Levin DL. Effects of inhibition of prostaglandin synthesis on fetal development, oxygenation, and the fetal circulation. Semin Perinatol 1980; 4:35.

103. Witter FR, Niebyl JR. Inhibition of arachidonic acid metabolism in the perinatal period: pharmacology, clinical application, and potential adverse effects. Semin Perinatol 1986; 10:316.

104. Kawai N, Bloch DB, Filippov G, et al. Constitutive endothelial nitric oxide synthase gene expression is regulated during lung development. Am J Physiol 1995; 268:L589.

105. Villamor E, Le Cras TD, Horan MP, et al. Chronic intrauterine pulmonary hypertension impairs endothelial nitric oxide synthase in the ovine fetus. Am J Physiol 1997; 272:L1013.

106. Sheffield M, Mabry S, Thibeault DW, et al. Pulmonary nitric oxide synthases and nitrotyrosine: findings during lung development and in chronic lung disease of prematurity. Pediatrics 2006; 118:1056.

107. Abman SH, Chatfield BA, Rodman DM, et al. Maturational changes in endothelium-derived relaxing factor activity of ovine pulmonary arteries in vitro. Am J Physiol 1991; 260:L280.

108. Shaul PW, Farrar MA, Magness RR. Pulmonary endothelial nitric oxide production is developmentally regulated in the fetus and newborn. Am J Physiol 1993; 265:H1056.

109. Fineman JR, Wong J, Morin FC, III, et al. Chronic nitric oxide inhibition in utero produces persistent pulmonary hypertension in newborn lambs. J Clin Invest 1994; 93:2675.

110. Miller AA, Hislop AA, Vallance PJ, et al. Deletion of the eNOS gene has a greater impact on the pulmonary circulation of male than female mice. Am J Physiol Lung Cell Mol Physiol 2005; 289:L299.

111. Shaul PW, Yuhanna IS, German Z, et al. Pulmonary endothelial NO synthase gene expression is decreased in fetal lambs with pulmonary hypertension. Am J Physiol 1997; 272:L1005.

112. Black SM, Fineman JR, Steinhorn RH, et al. Increased endothelial NOS in lambs with increased pulmonary blood flow and pulmonary hypertension. Am J Physiol 1998; 275:H1643.

113. Ivy DD, Le Cras TD, Horan MP, et al. Increased lung preproET-1 and decreased ETB-receptor gene expression in fetal pulmonary hypertension. Am J Physiol 1998; 274:L535.

114. Black SM, Bekker JM, Johengen MJ, et al. Altered regulation of the ET-1 cascade in lambs with increased pulmonary blood flow and pulmonary hypertension. Pediatr Res 2000; 47:97.

115. Kumar P, Kazzi NJ, Shankaran S. Plasma immunoreactive endothelin-1 concentrations in infants with persistent pulmonary hypertension of the newborn. Am J Perinatol 1996; 13:335.

116. Rosenberg AA, Kennaugh J, Koppenhafer SL, et al. Elevated immunoreactive endothelin-1 levels in newborn infants with persistent pulmonary hypertension. J Pediatr 1993; 123:109.

117. Winters JW, Wong J, Van DD, et al. Endothelin receptor blockade does not alter the increase in pulmonary blood flow due to oxygen ventilation in fetal lambs. Pediatr Res 1996; 40:152.

118. Dobyns EL, Wescott JY, Kennaugh JM, et al. Eicosanoids decrease with successful extracorporeal membrane oxygenation therapy in neonatal pulmonary hypertension. Am J Respir Crit Care Med 1994; 149:873.

119. Ford WD, James MJ, Walsh JA. Congenital diaphragmatic hernia: association between pulmonary vascular resistance and plasma thromboxane concentrations. Arch Dis Child 1984; 59:143.

120. Stenmark KR, James SL, Voelkel NF, et al. Leukotriene C4 and D4 in neonates with hypoxemia and pulmonary hypertension. N Engl J Med 1983; 309:77.
121. Fike CD, Hansen TN. Hypoxic vasoconstriction increases with postnatal age in lungs from newborn rabbits. Circ Res 1987; 60:297.
122. Gordon JB, Hortop J, Hakim TS. Developmental effects of hypoxia and indomethacin on distribution of vascular resistances in lamb lungs. Pediatr Res 1989; 26:325.
123. Owen-Thomas JB, Reeves JT. Hypoxia and pulmonary arterial pressure in the rabbit. J Physiol 1969; 201:665.
124. Rendas A, Branthwaite M, Lennox S, et al. Response of the pulmonary circulation to acute hypoxia in the growing pig. J Appl Physiol 1982; 52:811.
125. Rudolph AM, Yuan S. Response of the pulmonary vasculature to hypoxia and H+ ion concentration changes. J Clin Invest 1966; 45:399.
126. Lyrene RK, Welch KA, Godoy G, et al. Alkalosis attenuates hypoxic pulmonary vasoconstriction in neonatal lambs. Pediatr Res 1985; 19:1268.
127. Morin FC, III. Hyperventilation, alkalosis, prostaglandins, and pulmonary circulation of the newborn. J Appl Physiol 1986; 61:2088.
128. Fike CD, Hansen TN. The effect of alkalosis on hypoxia-induced pulmonary vasoconstriction in lungs of newborn rabbits. Pediatr Res 1989; 25:383.
129. Farrukh IS, Gurtner GH, Terry PB, et al. Effect of pH on pulmonary vascular tone, reactivity, and arachidonate metabolism. J Appl Physiol 1989; 67:445.
130. Gordon JB, Martinez FR, Keller PA, et al. Differing effects of acute and prolonged alkalosis on hypoxic pulmonary vasoconstriction. Am Rev Respir Dis 1993; 148:1651.
131. Redding GJ, Gibson RL, Davis CB, et al. Effects of respiratory alkalosis on thromboxane-induced pulmonary hypertension in piglets. Pediatr Res 1988; 24:558.
132. Hammerman C, Aramburo MJ. Effects of hyperventilation on prostacyclin formation and on pulmonary vasodilation after group B beta-hemolytic streptococci-induced pulmonary hypertension. Pediatr Res 1991; 29:282.
133. Schreiber MD, Heymann MA, Soifer SJ. Increased arterial pH, not decreased PaCO$_2$, attenuates hypoxia-induced pulmonary vasoconstriction in newborn lambs. Pediatr Res 1986; 20:113.
134. Gersony WM. Neonatal pulmonary hypertension: pathophysiology, classification, and etiology. Clin Perinatol 1984; 11:517.
135. Bland RD, Albertine KH, Carlton DP, et al. Chronic lung injury in preterm lambs: abnormalities of the pulmonary circulation and lung fluid balance. Pediatr Res 2000; 48:64.
136. Mulrooney N, Champion Z, Moss TJ, et al. Surfactant and physiologic responses of preterm lambs to continuous positive airway pressure. Am J Respir Crit Care Med 2005; 171:488.
137. Murphy JD, Rabinovitch M, Goldstein JD, et al. The structural basis of persistent pulmonary hypertension of the newborn infant. J Pediatr 1981; 98:962.
138. Murphy JD, Vawter GF, Reid LM. Pulmonary vascular disease in fatal meconium aspiration. J Pediatr 1984; 104:758.
139. Abman SH, Shanley PF, Accurso FJ. Failure of postnatal adaptation of the pulmonary circulation after chronic intrauterine pulmonary hypertension in fetal lambs. J Clin Invest 1989; 83:1849.
140. Belik J, Keeley FW, Baldwin F, et al. Pulmonary hypertension and vascular remodeling in fetal sheep. Am J Physiol 1994; 266:H2303.
141. Wild LM, Nickerson PA, Morin FC, III. Ligating the ductus arteriosus before birth remodels the pulmonary vasculature of the lamb. Pediatr Res 1989; 25:251.
142. Reddy VM, Meyrick B, Wong J, et al. In utero placement of aortopulmonary shunts. A model of postnatal pulmonary hypertension with increased pulmonary blood flow in lambs. Circulation 1995; 92:606.
143. Jouannic JM, Roussin R, Hislop AA, et al. Systemic arteriovenous fistula leads to pulmonary artery remodeling and abnormal vasoreactivity in the fetal lamb. Am J Physiol Lung Cell Mol Physiol 2003; 285:L701.
144. Suzuki K, Hooper SB, Cock ML, et al. Effect of lung hypoplasia on birth-related changes in the pulmonary circulation in sheep. Pediatr Res 2005; 57:530.
145. Levin DL. Morphologic analysis of the pulmonary vascular bed in congenital left-sided diaphragmatic hernia. J Pediatr 1978; 92:805.
146. Belik J, Halayko AJ, Rao K, et al. Fetal ductus arteriosus ligation. Pulmonary vascular smooth muscle biochemical and mechanical changes. Circ Res 1993; 72:588.
147. Kelly DA, Hislop AA, Hall SM, et al. Relationship between structural remodeling and reactivity in pulmonary resistance arteries from hypertensive piglets. Pediatr Res 2005; 58:525.
148. Belik J, Majumdar R, Fabris VE, et al. Myosin light chain phosphatase and kinase abnormalities in fetal sheep pulmonary hypertension. Pediatr Res 1998; 43:57.
149. McQueston JA, Kinsella JP, Ivy DD, et al. Chronic pulmonary hypertension in utero impairs endothelium-dependent vasodilation. Am J Physiol 1995; 268:H288.
150. Reddy VM, Wong J, Liddicoat JR, et al. Altered endothelium-dependent responses in lambs with pulmonary hypertension and increased pulmonary blood flow. Am J Physiol 1996; 271:H562.
151. Wojciak-Stothard B, Haworth SG. Perinatal changes in pulmonary vascular endothelial function. Pharmacol Ther 2006; 109:78.
152. Boels PJ, Deutsch J, Gao B, et al. Perinatal development influences mechanisms of bradykinin-induced relaxations in pulmonary resistance and conduit arteries differently. Cardiovasc Res 2001; 51:140.

153. Black SM, Bekker JM, McMullan DM, et al. Alterations in nitric oxide production in 8-week-old lambs with increased pulmonary blood flow. Pediatr Res 2002; 52:233.

154. Fike CD, Kaplowitz MR. Effect of chronic hypoxia on pulmonary vascular pressures in isolated lungs of newborn pigs. J Appl Physiol 1994; 77:2853.

155. Bland RD, Ling CY, Albertine KH, et al. Pulmonary vascular dysfunction in preterm lambs with chronic lung disease. Am J Physiol Lung Cell Mol Physiol 2003; 285:L76.

156. Fike CD, Aschner JL, Zhang Y, et al. Impaired NO signaling in small pulmonary arteries of chronically hypoxic newborn piglets. Am J Physiol Lung Cell Mol Physiol 2004; 286:L1244.

157. Walsh-Sukys MC, Bauer RE, Cornell DJ, et al. Severe respiratory failure in neonates: mortality and morbidity rates and neurodevelopmental outcomes. J Pediatr 1994; 125:104.

158. Angus DC, Linde-Zwirble WT, Clermont G, et al. Epidemiology of neonatal respiratory failure in the United States: projections from California and New York. Am J Respir Crit Care Med 2001; 164:1154.

159. Pearson DL, Dawling S, Walsh WF, et al. Neonatal pulmonary hypertension–urea-cycle intermediates, nitric oxide production, and carbamoyl-phosphate synthetase function. N Engl J Med 2001; 344:1832.

160. Walsh-Sukys MC, Tyson JE, Wright LL, et al. Persistent pulmonary hypertension of the newborn in the era before nitric oxide: practice variation and outcomes. Pediatrics 2000; 105:14.

161. Fox WW, Gewitz MH, Dinwiddie R, et al. Pulmonary hypertension in the perinatal aspiration syndromes. Pediatrics 1977; 59:205.

162. Konduri GG. New approaches for persistent pulmonary hypertension of newborn. Clin Perinatol 2004; 31:591.

163. Steinhorn RH, Fineman JR. The pathophysiology of pulmonary hypertension in congenital heart disease. Artif Organs 1999; 23:970.

164. Barr FE, Beverley H, VanHook K, et al. Effect of cardiopulmonary bypass on urea cycle intermediates and nitric oxide levels after congenital heart surgery. J Pediatr 2003; 142:26.

165. Alano MA, Ngougmna E, Ostrea EM, Jr., et al. Analysis of nonsteroidal antiinflammatory drugs in meconium and its relation to persistent pulmonary hypertension of the newborn. Pediatrics 2001; 107:519.

166. Chambers CD, Hernandez-Diaz S, Van Marter LJ, et al. Selective serotonin-reuptake inhibitors and risk of persistent pulmonary hypertension of the newborn. N Engl J Med 2006; 354:579.

167. Gournay V, Savagner C, Thiriez G, et al. Pulmonary hypertension after ibuprofen prophylaxis in very preterm infants. Lancet 2002; 359:1486.

168. Lakshminrusimha S, Russell JA, Steinhorn RH, et al. Pulmonary arterial contractility in neonatal lambs increases with 100% oxygen resuscitation. Pediatr Res 2006; 59:137.

169. Lakshminrusimha S, Russell JA, Wedgwood S, et al. Superoxide dismutase improves oxygenation and reduces oxidation in neonatal pulmonary hypertension. Am J Respir Crit Care Med 2006; 174:1370.

170. Vento M, Asensi M, Sastre J, et al. Resuscitation with room air instead of 100% oxygen prevents oxidative stress in moderately asphyxiated term neonates. Pediatrics 2001; 107:642.

171. Mourani PM, Ivy DD, Gao D, et al. Pulmonary vascular effects of inhaled nitric oxide and oxygen tension in bronchopulmonary dysplasia. Am J Respir Crit Care Med 2004; 170:1006.

172. Wung JT, James LS, Kilchevsky E, et al. Management of infants with severe respiratory failure and persistence of the fetal circulation, without hyperventilation. Pediatrics 1985; 76:488.

173. Peckham GJ, Fox WW. Physiologic factors affecting pulmonary artery pressure in infants with persistent pulmonary hypertension. J Pediatr 1978; 93:1005.

174. Drummond WH, Gregory GA, Heymann MA, et al. The independent effects of hyperventilation, tolazoline, and dopamine on infants with persistent pulmonary hypertension. J Pediatr 1981; 98:603.

175. Heymann MA. Control of the pulmonary circulation in the perinatal period. J Dev Physiol 1984; 6:281.

176. Morray JP, Lynn AM, Mansfield PB. Effect of pH and PCO_2 on pulmonary and systemic hemodynamics after surgery in children with congenital heart disease and pulmonary hypertension. J Pediatr 1988; 113:474.

177. Dworetz AR, Moya FR, Sabo B, et al. Survival of infants with persistent pulmonary hypertension without extracorporeal membrane oxygenation. Pediatrics 1989; 84:1.

178. Bifano EM, Pfannenstiel A. Duration of hyperventilation and outcome in infants with persistent pulmonary hypertension. Pediatrics 1988; 81:657.

179. Hendricks-Munoz KD, Walton JP. Hearing loss in infants with persistent fetal circulation. Pediatrics 1988; 81:650.

180. Stevenson DK, Kasting DS, Darnall RA, Jr., et al. Refractory hypoxemia associated with neonatal pulmonary disease: the use and limitations of tolazoline. J Pediatr 1979; 95:595.

181. Parida SK, Baker S, Kuhn R, et al. Endotracheal tolazoline administration in neonates with persistent pulmonary hypertension. J Perinatol 1997; 17:461.

182. Wu TJ, Teng RJ, Tsou KI. Persistent pulmonary hypertension of the newborn treated with magnesium sulfate in premature neonates. Pediatrics 1995; 96:472.

183. Weinberger B, Weiss K, Heck DE, et al. Pharmacologic therapy of persistent pulmonary hypertension of the newborn. Pharmacol Ther 2001; 89:67.

184. Abu-Osba YK, Galal O, Manasra K, et al. Treatment of severe persistent pulmonary hypertension of the newborn with magnesium sulphate. Arch Dis Child 1992; 67:31.

185. Patole SK, Finer NN. Experimental and clinical effects of magnesium infusion in the treatment of neonatal pulmonary hypertension. Magnes Res 1995; 8:373.

186. Inhaled nitric oxide and hypoxic respiratory failure in infants with congenital diaphragmatic hernia. The Neonatal Inhaled Nitric Oxide Study Group (NINOS). Pediatrics 1997; 99:838.

187. Inhaled nitric oxide in term and near-term infants: neurodevelopmental follow-up of the neonatal inhaled nitric oxide study group (NINOS). J Pediatr 2000; 136:611.

188. Clark RH, Kueser TJ, Walker MW, et al. Low-dose nitric oxide therapy for persistent pulmonary hypertension of the newborn. Clinical Inhaled Nitric Oxide Research Group. N Engl J Med 2000; 342:469.

189. Wessel DL, Adatia I, Van Marter LJ, et al. Improved oxygenation in a randomized trial of inhaled nitric oxide for persistent pulmonary hypertension of the newborn. Pediatrics 1997; 100:E7.

190. Kinsella JP, Abman SH. Inhaled nitric oxide and high frequency oscillatory ventilation in persistent pulmonary hypertension of the newborn. Eur J Pediatr. 1998; 157(Suppl 1):S28.

191. Roberts JD, Jr., Fineman JR, Morin FC, III, et al. Inhaled nitric oxide and persistent pulmonary hypertension of the newborn. The Inhaled Nitric Oxide Study Group. N Engl J Med 1997; 336:605.

192. Barefield ES, Karle VA, Phillips JB, III, et al. Inhaled nitric oxide in term infants with hypoxemic respiratory failure. J Pediatr 1996; 129:279.

193. Christou H, Van Marter LJ, Wessel DL, et al. Inhaled nitric oxide reduces the need for extracorporeal membrane oxygenation in infants with persistent pulmonary hypertension of the newborn. Crit Care Med 2000; 28:3722.

194. Davidson D, Barefield ES, Kattwinkel J, et al. Inhaled nitric oxide for the early treatment of persistent pulmonary hypertension of the term newborn: a randomized, double-masked, placebo-controlled, dose-response, multicenter study. The I-NO/PPHN Study Group. Pediatrics 1998; 101:325.

195. Finer NN, Barrington KJ. Nitric oxide for respiratory failure in infants born at or near term. Cochrane Database Syst 2006; Rev. CD000399.

196. Lipkin PH, Davidson D, Spivak L, et al. Neurodevelopmental and medical outcomes of persistent pulmonary hypertension in term newborns treated with nitric oxide. J Pediatr 2002; 140:306.

197. Schreiber MD, Gin-Mestan K, Marks JD, et al. Inhaled nitric oxide in premature infants with the respiratory distress syndrome. N Engl J Med 2003; 349:2099.

198. Van Meurs KP, Wright LL, Ehrenkranz RA, et al. Inhaled nitric oxide for premature infants with severe respiratory failure. N Engl J Med 2005; 353:13.

199. Kinsella JP, Cutter GR, Walsh WF, et al. Early inhaled nitric oxide therapy in premature newborns with respiratory failure. N Engl J Med 2006; 355:354.

200. Ballard RA, Truog WE, Cnaan A, et al. Inhaled nitric oxide in preterm infants undergoing mechanical ventilation. N Engl J Med 2006; 355:343.

201. Kinsella JP, Parker TA, Ivy DD, et al. Noninvasive delivery of inhaled nitric oxide therapy for late pulmonary hypertension in newborn infants with congenital diaphragmatic hernia. J Pediatr 2003; 142:397.

202. Banks BA, Seri I, Ischiropoulos H, et al. Changes in oxygenation with inhaled nitric oxide in severe bronchopulmonary dysplasia. Pediatrics 1999; 103:610.

203. Channick RN, Newhart JW, Johnson FW, et al. Pulsed delivery of inhaled nitric oxide to patients with primary pulmonary hypertension: an ambulatory delivery system and initial clinical tests. Chest 1996; 109:1545.

204. Day RW, Hawkins JA, McGough EC, et al. Randomized controlled study of inhaled nitric oxide after operation for congenital heart disease. Ann Thorac Surg 2000; 69:1907.

205. Dobyns EL, Cornfield DN, Anas NG, et al. Multicenter randomized controlled trial of the effects of inhaled nitric oxide therapy on gas exchange in children with acute hypoxemic respiratory failure. J Pediatr 1999; 134:406.

206. Kinsella JP, Abman SH. Inhaled nitric oxide therapy in children. Paediatr Respir Rev 2005; 6:190.

207. Miller OI, Tang SF, Keech A, et al. Inhaled nitric oxide and prevention of pulmonary hypertension after congenital heart surgery: a randomised double-blind study. Lancet 2000; 356:1464.

208. Weiner DL, Hibberd PL, Betit P, et al. Preliminary assessment of inhaled nitric oxide for acute vaso-occlusive crisis in pediatric patients with sickle cell disease. JAMA 2003; 289:1136.

209. Konduri GG, Solimano A, Sokol GM, et al. A randomized trial of early versus standard inhaled nitric oxide therapy in term and near-term newborn infants with hypoxic respiratory failure. Pediatrics 2004; 113:559.

210. Early compared with delayed inhaled nitric oxide in moderately hypoxaemic neonates with respiratory failure: a randomised controlled trial. The Franco-Belgium Collaborative NO Trial Group. Lancet 1999; 354:1066.

211. Rossaint R, Falke KJ, Lopez F, et al. Inhaled nitric oxide for the adult respiratory distress syndrome. N Engl J Med 1993; 328:399.

212. Inhaled nitric oxide in full-term and nearly full-term infants with hypoxic respiratory failure. The Neonatal Inhaled Nitric Oxide Study Group. N Engl J Med 1997; 336:597.

213. Kinsella JP, Truog WE, Walsh WF, et al. Randomized, multicenter trial of inhaled nitric oxide and high-frequency oscillatory ventilation in severe, persistent pulmonary hypertension of the newborn. J Pediatr 1997; 131:55.

214. Karamanoukian HL, Glick PL, Zayek M, et al. Inhaled nitric oxide in congenital hypoplasia of the lungs due to diaphragmatic hernia or oligohydramnios. Pediatrics 1994; 94:715.

215. Finer NN, Etches PC, Kamstra B, et al. Inhaled nitric oxide in infants referred for extracorporeal membrane oxygenation: dose response. J Pediatr 1994; 124:302.

216. Robbins CG, Davis JM, Merritt TA, et al. Combined effects of nitric oxide and hyperoxia on surfactant function and pulmonary inflammation. Am J Physiol 1995; 269:L545.

217. Beckman JS, Beckman TW, Chen J, et al. Apparent hydroxyl radical production by peroxynitrite: implications for endothelial injury from nitric oxide and superoxide. Proc Natl Acad Sci USA 1990; 87:1620.

218. Guthrie SO, Walsh WF, Auten K, et al. Initial dosing of inhaled nitric oxide in infants with hypoxic respiratory failure. J Perinatol 2004; 24:290.

219. Goldman AP, Tasker RC, Haworth SG, et al. Four patterns of response to inhaled nitric oxide for persistent pulmonary hypertension of the newborn. Pediatrics 1996; 98:706.

220. Lotze A, Mitchell BR, Bulas DI, et al. Multicenter study of surfactant (beractant) use in the treatment of term infants with severe respiratory failure. Survanta in Term Infants Study Group. J Pediatr 1998; 132:40.

221. Aly H, Sahni R, Wung JT. Weaning strategy with inhaled nitric oxide treatment in persistent pulmonary hypertension of the newborn. Arch Dis Child Fetal Neonatal Ed 1997; 76:F118.

222. Cueto E, Lopez-Herce J, Sanchez A, et al. Life-threatening effects of discontinuing inhaled nitric oxide in children. Acta Paediatr 1997; 86:1337.

223. Davidson D, Barefield ES, Kattwinkel J, et al. Safety of withdrawing inhaled nitric oxide therapy in persistent pulmonary hypertension of the newborn. Pediatrics 1999; 104:231.

224. Ivy DD, Kinsella JP, Ziegler JW, et al. Dipyridamole attenuates rebound pulmonary hypertension after inhaled nitric oxide withdrawal in postoperative congenital heart disease. J Thorac Cardiovasc Surg 1998; 115:875.

225. Kinsella JP, Abman SH. Recent developments in the pathophysiology and treatment of persistent pulmonary hypertension of the newborn. J Pediatr 1995; 126:853.

226. Black SM, Heidersbach RS, McMullan DM, et al. Inhaled nitric oxide inhibits NOS activity in lambs: potential mechanism for rebound pulmonary hypertension. Am J Physiol 1999; 277:H1849.

227. Buga GM, Griscavage JM, Rogers NE, et al. Negative feedback regulation of endothelial cell function by nitric oxide. Circ Res 1993; 73:808.

228. McMullan DM, Bekker JM, Johengen MJ, et al. Inhaled nitric oxide-induced rebound pulmonary hypertension: role for endothelin-1. Am J Physiol Heart Circ Physiol 2001; 280:H777.

229. Wedgwood S, McMullan DM, Bekker JM, et al. Role for endothelin-1-induced superoxide and peroxynitrite production in rebound pulmonary hypertension associated with inhaled nitric oxide therapy. Circ Res 2001; 89:357.

230. Sokol GM, Fineberg NS, Wright LL, et al. Changes in arterial oxygen tension when weaning neonates from inhaled nitric oxide. Pediatr Pulmonol 2001; 32:14.

231. Gianetti J, Bevilacqua S, De CR. Inhaled nitric oxide: more than a selective pulmonary vasodilator. Eur J Clin Invest 2002; 32:628.

232. Guidot DM, Repine MJ, Hybertson BM, et al. Inhaled nitric oxide prevents neutrophil-mediated, oxygen radical-dependent leak in isolated rat lungs. Am J Physiol 1995; 269:L2.

233. Kinsella JP, Parker TA, Galan H, et al. Effects of inhaled nitric oxide on pulmonary edema and lung neutrophil accumulation in severe experimental hyaline membrane disease. Pediatr Res 1997; 41:457.

234. Williams LJ, Shaffer TH, Greenspan JS. Inhaled nitric oxide therapy in the near-term or term neonate with hypoxic respiratory failure. Neonatal Netw 2004; 23:5.

235. Abman SH, Wolfe RR, Accurso FJ, et al. Pulmonary vascular response to oxygen in infants with severe bronchopulmonary dysplasia. Pediatrics 1985; 75:80.

236. American Academy of Pediatrics. Committee on Fetus and Newborn. Use of inhaled nitric oxide. Pediatrics 2000; 106:344.

237. Ellington M, Jr., O'Reilly D, Allred EN, et al. Child health status, neurodevelopmental outcome, and parental satisfaction in a randomized, controlled trial of nitric oxide for persistent pulmonary hypertension of the newborn. Pediatrics 2001; 107:1351.

238. Rosenberg AA, Kennaugh JM, Moreland SG, et al. Longitudinal follow-up of a cohort of newborn infants treated with inhaled nitric oxide for persistent pulmonary hypertension. J Pediatr 1997; 131:70.

239. Rosenberg AA. Outcome in term infants treated with inhaled nitric oxide. J Pediatr 2002; 140:284.

240. Hallman M, Kankaanpaa K. Evidence of surfactant deficiency in persistence of the fetal circulation. Eur J Pediatr 1980; 134:129.

241. Lotze A, Whitsett JA, Kammerman LA, et al. Surfactant protein A concentrations in tracheal aspirate fluid from infants requiring extracorporeal membrane oxygenation. J Pediatr 1990; 116:435.

242. Auten RL, Notter RH, Kendig JW, et al. Surfactant treatment of full-term newborns with respiratory failure. Pediatrics 1991; 87:101.

243. Lotze A, Knight GR, Martin GR, et al. Improved pulmonary outcome after exogenous surfactant therapy for respiratory failure in term infants requiring extracorporeal membrane oxygenation. J Pediatr 1993; 122:261.

244. Moya MP, Gow AJ, Califf RM, et al. Inhaled ethyl nitrite gas for persistent pulmonary hypertension of the newborn. Lancet 2002; 360:141.

245. Fink TL, Francis SH, Beasley A, et al. Expression of an active, monomeric catalytic domain of the cGMP-binding cGMP-specific phosphodiesterase (PDE5). J Biol Chem 1999; 274:34613.

246. Wharton J, Strange JW, Moller GM, et al. Antiproliferative effects of phosphodiesterase type 5 inhibition in human pulmonary artery cells. Am J Respir Crit Care Med 2005; 172:105.

247. Black SM, Sanchez LS, Mata-Greenwood E, et al. sGC and PDE5 are elevated in lambs with increased pulmonary blood flow and pulmonary hypertension. Am J Physiol Lung Cell Mol Physiol 2001; 281:L1051.

248. Buysse C, Fonteyne C, Dessy H, et al. The use of dipyridamole to wean from inhaled nitric oxide in congenital diaphragmatic hernia. J Pediatr Surg 2001; 36:1864.

249. Kinsella JP, Torielli F, Ziegler JW, et al. Dipyridamole augmentation of response to nitric oxide. Lancet 1995; 346:647.

250. Binns-Loveman KM, Kaplowitz MR, Fike CD. Sildenafil and an early stage of chronic hypoxia-induced pulmonary hypertension in newborn piglets. Pediatr Pulmonol 2005; 40:72.

251. Sastry BK, Narasimhan C, Reddy NK, et al. Clinical efficacy of sildenafil in primary pulmonary hypertension: a randomized, placebo-controlled, double-blind, crossover study. J Am Coll Cardiol 2004; 43:1149.

252. Michelakis E, Tymchak W, Lien D, et al. Oral sildenafil is an effective and specific pulmonary vasodilator in patients with pulmonary arterial hypertension: comparison with inhaled nitric oxide. Circulation 2002; 105:2398.

253. Lepore JJ, Maroo A, Pereira NL, et al. Effect of sildenafil on the acute pulmonary vasodilator response to inhaled nitric oxide in adults with primary pulmonary hypertension. Am J Cardiol 2002; 90:677.

254. Ghofrani HA, Wiedemann R, Rose F, et al. Sildenafil for treatment of lung fibrosis and pulmonary hypertension: a randomised controlled trial. Lancet 2002; 360:895.

255. Galie N, Ghofrani HA, Torbicki A, et al. Sildenafil citrate therapy for pulmonary arterial hypertension. N Engl J Med 2005; 353:2148.

256. Atz AM, Wessel DL. Sildenafil ameliorates effects of inhaled nitric oxide withdrawal. Anesthesiology 1999; 91:307.

257. Juliana AE, Abbad FC. Severe persistent pulmonary hypertension of the newborn in a setting where limited resources exclude the use of inhaled nitric oxide: successful treatment with sildenafil. Eur J Pediatr 2005; 164:626.

258. Baquero H, Soliz A, Neira F, et al. Oral sildenafil in infants with persistent pulmonary hypertension of the newborn: a pilot randomized blinded study. Pediatrics 2006; 117:1077.

259. Travadi JN, Patole SK. Phosphodiesterase inhibitors for persistent pulmonary hypertension of the newborn: a review. Pediatr Pulmonol 2003; 36:529.

260. Marsh CS, Marden B, Newsom R. Severe retinopathy of prematurity (ROP) in a premature baby treated with sildenafil acetate (Viagra) for pulmonary hypertension. Br J Ophthalmol 2004; 88:306.

261. Pierce CM, Petros AJ, Fielder AR. No evidence for severe retinopathy of prematurity following sildenafil. Br J Ophthalmol 2005; 89:250.

262. Van Staveren WC, Steinbusch HW, Markerink-Van IM, et al. mRNA expression patterns of the cGMP-hydrolyzing phosphodiesterases types 2, 5, and 9 during development of the rat brain. J Comp Neurol 2003; 467:566.

263. Zhang L, Zhang RL, Wang Y, et al. Functional recovery in aged and young rats after embolic stroke: treatment with a phosphodiesterase type 5 inhibitor. Stroke 2005; 36:847.

264. Namachivayam P, Theilen U, Butt WW, et al. Sildenafil prevents rebound pulmonary hypertension after withdrawal of nitric oxide in children. Am J Respir Crit Care Med 2006; 174:1042.

265. Harrison DG. Cellular and molecular mechanisms of endothelial cell dysfunction. J Clin Invest 1997; 100:2153.

266. Mitani Y, Maruyama K, Sakurai M. Prolonged administration of L-arginine ameliorates chronic pulmonary hypertension and pulmonary vascular remodeling in rats. Circulation 1997; 96:689.

267. Fike CD, Kaplowitz MR, Rehorst-Paea LA, et al. L-Arginine increases nitric oxide production in isolated lungs of chronically hypoxic newborn pigs. J Appl Physiol 2000; 88:1797.

268. Mehta S, Stewart DJ, Langleben D, et al. Short-term pulmonary vasodilatation with L-arginine in pulmonary hypertension. Circulation 1995; 92:1539.

269. Nagaya N, Uematsu M, Oya H, et al. Short-term oral administration of L-arginine improves hemodynamics and exercise capacity in patients with precapillary pulmonary hypertension. Am J Respir Crit Care Med 2001; 163:887.

270. Schulze-Neick I, Penny DJ, Rigby ML, et al. L-arginine and substance P reverse the pulmonary endothelial dysfunction caused by congenital heart surgery. Circulation 1999; 100:749.

271. McCaffrey MJ, Bose CL, Reiter PD, et al. Effect of L-arginine infusion on infants with persistent pulmonary hypertension of the newborn. Biol Neonate 1995; 67:240.

272. Morris CR, Morris SM Jr., Hagar W, et al. Arginine therapy: a new treatment for pulmonary hypertension in sickle cell disease? Am J Respir Crit Care Med 2003; 168:63.

273. Gorenflo M, Zheng C, Werle E, et al. Plasma levels of asymmetrical dimethyl-L-arginine in patients with congenital heart disease and pulmonary hypertension. J Cardiovasc Pharmacol 2001; 37:489.

274. Bulau P, Zakrzewicz D, Kitowska K, et al. Analysis of methylarginine metabolism in the cardiovascular system identifies the lung as a major source of ADMA. Am J Physiol Lung Cell Mol Physiol 2007; 292:L18.

275. Dweik RA. The lung in the balance: arginine, methylated arginines, and nitric oxide. Am J Physiol Lung Cell Mol Physiol 2007; 292:L15.

276. Raiha NC, Suihkonen J. Factors influencing the development of urea-synthesizing enzymes in rat liver. Biochem J 1968; 107:793.

277. Raiha NC, Suihkonen J. Development of urea-synthesizing enzymes in human liver. Acta Paediatr Scand 1968; 57:121.

278. Mukarram Ali BM, Habibullah CM, Swamy M, et al. Studies on urea cycle enzyme levels in the human fetal liver at different gestational ages. Pediatr Res 1992; 31:143.

279. Pearson DL, Dawling S, Walsh WF, et al. Neonatal pulmonary hypertension–urea-cycle intermediates, nitric oxide production, and carbamoyl-phosphate synthetase function. N Engl J Med 2001; 344:1832.

280. Summar M. Current strategies for the management of neonatal urea cycle disorders. J Pediatr 2001; 138:S30.

281. Kuhn KP, Harris PA, Cunningham GR, et al. Oral citrulline effectively elevates plasma arginine levels for 24 hours in normal volunteers. Circulation 2002; 106:II–339.

282. Hartman WJ, Torre PM, Prior RL. Dietary citrulline but not ornithine counteracts dietary arginine deficiency in rats by increasing splanchnic release of citrulline. J Nutr 1994; 124:1950.

283. Batshaw ML, Brusilow S, Waber L, et al. Treatment of inborn errors of urea synthesis: activation of alternative pathways of waste nitrogen synthesis and excretion. N Engl J Med. 1982; 306:1387.

284. Batshaw ML, Wachtel RC, Thomas GH, et al. Arginine-responsive asymptomatic hyperammonemia in the premature infant. J Pediatr 1984; 105:86.

285. Smith HA, Canter JA, Christian KG, et al. Nitric oxide precursors and congenital heart surgery: a randomized controlled trial of oral citrulline. J Thorac Cardiovasc Surg 2006; 132:58.

286. Cracowski JL, Cracowski C, Bessard G, et al. Increased lipid peroxidation in patients with pulmonary hypertension. Am J Respir Crit Care Med 2001; 164:1038.

287. Brennan LA, Steinhorn RH, Wedgwood S, et al. Increased superoxide generation is associated with pulmonary hypertension in fetal lambs: a role for NADPH oxidase. Circ Res 2003; 92:683.

288. Mata-Greenwood E, Jenkins C, Farrow KN, et al. eNOS function is developmentally regulated: uncoupling of eNOS occurs postnatally. Am J Physiol Lung Cell Mol Physiol 2006; 290:L232.

289. Konduri GG, Ou J, Shi Y, et al. Decreased association of HSP90 impairs endothelial nitric oxide synthase in fetal lambs with persistent pulmonary hypertension. Am J Physiol Heart Circ Physiol 2003; 285:H204.

290. Konduri GG, Bakhutashvili I, Eis A, et al. Oxidant stress from uncoupled nitric oxide synthase impairs vasodilatation in fetal lambs with persistent pulmonary hypertension. Am J Physiol Heart Circ Physiol 2007; 292:H1812.

291. Faraci FM, Didion SP. Vascular protection: superoxide dismutase isoforms in the vessel wall. Arterioscler Thromb Vasc Biol 2004; 24:1367.

292. Belik J, Jankov RP, Pan J, et al. Peroxynitrite inhibits relaxation and induces pulmonary artery muscle contraction in the newborn rat. Free Radic Biol Med 2004; 37:1384.

293. Sheehan DW, Giese EC, Gugino SF, et al. Characterization and mechanisms of H_2O_2-induced contractions of pulmonary arteries. Am J Physiol 1993; 264:H1542.

294. Janssen LJ. Isoprostanes: an overview and putative roles in pulmonary pathophysiology. Am J Physiol Lung Cell Mol Physiol 2001; 280:L1067.

295. Belik J, Jankov RP, Pan J, et al. Chronic O_2 exposure in the newborn rat results in decreased pulmonary arterial nitric oxide release and altered smooth muscle response to isoprostane. J Appl Physiol 2004; 96:725.

296. Aikio O, Vuopala K, Pokela ML, et al. Nitrotyrosine and NO synthases in infants with respiratory failure: influence of inhaled NO. Pediatr Pulmonol 2003; 35:8.

297. Goil S, Truog WE, Barnes C, et al. Eight-epi-PGF2alpha: a possible marker of lipid peroxidation in term infants with severe pulmonary disease. J Pediatr 1998; 132:349.

298. Wedgwood S, Black SM. Role of reactive oxygen species in vascular remodeling associated with pulmonary hypertension. Antioxid Redox Signal 2003; 5:759.

299. Steinhorn RH, Albert G, Swartz DD, et al. Recombinant human superoxide dismutase enhances the effect of inhaled nitric oxide in persistent pulmonary hypertension. Am J Respir Crit Care Med 2001; 164:834.

300. Villamor E, Perez-Vizcaino F, Cogolludo AL, et al. Relaxant effects of carbon monoxide compared with nitric oxide in pulmonary and systemic vessels of newborn piglets. Pediatr Res 2000; 48:546.

301. Villamor E, Perez-Vizcaino F, Cogolludo AL, et al. Relaxant effects of carbon monoxide compared with nitric oxide in pulmonary and systemic vessels of newborn piglets. Pediatr Res 2000; 48:546.

302. Kinsella JP, Parker TA, Davis JM, et al. Superoxide dismutase improves gas exchange and pulmonary hemodynamics in premature lambs. Am J Respir Crit Care Med 2005; 172:745.

303. Davis JM, Rosenfeld WN, Richter SE, et al. Safety and pharmacokinetics of multiple doses of recombinant human CuZn superoxide dismutase administered intratracheally to premature neonates with respiratory distress syndrome. Pediatrics 1997; 100:24.

304. Davis JM, Parad RB, Michele T, et al. Pulmonary outcome at 1 year corrected age in premature infants treated at birth with recombinant human CuZn superoxide dismutase. Pediatrics 2003; 111:469.

305. Fike CD, Kaplowitz MR, Pfister SL. Arachidonic acid metabolites and an early stage of pulmonary hypertension in chronically hypoxic newborn pigs. Am J Physiol Lung Cell Mol Physiol 2003; 284:L316.

306. Galie N, Manes A, Branzi A. Medical therapy of pulmonary hypertension. The prostacyclins. Clin Chest Med 2001; 22:529.

307. Widlitz A, Barst RJ. Pulmonary arterial hypertension in children. Eur Respir J 2003; 21:155.

308. Max M, Rossaint R. Inhaled prostacyclin in the treatment of pulmonary hypertension. Eur J Pediatr 1999; 158(Suppl 1):S23.

309. Kelly LK, Porta NF, Goodman DM, et al. Inhaled prostacyclin for term infants with persistent pulmonary hypertension refractory to inhaled nitric oxide. J Pediatr 2002; 141:830.

310. Christman BW, McPherson CD, Newman JH, et al. An imbalance between the excretion of thromboxane and prostacyclin metabolites in pulmonary hypertension. N Engl J Med 1992; 327:70.

311. Fike CD, Zhang Y, Kaplowitz MR. Thromboxane inhibition reduces an early stage of chronic hypoxia-induced pulmonary hypertension in piglets. J Appl Physiol 2005; 99:670.

312. Langleben D, Christman BW, Barst RJ, et al. Effects of the thromboxane synthetase inhibitor and receptor antagonist terbogrel in patients with primary pulmonary hypertension. Am Heart J 2002; 143:E4.

313. Kataoka M, Nagaya N, Satoh T, et al. A long-acting prostacyclin agonist with thromboxane inhibitory activity for pulmonary hypertension. Am J Respir Crit Care Med 2005; 172:1575.

314. Channick RN, Simonneau G, Sitbon O, et al. Effects of the dual endothelin-receptor antagonist bosentan in patients with pulmonary hypertension: a randomised placebo-controlled study. Lancet 2001; 358:1119.

315. Badesch DB, Bodin F, Channick RN, et al. Complete results of the first randomized placebo-controlled study of bosentan, a dual endothelin receptor antagonist, in pulmonary arterial hypertension. Curr Ther Res 2002; 63:227.

316. Rubin LJ, Badesch DB, Barst RJ, et al. Bosentan therapy for pulmonary arterial hypertension. N Engl J Med 2002; 346:896.

317. Barst RJ, Ivy D, Dingemanse J, et al. Pharmacokinetics, safety, and efficacy of bosentan in pediatric patients with pulmonary arterial hypertension. Clin Pharmacol Ther 2003; 73:372.

318. Ivy DD, Doran A, Claussen L, et al. Weaning and discontinuation of epoprostenol in children with idiopathic pulmonary arterial hypertension receiving concomitant bosentan. Am J Cardiol 2004; 93:943.

319. Gilbert N, Luther YC, Miera O, et al. Initial experience with bosentan (Tracleer) as treatment for pulmonary arterial hypertension (PAH) due to congenital heart disease in infants and young children. Z Kardiol 2005; 94:570.

320. Rugolotto S, Errico G, Beghini R, et al. Weaning of epoprostenol in a small infant receiving concomitant bosentan for severe pulmonary arterial hypertension secondary to bronchopulmonary dysplasia. Minerva Pediatr 2006; 58:491.

321. Barst RJ, Langleben D, Badesch D, et al. Treatment of pulmonary arterial hypertension with the selective endothelin-A receptor antagonist sitaxsentan. J Am Coll Cardiol 2006; 47:2049.

322. Ghofrani HA, Rose F, Schermuly RT, et al. Oral sildenafil as long-term adjunct therapy to inhaled iloprost in severe pulmonary arterial hypertension. J Am Coll Cardiol 2003; 42:158.

323. Humbert M, Barst RJ, Robbins IM, et al. Combination of bosentan with epoprostenol in pulmonary arterial hypertension: BREATHE-2. Eur Respir J 2004; 24:353.

324. Mathai SC, Girgis RE, Fisher MR, et al. Addition of sildenafil to bosentan monotherapy in pulmonary arterial hypertension. Eur Respir J 2007; 29:469.

325. Hoeper M, Leuchte H, Halank M, et al. Combining inhaled iloprost with bosentan in patients with idiopathic pulmonary arterial hypertension. Eur J Pediatr 2006; 28(4):691.

326. Hoeper MM, Markevych I, Spiekerkoetter E, et al. Goal-oriented treatment and combination therapy for pulmonary arterial hypertension. Eur Respir J 2005; 26:858.

327. Rubin LJ. Therapy of pulmonary hypertension: the evolution from vasodilators to antiproliferative agents. Am J Respir Crit Care Med 2002; 166:1308.

328. Rabinovitch M. Elastase and the pathobiology of unexplained pulmonary hypertension. Chest 1998; 114:213S.

329. Stenmark KR, Mecham RP. Cellular and molecular mechanisms of pulmonary vascular remodeling. Annu Rev Physiol 1997; 59:89.

330. Gibbons GH, Dzau VJ. The emerging concept of vascular remodeling. N Engl J Med 1994; 330:1431.

331. Voelkel NF, Tuder RM. Cellular and molecular biology of vascular smooth muscle cells in pulmonary hypertension. Pulm Pharmacol Ther 1997; 10:231.

332. Archer S, Rich S. Primary pulmonary hypertension: a vascular biology and translational research "Work in progress." Circulation 2000; 102:2781.

333. Stenmark KR, Fagan KA, Frid MG. Hypoxia-induced pulmonary vascular remodeling: cellular and molecular mechanisms. Circ Res 2006; 99:675.

334. Todorovich-Hunter L, Johnson DJ, Ranger P, et al. Altered elastin and collagen synthesis associated with progressive pulmonary hypertension induced by monocrotaline. A biochemical and ultrastructural study. Lab Invest 1988; 58:184.

335. Prosser IW, Stenmark KR, Suthar M, et al. Regional heterogeneity of elastin and collagen gene expression in intralobar arteries in response to hypoxic pulmonary hypertension as demonstrated by in situ hybridization. Am J Pathol 1989; 135:1073.

336. Jones PL, Rabinovitch M. Tenascin-C is induced with progressive pulmonary vascular disease in rats and is functionally related to increased smooth muscle cell proliferation. Circ Res 1996; 79:1131.

337. Jones PL, Cowan KN, Rabinovitch M. Tenascin-C, proliferation and subendothelial fibronectin in progressive pulmonary vascular disease. Am J Pathol 1997; 150:1349.

338. Reeve HL, Michelakis E, Nelson DP, et al. Alterations in a redox oxygen sensing mechanism in chronic hypoxia. J Appl Physiol 2001; 90:2249.

339. Yuan XJ, Wang J, Juhaszova M, et al. Attenuated K+ channel gene transcription in primary pulmonary hypertension. Lancet 1998; 351:726.

340. McMurtry MS, Archer SL, Altieri DC, et al. Gene therapy targeting survivin selectively induces pulmonary vascular apoptosis and reverses pulmonary arterial hypertension. J Clin Invest 2005; 115:1479.

341. Guignabert C, Raffestin B, Benferhat R, et al. Serotonin transporter inhibition prevents and reverses monocrotaline-induced pulmonary hypertension in rats. Circulation 2005; 111:2812.

342. Cowan KN, Leung WC, Mar C, et al. Caspases from apoptotic myocytes degrade extracellular matrix: a novel remodeling paradigm. FASEB J 2005; 19:1848.

343. Strauss BH, Rabinovitch M. Adventitial fibroblasts: defining a role in vessel wall remodeling. Am J Respir Cell Mol Biol 2000; 22:1.

344. Bonnet S, Michelakis ED, Porter CJ, et al. An abnormal mitochondrial-hypoxia inducible factor-1alpha-Kv channel pathway disrupts oxygen sensing and triggers pulmonary arterial hypertension in fawn hooded rats: similarities to human pulmonary arterial hypertension. Circulation 2006; 113:2630.

345. Cowan KN, Heilbut A, Humpl T, et al. Complete reversal of fatal pulmonary hypertension in rats by a serine elastase inhibitor. Nat Med 2000; 6:698.

346. Pollman MJ, Yamada T, Horiuchi M, et al. Vasoactive substances regulate vascular smooth muscle cell apoptosis. Countervailing influences of nitric oxide and angiotensin II. Circ Res 1996; 79:748.

347. Cattaruzza M, Dimigen C, Ehrenreich H, et al. Stretch-induced endothelin B receptor-mediated apoptosis in vascular smooth muscle cells. FASEB J 2000; 14:991.

348. Irani K. Oxidant signaling in vascular cell growth, death, and survival: a review of the roles of reactive oxygen species in smooth muscle and endothelial cell mitogenic and apoptotic signaling. Circ Res 2000; 87:179.

349. Jones PL, Crack J, Rabinovitch M. Regulation of tenascin-C, a vascular smooth muscle cell survival factor that interacts with the alpha v beta 3 integrin to promote epidermal growth factor receptor phosphorylation and growth. J Cell Biol 1997; 139:279.

350. Ye CL, Rabinovitch M. Inhibition of elastolysis by SC-37698 reduces development and progression of monocrotaline pulmonary hypertension. Am J Physiol 1991; 261:H1255.

351. Zaidi SH, You XM, Ciura S, et al. Overexpression of the serine elastase inhibitor elafin protects transgenic mice from hypoxic pulmonary hypertension. Circulation 2002; 105:516.

352. Maruyama K, Ye CL, Woo M, et al. Chronic hypoxic pulmonary hypertension in rats and increased elastolytic activity. Am J Physiol 1991; 261:H1716.

353. Cowan KN, Jones PL, Rabinovitch M. Elastase and matrix metalloproteinase inhibitors induce regression, and tenascin-C antisense prevents progression, of vascular disease. J Clin Invest 2000; 105:21.

354. Merklinger SL, Jones PL, Martinez EC, et al. Epidermal growth factor receptor blockade mediates smooth muscle cell apoptosis and improves survival in rats with pulmonary hypertension. Circulation 2005; 112:423.

355. Yuan XJ, Goldman WF, Tod ML, et al. Hypoxia reduces potassium currents in cultured rat pulmonary but not mesenteric arterial myocytes. Am J Physiol 1993; 264:L116.

356. Post JM, Hume JR, Archer SL, et al. Direct role for potassium channel inhibition in hypoxic pulmonary vasoconstriction. Am J Physiol 1992; 262:C882.

357. Moudgil R, Michelakis ED, Archer SL. The role of k+ channels in determining pulmonary vascular tone, oxygen sensing, cell proliferation, and apoptosis: implications in hypoxic pulmonary vasoconstriction and pulmonary arterial hypertension. Microcirculation 2006; 13:615.

358. Weir EK, Lopez-Barneo J, Buckler KJ, et al. Acute oxygen-sensing mechanisms. N Engl J Med 2005; 353:2042.

359. Yuan XJ, Wang J, Juhaszova M, et al. Molecular basis and function of voltage-gated K+ channels in pulmonary arterial smooth muscle cells. Am J Physiol 1998; 274:L621.

360. Michelakis ED, Hampl V, Nsair A, et al. Diversity in mitochondrial function explains differences in vascular oxygen sensing. Circ Res 2002; 90:1307.

361. Reeve HL, Weir EK, Nelson DP, et al. Opposing effects of oxidants and antioxidants on K+ channel activity and tone in rat vascular tissue. Exp Physiol 1995; 80:825.

362. Hasunuma K, Rodman DM, McMurtry IF. Effects of K+ channel blockers on vascular tone in the perfused rat lung. Am Rev Respir Dis 1991; 144:884.

363. Robertson TP, Ward JP, Aaronson PI. Hypoxia induces the release of a pulmonary-selective, Ca(2+)-sensitising, vasoconstrictor from the perfused rat lung. Cardiovasc Res 2001; 50:145.

364. Archer SL, Nelson DP, Weir EK. Simultaneous measurement of O_2 radicals and pulmonary vascular reactivity in rat lung. J Appl Physiol 1989; 67:1903.

365. Archer SL, Reeve HL, Michelakis E, et al. O_2 sensing is preserved in mice lacking the gp91 phox subunit of NADPH oxidase. Proc Natl Acad Sci USA 1999; 96:7944.

366. Paky A, Michael JR, Burke-Wolin TM, et al. Endogenous production of superoxide by rabbit lungs: effects of hypoxia or metabolic inhibitors. J Appl Physiol 1993; 74:2868.

367. Liu JQ, Sham JS, Shimoda LA, et al. Hypoxic constriction and reactive oxygen species in porcine distal pulmonary arteries. Am J Physiol Lung Cell Mol Physiol 2003; 285:L322.

368. Waypa GB, Chandel NS, Schumacker PT. Model for hypoxic pulmonary vasoconstriction involving mitochondrial oxygen sensing. Circ Res 2001; 88:1259.

369. Archer SL, Huang J, Henry T, et al. A redox-based O_2 sensor in rat pulmonary vasculature. Circ Res 1993; 73:1100.

370. Jones RD, Thompson JS, Morice AH. The NADPH oxidase inhibitors iodonium diphenyl and cadmium sulphate inhibit hypoxic pulmonary vasoconstriction in isolated rat pulmonary arteries. Physiol Res 2000; 49:587.

371. Mohazzab KM, Fayngersh RP, Kaminski PM, et al. Potential role of NADH oxidoreductase-derived reactive O_2 species in calf pulmonary arterial PO_2-elicited responses. Am J Physiol 1995; 269:L637.

372. Mohazzab KM, Wolin MS. Properties of a superoxide anion-generating microsomal NADH oxidoreductase, a potential pulmonary artery PO_2 sensor. Am J Physiol 1994; 267:L823.

373. Weissmann N, Tadic A, Hanze J, et al. Hypoxic vasoconstriction in intact lungs: a role for NADPH oxidase-derived H(2)O(2)? Am J Physiol Lung Cell Mol Physiol 2000; 279:L683.

374. Archer SL, Wu XC, Thebaud B, et al. Preferential expression and function of voltage-gated, O_2-sensitive K+ channels in resistance pulmonary arteries explains regional heterogeneity in hypoxic pulmonary vasoconstriction: ionic diversity in smooth muscle cells. Circ Res 2004; 95:308.

375. Pozeg ZI, Michelakis ED, McMurtry MS, et al. In vivo gene transfer of the O_2-sensitive potassium channel Kv1.5 reduces pulmonary hypertension and restores hypoxic pulmonary vasoconstriction in chronically hypoxic rats. Circulation 2003; 107:2037.

376. Archer SL, London B, Hampl V, et al. Impairment of hypoxic pulmonary vasoconstriction in mice lacking the voltage-gated potassium channel Kv1.5. FASEB J 2001; 15:1801.

377. Archer SL, Souil E, nh-Xuan AT, et al. Molecular identification of the role of voltage-gated K+ channels, Kv1.5 and Kv2.1, in hypoxic pulmonary vasoconstriction and control of resting membrane potential in rat pulmonary artery myocytes. J Clin Invest 1998; 101:2319.

378. Perchenet L, Hilfiger L, Mizrahi J, et al. Effects of anorexinogen agents on cloned voltage-gated K(+) channel hKv1.5. J Pharmacol Exp Ther 2001; 298:1108.

379. Weir EK, Reeve HL, Johnson G, et al. A role for potassium channels in smooth muscle cells and platelets in the etiology of primary pulmonary hypertension. Chest 1998; 114:200S.

380. Michelakis ED, McMurtry MS, Wu XC, et al. Dichloroacetate, a metabolic modulator, prevents and reverses chronic hypoxic pulmonary hypertension in rats: role of increased expression and activity of voltage-gated potassium channels. Circulation 2002; 105:244.

381. McMurtry MS, Bonnet S, Wu X, et al. Dichloroacetate prevents and reverses pulmonary hypertension by inducing pulmonary artery smooth muscle cell apoptosis. Circ Res 2004; 95:830.

382. Sato K, Webb S, Tucker A, et al. Factors influencing the idiopathic development of pulmonary hypertension in the fawn hooded rat. Am Rev Respir Dis 1992; 145:793.

383. Le Cras TD, Kim DH, Markham NE, et al. Early abnormalities of pulmonary vascular development in the Fawn-Hooded rat raised at Denver's altitude. Am J Physiol Lung Cell Mol Physiol 2000; 279:L283.

384. Huang LE, Arany Z, Livingston DM, et al. Activation of hypoxia-inducible transcription factor depends primarily upon redox-sensitive stabilization of its alpha subunit. J Biol Chem 1996; 271:32253.

385. Stacpoole PW, Nagaraja NV, Hutson AD. Efficacy of dichloroacetate as a lactate-lowering drug. J Clin Pharmacol 2003; 43:683.

386. Schermuly RT, Dony E, Ghofrani HA, et al. Reversal of experimental pulmonary hypertension by PDGF inhibition. J Clin Invest 2005; 115:2811.

387. Balasubramaniam V, Le Cras TD, Ivy DD, et al. Role of platelet-derived growth factor in vascular remodeling during pulmonary hypertension in the ovine fetus. Am J Physiol Lung Cell Mol Physiol 2003; 284:L826.

388. Ghofrani HA, Seeger W, Grimminger F. Imatinib for the treatment of pulmonary arterial hypertension. N Engl J Med 2005; 353:1412.

389. Patterson KC, Weissmann A, Ahmadi T, et al. Imatinib mesylate in the treatment of refractory idiopathic pulmonary arterial hypertension. Ann Intern Med 2006; 145:152.

390. Souza R, Sitbon O, Parent F, et al. Long term imatinib treatment in pulmonary arterial hypertension. Thorax 2006; 61:736.

391. Zhang S, Fantozzi I, Tigno DD, et al. Bone morphogenetic proteins induce apoptosis in human pulmonary vascular smooth muscle cells. Am J Physiol Lung Cell Mol Physiol 2003; 285:L740.

392. Morrell NW, Yang X, Upton PD, et al. Altered growth responses of pulmonary artery smooth muscle cells from patients with primary pulmonary hypertension to transforming growth factor-beta(1) and bone morphogenetic proteins. Circulation 2001; 104:790.

393. Lane KB, Machado RD, Pauciulo MW, et al. Heterozygous germline mutations in BMPR2, encoding a TGF-beta receptor, cause familial primary pulmonary hypertension. The International PPH Consortium. Nat Genet 2000; 26:81.

394. Altieri DC. Validating survivin as a cancer therapeutic target. Nat Rev Cancer 2003; 3:46.

395. Blanc-Brude OP, Yu J, Simosa H, et al. Inhibitor of apoptosis protein survivin regulates vascular injury. Nat Med 2002; 8:987.

396. Newman JH, Fanburg BL, Archer SL, et al. Pulmonary arterial hypertension: future directions: report of a National Heart, Lung and Blood Institute/Office of Rare Diseases workshop. Circulation 2004; 109:2947.

397. Laufs U, Marra D, Node K, et al. 3-Hydroxy-3-methylglutaryl-CoA reductase inhibitors attenuate vascular smooth muscle proliferation by preventing rho GTPase-induced down-regulation of p27(Kip1). J Biol Chem 1999; 274:21926.

398. Indolfi C, Cioppa A, Stabile E, et al. Effects of hydroxymethylglutaryl coenzyme A reductase inhibitor simvastatin on smooth muscle cell proliferation in vitro and neointimal formation in vivo after vascular injury. J Am Coll Cardiol 2000; 35:214.

399. Nishimura T, Vaszar LT, Faul JL, et al. Simvastatin rescues rats from fatal pulmonary hypertension by inducing apoptosis of neointimal smooth muscle cells. Circulation 2003; 108:1640.

400. Girgis RE, Li D, Zhan X, et al. Attenuation of chronic hypoxic pulmonary hypertension by simvastatin. Am J Physiol Heart Circ Physiol 2003; 285:H938.

401. Laufs U, Fata VL, Liao JK. Inhibition of 3-hydroxy-3-methylglutaryl (HMG)-CoA reductase blocks hypoxia-mediated down-regulation of endothelial nitric oxide synthase. J Biol Chem 1997; 272:31725.

402. Dimmeler S, Aicher A, Vasa M, et al. HMG-CoA reductase inhibitors (statins) increase endothelial progenitor cells via the PI 3-kinase/Akt pathway. J Clin Invest 2001; 108:391.

403. Takemoto M, Sun J, Hiroki J, et al. Rho-kinase mediates hypoxia-induced downregulation of endothelial nitric oxide synthase. Circulation 2002; 106:57.

404. Gurbanov E, Shiliang X. The key role of apoptosis in the pathogenesis and treatment of pulmonary hypertension. Eur J Cardiothorac Surg 2006; 30:499.

405. Abe K, Shimokawa H, Morikawa K, et al. Long-term treatment with a Rho-kinase inhibitor improves monocrotaline-induced fatal pulmonary hypertension in rats. Circ Res 2004; 94:385.

406. Fagan KA, Oka M, Bauer NR, et al. Attenuation of acute hypoxic pulmonary vasoconstriction and hypoxic pulmonary hypertension in mice by inhibition of Rho-kinase. Am J Physiol Lung Cell Mol Physiol 2004; 287:L656.

407. Nagaoka T, Fagan KA, Gebb SA, et al. Inhaled Rho kinase inhibitors are potent and selective vasodilators in rat pulmonary hypertension. Am J Respir Crit Care Med 2005; 171:494.

408. Nagaya N, Kangawa K, Kanda M, et al. Hybrid cell-gene therapy for pulmonary hypertension based on phagocytosing action of endothelial progenitor cells. Circulation 2003; 108:889.

409. Baber SR, Deng W, Master RG, et al. Intratracheal mesenchymal stem cell administration attenuates monocrotaline-induced pulmonary hypertension and endothelial dysfunction. Am J Physiol Heart Circ Physiol 2007; 292:H1120.

410. Kanki-Horimoto S, Horimoto H, Mieno S, et al. Implantation of mesenchymal stem cells overexpressing endothelial nitric oxide synthase improves right ventricular impairments caused by pulmonary hypertension. Circulation 2006; 114:I181.

411. Okoye BO, Losty PD, Lloyd DA, et al. Effect of prenatal glucocorticoids on pulmonary vascular muscularisation in nitrofen-induced congenital diaphragmatic hernia. J Pediatr Surg 1998; 33:76.

412. Yamataka T, Puri P. Active collagen synthesis by pulmonary arteries in pulmonary hypertension complicated by congenital diaphragmatic hernia. J Pediatr Surg 1997; 32:682.

413. Sakai M, Unemoto K, Solari V, et al. Decreased expression of voltage-gated K+ channels in pulmonary artery smooth muscle cells in nitrofen-induced congenital diaphragmatic hernia in rats. Pediatr Surg Int 2004; 20:192.

414. Anderson DH. Incidence of congenital diaphragmatic hernia in the young of rats bred on a diet deficient in Vitamin A. Am J Dis Child 1941; 62:888.

415. Anderson DH. Effect of diet during pregnancy upon the incidence of congenital hereditary diaphragmatic hernia in the rat. Am J Path 1949; 25:163.

416. Wilson JG, Roth CB, Warkany J. An analysis of the syndrome of malformations induced by maternal vitamin A deficiency. Effects of restoration of vitamin A at various times during gestation. Am J Anat 1953; 92:189.

417. Mendelsohn C, Lohnes D, Decimo D, et al. Function of the retinoic acid receptors (RARs) during development (II). Multiple abnormalities at various stages of organogenesis in RAR double mutants. Development 1994; 120:2749.

418. Lohnes D, Mark M, Mendelsohn C, et al. Developmental roles of the retinoic acid receptors. J Steroid Biochem Mol Biol 1995; 53:475.

419. Ambrose AM, Larson PS, Borzelleca JF, et al. Toxicologic studies on 2,4-dichlorophenyl-p-nitrophenyl ether. Toxicol Appl Pharmacol 1971; 19:263.

420. Costlow RD, Manson JM. The heart and diaphragm: target organs in the neonatal death induced by nitrofen (2,4-dichlorophenyl-p-nitrophenyl ether). Toxicology 1981; 20:209.

421. Kluth D, Kangah R, Reich P, et al. Nitrofen-induced diaphragmatic hernias in rats: an animal model. J Pediatr Surg 1990; 25:850.

422. Migliazza L, Xia H, ez-Pardo JA, et al. Skeletal malformations associated with congenital diaphragmatic hernia: experimental and human studies. J Pediatr Surg 1999; 34:1624.

423. Thebaud B, Tibboel D, Rambaud C, et al. Vitamin A decreases the incidence and severity of nitrofen-induced congenital diaphragmatic hernia in rats. Am J Physiol 1999; 277:L423.

424. Mey J, Babiuk RP, Clugston R, et al. Retinal dehydrogenase-2 is inhibited by compounds that induce congenital diaphragmatic hernias in rodents. Am J Pathol 2003; 162:673.

425. Thebaud B, Barlier-Mur AM, Chailley-Heu B, et al. Restoring effects of vitamin A on surfactant synthesis in nitrofen-induced congenital diaphragmatic hernia in rats. Am J Respir Crit Care Med 2001; 164:1083.

426. Major D, Cadenas M, Fournier L, et al. Retinol status of newborn infants with congenital diaphragmatic hernia. Pediatr Surg Int 1998; 13:547.

427. Greer JJ, Babiuk RP, Thebaud B. Etiology of congenital diaphragmatic hernia: the retinoid hypothesis. Pediatr Res 2003; 53:726.

428. Wilcox DT, Glick PL, Karamanoukian HL, et al. Contributions by individual lungs to the surfactant status in congenital diaphragmatic hernia. Pediatr Res 1997; 41:686.

429. Mysore MR, Margraf LR, Jaramillo MA, et al. Surfactant protein A is decreased in a rat model of congenital diaphragmatic hernia. Am J Respir Crit Care Med 1998; 157:654.

430. Asabe K, Tsuji K, Handa N, et al. Immunohistochemical distribution of surfactant apoprotein-A in congenital diaphragmatic hernia. J Pediatr Surg 1997; 32:667.
431. Lotze A, Knight GR, Anderson KD, et al. Surfactant (beractant) therapy for infants with congenital diaphragmatic hernia on ECMO: evidence of persistent surfactant deficiency. J Pediatr Surg 1994; 29:407.
432. O'Toole SJ, Karamanoukian HL, Morin FC, III, et al. Surfactant decreases pulmonary vascular resistance and increases pulmonary blood flow in the fetal lamb model of congenital diaphragmatic hernia. J Pediatr Surg 1996; 31:507.
433. Coalson JJ. Pathology of chronic lung disease of early infancy. In: Bland RD, Coalson JJ, eds., Chronic lung disease in early infancy. Informa Healthcare: 1999: 85–124.
434. Coalson JJ, Winter VT, Siler-Khodr T, et al. Neonatal chronic lung disease in extremely immature baboons. Am J Respir Crit Care Med 1999; 160:1333.
435. Jobe AH, Bancalari E. Bronchopulmonary dysplasia. Am J Respir Crit Care Med 2001; 163:1723.
436. Jobe AJ. The new BPD: an arrest of lung development. Pediatr Res 1999; 46:641.
437. McCurnin DC, Pierce RA, Chang LY, et al. Inhaled NO improves early pulmonary function and modifies lung growth and elastin deposition in a baboon model of neonatal chronic lung disease. Am J Physiol Lung Cell Mol Physiol 2005; 288:L450.
438. Bland RD, Albertine KH, Carlton DP, et al. Inhaled nitric oxide effects on lung structure and function in chronically ventilated preterm lambs. Am J Respir Crit Care Med 2005; 172:899.
439. Lin YJ, Markham NE, Balasubramaniam V, et al. Inhaled nitric oxide enhances distal lung growth after exposure to hyperoxia in neonatal rats. Pediatr Res 2005; 58:22.
440. Balasubramaniam V, Maxey AM, Morgan DB, et al. Inhaled NO restores lung structure in eNOS-deficient mice recovering from neonatal hypoxia. Am J Physiol Lung Cell Mol Physiol 2006; 291:L119.
441. Tang JR, Markham NE, Lin YJ, et al. Inhaled nitric oxide attenuates pulmonary hypertension and improves lung growth in infant rats after neonatal treatment with a VEGF receptor inhibitor. Am J Physiol Lung Cell Mol Physiol 2004; 287:L344.
442. Maniscalco WM, Watkins RH, Finkelstein JN, et al. Vascular endothelial growth factor mRNA increases in alveolar epithelial cells during recovery from oxygen injury. Am J Respir Cell Mol Biol 1995; 13:377.
443. Papapetropoulos A, Garcia-Cardena G, Madri JA, et al. Nitric oxide production contributes to the angiogenic properties of vascular endothelial growth factor in human endothelial cells. J Clin Invest 1997; 100:3131.
444. Kroll J, Waltenberger J. A novel function of VEGF receptor-2 (KDR): rapid release of nitric oxide in response to VEGF-A stimulation in endothelial cells. Biochem Biophys Res Commun 1999; 265:636.
445. Le Cras TD, Markham NE, Tuder RM, et al. Treatment of newborn rats with a VEGF receptor inhibitor causes pulmonary hypertension and abnormal lung structure. Am J Physiol Lung Cell Mol Physiol 2002; 283:L555.
446. Bhatt AJ, Pryhuber GS, Huyck H, et al. Disrupted pulmonary vasculature and decreased vascular endothelial growth factor, Flt-1, and TIE-2 in human infants dying with bronchopulmonary dysplasia. Am J Respir Crit Care Med 2001; 164:1971.
447. Maniscalco WM, Watkins RH, Pryhuber GS, et al. Angiogenic factors and alveolar vasculature: development and alterations by injury in very premature baboons. Am J Physiol Lung Cell Mol Physiol 2002; 282:L811.
448. Fouron JC, Le Guennec JC, Villemant D, et al. Value of echocardiography in assessing the outcome of bronchopulmonary dysplasia of the newborn. Pediatrics 1980; 65:529.
449. Abman SH, Accurso FJ, Bowman CM. Unsuspected cardiopulmonary abnormalities complicating bronchopulmonary dysplasia. Arch Dis Child 1984; 59:966.
450. Nagaya N, Nishikimi T, Uematsu M, et al. Plasma brain natriuretic peptide as a prognostic indicator in patients with primary pulmonary hypertension. Circulation 2000; 102:865.

Chapter 13

Impact of Perinatal Lung Injury in Later Life

Lex W. Doyle. MD FRACP • Peter J. Anderson PhD

Respiratory Outcomes of BPD

Neurological Outcomes

Conclusions

Before the 1970s very few extremely low birthweight (ELBW, birthweight < 1000 g) infants survived. At the Royal Women's Hospital in Melbourne survival rates for inborn babies of birthweight 500–999 g averaged 6% through the 1960s. Survival rates for very low birthweight (VLBW, birthweight < 1500 g) infants were also relatively low, with only approximately 1 in 3 surviving long-term at this time (1). Intensive care in Melbourne was rudimentary by today's standards, and comprised the ability to administer oxygen, to monitor blood gases intermittently through an indwelling umbilical arterial catheter, and to infuse glucose and bicarbonate; there was no assisted ventilation. In other parts of the world mechanical ventilation was introduced around this time, and with it the first reports of lung injury, called bronchopulmonary dysplasia (BPD) (2).

Assisted ventilation in the form of intermittent positive pressure ventilation via an endotracheal tube was introduced at the Royal Women's Hospital in the early 1970s (3), and antenatal corticosteroids to accelerate lung maturation began later in the decade (4, 5). These innovations were associated with big increases in survival rates of ELBW infants up to 25–30% and of VLBW infants up to 65–70% by the end of the 1970s. During the 1980s assisted ventilation and antenatal corticosteroids increased along with survival rates, but it was the introduction of exogenous surfactant in 1991 that was associated with the next large increase in survival rates, up to 70% for ELBW infants and to 90% for VLBW infants. As would be expected after the introduction of assisted ventilation, some survivors had BPD, the rate of which has increased over time.

BPD has implications for long-term health, particularly affecting the lung and the brain. The aim of this review is to synthesize the data on long-term respiratory and neurological outcomes of BPD and discuss some of the controversies concerning the impact of BPD in later life. The review will, where possible, focus on outcomes to school-age and beyond.

RESPIRATORY OUTCOMES OF BPD

Methodological Issues

There are several methodological issues to consider when synthesizing data on respiratory health. First, the later that respiratory outcomes are reported, the more certain it is that the respiratory health at that point is likely to persist through the remainder of the subjects' lives. On the other hand, the older the subjects, the less relevant might be the results to babies in nurseries today. However, any results are relevant to contemporaneous survivors and remain the best estimates of what might confront today's babies until superseded by more up-to-date data. Second, there must be a basis for comparison to consider the long-term respiratory outcome for the tiniest survivors with BPD. Two possible comparison groups include survivors of similar size or gestational age without BPD, or those with normal birth-weight (NBW, birthweight > 2499 g) or who were not preterm. Third, the types of respiratory outcomes could relate to clinical outcomes, such as the frequency of asthma or pneumonia, or to exercise tolerance, or could relate to the results of respiratory function tests. Of respiratory function tests, there are those variables reflecting obstruction to airflow, or those reflecting air trapping. Variables reflecting airflow include the forced expired volume in 1 s (FEV_1), the FEV_1/forced vital capacity (FVC) ratio, instantaneous flows at various % of vital capacity (VC), such as the flow rate at 75% of VC ($V'_{EMAX75\%}$), at 50% of vital capacity ($V'_{EMAX50\%}$), or at 25% of vital capacity ($V'_{EMAX25\%}$), the maximum forced expiratory flow between 25% and 75% of vital capacity ($FEF_{25-75\%}$), or the peak expiratory flow rate (PEFR). Variables reflecting air trapping include the residual volume (RV), or the RV/total lung capacity (TLC) ratio. Values for respiratory function variables are usually reported as % predicted for age, height and gender, and hence they might vary between studies because of differences in selection criteria of the reference population. However, the FEV_1/FVC and the RV/TLC can be interpreted just as ratios, but do change with age in healthy children (6). Not all studies report all of these variables, but the most commonly reported variable reflecting airflow would be the FEV_1. Finally, there are various definitions of BPD in the studies that have reported on long-term outcomes, and these variations need to be considered when comparing results from these studies. A workshop convened in 2000 to clarify the criteria for a diagnosis of BPD (7) will not have much effect on long-term outcome studies for many years.

Controversies

Some of the controversies regarding respiratory outcomes of BPD include the following. What are the pulmonary outcomes for the oldest survivors of BPD? How does the respiratory function of BPD survivors change with increasing age of survivors? How has the respiratory outcome for BPD survivors changed with the introduction of exogenous surfactant? What are the effects of cigarette smoking on survivors with BPD? What other health issues are related to BPD?

What are the Pulmonary Outcomes for the Oldest Survivors of BPD?

The oldest subjects with BPD to have respiratory function data reported have been in the late teens or early 20s, and there are only three studies of subjects of that age (8–10). Northway et al. (8) described the respiratory function in late adolescence of 26 subjects who had BPD and who were born between 1964 and 1973. BPD was diagnosed in those who had been ventilated for respiratory distress, who were oxygen dependent at 28 days, and who had Northway stages 3 or 4 on chest X-ray (2). Results were compared with 26 age-matched controls of similar birthweight and gestational age who had not been ventilated as infants, and 53 age-matched normal subjects who were not born prematurely, who had no history of chronic lung disease and who were non-smokers. The mean birthweights of the 2 preterm groups were 1894 g and 1978 g, their mean gestational ages were 33.2 weeks and 34.5 weeks, and they were assessed at mean ages of 18.3 years and 18.8 years, respectively. Northway et al. found that 68% of BPD subjects had

Table 13-1	Forced Expired Volume in 1 s (FEV1 –% predicted) for Three Studies with Respiratory Function Reported in Late Adolescence/Early Adulthood		
	PRETERM GROUPS		
Study	**BPD**	**No BPD**	**NBW controls**
Northway	74.8 (14.5) $n=25^*$	96.6 (10.2) $n=26$	100.4 (10.9) $n=53$
Halvorsen	87.8 (13.8) $n=12^\dagger$	97.7 (12.9) $n=34$	108.1 (13.8) $n=46$
Doyle	81.6 (18.7) $n=33^*$	92.9 (12.8) $n=114$	99.4 (9.5) $n=37$

*BPD determined by ventilator dependency, oxygen requirement > 28 days and chest X-ray consistent with Northway Stage 3 or 4 changes (2).
†BPD group had oxygen requirement at 36 weeks; the remainder in this table are considered to have no BPD.

airway obstruction; this was reversible in most, but fixed in 24%. In addition those with BPD had reductions in variables reflecting airflow (lower FEV_1, FVC, $FEF_{25-75\%}$, $V'_{EMAX50\%}$, and PEFR) and increased gas trapping (higher RV/TLC) compared with both the preterm controls and the normal controls; 24% had one or more severe abnormalities in respiratory function. Respiratory function in BPD subjects was also worse than in normal controls; values for FEV_1 in the BPD group, the non-BPD preterm group, and the normal controls are shown in Table 13-1. Within the preterm group the FEV_1 (% predicted) was 21.8% (95% confidence interval [CI] 14.9–28.7%) lower in the BPD subjects compared with the matched controls. BPD subjects had more wheezing, episodes of pneumonia, limitation of exercise capacity and long-term medication use than either control group, but precise rates of these outcomes were not reported. They also had more chronic changes on chest X-ray. Few subjects in either preterm group were smokers so the effect of smoking was not reported separately.

Halvorsen et al. (9) reported the pulmonary outcomes for 46 subjects of birthweight < 1001 g or gestational ages < 29 weeks at a mean age of 17.7 years from a geographically based cohort of births between 1982 and 1985 in Western Norway. Twelve (26%) of the subjects had moderate or severe BPD based on oxygen requirement at 36 weeks postmenstrual age, 24 (52%) had mild BPD based on oxygen requirement at 28 days but not 36 weeks, and 10 (22%) had no BPD. They compared results with 46 temporally related controls who were born at term and of the same gender; the controls were not randomly selected, however, as they had to ask 40% more controls to participate to get the required number of 46, raising the possibility of volunteer bias influencing the results. In their study the preterm group had reductions in variables reflecting flow, and these were lower with increasing severity of BPD; Table 13-1 shows the data for the moderate/severe BPD group, the remainder of the preterm group, and the controls. Within the preterm group the FEV_1 (% predicted) was 9.9% (95% CI 1.0–18.8%) lower in the moderate/severe BPD subjects compared with the remainder. Rates of asthma were reported to be higher in the preterm cohort compared with the controls, but the rates were not reported separately for BPD and non-BPD preterm subjects.

Doyle et al. (10) studied 147 survivors of birthweight < 1500 g from the Royal Women's Hospital, Melbourne, who were born during 1977–1982 and who had respiratory function tests at a mean age of 18.9 (SD 1.1) years. Of the 147 subjects, 33 (22%) had BPD in the newborn period, defined as in the original Northway study (2). There were also 37 NBW controls with respiratory function tests. All respiratory function variables reflecting airflow were substantially diminished in the BPD group, but lung volumes were not significantly different. Within the preterm group the FEV_1 (% predicted) was 11.3% (95% CI 5.7–16.9%) lower in the BPD subjects than in preterm controls, and both groups were lower than NBW controls (Table 13-1). More subjects in the BPD group had reductions in airflow in the clinically significant range (e.g., FEV_1 <75% predicted, BPD 30.3%, no BPD 7.9%, $\chi^2 = 11.4$, $P = 0.001$; FEV_1/FVC <75%, BPD 42.4%, no BPD 15.8%, $\chi^2 = 10.7$, $P = 0.001$). Importantly in this study respiratory function results varied little with different definitions of BPD, ranging from the milder definition of oxygen dependency at 28 days, through to the more severe definition of oxygen dependency at 36 weeks postmenstrual age. The rates of asthma were similar in those with BPD (24.2%) and no BPD (21.9%), but active smoking was less frequent in those with BPD (18.2%) than in those with no BPD (37.7%) ($\chi^2 = 4.4$, $P = 0.036$). Active smoking did not account for the differences in respiratory function between those with and without BPD, as adjustment for smoking did not affect the differences between the groups.

Summarizing this controversy, BPD survivors into late adolescence or early adulthood have substantial reductions in airflow compared with both normal birthweight controls, as well as controls of similar birthweight or gestational ages. Clearly respiratory function tests should be repeated later in adulthood in these subjects.

How does Respiratory Function Change with Increasing Age in BPD Survivors?

There are few studies with longitudinal data in the same subjects, and only one that has reported changes from early school age up to late adolescence/early adulthood (10). In this study data at 8 years and 18+ years of age in 129 subjects of birthweight < 1500 g were described; 29 of the 129 subjects had BPD. Compared with respiratory function variables measured at 8 years, the only variable with a statistically significant difference over time in BPD subjects was a larger fall in the FEV_1/FVC ratio between 8 and 18 years of age compared with non-BPD preterm subjects (mean reduction 3.4%, 95% CI 0.2–6.7%). Active smoking was associated with a statistically significant reduction, and birthweight SD score was associated with a significant increase in the FEV_1/FVC ratio between 8 and 18 years. Adjusting for these variables augmented the statistical significance of the difference in the reduction in the FEV_1/FVC ratio between BPD and non-BPD subjects (adjusted mean reduction 4.8%, 95% CI 1.7–7.9%). Of note, gender was not associated with a significant change in FEV_1/FVC ratio between 8 and 18 years in this study.

In a subset of 120 of the same VLBW cohort there were no statistically significant changes in respiratory function between 8 and 11 years of age in the BPD and non-BPD subjects, but the time interval was relatively short (11). The respiratory function changes between 8 and 14 years of age have also been reported on 153 of the complete cohort (12). Overall respiratory function in these children at both 8 and 14 years was similar to predicted values. However, there were some changes, mostly improvements, in respiratory function between 8 to 14 years relative to predicted values. Variables reflecting flow were increased and closer to predicted values by age 14 when compared to age 8. The mean FEV_1 for the cohort at 8 years was 88.5% predicted, and at 14 years was 94.9% predicted, a mean increase of 6.4% (95% confidence interval 4.4–8.3%). Moreover, variables reflecting air trapping (RV, RV/TLC) were reduced and closer to expected values by 14 years of age. Again there were no significant differences in the rate of change between those with and without BPD.

Others have suggested that respiratory function in survivors with BPD might improve as they grow older. Blayney et al. (13) studied 32 children with BPD at both 7 and 10 years of age. The 19 with an FEV_1 <80% predicted at age 7 years improved by 10 years of age, but this may just reflect regression towards the mean. In another study where respiratory function tests were repeated in 17 subjects with BPD between 8 and 15 years, Koumbourlis et al. (14) reported that reductions in airflow persisted over time, although there was improvement in air trapping. It should be noted that both of these studies were on selected children with BPD, rather than complete cohorts of VLBW survivors.

In summary it is not clear whether respiratory function in the same subjects with BPD changes substantially over time. However, given that respiratory function begins to deteriorate in everyone after the mid-20s, it is vital that respiratory function be measured later in adult life in those with BPD. The more rapid decline in the FEV_1/FVC ratio in BPD subjects between 8 and 18 years of age observed in one study (10) is concerning.

How has the Respiratory Outcome for BPD Survivors Changed with the Introduction of Exogenous Surfactant?

Respiratory function in ELBW or very preterm (< 28 weeks) children born before surfactant was available was not as good as in NBW children, particularly with reductions in variables reflecting airflow (15–19). Within ELBW/very preterm survivors born before surfactant was available, those with BPD had more abnormal respiratory function than those without BPD (11, 20–22). With the introduction of surfactant in the 1990s survival rates in ELBW/very preterm babies have increased dramatically (23). The effect of surfactant administered soon after birth on respiratory function in small numbers of children enrolled in clinical trials has been reported to be minimal (24), or possibly beneficial (25). Moreover, the nature of BPD has also changed in recent times, with the advent of the "new BPD" (7), which is characterized more by alveolar arrest rather than by pulmonary fibrosis and cyst formation typical of BPD in earlier times.

The effect of BPD in the surfactant era on respiratory function has been reported to be similar to that before surfactant was available in several studies (26, 27). Korhonen et al. (26) studied 34 VLBW children at 7–8 years of age who had BPD diagnosed by oxygen dependency at 28 days of age, 14 of whom still had oxygen dependency at 36 weeks postmenstrual age. Results were compared with age- and sex-matched controls comprising 34 VLBW cases without BPD and 34 term children. Compared with term controls, the BPD cases had lower FEV_1, and those with oxygen dependency had lower FEV_1 than both control groups.

Doyle et al. (27) reported the results of a geographical cohort study of 298 consecutive ELBW/very preterm survivors born in Victoria in 1991–92. Exogenous surfactant was first used in Victoria in March 1991. It was initially restricted to rescue therapy, and limited to those with established lung disease requiring assisted ventilation via an endotracheal tube and more than 50% oxygen. After the first year surfactant could be given more liberally, but was still confined to rescue therapy. Respiratory function was measured in 81% (240/298) ELBW/very preterm children at a mean age of 8.7 (SD 0.3) years, and in 79% (208/262) NBW controls at a mean age of 8.9 (SD 0.4) years. Of the 240 ELBW/very preterm children cohort, 89 (37%) had BPD in the newborn period, defined as oxygen dependency at 36 weeks postmenstrual age in children who had received assisted ventilation via an endotracheal tube. Most children with BPD had respiratory function within the expected range. However, some variables reflecting airflow were reduced in children with BPD, compared with both ELBW/very preterm children without BPD, as well as with NBW controls, but the differences were not as marked as in the pre-surfactant era. For example, within the ELBW/very preterm group, the mean (SD) for FEV_1 (% predicted) was 81.1% (13.7%) in the BPD group, and 87.1% (11.5%) in the non-BPD group, a mean difference of 6.0% (95% CI 2.7–9.3%). This is approximately half the difference of 11.3% (95% CI 5.7–16.9%) described above for the pre-surfactant era, although the definition of BPD was different, and the subjects were older in the early study (10). The smaller difference was related more to a reduction in FEV_1 in the non-BPD group in the latter era compared with the earlier era (Table 13-1) as the mean FEV_1 for the BPD groups in both eras

Table 13-2 **Selected Respiratory Function Variables at 8 years of age in Children Born at the Royal Women's Hospital, Melbourne, with Birthweights < 1000 g from Two Different Eras – Before Surfactant (1977–82) and After Surfactant (1991–92)**

Years of birth	BPD	No BPD	Mean difference (95% CI)	
FEV$_1$ (% predicted)				
1977–82	80.0 (15.9) $n=31$	83.1 (12.5) $n=42$	–3.1 (–9.7, 3.5)	$t=-0.9$, $P=0.35$
1991–92	82.1 (9.7) $n=27$	86.3 (12.4) $n=52$	–4.2 (–9.6, 1.3)	$t=-1.5$, $P=0.13$
FEV$_1$/FVC (%)				
1977–82	84.3 (10.5) $n=31$	85.9 (8.4) $n=42$	–1.6 (–6.0, 2.8)	$t=-0.7$, $P=0.48$
1991–92	88.3 (8.6) $n=27$	88.4 (8.9) $n=52$	–0.1 (–4.3, 4.0)	$t=-0.1$, $P=0.95$
RV/TLC (%)				
1977–82	38.0 (9.9) $n=29$	36.3 (9.6) $n=37$	1.6 (–3.1, 6.5)	$t=0.7$, $P=0.50$
1991–92	34.8 (6.5) $n=27$	33.6 (8.0) $n=50$	1.1 (–2.4, 4.7)	$t=0.6$, $P=0.53$

CI = confidence interval; FEV$_1$ = forced expired volume in 1 s; FEV$_1$/FVC = forced expired volume in 1 s/forced vital capacity ratio; RV/TLC = residual volume/total lung capacity ratio.

was similar. In this study there were no substantial differences in respiratory function results between the 92 subjects treated and the 148 not treated with surfactant.

The results of selected respiratory function variables at 8 years of age in two more comparable groups pre- and post-surfactant are shown in Table 13-2. Both groups weighed < 1000 g, were born in the Royal Women's Hospital, Melbourne, and had respiratory function measured in the same laboratory. These are subsets of the groups described above (10, 27). There are only small differences in flow rates and lung volumes between BPD and non-BPD subjects, and between eras, suggesting little effect of the introduction of surfactant on respiratory function.

In summary it appears that respiratory function at early school age in ELBW/ very preterm children who had BPD in the newborn period has probably not changed much between eras with the introduction of exogenous surfactant; at least it is not worse than in earlier eras. However, the longer-term effects of the "new BPD" and of surfactant into adulthood remain to be determined.

What are the Effects of Cigarette Smoking on Survivors with BPD?

Respiratory function in ELBW subjects who smoke in early adulthood has been reported to be worse than in those who do not smoke; Doyle et al. (28) reported the results of respiratory function at a mean age of 20.2 years of a cohort of 44 of 60 consecutive ELBW subjects born during 1977–1980 at the Royal Women's Hospital, Melbourne, Australia. Respiratory function had also been measured in 42 of the 44 subjects at 8 years of age. Respiratory function was compared between the 14 smokers and the 30 nonsmokers. Several respiratory function variables reflecting airflow (FEV$_1$/FVC, V$'_{EMAX75\%}$, V$'_{EMAX50\%}$, V$'_{EMAX25\%}$ and FEF$_{25-75\%}$) were significantly diminished in smokers. The proportion with a clinically important reduction in the FEV$_1$/FVC ($< 75\%$) was significantly higher in smokers (64%) than in nonsmokers (20%) ($\chi^2 = 8.3$, $P < 0.01$). There was a significantly larger decrease in the FEV$_1$/FVC ratio between ages 8 and 20 years in the smokers compared with the non-smokers (mean difference in rate of change: -8.2%; 95% CI -14.1% to -2.4%). There were too few subjects with BPD who were also smokers in this study to test whether smoking was even worse in ELBW subjects with BPD. However, given that the rate of deterioration in respiratory function is more rapid in ELBW smokers up to age 20 years, and the fact that cigarette smoking is detrimental to respiratory function in all subjects in adulthood

(29, 30), adults with BPD and who smoke should have repeat respiratory function tests well into adulthood, to establish whether chronic obstructive airway disease develops more rapidly and at earlier ages.

What other Respiratory Health Issues are Related to BPD?

In most studies high rehospitalization rates are reported in children with BPD, with rates varying from 40% to 60% in the first two years of life (22, 31–39). Rates of rehospitalization are generally higher in early life in children with BPD; in one study Gross et al. (22) reported that 53% of children < 32 weeks gestational age with BPD required rehospitalization during the first 2 years of life compared with 26% in those with no BPD ($P < 0.01$). As well as having higher rehospitalization rates, children with BPD are also more likely to require multiple rehospitalizations and longer hospital stays. Cunningham et al. (34) reported 26% of the BPD group versus 5% of the non-BPD group had multiple rehospitalizations, as well as a cumulative hospital stay of > 31 days in 12% of the BPD group compared with 5% in the non-BPD group. Chien et al. (39) found a significant difference in the length of hospital stay in infants with BPD compared with no BPD (median 10 days versus 3 days).

As children with a history of BPD enter school age it appears that the risk of rehospitalization may be similar to their non-BPD peers. In a study of VLBW children at ages 8–10 years, McCormick et al. (40) reported that the risk of rehospitalization in the preceding year was similar for BPD (6%) and non-BPD (7%) groups. Doyle et al. (41) reported the respiratory outcome of the previously described VLBW and NBW cohorts at 14 years of age; rehospitalization for respiratory illness was infrequent in all groups, including those with BPD.

Rates of wheezing or asthma, or of bronchial hyper-responsiveness, are generally reported to be higher in BPD survivors (9, 22, 42–44). However, we have not found this consistently in our studies; as indicated above the rates of asthma (defined as requiring bronchodilators for recurrent wheezing in the previous 12 months) were similar in the late adolescents/young adults with BPD (24.2%) and no BPD (21.9%) (10).

The effect of surfactant therapy on rates of asthma in children with BPD is not clear. In an epidemiological study of 384 VLBW children from Wisconsin and Iowa followed to 8 years of age, the rate of reported wheezing fell from 50% to 16% in children with BPD with the introduction of surfactant therapy (43). However, we have not observed a decrease in rates of asthma after the introduction of surfactant; in our regional cohort of ELBW/very preterm children at 8 years of age described above (27), the rates of asthma were 31.7% (32/101) in the BPD group and 27.8% in the no-BPD group (unpublished data). These are higher rates than we have observed before surfactant was available; in the VLBW cohort born in 1977–1982 described above, 16.6% of BPD and 15.5% of non-BPD children had asthma at 8 years of age (unpublished data).

In summary, BPD survivors require more hospital readmissions in the first few years after discharge, predominantly for respiratory reasons, but this is less of a problem as they grow older. Asthma is possibly more frequent in BPD children, but the effects of the new BPD and of surfactant on respiratory health into adulthood remain to be determined.

Summary of Controversies and Respiratory Outcomes

- BPD survivors into late adolescence or early adulthood have substantial reductions in airflow on respiratory function tests.
- Respiratory function in the same subjects with BPD does not change substantially over time.

- Respiratory function at early school age in children who had BPD has probably not changed much between eras with the introduction of exogenous surfactant.
- The effects of cigarette smoking on BPD survivors are not clear, but must remain a concern.
- Hospital readmissions are more common in the first few years after discharge, predominantly for respiratory reasons.
- Asthma is possibly more frequent in BPD children.
- Respiratory function and respiratory health into later life must be determined, not only for those with "old BPD," but also for those with the "new BPD."

NEUROLOGICAL OUTCOMES

Apart from respiratory health, the other major long-term problem for survivors with BPD is adverse neurological outcomes. This is partly because corticosteroids after birth have been one therapy for BPD, and these are known to be neurotoxic (45, 46). On the other hand, BPD without corticosteroids is also associated with adverse neurological outcomes, as outlined in survivors of BPD born before corticosteroids were prescribed widely in the 1970s and early 1980s in a review by Saigal and O'Brodovich (47), and also in other studies (48).

Methodological Issues

Some of the methodological issues relevant to data on respiratory health also apply to synthesizing data on neurological outcomes. These include the balance between certainty in outcomes related to age when assessed versus relevance to contemporary nursery management, the choice of comparison groups, and the differing definitions of BPD in the studies that have reported on long-term neurological outcomes. More specifically, while there has been substantial research exploring the relationship between BPD and later development, most of the studies have been cross-sectional and have employed general outcome measures such as IQ. To date, few studies have adopted a neuropsychological approach, and as such there is limited information on how BPD affects specific cognitive domains. Furthermore, given that BPD often occurs in conjunction with other serious medical complications, the independent effect of BPD is difficult to gauge.

Controversies

The controversies regarding neurological outcomes of BPD are: Are neurosensory problems more common, and, if so, what are they? Are there specific effects of BPD on psychological outcomes, such as attention, language, memory and learning, visual-spatial function, executive skills, academic performance or behavior?

The cognitive, educational and behavioral impairments displayed by children with BPD have been recently reviewed (49), and will be summarized here.

Are Neurosensory Problems more Common in BPD Survivors?

Cerebral palsy occurs more frequently in ELBW (23) or very preterm children (50) than in NBW controls, and is usually even more common in children with BPD. In one study of infants of birthweight < 1500 g, 15% of survivors of BPD, defined as oxygen dependence > 27 days, had cerebral palsy compared with 3–4% in those treated with oxygen for < 28 days (51). In a report from the NICHD Network of 827 infants < 25 weeks born between 1993 and 1999, BPD was a significant risk factor for cerebral palsy at 18–22 months corrected age (odds ratio 1.66, 95% confidence interval 1.01–2.74), after adjustment for other confounding variables such as major intraventricular hemorrhage and cystic periventricular leucomalacia (52). In an overlapping NICHD Network study of births < 33 weeks in 1993–1998, BPD was again a significant independent risk factor for moderate or severe cerebral palsy (53).

Apart from cerebral palsy, a movement disorder specific to infants with BPD has been described, affecting the limbs, neck, trunk and oral-buccal-lingual movements (54). Children with BPD also exhibit poorer fine and gross motor skills than VLBW children without BPD (55, 56).

Blindness and deafness are uncommon events in survivors in recent times. However, other less-severe visual and hearing problems occur more frequently. BPD is a major risk factor for strabismus (57), and is associated with conductive deafness (58).

In summary, BPD is associated with abnormal movement disorders, including cerebral palsy, as well as with less severe visual and auditory problems.

Are there Specific Effects of BPD on Psychological Outcomes?

GENERAL COGNITIVE FUNCTIONING

Children with BPD score lower on tests of early development (59–62). Singer et al. (61) reported that the rate of cognitive and motor delay in a large cohort of VLBW preschoolers with BPD was more than double that of VLBW peers without BPD. Developmental delay is often an early marker for later cognitive deficits, learning disabilities and behavioral problems, but for many children early developmental delay is a reflection of maturational lag and they will eventually catch-up to peers (60). In general, school-aged children with BPD have lower IQs than VLBW children without BPD (56, 63–67), although some studies have failed to find significant differences between groups (55, 68). The mean IQ for school-aged children with BPD generally falls in the low-average range (80–90) (56, 63–67), and the difference in IQ between VLBW children with and without BPD ranges from 1/4 to 2/3 of a standard deviation (56, 64–67). In a recent Australian study, Gray et al. (67) reported that 40% of children with BPD had a full-scale IQ which was more than 1 SD below the normative mean (i.e., IQ < 85), while in another study the rate of children with significant intellectual impairment (i.e. IQ < 70) was reported to be 20% (56).

ATTENTION

There are few reports examining attentional skills in children with BPD. However, there is some evidence to suggest that attentional impairments are more frequent and severe in this high-risk population. Farel et al. (69) recently reported that children with BPD scored lower on an attention composite than non-BPD children, although the group differences failed to reach significance. When they examined the proportion of children who displayed an attentional impairment (i.e. scores > 1 SD below normal expectations) 59% of the BPD sample were classified as having an attentional impairment, significantly greater than VLBW children without BPD (32%). Similarly, on a Continuous Performance Task, Short et al. (56) found BPD children made more errors than controls, suggestive of impaired sustained attention. Consistent with these findings, the rate of ADHD in 8-year-old VLBW children with BPD has been reported to be 15%, double that of non-BPD VLBW children (56). More research is required to determine the impact of BPD on later attention skills; however, the research that has been conducted implies that these children tend to have problems focusing and sustaining attention.

LANGUAGE

Speech and language disorders are more common in preterm children than children born at term (70–72), with impairments more prevalent in children who experience medical complications such as BPD (70). Singer and associates reported that children with BPD at preschool age displayed less-developed receptive and expressive language skills than VLBW children without BPD. In relation to receptive language development 49% of the BPD preschoolers were significantly delayed, while for expressive language 43% were significantly delayed (73). Studies with school-age cohorts have also found receptive language impairments to be more frequent and severe in VLBW children with BPD (63, 69, 74). Furthermore, reduced articulation skills have been described in children with BPD, which may be secondary to a general motor deficit (74). In terms of severity, it has been reported that approximately 15% of children with BPD have a significant receptive language impairment and 9% have a significant expressive language impairment, more than double that of non-BPD VLBW peers (74). Two recent cohort studies have found that approximately 50% of school-aged children with BPD were enrolled in speech-language therapy, in contrast to about 20% of VLBW children without BPD (56, 74).

Thus, there is a strong possibility that children with BPD will display delayed language development, particularly in receptive language skills. Given the lack of long-term outcome studies, it is not clear whether these deficits persist into adolescence and adulthood. However, speech and language problems are common in BPD children during the early school years, which may subsequently compromise the acquisition of early literacy skills and social-emotional development.

MEMORY AND LEARNING

While few studies have specifically assessed memory and learning in children with BPD, there is some indication that these children exhibit memory difficulties that are greater than that associated with prematurity per se. In a study of 17 VLBW children with BPD and 28 non-BPD peers, Farel et al. (69) found that 65% of the BPD group exhibited a memory impairment (> 1 SD below expectations) compared with 29% of the non-BPD group. Further analyses revealed that these children had particular difficulty with immediate auditory memory and working memory. In addition, Taylor et al. (75) found that duration of oxygen requirement was negatively associated with memory and learning; however, in general, these associations were weak and failed to reach statistical significance.

VISUAL-SPATIAL PERCEPTION

Children with BPD perform more poorly on tests of visual-spatial perception than VLBW children without BPD. A number of studies have found children with BPD to perform significantly below VLBW controls on the Developmental Test of Visual-Motor Integration (VMI) (63, 66, 67), suggesting visual-spatial perceptual deficits. Nearly 30% of children with BPD are reported to perform below age expectations on the VMI (67). Consistent with these findings, a longitudinal study by Taylor and colleagues (65, 75) reported an association between perceptual difficulties and BPD. They found elementary school-aged children with BPD had a specific impairment on perceptual motor tasks (65), while a later follow-up (mean age of 16 years) revealed that weeks of oxygen requirement was strongly associated with a number of measures that tap visual-spatial perceptual skills (75), including the VMI, Rey Complex Figure and Judgement of Line Orientation Test.

EXECUTIVE SKILLS

Executive function refers to a collection of inter-related processes responsible for purposeful, goal-directed behavior, and is important in a child's cognitive functioning, behavior, emotional control and social interaction (76). The principal components of executive function include anticipation, goal selection, planning and organization, initiation of activity, self-regulation, mental flexibility, deployment of attention, working memory, and utilization of feedback (77). Executive deficits have been reported in very preterm children (75, 78, 79), but again research examining the long-term effects of BPD on executive functioning is lacking. A study by Taylor et al. (75) found measures of planning ability, mental flexibility, working memory, and self-monitoring to be negatively correlated with duration of oxygen requirement in VLBW children, suggesting that children with BPD may be at increased risk for executive dysfunction.

ACADEMIC PERFORMANCE

Children with a history of BPD have greater school-based problems than those without BPD (55, 56, 63, 66, 67). For example, in a large cohort study Hughes et al. (66) found children with BPD performed significantly below VLBW children without BPD and full-term controls on tests of reading and mathematics. Poorer spelling skills have also been reported in school-aged children with BPD (63). The rate of problems in reading and mathematics has been reported to be as high as 47% (69). Further, it has been reported that children with BPD are more likely to require educational assistance (55, 69), with one study reporting that over 50% of children with BPD were receiving special education services (56).

BEHAVIORAL PROBLEMS

Preterm children who experience medical complications, such as BPD, tend to exhibit more behavioral problems than peers without complications (63, 65). BPD is a strong predictor for attention deficit–hyperactivity disorder ADHD symptoms (56, 63, 69, 80); Farel et al. (69) reported that 75% of their BPD sample exhibited hyperactivity.

Summary of Controversies and Neurological Outcomes

- BPD is an additional risk factor for adverse neurological outcomes.
- BPD is associated with abnormal movement disorders, including cerebral palsy, as well as with less severe visual and auditory problems.
- Children with BPD exhibit low average IQ, academic difficulties, delayed speech and language development, visual-motor integration impairments, and behavior problems.
- There is also some evidence that children with BPD display attention problems, memory and learning deficits and executive dysfunction.
- BPD does not appear to be associated with a specific neuropsychological impairment, but rather a global cognitive impairment.

Effect of Treatment with Postnatal Corticosteroids for BPD on Neurological Outcomes

From the mid-1980s postnatal corticosteroids were increasingly prescribed for prevention or treatment of BPD, supported by evidence of short-term benefits from randomized controlled trials (RCTs), including earlier weaning from mechanical ventilation and a reduction in rates of BPD (81–83). However, corticosteroids have direct toxic effects on the developing brain, including neuronal necrosis, interference with healing and inhibition of brain growth (45, 46). There is little doubt that postnatal corticosteroids can cause cerebral palsy, having been reported to occur more frequently in some individual RCTs (84–86) and meta-analyses of RCTs (81, 87, 88). Reports of the adverse effects of corticosteroids on cerebral palsy are mostly limited to studies where treatment started in the first week of life (81, 87). Moreover, the risk for cerebral palsy from corticosteroids may be outweighed by the risk of BPD causing cerebral palsy in those who are particularly at high risk of cerebral palsy when treatment is started (87). In addition to cerebral palsy postnatal corticosteroids have been associated with other neurological and cognitive deficits (89).

CONCLUSIONS

Subjects with BPD have worse respiratory function and more respiratory ill-health than those of similar size and gestational age who did not have BPD. They also have higher rates of adverse neurological sequelae, only partly because of the additional therapies that they require, such as postnatal corticosteroids. As survival rates of ELBW and very preterm babies are increasing dramatically, with no decrease in the rate of BPD in survivors, the increasing number of children with BPD is going to add to the burden of respiratory and neurological disease into later life. It is clear that reducing the rate of BPD remains one of the biggest challenges in neonatal care today (7).

REFERENCES

1. Kitchen WH, Campbell DG. Controlled trial of intensive care for very low birth weight infants. Pediatrics 1971; 48:711–714.
2. Northway WH, Jr, Rosan RC, Porter DY. Pulmonary disease following respirator therapy of hyaline-membrane disease. Bronchopulmonary dysplasia. N Engl J Med 1967; 276:357–368.
3. Doyle LW, Davis P, Dharmalingam A, Bowman E. Assisted ventilation and survival of extremely low birthweight infants. J Paediatr Child Health 1996; 32:138–142.
4. Eggers TR, Doyle LW, Pepperell RJ. Premature labour. Med J Aust 1979; 1:213–216.
5. Eggers TR, Doyle LW, Pepperell RJ. Premature rupture of the membranes. Med J Aust 1979; 1:209–213.
6. Hibbert ME, Lannigan A, Landau LI, Phelan PD. Lung function values from a longitudinal study of healthy children and adolescents. Pediatr Pulmonol 1989; 7:101–109.
7. Jobe AH, Bancalari E. Bronchopulmonary dysplasia. Am J Respir Crit Care Med 2001; 163:1723–1729.
8. Northway WH, Jr., Moss RB, Carlisle KB, et al. Late pulmonary sequelae of bronchopulmonary dysplasia. N Engl J Med 1990; 323:1793–1799.
9. Halvorsen T, Skadberg BT, Eide GE, et al. Pulmonary outcome in adolescents of extreme preterm birth: a regional cohort study. Acta Paediatr 2004; 93:1294–1300.
10. Doyle LW, Faber B, Callanan C, et al. Bronchopulmonary dysplasia in very low birth weight subjects and lung function in late adolescence. Pediatrics 2006; 118:108–113.
11. Doyle LW, Ford GW, Olinsky A, et al. Bronchopulmonary dysplasia and very low birthweight: lung function at 11 years of age. J Paediatr Child Health 1996; 32:339–343.
12. Doyle LW, Chavasse R, Ford GW, et al. Changes in lung function between age 8 and 14 years in children with birth weight of less than 1,501 g. Pediatr Pulmonol 1999; 27:185–190.
13. Blayney M, Kerem E, Whyte H, O'Brodovich H. Bronchopulmonary dysplasia: improvement in lung function between 7 and 10 years of age. J Pediatr 1991; 118:201–206.
14. Koumbourlis AC, Motoyama EK, Mutich RL, et al. Longitudinal follow-up of lung function from childhood to adolescence in prematurely born patients with neonatal chronic lung disease. Pediatr Pulmonol 1996; 21:28–34.
15. Chan KN, Noble-Jamieson CM, Elliman A, et al. Lung function in children of low birth weight. Arch Dis Child 1989; 64:1284–1293.
16. Kitchen WH, Olinsky A, Doyle LW, et al. Respiratory health and lung function in 8-year-old children of very low birth weight: a cohort study. Pediatrics 1992; 89:1151–1158.
17. McLeod A, Ross P, Mitchell S, et al. Respiratory health in a total very low birthweight cohort and their classroom controls. Arch Dis Child 1996; 74:188–194.
18. Kennedy JD, Edward LJ, Bates DJ, et al. Effects of birthweight and oxygen supplementation on lung function in late childhood in children of very low birth weight. Pediatr Pulmonol 2000; 30:32–40.
19. Siltanen M, Savilahti E, Pohjavuori M, Kajosaari M. Respiratory symptoms and lung function in relation to atopy in children born preterm. Pediatr Pulmonol 2004; 37:43–49.
20. Chan KN, Wong YC, Silverman M. Relationship between infant lung mechanics and childhood lung function in children of very low birthweight. Pediatr Pulmonol 1990; 8:74–81.
21. Doyle LW, Kitchen WH, Ford GW, et al. Outcome to 8 years of infants less than 1000 g birthweight: relationship with neonatal ventilator and oxygen therapy. J Paediatr Child Health 1991; 27:184–188.
22. Gross SJ, Iannuzzi DM, Kveselis DA, Anbar RD. Effect of preterm birth on pulmonary function at school age: a prospective controlled study. J Pediatr 1998; 133:188–192.

23. Doyle LW, and the Victorian Infant Collaborative Study Group. Evaluation of neonatal intensive care for extremely low birth weight infants in Victoria over two decades: I. Effectiveness. Pediatrics 2004; 113:505–509.

24. Gappa M, Berner MM, Hohenschild S, et al. Pulmonary function at school-age in surfactant-treated preterm infants. Pediatr Pulmonol 1999; 27:191–198.

25. Pelkonen AS, Hakulinen AL, Turpeinen M, Hallman M. Effect of neonatal surfactant therapy on lung function at school age in children born very preterm. Pediatr Pulmonol 1998; 25:182–190.

26. Korhonen P, Laitinen J, Hyodynmaa E, Tammela O. Respiratory outcome in school-aged, very-low-birth-weight children in the surfactant era. Acta Paediatr 2004; 93:316–321.

27. Doyle LW, and the Victorian Infant Collaborative Study Group. Respiratory function at age 8–9 years in extremely low birthweight/very preterm children born in Victoria in 1991–92. Pediatr Pulmonol 2006; 41:570–576.

28. Doyle LW, Olinsky A, Faber B, Callanan C. Adverse effects of smoking on respiratory function in young adults born weighing less than 1000 grams. Pediatrics 2003; 112:565–569.

29. Higgins MW, Enright PL, Kronmal RA, et al. Smoking and lung function in elderly men and women. The Cardiovascular Health Study. JAMA 1993; 269:2741–2748.

30. Dockery DW, Speizer FE, Ferris BGJ, et al. Cumulative and reversible effects of lifetime smoking on simple tests of lung function in adults. Am Rev Respir Dis 1988; 137:286–292.

31. Markestad T, Fitzhardinge PM. Growth and development in children recovering from bronchopulmonary dysplasia. J Pediatr 1981; 98:597–602.

32. Astbury J, Orgill AA, Bajuk B, Yu VY. Determinants of developmental performance of very low-birthweight survivors at one and two years of age. Dev Med Child Neurol 1983; 25:709–716.

33. Sauve RS, Singhal N. Long-term morbidity of infants with bronchopulmonary dysplasia. Pediatrics 1985; 76:725–733.

34. Cunningham CK, McMillan JA, Gross SJ. Rehospitalization for respiratory illness in infants of less than 32 weeks' gestation. Pediatrics 1991; 88:527–532.

35. Chye JK, Gray PH. Rehospitalization and growth of infants with bronchopulmonary dysplasia: a matched control study. J Paediatr Child Health 1995; 31:105–111.

36. Furman L, Hack M, Watts C, et al. Twenty-month outcome in ventilator-dependent, very low birth weight infants born during the early years of dexamethasone therapy. J Pediatr 1995; 126:434–440.

37. Furman L, Baley J, Borawski-Clark E, et al. Hospitalization as a measure of morbidity among very low birth weight infants with chronic lung disease. J Pediatr 1996; 128:447–452.

38. Gregoire MC, Lefebvre F, Glorieux J. Health and developmental outcomes at 18 months in very preterm infants with bronchopulmonary dysplasia. Pediatrics 1998; 101:856–860.

39. Chien YH, Tsao PN, Chou HC, et al. Rehospitalization of extremely-low-birth-weight infants in first 2 years of life. Early Hum Dev 2002; 66:33–40.

40. McCormick MC, Workman-Daniels K, Brooks-Gunn J, Peckham GJ. Hospitalization of very low birth weight children at school age. J Pediatr 1993; 122:360–365.

41. Doyle LW, Cheung MM, Ford GW, Olinsky A, Davis NM, Callanan C. Birth weight < 1501 g and respiratory health at age 14. Arch Dis Child 2001; 84:40–44.

42. Ng DK, Lau WY, Lee SL. Pulmonary sequelae in long-term survivors of bronchopulmonary dysplasia. Pediatr Int 2000; 42:603–607.

43. Palta M, Sadek-Badawi M, Sheehy M, et al. Respiratory symptoms at age 8 years in a cohort of very low birth weight children. Am J Epidemiol 2001; 154:521–529.

44. Halvorsen T, Skadberg BT, Eide GE, et al. Characteristics of asthma and airway hyper-responsiveness after premature birth. Pediatr Allergy Immunol 2005; 16:487–494.

45. Taeusch HW, Jr. Glucocorticoid prophylaxis for respiratory distress syndrome: a review of potential toxicity. J Pediatr 1975; 87:617–623.

46. Weichsel ME, Jr. The therapeutic use of glucocorticoid hormones in the perinatal period: potential neurological hazards. Ann Neurol 1977; 2:364–366.

47. Saigal S, O'Brodovich H. Long-term outcome of preterm infants with respiratory disease. Clin Perinatol 1987; 14:635–650.

48. Teberg AJ, Pena I, Finello K, et al. Prediction of neurodevelopmental outcome in infants with and without bronchopulmonary dysplasia. Am J Med Sci 1991; 301:369–374.

49. Anderson PJ, Doyle LW. Neurodevelopmental outcome of bronchopulmonary dysplasia. Semin Fetal Neonatal Med 2006; 30:227–232.

50. Doyle LW, and the Victorian Infant Collaborative Study Group. Neonatal intensive care at border-line viability – is it worth it? Early Hum Dev 2004; 80:103–113.

51. Skidmore MD, Rivers A, Hack M. Increased risk of cerebral palsy among very-low-birthweight infants with chronic lung disease. Dev Med Child Neurol 1990; 32:325–332.

52. Hintz SR, Kendrick DE, Stoll BJ, et al. Neurodevelopmental and growth outcomes of extremely low birth weight infants after necrotizing enterocolitis. Pediatrics 2005; 115:696–703.

53. Vohr BR, Wright LL, Poole WK, McDonald SA. Neurodevelopmental outcomes of extremely low birth weight infants < 32 weeks' gestation between 1993 and 1998. Pediatrics 2005; 116:635–643.

54. Perlman JM, Volpe JJ. Movement disorder of premature infants with severe bronchopulmonary dysplasia: a new syndrome. Pediatrics 1989; 84:215–218.

55. Vohr BR, Coll CG, Lobato D, et al. Neurodevelopmental and medical status of low-birthweight survivors of bronchopulmonary dysplasia at 10 to 12 years of age. Dev Med Child Neurol 1991; 33:690–697.

56. Short EJ, Klein NK, Lewis BA, et al. Cognitive and academic consequences of bronchopulmonary dysplasia and very low birth weight: 8-year-old outcomes. Pediatrics 2003; 112:e359.

57. McGinnity FG, Halliday HL. Perinatal predictors of ocular morbidity in school children who were very low birthweight. Paediatr Perinat Epidemiol 1993; 7:417–425.

58. Gray PH, Sarkar S, Young J, Rogers YM. Conductive hearing loss in preterm infants with bronchopulmonary dysplasia. J Paediatr Child Health 2001; 37:278–282.

59. Goldson E. Severe bronchopulmonary dysplasia in the very low birth weight infant: its relationship to developmental outcome. J Dev Behav Pediatr 1984; 5:165–168.

60. Landry SH, Fletcher JM, Denson SE, Chapieski ML. Longitudinal outcome for low birth weight infants: effects of intraventricular hemorrhage and bronchopulmonary dysplasia. J Clin Exp Neuropsychol 1993; 15:205–218.

61. Singer L, Yamashita T, Lilien L, et al. A longitudinal study of developmental outcome of infants with bronchopulmonary dysplasia and very low birth weight. Pediatrics 1997; 100:987–993.

62. Schmidt B, Asztalos EV, Roberts RS, et al. Impact of bronchopulmonary dysplasia, brain injury, and severe retinopathy on the outcome of extremely low-birth-weight infants at 18 months: results from the trial of indomethacin prophylaxis in preterms. JAMA 2003; 289:1124–1129.

63. Robertson CM, Etches PC, Goldson E, Kyle JM. Eight-year school performance, neurodevelopmental, and growth outcome of neonates with bronchopulmonary dysplasia: a comparative study. Pediatrics 1992; 89:365–372.

64. O'Shea TM, Goldstein DJ, deRegnier RA, et al. Outcome at 4 to 5 years of age in children recovered from neonatal chronic lung disease. Dev Med Child Neurol 1996; 38:830–839.

65. Taylor HG, Klein N, Schatschneider C, Hack M. Predictors of early school age outcomes in very low birth weight children. J Dev Behav Pediatr 1998; 19:235–243.

66. Hughes CA, O'Gorman LA, Shyr Y, et al. Cognitive performance at school age of very low birth weight infants with bronchopulmonary dysplasia. J Dev Behav Pediatr 1999; 20:1–8.

67. Gray PH, O'Callaghan MJ, Rogers YM. Psychoeducational outcome at school age of preterm infants with bronchopulmonary dysplasia. J Paediatr Child Health 2004; 40:114–120.

68. Bohm B, Katz-Salamon M. Cognitive development at 5.5 years of children with chronic lung disease of prematurity. Arch Dis Child Fetal Neonatal Ed 2003; 88:F101–F105.

69. Farel AM, Hooper SR, Teplin SW, et al. Very-low-birthweight infants at seven years: an assessment of the health and neurodevelopmental risk conveyed by chronic lung disease. J Learn Disabil 1998; 31:118–126.

70. Casiro OG, Moddemann DM, Stanwick RS, et al. Language development of very low birth weight infants and fullterm controls at 12 months of age. Early Hum Dev 1990; 24:65–77.

71. Aram DM, Hack M, Hawkins S, et al. Very-low-birthweight children and speech and language development. J Speech Hear Res 1991; 34:1169–1179.

72. Breslau N, Chilcoat H, DelDotto J, et al. Low birth weight and neurocognitive status at six years of age. Biol Psychiatry 1996; 40:389–397.

73. Singer LT, Siegel AC, Lewis B, et al. Preschool language outcomes of children with history of bronchopulmonary dysplasia and very low birth weight. J Dev Behav Pediatr 2001; 22:19–26.

74. Lewis BA, Singer LT, Fulton S, et al. Speech and language outcomes of children with bronchopulmonary dysplasia. J Commun Disord 2002; 35:393–406.

75. Taylor HG, Minich N, Bangert B, et al. Long-term neuropsychological outcomes of very low birth weight: associations with early risks for periventricular brain insults. J Int Neuropsychol Soc 2004; 10:987–1004.

76. Gioia G, Isquith P, Guy S. Assessment of executive functions in children with neurological impairment. In: Simeonsson R, Rosenthal S, eds. Psychological and developmental assessment: children with disabilities and chronic conditions. New York: The Guilford Press; 2001:316–317.

77. Anderson P. Assessment and development of executive function (EF) during childhood. Child Neuropsychol 2002; 8:71–82.

78. Espy KA, Stalets MM, McDiarmid MM, et al. Executive functions in preschool children born preterm: application of cognitive neuroscience paradigms. Neuropsychol Dev Cogn Sect C Child Neuropsychol 2002; 8:83–92.

79. Anderson PJ, Doyle LW, for the Victorian Infant Collaborative Study Group. Executive functioning in school-aged children who were born very preterm or with extremely low birth weight in the 1990s. Pediatrics 2004; 114:50–57.

80. Astbury J, Orgill AA, Bajuk B, Yu VY. Neonatal and neurodevelopmental significance of behaviour in very low birthweight children. Early Hum Dev 1985; 11:113–121.

81. Halliday HL, Ehrenkranz RA, Doyle LW. Early postnatal (< 96 hours) corticosteroids for preventing chronic lung disease in preterm infants (Cochrane Review). In: The Cochrane Library, Issue 1, 2004. Chichester, UK: John Wiley; 2004.

82. Halliday HL, Ehrenkranz RA, Doyle LW. Moderately early (7–14 days) postnatal corticosteroids for preventing chronic lung disease in preterm infants (Cochrane Review). In: The Cochrane Library, Issue 1. Chichester, UK: John Wiley; 2004.

83. Halliday HL, Ehrenkranz RA, Doyle LW. Delayed (> 3 weeks) postnatal corticosteroids for chronic lung disease in preterm infants (Cochrane Review). In: The Cochrane Library, Issue 1, 2004. Chichester, UK: John Wiley; 2004.

84. Yeh TF, Lin YJ, Huang CC, et al. Early dexamethasone therapy in preterm infants: a follow up study. Pediatrics 1998; 101:E7.

85. O'Shea TM, Kothadia JM, Klinepeter KL, et al. Randomized placebo-controlled trial of a 42-day tapering course of dexamethasone to reduce the duration of ventilator dependency in very low birth weight infants: outcome of study participants at 1-year adjusted age. Pediatrics 1999; 104:15–21.

86. Shinwell ES, Karplus M, Reich D, et al. Early postnatal dexamethasone treatment and increased incidence of cerebral palsy. Arch Dis Child Fetal Neonatal Ed 2000; 83:F177–F181.

87. Doyle LW, Halliday HL, Ehrenkranz RA, et al. Impact of postnatal systemic corticosteroids on mortality and cerebral palsy in preterm infants: effect modification by risk of chronic lung disease. Pediatrics 2005; 115:655–661.

88. Barrington KJ. The adverse neuro-developmental effects of postnatal steroids in the preterm infant: a systematic review of RCTs. BMC Pediatr 2001; 1:1.

89. The Victorian Infant Collaborative Study Group. Postnatal corticosteroids and sensorineural outcome at 5 years of age. J Paediatr Child Health 2000; 36:256–261.

Section III

Management of Respiratory Failure

Chapter 14

The Oxygen Versus Room Air Controversy for Neonatal Resuscitation

Peter W. Fowlie MB ChB MSc DRCOG MRCGP
FRCPCH • Hannah Shore MB ChB MRCPCH

Basic Science and Animal Data

The Human Data

Can We Believe What We See Here?

Can We Use This Information Now?

The Potential Clinical Impact

The Way Forward?

Conclusion

Ever since the lay preacher and scientist Joseph Priestley discovered oxygen in the 18th century (1), scientists, health professionals and other "healers" have been extolling its virtues. Given the apparent life-giving properties associated with the use of oxygen, it is not difficult to appreciate how the use of oxygen became inextricably linked with the active resuscitation of collapsed newborn infants, which itself has been described since biblical times (2). Through most of the 20th century, the use of 100% oxygen for the resuscitation of newborn infants has been simply accepted as "best practice": the basic premise has been that by giving high concentrations of oxygen to hypoxic newborn infants, any hypoxic/ischemic damage might be limited. However, the potential for a toxic effect caused by the resulting hyperoxia has recently been postulated. In this chapter we will explore the reasons that have led to a more critical review of the use of 100% oxygen as part of newborn resuscitation. We will then describe and discuss the clinical evidence that has accumulated in recent years that might well question what has been accepted for years as "best practice."

BASIC SCIENCE AND ANIMAL DATA

There are a variety of mechanisms that help to explain the potential toxicity associated with hyperoxia resulting from the acute resuscitation of "flat" or asphyxiated newborn infants using 100% oxygen. Free radical damage is most commonly cited along with potential changes in cerebral blood flow, including "reperfusion" injury.

Free radicals were first described in the 1960s: reduction of oxygen in the respiratory chain of mitochondria gives rise to the formation of free radicals via the nicotinamide adenosine dinucleotide phosphate (NADPH) oxidase and xanthene oxidase pathways. Initially, free radicals were not felt to be involved in biological processes due to their reactivity but the discovery of superoxide dismutase suggested that, as well as being potentially toxic, they may have a vital role to play in many key biological processes (3). For example, free radicals appear to be essential in antimicrobial function, especially within macrophages and neutrophils that contain NADPH oxidase, and they are also present in certain endothelial cells, thus contributing to the integrity of the blood-brain barrier. Usually, only about 5% of the oxygen passing through the respiratory chain forms free radicals and this is controlled well by antioxidant systems, especially glutathione. However, toxic effects may occur if this mechanism gets saturated.

Free radicals exert some of their detrimental effect through peroxidation of lipid within cell membranes leading to increased microvascular permeability, oedema, inflammation and cell death. The normal function of membrane receptors, enzymes and ion channels may also be disturbed. In addition while nitric oxide in low concentrations is a useful biological agent involved in cellular signaling and regulation of vascular tone, in higher quantities it reacts with the superoxide radical to form the highly toxic molecule peroxynitrite (4). Free radicals are also known to affect the expression of genes controlling antioxidant pathways. Depolarization of the mitochondrial membrane follows loss of control of these pathways, releasing cytochrome c and a rush of pro-inflammatory cytokines. This leads to uncontrolled apoptosis and the start of cell death (5).

Different cells demonstrate varying responses to free radical insult. Although this is primarily related to the amount of antioxidants present, the response is also affected by other factors. For example, superoxide radicals will react with free iron resulting in the hydroxyl radical via the Fenton reaction. This reaction occurs preferentially in oligodendrocytes, as these cells possess significant amounts of free iron, thus explaining one possible mechanism accounting for white matter damage. Premature infants appear to be at an especially high risk of this mechanism of injury as their antioxidant defenses are immature and consequently less effective (6).

There is a range of recognized animal models depicting hypoxic/ischemic injury and hyperoxic insult. These models involve different techniques to induce the clinical scenario to be replicated and use a range of animal species. The rat pup at birth is the equivalent to a 26-week-gestation infant in terms of retinal and neurological development. Each day in the life of a rat pup is equivalent to 1.3 weeks in a human and by day 14 of life the rat pup is therefore comparable to a post-term infant. A newborn piglet brain, however, is comparable, histologically and electrophysiologically, to a human infant between 36 and 38 weeks gestation (7). The precise age of the animal used in such studies should therefore be considered when assessing the potential implications for the newborn human.

Hypoxic/ischemic insults and hyperoxic states can be generated in a number of ways. Animals can be rendered hypoxic by ventilation in 8% oxygen for varying periods, with some models inducing bilateral pneumothoraces to provide a more acute insult. When brain injury is to be studied, ischemia has been induced by occlusion of one of the common carotid arteries. This has the advantage of allowing administration of a unilateral insult, which enables a comparison to be made between the hemispheres of the brain.

Hyperoxic states can be created simply by placing animals in chambers of varying amounts of pure oxygen. Experiments can be run over many hours but usually no more than 48 h, in order to allow the adult female who is suckling the young to recover. Constant levels of hyperoxia induced in this way may not be relevant to current neonatal clinical practice, however, as clinicians will tend to alter the amount of oxygen given to a neonate on the basis of perceived clinical need. An alternative model of hyperoxia developed in Edinburgh relies on a more "physiological" oxygen profile that precisely mimics the actual inspired oxygen profile of infants born at 26 weeks who subsequently develop retinopathy of prematurity (8). In addition, a hyperoxic state sustained over many hours, however created, might not best mimic the relatively brief hyperoxic state likely to be induced during acute resuscitation, and the effect of shorter exposures has also been explored.

A variety of outcome measures have been used in animal (and human) studies examining the effect of hyperoxia after a period of hypoxia/ischemia. Common biochemical markers found in blood, cerebrospinal fluid or in tissue sections include glutathione (a natural antioxidant), oxidized glutathione (an end product of free radical damage), nitric oxide synthase (an enzyme that is induced at times of injury to increase the formation of nitric oxide which, in return, reacts with the superoxide radical to form the highly reactive peroxynitrite) and nitrotyrosine (the end product of the free-radical-induced injury caused by peroxynitrite). Less specific biochemical markers of "stress" such as acid base balance, PaO_2, and $PaCO_2$ can also be studied along with physiological parameters such as heart rate, mean arterial blood pressure and cerebral blood flow. Scoring schemes have been used to assess the general behavior and neurological outcome of study subjects following hyperoxic insult. Pathological outcomes are also used when animals are sacrificed at the end of the experiment. Post-mortem examination of tissue can quantify the extent of cell death. More specific immuno-cytochemistry can be performed to identify the presence of products from free radical reactions (e.g. nitrotyrosine) or to highlight specific neuronal cell damage such as the reduction in myelin basic protein expression in damaged white matter or the presence of glial fibrillary acid protein in reactive asytrocytosis.

Exposure to hyperoxia over a prolonged period of time is associated with adverse effects in animal models (Fig. 14-1). In rat pups exposed to increasing concentrations of oxygen over increasing exposure times, cell death was seen in brains exposed for just 2 h (9, 10). Levels of nitric oxide synthase, an enzyme essential for the production of the potent free radical peroxynitrite, were also shown to rise in the brain. This finding was in keeping with the significant increase in free radical damage seen on pathological examination of the hyperoxic brains. Prolonged hyperoxia (hours) may not mimic the far briefer exposure times occurring during active resuscitation, however, and the effect of briefer exposure to hyperoxia (minutes) needs to be reviewed as well.

In the early 1990s, Poulsen et al. found no difference in physiological parameters and in markers of hypoxic injury (hypoxanthine, xanthene and uric acid) in pigs rendered hypoxic and then resuscitated in room air or 100% oxygen. However, PaO_2 was grossly elevated in the group resuscitated with 100% oxygen (11). Temesvari and Karg then showed that in piglets rendered hypoxic by inducing a pneumothorax, neurological outcome was significantly worse in those resuscitated with 100% oxygen compared to those resuscitated in air (7). A few years later, using a more relevant model of a shortened resuscitation period, Solas et al. compared 5 and 20 min at 100% oxygen against room air following an hypoxic/ischemic insult induced in piglets. Again there was no difference between the groups in terms of biochemical and physiological markers of hypoxic/ischemic damage but again PaO_2 was grossly elevated in the groups resuscitated with 100% oxygen (12). The same group went on to examine oxidative stress in piglet brains that had been exposed to hypoxia and subsequently resuscitated with either 21% or 100% oxygen for 30 min and showed a significant increase in the amount of glycerol present in the brains of those resuscitated in 100% oxygen along with a reduced antioxidant capacity (13).

The gut has also been studied in relation to hypoxic/ischemic recovery and hyperoxic damage in a piglet model developed to test the hypothesis that the pathogenesis of necrotizing enterocolitis is related to hypoxia/reperfusion injury leading to the formation of free radicals. A significant increase in blood flow to the gut, evidence of tissue damage, and also an increase in the biochemical markers of

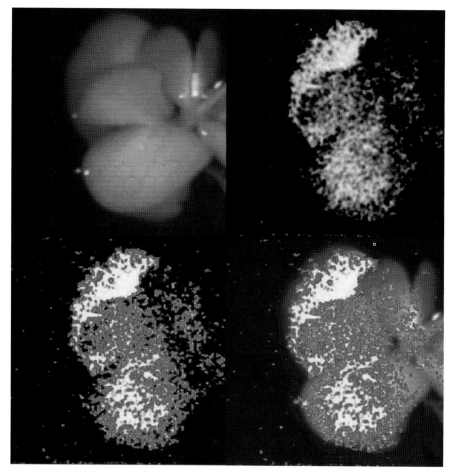

Figure 14-1 Free oxygen radical formation (detected by means of the chemiluminescence) in rat liver subjected to oxidative stress. With permission from Prof. A Roda (www.anchem.unibo.it/.../ Gallery/Gallery13.htm).

oxidative processes were seen in those piglets resuscitated in higher concentrations of oxygen as compared to those resuscitated in room air. As well as the damage increasing in accordance with the increase in oxygen concentration, there was also a greater reduction in the presence of antioxidants found when the higher concentrations of oxygen were used (14).

The animal data exploring the effect of hypoxia/ischemia tend to show little difference in markers of hypoxic/ischemic damage whether the animal is resuscitated in room air or is exposed to hyperoxic "resuscitation" either over several hours or over shorter periods that may be more akin to the acute clinical situation. The data do, however, suggest even brief exposure to higher concentrations of oxygen is associated with significantly raised PaO_2, leading to reduced antioxidant capacity and increased risk of exposure to toxic levels of free radicals. This supports the hypothesis that resuscitation in higher concentrations of oxygen may increase the potential for hyperoxic damage in the face of little or no perceived benefit in terms of hypoxic/ischemic recovery.

THE HUMAN DATA

In neonatology, we need look no further than the 1950s for perhaps one of the clearest and most dramatic clinical examples of oxygen toxicity and its devastating effects. The well-meaning but overzealous use of oxygen in treating apnoeic/cyanosed infants led to the explosion of retrolental fibroplasias, causing significant visual impairment in huge numbers of surviving preterm and otherwise vulnerable newborn infants (15). This "epidemic" could arguably have been prevented by a more rigorous and methodical evaluation of the therapy long before it was accepted into routine practice. In the clinical situation under scrutiny here, the resuscitation of human newborns in 100% oxygen could potentially result in a sudden burst in availability of oxygen due to both its high concentration of administration and the reperfusion that occurs following the initial hypoxic/ischemic insult. Could this sudden brief period of hyperoxia overwhelm antioxidant defenses, even in a term infant, and potentially lead to free-radical-related damage? Could this be another example of well-meaning clinicians inadvertently causing more harm than good?

A number of well-conducted observational studies provide human data supporting this worrying hypothesis – that hyperoxia may be associated with adverse outcome. In both preterm and term infants, hyperoxia has been associated with disrupted cerebral blood flow (16) which is clearly associated with white matter injury and germinal matrix hemorrhage (17). Mortola et al. prospectively examined ventilatory responses to hyperoxia in healthy newborn infants exposed to room air ventilation and 100% oxygen for 5 min each and showed that hyperoxia led to an increase in minute ventilation, thereby increasing the infants' oxygen consumption by 25% and carbon dioxide production by 17% (18). And in a retrospective study using data recorded between 1985 and 1995 on all asphyxiated babies admitted to one tertiary neonatal unit in Toronto, Klinger et al. concluded that hyperoxemia led to a 3-fold increase in adverse neurological outcome (19). In addition to these observational studies that examine short-term effects of hyperoxia, longer-term effects of hyperoxia have been postulated with two large retrospective case control studies from Sweden and the USA, suggesting that exposure to oxygen during the immediate post-natal period may as much as double the chances of an infant developing childhood leukemia or malignancy (20, 21).

The strength or validity of the data from non-randomized observational studies is perhaps limited by the potential for the findings to be biased (22). As a result, it has been proposed that clinical questions exploring the effects of any given "intervention" should, if possible, be addressed using the most appropriate robust methodology, namely the randomized clinical trial (23). Although the clinical situation relevant here – the acute resuscitation of "flat" or asphyxiated newborn infants – throws up enormous practical and ethical challenges (Box 14-1), a number of determined individuals have endeavored to conduct appropriate clinical trials in order to provide more robust evidence (see Appendix).

Box 14-1   *Issues around Clinical Trials Exploring the Resuscitation of "Flat" Newborn Infants*

- Is it ever ethical to conduct an "experiment" in a life-and-death situation?
- Can meaningful informed consent ever be obtained in such situations and if so when should it be taken?
- How might the "asphyxiated" or "flat" newborn infant be defined and how would inclusion criteria be assessed in the acute setting?
- Can patients ever be "randomized" during acute life-threatening episodes and if so when should they be assigned?
- Can carers and those assessing outcomes to such interventions remain blind to treatment allocation?
- What are the clinically important outcomes to measure and will these outcomes be viewed in the same way by parents as they are by clinicians?

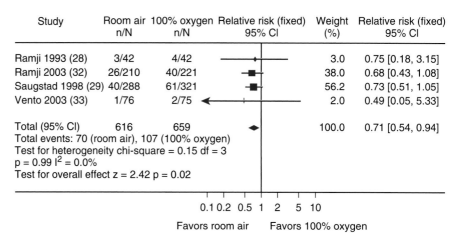

Study	Room air n/N	100% oxygen n/N	Relative risk (fixed) 95% CI	Weight (%)	Relative risk (fixed) 95% CI
Ramji 1993 (28)	3/42	4/42		3.0	0.75 [0.18, 3.15]
Ramji 2003 (32)	26/210	40/221		38.0	0.68 [0.43, 1.08]
Saugstad 1998 (29)	40/288	61/321		56.2	0.73 [0.51, 1.05]
Vento 2003 (33)	1/76	2/75		2.0	0.49 [0.05, 5.33]
Total (95% CI)	616	659		100.0	0.71 [0.54, 0.94]

Total events: 70 (room air), 107 (100% oxygen)
Test for heterogeneity chi-square = 0.15 df = 3
p = 0.99 I^2 = 0.0%
Test for overall effect z = 2.42 p = 0.02

0.1 0.2 0.5 1   2   5 10

Favors room air   Favors 100% oxygen

Figure 14-2 Mortality in relation to air vs. 100% oxygen for resuscitation. With permission from: Tan A, Schulze A, O'Donnell CP, et al. Air versus oxygen for resuscitation of infants at birth. Cochrane Database Syst Rev 2005; (2):CD002273.

There are at least three published systematic reviews examining the use of room air versus 100% oxygen for resuscitating "asphyxiated" newborn infants (24–26). Currently the Cochrane Review (25) and the review appearing in the Lancet (24) are essentially the same review published in different media (27). Although in due course the Cochrane Review is likely to be updated as new data become available, for the moment there are therefore in essence just two systematic reviews, both conducted rigorously, available for scrutiny.

On the basis of well over 1000 infants contributing data from the various trials, both reviews suggest that there is a clear and important reduction in death rate by perhaps as much as 30% when air is used for initial resuscitation rather than 100% oxygen (Fig. 14-2). One of the reviews (26) was conducted by three researchers who, with others, have led most of the clinical trial work in this area. They had access to much of the original trial data and were therefore able to conduct several sub-group analyses including looking for potential differences between any effect(s) seen in preterm vs. term infants and any relationship between treatment effect(s) and the severity of asphyxia. It is suggested that the apparent reduction in mortality favoring the use of air is seen across both term and preterm infants: OR (95% confidence interval) for death in term infants = 0.59 (0.40, 0.87); OR for preterm infants = 0.51 (0.28, 0.90). In more severely asphyxiated infants, Apgar score < 4, the mortality rate was the same regardless of resuscitation gas used. (Note that since the individual trials did not randomize babies on the basis of gestation or severity of asphyxia, it is not clear how the authors conducted these subgroup analyses and the results should perhaps be interpreted with caution.)

Even in rigorously conducted systematic reviews, the *interpretation* of the data and any *conclusions* drawn depend heavily on the quality of the individual studies included in the review. We must therefore explore the likely validity of the data arising from the individual studies and the study profiles in order to determine the generalizability of the results to populations other than the study populations.

The first published human data arising from a randomized clinical trial appeared in 1993 (28). Ramji and his colleagues carried out their study at Maudlana Azad Medical College in New Delhi. Infants with a heart rate less than 80 beats per min and/or apnea at birth were randomized on an "even versus odd" date basis to be resuscitated with either air or 100% oxygen. Those being resuscitated in air could switch to 100% oxygen if it was felt clinically indicated because of lack of response to air. The primary outcomes assessed were 5 min Apgar and heart rate at 5 min (itself a part of the Apgar score). Secondary outcomes presented included other physiological variables at 10 and 30 min along with some basic neurological outcomes at 28 days. Observers recording the outcomes were not blinded to the intervention received. The study was powered to detect a difference between the groups of 1 point in the mean Apgar score at 5 min.

Eighty-four infants were enrolled. It is not possible to determine what proportion was preterm but the mean gestational age at birth was 38 weeks. Only 50% of mothers had received any antenatal care. In keeping with the trial entry criteria indicating "asphyxia," the infants were significantly acidotic at birth, with an average cord pH of 7.16 and base deficit of 15 mmol/L in the infants receiving air and an average cord pH of 7.17 and base deficit of 13 mmol/L in those receiving 100% oxygen. Six of 42 infants (14%) originally receiving air switched to receive 100% oxygen during the resuscitation.

No differences were found between the groups in either the primary outcome or any of the secondary outcomes measured. Mean 5 min Apgar score in both groups was 7, with a heart rate around 140 beats per min. A total of 7 infants died (8%), three in the group initially receiving air.

In 1998, Saugstad and his colleagues published the results of "The Resair 2" study (29). This multicenter study was conducted in the mid 1990s in 10 centers in 6 countries spread across Europe and South East Asia. Efforts were again made to define the "asphyxiated" newborn by stipulating virtually the same entry criteria as Ramji et al. (28). Infants were again similarly randomized on the basis of birth date and the study was again not blinded. The primary outcome measure in this study, however, was death within the first week of life and/or hypoxic ischemic encephalopathy (HIE). Multiple acute physiological variables were recorded as secondary outcomes. A proportion of the original study group was assessed for evidence of neurodisability at 18–24 months of age (30).

Six hundred and nine babies were included in the overall analysis. Median gestational age was 38 weeks with a range of 27–44 weeks, about a quarter being preterm in total. Over half the infants enrolled were born in Indian centers. About a quarter of those infants originally assigned to receive room air switched to being given 100% oxygen during the resuscitation.

There was no statistically significant difference between the groups in terms of the primary outcome measure, death within first week and/or HIE. One hundred and two infants of 601 survivors at the end of the first week showed signs of HIE (17%, no statistical difference between groups). One hundred and one babies died within the first 28 days (17%, no significant difference between groups) although none of the 33 infants enrolled in European countries failed to survive. A few of the multiple secondary physiological outcome measures reached statistical significance but it is arguable whether any of the differences detected were clinically important.

Seven out of the original 11 centers participated in the 18–24 month neurological follow-up and only about two-thirds of the original cohort (213/591) of babies contributed data (30). Examiners were not blinded to treatment allocation and a pragmatic clinical examination was used rather than any objective tools or measures of neurological impairment or development. There was no statistically significant difference in terms of motor or sensory impairment between the groups; nor was there any statistically significant difference between the rates of cerebral palsy (10% air vs. 7% oxygen, odds ratio 1.38, 95% confidence interval 0.52–3.62) or "abnormal development" (15% air vs. 10% oxygen, odds ratio 1.67, 95% confidence interval 0.73–3.80).

In 2001, Vento and his colleagues in Spain published the results of their randomized clinical trial conducted in the Hospital Virgen del Consuelo in Valencia (31). This was a small study of 40 "asphyxiated" term infants. The definition of "asphyxia" (and thereby the entry criteria) was again similar to earlier studies using clinical findings such as bradycardia and non-responsive apnea but also included umbilical cord gas criteria. The randomization procedure appears to have been concealed and carers/researchers blinded to treatment allocation. (A "control" group of non-asphyxiated infants was included to allow potential biochemical markers of asphyxia to be explored.) No primary outcome was stipulated and the results of multiple surrogate physiological markers of acute recovery (Apgar scores, onset of first cry etc.) were presented along with a variety of biochemical indices (blood gas parameters, blood glutathione and erythrocyte antioxidant enzyme levels). Clinical neurological examination, cranial ultrasound and electroencephalogram findings at 28 days were also presented.

Forty out of 245 eligible infants were enrolled. None of the babies was preterm. Average birth weight was 3.3 kg. Mean arterial pH at birth (umbilical artery) was 7.11 in the infants resuscitated using room air and 7.09 in those resuscitated using 100% oxygen. The median 1 min Apgar score in each group was 4. There was no statistically significant difference found in any of the outcomes presented. None of the babies died.

Two years after Vento's results appeared, Ramji and his colleagues published the results of a four-center study in India conducted in the mid 1990s (32). "Asphyxiated" infants weighing over 1000 g were randomized on an odd/even date basis. Treatment allocation was not blinded. The study was powered to detect a difference of 1 in the 5 min Apgar score, the primary outcome measure. Secondary outcomes included mortality and HIE.

Four hundred and thirty-one babies were reported on. Mean birthweight in both groups was around 2.5 kg and mean gestation around 38 weeks. Thirty-nine percent of the infants initially resuscitated in room air "switched" to be resuscitated in 100% oxygen. (The authors point out, however, that a similar number of infants in the group starting off in the 100% oxygen group also met the criteria for "failed resuscitation.") The median 5 min Apgar score was 7 in both groups (no statistical difference) and no differences could be detected in any of the secondary outcomes examined. Mortality was around 12% in the infants resuscitated in air vs. around 18% in those resuscitated using 100% oxygen (odds ratio 0.64, 95% confidence interval 0.36–1.13).

In 2003 Vento published a clinical trial (33) very similar in methodology used to the one he and his colleagues reported in 2001. In this case, however, the aim appears to have been to explore the relationship between the duration of resuscitation in 100% oxygen and the degree of oxidative stress as defined by recognized biochemical markers. Some clinical data are available, however.

The trial was randomized on the basis of concealed random-number generation. Of 151 term "asphyxiated" infants who were eligible for inclusion, 106 were enrolled. The babies studied weighed on average just over 3 kg.

Apgar scores were similar between those infants resuscitated in air compared to those receiving 100% oxygen. The time elapsed to first cry was shorter in the air group by around 30 s, as was the time to spontaneous sustained respiration shorter by about 90 s. Although these differences were both statistically significant it is less certain how clinically important they might be, given that no clinical data on mortality or longer-term morbidity were presented other than a statement suggesting that "follow-up studies at the end of the first week of life and 4 weeks of age did not reveal any differences between either experimental groups."

More recently, Bajaj and his colleagues reported a randomized trial enrolling over 200 "asphyxiated" infants weighing more than 1000 g (34). The study was carried out in a single tertiary center in Mumbai, India, in 2001–02. The definition of "asphyxia" and the interventions used were very similar to those used in the previous trials described but the primary endpoint was a composite outcome – hypoxic ischemic encephalopathy and/or death. The mean birthweight of the infants was around 2.4 kg with an associated average gestation of around 37 weeks. There was no difference seen in the primary outcome in those resuscitated in air compared to those resuscitated in 100% oxygen. Just over 40% of babies in each group had either HIE or died – OR = 0.92 (95% CI 0.52–1.60). This study also reported on "asphyxial related mortality" and again found no difference between the groups – OR = 0.79 (95% CI 0.29–2.14). More of the infants initially resuscitated in room air had an "abnormal neurological examination at discharge" although the difference did not reach statistical significance (20% vs. 14%, $P = 0.60$).

Another recent paper described a randomized clinical trial, conducted in a UK tertiary center, that explored the potential difference in using 50% oxygen as the resuscitation gas compared with 100% oxygen in premature infants (less than 31 weeks gestation) along with other different resuscitation practices by using a factorial design (35). The primary outcome measures were inflammatory markers – cytokines IL6, IL10 and IL1ß and tumor necrosis factor in bronchoalveolar lavage, but secondary outcome measures included major neonatal morbidities such as bronchopulmonary dysplasia, retinopathy of prematurity, patent ductus arteriosus and cranial ultrasound abnormality. There were no significant differences in levels of inflammatory markers or in rates of the clinical outcomes between the two groups, although this small study (52 infants) was probably relatively under-powered to detect differences in any of the clinical outcomes.

CAN WE BELIEVE WHAT WE SEE HERE?

There is clearly an amount of evidence to consider here. However, in recent years, when trial data have been discussed, greater emphasis has been placed on the critical assessment of how clinical trials are conducted. This is based on the understanding that "flawed" methodology may skew study results in one direction or the other. If such bias is perceived, it is sometimes possible to predict in which direction the bias might affect the results: indeed there is some empirical evidence that certain methodological threats to the validity of the data tend to inflate the effect of any treatment under consideration (36). However, it is clear that it is not always possible to determine the direction of any potential bias let alone quantify its impact.

One of the main potential threats to the validity of clinical trial data is failed randomization or more particularly failure to conceal the randomization process. This is because of theoretical and some empirical evidence that this leads to selection bias by unequally assigning patients with certain characteristics to one group or another (37). In the quasi-randomized trials that used birth date to determine treatment group, it can be argued that it would clearly be possible to determine which group – air or 100% oxygen – any given baby would be entered into. This would only be important if certain infants, e.g. particularly sick infants, were deliberately not entered into the trial on the basis of whether air or oxygen was being used that day. There is not much evidence of this happening in that the data presented from all the clinical trials show that the numbers in each group are appropriately similar (the authors who reported the quasi-randomized trials even explained that because there are more odd dates than even dates, the numbers are not likely to be the same in each group) and baseline characteristics that have been assessed are similar between the groups. In addition, analyses within one of the systematic reviews of this evidence (25) did not detect any significant heterogeneity between the results to date from trials using different methods of randomization. We believe the randomization procedures used in this series of clinical trials, including the quasi-randomization method based on birth date, are unlikely to threaten the validity of the results to a significant extent.

If the treatment group to which an individual baby has been assigned is known to carers or those assessing outcomes, i.e. the trial is not sufficiently blinded, it is again possible that the babies in the different treatment groups will be treated differently or the outcomes assessed differently. This again therefore has the potential to introduce bias. Although some of the studies were unblinded, it is again hard to see how this might bias results in the case of physiological data that are measured automatically or electronically and we would have to argue against any purists who might suggest that clinicians would subsequently care for infants differently (either knowingly or unwittingly) depending on whether they received oxygen or air during resuscitation to such an extent that it might impact on survival chances or neurological outcome. It would seem unlikely therefore, though not impossible, that lack of blinding would lead to significant bias in the trials under consideration here.

Outcome data are available for the vast majority of the babies, although in the one trial providing longer-term neurodevelopmental follow-up data (30) there was significant loss to follow-up, which might lead to biased or inaccurate results for this outcome (38). Even then, the proportion of infants lost to follow-up was similar in each group and baseline characteristics of those assessed were similar, perhaps making it harder to completely discount these data.

Certain statistical analyses of trial data can provide empirical evidence of potential bias, but assessing the validity of trial data is still to a large extent an inexact science and an element of personal judgment has to come into any final assessment. We believe that on the whole the data available are remarkably robust. It is difficult to determine in which direction any methodological issues might bias the results and even then we think the risk of significant bias is relatively low. We must now explore whether or not these data can be extrapolated to the wider clinical arena and whether or not they are clinically important.

CAN WE USE THIS INFORMATION NOW?

Let us assume that we do "believe" the trial data and want to consider a move to using air instead of 100% oxygen for resuscitation. We must then ask whether, if the same intervention were to be used in our own clinical setting, we would see the same effect(s)

First let us consider whether or not we could ever hope to replicate the intervention described in the trial protocol(s) within the "real-life" clinical setting. At first glance, this issue is clearly easy. Right across the world we could all stop using 100% oxygen tomorrow and, where no oxygen is available, we could be reassured that we have been doing the right thing all along. However on closer scrutiny, in all trials to date the intervention assessed has been 100% oxygen versus ambient air *with oxygen backup* with up to 1/4 of the study infants switching to back-up 100% oxygen. While a reduced reliance on oxygen may be justified, these data cannot begin to support the wholesale abandonment of oxygen being available at birth. The potential applicability and impact therefore in resource-poor countries, where there may not be access to oxygen in the first place, may be limited and many other factors such as antenatal care, intrapartum care and basic resuscitation skill may be far more important than the availability or otherwise of oxygen.

Next, are the babies described in the trials and the condition of interest likely to be similar in all clinical settings? The definition of "asphyxia" is always difficult but in all the trials to date we believe that a perfectly reasonable pragmatic approach has been taken to enrolling appropriate babies. We must all recognize the blue, floppy baby who simply lies on the resuscitaire making no attempt to breath and who is bradycardic. The babies may in some of the trials be a bit smaller than those we see but otherwise are similar to those we see every day on the labor ward.

The available data come from a variety of clinical settings in Europe, North Africa and South East Asia, with a significant proportion of the babies enrolled in Indian hospitals. While many of these settings may in some ways be different to our own labor wards in the UK and elsewhere, the real issue is whether or not "asphyxiated" infants in these countries will respond to resuscitation, and in particular this intervention, differently to the babies we see. We would argue that this is unlikely. Despite possible differences in antenatal care and intrapartum care, the physiological events occurring will be the same across the world and the babies seen in other settings will respond similarly.

However, even though a number of preterm infants are included in the trial data available, it is difficult to tease them out from the term infants and, despite the data presented in Saugstad et al.'s review (26), we believe that extreme caution is needed before beginning to consider this issue beyond term infants at present. There may well be different physiological adaptations at work and the "flat" preterm infant may not be the same as the "asphyxiated" term baby.

THE POTENTIAL CLINICAL IMPACT

Having considered issues of validity and generalizability, can we estimate the size of any treatment effect globally? The pooled estimate for reducing mortality found within the meta-analyses (24–26) suggests that perhaps 20 babies would need to be treated to save one additional life were we to move away from 100% oxygen (Number Needed to Treat (NNT) = 20). This would on the face of it seem to be a very powerful treatment. However, the NNT is dependent on the background incidence of the outcome of interest, here death. The overall mortality rate in the trial data is around 15%. This may be higher for a number of reasons than in other countries and settings and indeed the mortality in the Spanish study (31) is around 3.5%. This then will impact on the potential benefit of changing to air in these countries where the risk of dying from asphyxia might be less. However, if the babies themselves are similar and the "asphyxial" process and degree of "asphyxia" examined are similar there would seem to be no reason why these data cannot be extrapolated to other settings, albeit that the impact of any change in policy might vary. It could be argued that a change away from the use of 100% oxygen has the potential to save many hundreds of thousands of lives across the world.

Even in settings where the potential impact in terms of improved survival might be relatively small, this arguably only becomes an issue if the intervention is hugely expensive in terms of available resource (financial or otherwise) or if there are "adverse" outcomes that need to be balanced against the main benefits of the intervention. In this case, "asphyxia" is so common even in resource-rich countries that even a small effect would have a huge impact, and the "treatment" is "cheap" however it is looked at. There may, however, be another significant "adverse" outcome to consider in relation to long-term neurodevelopment.

We believe the biggest problem that prevents an immediate wholesale change to resuscitation practice is the lack of longer-term neurodevelopmental follow-up data. This would not be a particular problem if we could be assured that neurodevelopmental outcome mirrored survival data. Indeed, without further consideration, it may seem intuitive that if babies are not as likely to die when air is used, the damaging "asphyxial" process must be being interrupted and if that same "asphyxial process" is associated with brain damage in the longer term then surely the longer term neurodevelopmental outcome will be improved? But we would urge extreme caution here. There may be significant dissociation between acute outcomes around the time of birth and longer-term outcomes, particularly if the biological and physiological mechanisms at work are different (39). Indeed, there is a growing body of evidence that the duration of the "asphyxia" leading up to delivery varies enormously and that in a significant proportion of cases may have been going on for days or even weeks before delivery (40). A proportion of these babies will therefore have sustained significant irreversible damage long before

Table 14-1	Long-Term Neurodevelopmental Outcome Data are Limited		
Outcome	Air (n = 91)	100% oxygen (n = 122)	Odds ratio (95% confidence interval)
Cerebral palsy	10%	7%	1.38 (0.52–3.62)
"Abnormal development" at 18–24 months	15%	10%	1.67 (0.73–3.80)

From Saugstad et al. (30).

delivery and it becomes harder to accept that an acute intervention at the time of birth that might impact on survival might then have an impact on long-term neurodevelopmental outcome. When the possibility of "independent" hyperoxic damage is added to this model when 100% oxygen is used as part of acute resuscitation, the outcome in terms of disability-free survival becomes even harder to predict. Resuscitation initially with room air might limit the risk of death caused by hyperoxic pathology, but if these babies were already "brain-damaged" might we not then increase the number of babies (and families) growing up with significant neurodevelopmental disability/handicap?

The only long-term outcome data that are available come from a single study (30). The data are incomplete and neurodevelopmental outcome was clearly regarded as a secondary outcome. We believe, however, that since these are the only longer-term follow-up data available, they cannot be completely ignored when examining the overall picture of this proposed intervention – air for initial resuscitation.

The available data do not reach statistical significance (Table 14-1). This in itself is not surprising, since the study was not originally powered to detect differences in neurodevelopmental outcomes. The data do, however, point toward increased disability in those surviving infants who were resuscitated initially *in air*, and if the direction and size of effect seen here were to be confirmed in larger follow-up studies the use of room air would result in a huge increase in asphyxiated babies surviving with neurodisability and handicap.

Could this all suggest that by using 100% oxygen, we are inadvertently "killing" babies because of the impact of free radical damage etc. but that a proportion of these babies may have been destined to be disabled/handicapped? Choosing the "better" intervention under these circumstances will not be straightforward. Using an intervention that "kills" vulnerable babies (by using 100% oxygen for resuscitation) is an uncomfortable concept, while increased survival at the "expense" of increased rates of disability in those babies surviving (by using room air for initial resuscitation?) cannot automatically be regarded as "improved" outcome. How these options might be viewed might depend on how individuals and societies across the world view disability. If this finding was to be confirmed in larger follow-up studies – an increase in asphyxiated babies surviving with neurodisability and handicap following the use of room air for resuscitation – it would need to be acknowledged and taken into consideration by clinicians, health service managers and the public when planning future health service provision.

THE WAY FORWARD?

There is definite equipoise here. We do not believe it is possible to say at present which is the better treatment for "flat" term infants, and further trials are needed. Indeed it could be argued that we are behaving unethically as a profession if we do not explore this further given the potential consequences for so many babies and their families. The concern about increased disability in survivors needs to be confirmed (or refuted) and the size of any effect assessed more accurately. Further pragmatic trials could use a similar broad clinical definition of "asphyxia" along the lines used in the trials conducted to date. A variety of settings – "resource-rich" vs. "resource-poor" countries, primary/secondary/tertiary care centers – might also add to the external validity of any future data. Although subdividing infants on the basis of the possible cause or severity of the asphyxial insult may not be practical, a clear distinction between preterm and term infants needs to be made. Disability-free survival must be seen as the main primary outcome and trials should be powered to detect clinically important differences in rates of disability/handicap. Concealed randomization is theoretically more robust than quasi-randomized methods but is also practically more difficult. Given the arguments around the limited potential for bias already outlined, quasi-random methods might be justified. Varying degrees of blinding are clearly possible but may require additional resource.

But before going ahead with further such studies comparing resuscitation using air with resuscitation using 100% oxygen perhaps it should be considered whether or not this is the best comparison to explore. Might it not be that the answer lies somewhere in-between? Perhaps we should be providing the concentration of oxygen that the individual baby *needs* rather than what is easiest for us to provide. This of course throws up many different issues, not least of which is that there has long been and still is debate as to how best to assess oxygenation in newborn infants (41–43). (See Chapter 15: "Optimal levels of oxygenation in preterm infants.")

Although it is plausible therefore that individual babies may require an oxygen concentration tailored to their individual needs and while a number of studies have looked at the feasibility of assessing oxygenation during acute resuscitation procedures and shown it to be practical, we believe that the more fundamental issue around the meaning and interpretation of transcutaneuos oxygen saturation needs further clarification before it can be incorporated into pragmatic clinical trials. In addition, while the use of air instead of 100% oxygen would be likely to be "cheap" and might be dramatically effective, it can only ever be seen as part of the process of caring for "asphyxiated" infants. Improving standards of antenatal care and exploring other aspects of care of the newborn infant may well be equally important (44–49) and clearly merit consideration.

In the meantime, clinicians must be free to choose whichever approach to resuscitation they feel is most appropriate but they should do so in the clear knowledge that the overall picture remains uncertain. This is similar to the view taken by a number of professional bodies involved in this debate, although some individual clinicians and researchers have been more proscriptive (Box 14-2).

CONCLUSION

Managing the "asphyxiated" infant is a huge, world-wide health issue. The available clinical data, which we believe are unlikely to be significantly biased, point towards a clinically important reduction in the risk of death if room air is used (with oxygen backup available) instead of 100% oxygen for the resuscitation of "asphyxiated" or "flat" newborn term infants. There are no robust longer-term neurodevelopmental follow-up data and it is vital that such data are collected if we are to avoid the potential dilemma of this intervention – air instead of 100% oxygen – being adopted at the "expense" of infants surviving with increased rates of significant neurodisability. Pragmatic trials can and should be undertaken taking account of the potential difference between how term and preterm infants may respond to "asphyxia."

Box 14-2   *Practice Statements Published in the Past 2 Years*

- "For term and near-term infants, we can reasonably conclude that air should be used initially with oxygen as backup if initial resuscitation fails."
  *Systematic review by Davis et al. (24).**
- "... newborn infants in need of resuscitation at birth might benefit from avoiding the use of 100% oxygen immediately after birth."
  Systematic review by Saugstad et al. (26).
- "Ventilatory resuscitation may be started with air. However, where possible, additional oxygen should be available if there is not a rapid improvement in the infant's condition."
  UK Resuscitation Council Guidelines 2005 (50).
- "There is insufficient evidence at present on which to recommend a policy using room air over 100% oxygen, or vice versa, for newborn resuscitation."
  *Systematic review by Tan et al. (25).**
- "Standard resuscitation in delivery room should be made with 100% oxygen. However, lower concentrations are acceptable."
  European Resuscitation Council Guidelines for Resuscitation 2005 (51).
- "Some clinicians may begin resuscitation with an oxygen concentration of less than 100%, and some may start with no supplementary oxygen (i.e., room air). There is evidence that employing either of these practices during resuscitation of neonates is reasonable."
  American Heart Association 2005 Guidelines for CPR and ECC (52).

---

*It is interesting to note that these differing statements arise from the interpretation of the same data by the same authors. This issue generated significant debate about the interpretation and dual publishing of systematic reviews (53, 54).

Disability-free survival, not simply survival or surrogate physiological outcomes, must be the main endpoint. The possibility of varying oxygen provision depending on individual need should be explored but faces huge challenges. Clinicians must embrace and acknowledge the uncertainty. Depending on future results there may need to be a very difficult but necessary wider public debate that explores the social, moral, ethical and resource issues relating to disability and "euthanasia."

APPENDIX

While a comprehensive search of the literature was beyond the scope of this paper, a number of systematic reviews and clinical trials were identified by the authors searching the following sources for clinical "evidence": Cochrane Library (database of clinical trials and database of systematic reviews) (55), National Library of Medicine (Pubmed Clinical Queries: "systematic review" and "therapy" filters) (56), world wide web (Google Scholar: "medical" filter) (57).

REFERENCES

1. Priestley J. Experiments and observations on different kinds of air, St Paul's Church Yard, London, 1774.
2. 1 Kings Chapter 17, verses 17–23.
3. McCord JM, Fridovich I. Superoxide dismutase. An enzymic function for erythrocuprein (hemocuprein). J Biol Chem 1969; 244:6049–6055.
4. Squadrito GL, Pryor WA. The formation of peroxynitrite in vivo from nitric oxide and superoxide. Chem Biol Interact 1995; 96:203–206.
5. Saugstad OD. Resuscitation of the asphyxic newborn infant: new insight leads to new therapeutic possibilities. Biol Neonate 2001; 79:258–260.

6. Buonocore G, Perrone S, Bracci R. Free radicals and brain damage in the newborn. Biol Neonate. 2001; 79(3–4):180–186.

7. Temesvari P, Karg E, Bodi I, et al. Impaired early neurologic outcome in newborn piglets reoxygenated with 100% oxygen compared with room air after pneumothorax-induced asphyxia. Pediatr Res 2001; 49:812–819.

8. Cunningham S, McColm JR, Wade J, et al. A novel model of retinopathy of prematurity simulating preterm oxygen variability in the rat. Invest Ophthalmol Vis Sci 2000; 41:4275–4280.

9. Hoehn T, Felderhoff-Mueser U, Maschewski K, et al. Hyperoxia causes inducible nitric oxide synthase-mediated cellular damage to the immature rat brain. Pediatr Res 2003; 54:179–184.

10. Felderhoff-Mueser U, Bittigau P, Sifringer M, et al. Oxygen causes cell death in the developing brain. Neurobiol Dis 2004; 17:273–282.

11. Poulsen JP, Oyasaeter S, Saugstad OD. Hypoxanthine, xanthine, and uric acid in newborn pigs during hypoxemia followed by resuscitation with room air or 100% oxygen. Crit Care Med 1993; 21:1058–1065.

12. Solas AB, Munkeby BH, Saugstad OD. Comparison of short- and long-duration oxygen treatment after cerebral asphyxia in newborn piglets. Pediatr Res 2004; 56:125–131.

13. Munkeby BH, Borke WB, Bjornland K, et al. Resuscitation with 100% O_2 increases cerebral injury in hypoxemic piglets. Pediatr Res 2004; 56:783–790.

14. Haase E, Bigam DL, Nakonechny QB, et al. Resuscitation with 100% oxygen causes intestinal glutathione oxidation and reoxygenation injury in asphyxiated newborn piglets. Ann Surg 2004; 240:364–373.

15. Silverman WA. Retrolental fibroplasia: a modern parable. New York: Grune & Stratton; 1980. Available: www.neonatology.org/classics/parable/default.html

16. Niijima S, Shortland DB, Levene MI, et al. Transient hyperoxia and cerebral blood flow velocity in infants born prematurely and at full term. Arch Dis Child 1988; 63:1126–1130.

17. Pryds O. Low neonatal cerebral oxygen delivery is associated with brain injury in preterm infants. Acta Paediatr 1994; 83:1233–1236.

18. Mortola JP, Frappell PB, Dotta A, et al. Ventilatory and metabolic responses to acute hyperoxia in newborns. Am Rev Respir Dis 1992; 146:11–15.

19. Klinger G, Beyene J, Shah P, et al. Do hyperoxaemia and hypocapnia add to the risk of brain injury after intrapartum asphyxia? Arch Dis Child Fetal Neonatal Ed 2005; 90:F49–52.

20. Spector LG, Klebanoff MA, Feusner JH, et al. Childhood cancer following neonatal oxygen supplementation. J Pediatr 2005; 147:27–31.

21. Naumburg E, Bellocco R, Cnattingius S, et al. Supplementary oxygen and risk of childhood lymphatic leukaemia. Acta Paediatr 2002; 91:1328–1333.

22. Feinstein AR. Clinical epidemiology: the architecture of clinical research. Philadelphia: Saunders; 1985.

23. Kleijnen J, Gotzsche P, Kunz R, et al. So what's so special about randomisation? In: Maynard A, Chalmers I, eds. Non-random reflections on health services research. London: BMJ Publishing; 1997; 93–106.

24. Davis PG, Tan A, O'Donnell CP, et al. Resuscitation of newborn infants with 100% oxygen or air: a systematic review and meta-analysis. Lancet 2004; 364:1329–1333.

25. Tan A, Schulze A, O'Donnell CP, et al. Air versus oxygen for resuscitation of infants at birth. Cochrane Database Syst Rev 2005; (2):CD002273.

26. Saugstad OD, Ramji S, Vento M. Resuscitation of depressed newborn infants with ambient air or pure oxygen: a meta-analysis. Biol Neonate 2005; 87:27–34.

27. Clarke M, Horton R. Bringing it all together: Lancet-Cochrane collaboration on systematic review. Lancet 2001; 357:1728.

28. Ramji S, Ahuja S, Thirupuram S, et al. Resuscitation of asphyxic newborn infants with room air or 100% oxygen. Pediatr Research 1993; 34:809–812.

29. Saugstad OD, Rootwelt T, Aalen O. Resuscitation of asphyxiated newborn infants with room air or oxygen: an international controlled trial: the Resair 2 study. Pediatrics 1998; 102:e1.

30. Saugstad OD, Ramji S, Irani SF, et al. Resuscitation of newborn infants with 21% or 100% oxygen: follow-up at 18 to 24 months. Pediatrics 2003; 112:296–300.

31. Vento M, Asensi M, Sastre J, et al. Resuscitation with room air instead of 100% oxygen prevents oxidative stress in moderately asphyxiated term neonates. Pediatrics 2001; 107:642–647.

32. Ramji S, Rasaily R, Mishra PK, et al. Resuscitation of asphyxiated newborns with room air or 100% oxygen at birth: a multicentric clinical trial. Indian Pediatrics 2003; 40:510–517.

33. Vento M, Asensi M, Sastre J, et al. Oxidative stress in asphyxiated term infants resuscitated with 100% oxygen. J Pediatr 2003; 142:240–246.

34. Bajaj N, Udani RH, Nanavati RN. Room air vs. 100 per cent oxygen for neonatal resuscitation: a controlled clinical trial. J Trop Pediatr 2005; 51:206–211.

35. Harling AE, Beresford MW, Vince GS, et al. Does the use of 50% oxygen at birth in preterm infants reduce lung injury? Arch Dis Child Fetal Neonatal Ed 2005; 90:F401–405.

36. Schulz KF, Chalmers I, Hayes RJ, Altman DG. Empirical evidence of bias. Dimensions of methodological quality associated with estimates of treatment effects in controlled trials. JAMA 1995; 273:408–412.

37. Kunz R, Vist G, Oxman AD. Randomisation to protect against selection bias in healthcare trials. The Cochrane Database of Methodology Reviews 2002; (4):MR000012.

38. Wariyar UK, Richmond S. Morbidity and preterm delivery: importance of 100% follow-up. Lancet 1989; 1:387–388.

39. Fowlie P, Sinclair J. Resolution of insoluble dilemmas. In: Silverman WA, ed. Where's the evidence? Debates in modern medicine. Oxford: Oxford University Press; 1999; 142–144.

40. Becher JC, Bell JE, Keeling JW, et al. The Scottish perinatal neuropathology study: clinicopathological correlation in early neonatal deaths. Arch Dis Child Fetal Neonatal Ed 2004; 89:F399–407.

41. Wasunna A, Whitelaw AG. Pulse oximetry in preterm infants. Arch Dis Child 1987; 62:957–958.

42. Tin W, Walker S, Lacamp C. Oxygen monitoring in preterm babies: too high, too low? Paediatr Respir Rev 2003; 4:9–14.

43. Askie LM, Henderson-Smart DJ, Irwig L, et al. Oxygen-saturation targets and outcomes in extremely preterm infants. N Engl J Med 2003; 349:959–967.

44. McCall EM, Alderdice FA, Halliday HL, et al. Interventions to prevent hypothermia at birth in preterm and/or low birthweight babies. Cochrane Database Syst Rev 2005; (1):CD004210.

45. Gluckman PD, Wyatt JS, Azzopardi D, et al. Selective head cooling with mild systemic hypothermia after neonatal encephalopathy: multicentre randomised trial. Lancet 2005; 365:663–670.

46. Capasso L, Capasso A, Raimondi F, et al. A randomized trial comparing oxygen delivery on intermittent positive pressure with nasal cannulae versus facial mask in neonatal primary resuscitation. Acta Paediatr 2005; 94:197–200.

47. Vain NE, Szyld EG, Prudent LM, et al. Oropharyngeal and nasopharyngeal suctioning of meconium-stained neonates before delivery of their shoulders: multicentre, randomised controlled trial. Lancet 2004; 364:597–602.

48. Hutchison JH, Kerr MM, Inall JA, et al. Controlled trials of hyperbaric oxygen and tracheal intubation in asphyxia neonatorum. Lancet 1966; 1:935–939.

49. McGuire W, Fowlie PW, Evans DJ. Naloxone for preventing morbidity and mortality in newborn infants of greater than 34 weeks' gestation with suspected perinatal asphyxia. Cochrane Database Syst Rev 2004; (1):CD003955.

50. Resuscitation Council (UK). Resuscitation Guidelines 2005. Available: http://www.resus.org.uk/pages/guide.htm (accessed February 2006).

51. European Resuscitation Council Guidelines for Resuscitation 2005. Available: http://www.erc.edu/index.php/doclibrary/en/viewDoc/175/3/(accessed February 2006).

52. American Heart Association 2005 Guidelines for CPR and ECC. Part 13: Neonatal Resuscitation Guidelines. Circulation 2005; 112:IV188–IV195.

53. Shah PS. Resuscitation of newborn infants. Lancet 2005; 365:651–652.

54. Davis PG, O'Donnell CPF. Resuscitation of newborn infants. Lancet 2005; 365:652–653.

55. http://www3.interscience.wiley.com/cgi-bin/mrwhome/106568753/HOME (accessed February 2006).

56. http://www.ncbi.nlm.nih.gov/entrez/query/static/clinical.shtml (accessed February 2006).

57. http://scholar.google.com/advanced_scholar_search?hl=en&lr= (accessed February 2006).

Chapter 15

Optimal Levels of Oxygenation in Preterm Infants: Impact on Short- and Long-Term Outcomes

Win Tin MB BS FRCP FRCPCH • Samir Gupta MB BS MD MRCP(Ire) FRCPCH

Historical Perspectives

Physiological Considerations

The Critical Threshold of Fetal Oxygenation

Oxygenation During Fetal to Neonatal Transition

Oxygen Toxicity in Preterm Infants

"Normal" Levels of Oxygenation in Newborns

Optimal Levels of Oxygenation in Preterm Infants: Neonatal Period

Optimal Levels of Oxygenation in Preterm Infants: Post-Neonatal Period

Approaches to Oxygen Therapy and Clinical Outcomes

Controversies on Oxygen Therapy

Resolving the Uncertainty: the Way Forward

Multicenter Randomized Controlled Trials – "The Oxygen Saturation Trials"

"To put it bluntly, there has never been a shred of convincing evidence to guide limits for the rational use of supplemental oxygen in the care of extremely premature infants."

—William A. Silverman (2004)

Oxygen is the most commonly used therapy in the neonatal nurseries as an integral part of all the respiratory support. The goal of oxygen therapy is to achieve adequate delivery of oxygen to tissue without creating oxygen toxicity and oxidative stress. Oxygen must have been given to more newborn babies than any other medicinal product in the last 60 years. Despite that, we still know very little about how much oxygen these babies actually need, or how much it is safe to give. Given that we have also known for more than 50 years that it is easy to damage the eyes of preterm infants by giving too much oxygen, especially in the first few weeks of life (1–3), the depth of our ignorance is quite embarrassing.

HISTORICAL PERSPECTIVES

Joseph Priestley (4), Karl Scheele (5) and Anton Lavoisier (6) all contributed in the discovery that the air we breathe is really a mixture of dephlogisticated or "vital air" and "gas azote." Priestley was perceptive enough to write, in 1775, in his very first description of what we now call oxygen, that:

"From the greater strength and vivacity of the flame of a candle, in this pure air, it may be conjectured, that it might be peculiarly salutary to the lungs in certain morbid cases, when the common air would not be sufficient to carry off the phlogistic putrid effluvium fast enough. But, perhaps, we may also infer from these experiments, that though pure dephlogisticated air might be very useful as medicine, it might not be so proper for us in the usual healthy state of the body: for, as a candle burns out much faster in dephlogisticated than in common air, so we might, as might be said, live out too fast, and the animal powers be too soon exhausted in this pure kind of air. A moralist, at least, may say, that the air which nature has provided for us is as good as we deserve."

Whilst the use of oxygen as a medicinal product has a long history (7), the "routine" use of supplemental oxygen in the care of small or preterm infants had its origins in the 1940s. One report that had a marked influence on this practice was by Wilson et al. (8), who noted that the irregular pattern of periodic breathing commonly seen in babies of short gestation was largely abolished when these babies were given 70% oxygen or more to breathe. The authors at first commented: "We have no proof that the regular type of respiration which we are accustomed to call normal is better for the premature infant than the periodic type of breathing described. Likewise we have no convincing evidence that an increased oxygen content of arterial blood is beneficial or necessarily of importance. It is evident, however, that these healthy premature babies breathed in a more 'normal' manner in an oxygen enriched atmosphere." However, by 1949, Howard and Bauer were less cautious in their comments and were writing: "Irregular breathing in early infancy should be treated with a mixture of high oxygen even more than at present, as such an atmosphere regularly increases breathing volume and has a steadying effect on the rhythm of respiration. Oxygen is the most valuable single agent available for a premature or full term newborn infant who is showing any evidence of respiratory difficulty, and it should be used early and generously" (9). It was within this climate of opinion that the widespread practice of unrestricted oxygen supplementation for small or sick infants came into force in the early 1950s and the ensuing epidemic of severe eye disease and blindness is now well known (Fig. 15-1).

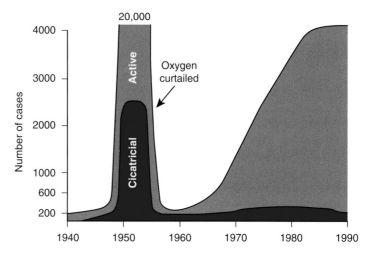

Figure 15-1 Incidence of ROP over time from the 1940s to the 1990s. Note that around 1955 the incidence of cicatricial and active ROP dropped significantly as this is the point in time when oxygen was curtailed. In the late 1960s through the 1990s, survival of very low birth weight infants increased along with the incidence of active ROP (red area). Note that the incidence of severe cicatricial ROP has remained relatively low during this period. (Reproduced with permission from: Wright K. Textbook of Ophthalmology Chapter 22, 1997. Lippincott Williams & Wilkins.)

The first person to suggest in print that oxygen could be responsible for the rising epidemic of severe retinopathy of prematurity (ROP), or retrolental fibroplasia as it was then known, was Kate Campbell in Melbourne, Australia, although she was generous enough to note that news of the idea came to her from colleagues returning from overseas, and that the idea arose from a comparison of the treatment of premature infants in America, where retrolental fibroplasia is a problem and where oxygen was used freely, with the treatment in England, where retrolental fibroplasia is rarely seen, and where oxygen was used sparingly. She concluded that "normal oxygen environment of the newborn full term infant is abnormal for the premature infant" (10). More convincing evidence came within a year from Mary Crosse in Birmingham, England (11), and from a randomized trial, started in 1948 by Arnall Patz (1) in Washington, USA, in which babies weighing less than 3.5 pounds were alternately assigned to high oxygen (65–70% for 4–7 weeks) or less than 40% oxygen for as short a time as possible (1–2 weeks) when 24 h old. Seven of the 28 babies nursed in high oxygen developed Stage 3–4 retinopathy, but none of the 37 nursed in as little oxygen as possible. The larger Cooperative Trial by Kinsey and his colleagues, designed to replicate the Washington trial and completed in 1955 (2), was widely interpreted at the time as suggesting that oxygen therapy was safe as long as the inspired oxygen concentration was not more than 40% (12). The fact that babies in one arm of the trial had not only had more oxygen but also had it for much longer was almost entirely overlooked. So too was the fact that some babies in the restricted exposure arm still developed eye damage. Even more seriously, it took a long time for clinicians to realize that a policy of restricting oxygen exposure rather than restricting arterial oxygen levels was almost certainly causing a rise in the number of early neonatal deaths (13–15).

Once it became clear from the Cooperative Trial that although excessive oxygen exposure was at least one of the causes of retinopathy, but there was no clarity as to how oxygen administration could be optimized, clinicians started to look for ways of monitoring arterial oxygen levels. Indwelling arterial lines were soon being widely used to monitor arterial oxygen tension, but no controlled trial has ever shown that their use reduces the risk of permanent retinal damage (16). Transcutaneous measurement of the partial pressure of oxygen ($TcPO_2$), a technology developed in the 1970s, appears to approximate actual arterial oxygen levels well in most circumstances (16). However, the anticipated benefits of this continuous, non-invasive oxygen monitoring method have not necessarily resulted in significant improvements in the outcomes that they were designed to affect, such as ROP (17). Some non-randomized studies have claimed a near abolition of retinopathy using $TcPO_2$ monitoring (18) whilst others have reported no difference in the incidence or severity of ROP attributable to $TcPO_2$ monitoring (19). The only randomized trial to date which has examined the effect of transcutaneous monitoring (continuous $TcPO_2$ monitoring versus standard care) on retinopathy incidence suggested a modest improvement in ROP rates for infants with greater than 1000 g birth weight, but no effect on smaller infants in whom ROP occurs more frequently and is more severe. Conversely there was a trend to higher mortality in the group receiving continuous transcutaneous monitoring, and the rates of the combined outcome, death or ROP, were nearly identical in the two groups (20). Analysis of some of the information collected during that trial later suggested that retinopathy occurred more often with longer exposure to $TcPO_2$ readings that reached or exceeded 80 mmHg (10.7 kPa) in the first 4 weeks of life (21). Oxygen saturation monitoring using pulse oximetry has gained widespread use in neonatal nurseries since the early 1980s (22) due to its ease of use and lack of heat-related side-effects, particularly in extremely preterm infants with sensitive skin, despite very little evidence of its effectiveness on clinically important outcomes (16). The evidence from non-randomized studies suggests that pulse oximetry is a reliable measure of

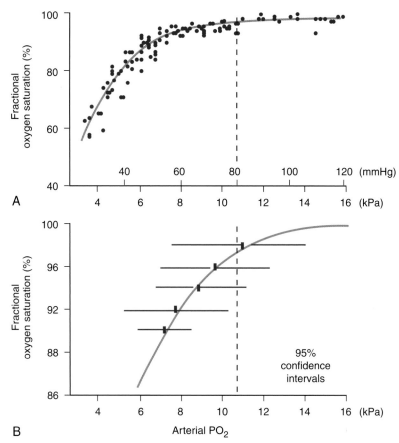

Figure 15-2 The relation between fractional oxygen saturation measured with a pulse oximeter, and arterial partial pressure in mmHg and kPa. The dashed line marks the transcutaneous PO$_2$ above which there was an increased risk of retinopathy in the study reported by Flynn et al. in 1992 (21). The bars in panel B show the range within which 95% of all measures of partial pressure varied when the oximeter read 90%, 92%, 94%, 96% and 98% in the study reported by Brockway and Hay in 1998 (28). (Reproduced with permission from: Neonatal Formulary 4, 2003, pp 187, BMJ Books.)

oxygenation in infants with chronic lung disease and prolonged oxygen dependency, particularly at lower PaO$_2$ levels (23, 24). However, the ability of pulse oximeters to reliably detect hyperoxia remains controversial (25–27), and it has been shown that fractional oxygen saturations of more than 92% can often be associated with hyperoxia as defined by arterial oxygen tension of more than 80 mmHg (28, 29) (Fig. 15-2).

Following the lessons learned from the oxygen-induced blindness epidemic in the 1950s and the ensuing proliferation of oxygen-monitoring devices, many studies have tried to define what constitutes a safe level of oxygenation for newborn babies over the past 50 years. Unfortunately very few studies in this area of medicine have used the methodology known to be the best way of reliably assessing the effects of interventions – "The Randomized Controlled Trial."

PHYSIOLOGICAL CONSIDERATIONS

Oxyhemoglobin Dissociation Curve

In its basic form, the oxyhemoglobin dissociation curve (Fig. 15-3) describes the relation between the partial pressure of oxygen (x axis) and the oxygen saturation

(y axis). The hemoglobin's affinity for oxygen increases in parallel with PO_2 until the maximum capacity is reached. As this limit is approached, very little additional binding occurs and the curve levels out as the hemoglobin becomes saturated with oxygen. This makes the curve a sigmoid or S-shaped. At pressures above ~60 mmHg, the standard oxyhemoglobin dissociation curve is relatively flat, which means that the oxygen content of the blood does not change significantly even with large increases in the oxygen partial pressure. To transport more oxygen to the tissue would require either an increase in the hemoglobin content to increase the oxygen-carrying capacity, or supplemental oxygen that would increase the oxygen dissolved in plasma (30).

The partial pressure of oxygen in the blood at which the hemoglobin is 50% saturated at temperature of 37°C and atmospheric pressure is known as the P_{50}. It is a conventional measure of hemoglobin affinity for oxygen. In the presence of disease or other conditions that change the hemoglobin's oxygen affinity, and consequently shift the curve to the right or left, the P_{50} changes accordingly. An increase in P_{50} indicates a rightward shift of the curve, which means that a larger partial pressure is necessary to maintain 50% oxygen saturation. This indicates a decreased affinity. Conversely, a lower P_{50} indicates a shift to the left (as with HbF) and a higher affinity of hemoglobin to oxygen. The shift of the oxygen dissociation curve to the right occurs in response to increase in the partial pressure of carbon dioxide (PCO_2), decrease in pH or both, which is known as "Bohr Effect." This effect is more pronounced at lower saturations, and is less remarkable when blood is depleted in 2,3-diphosphoglycerate (2,3-DPG) (31). This implies that the presence of HbF favors the performance of metabolic functions at the low intrauterine saturations.

Fetal Oxygenation

The oxygen delivery to the fetus is affected by placental circulation and the oxygen-carrying capacity of the HbF. Due to high oxygen-carrying capacity and increased oxygen affinity of HbF, the oxyhemoglobin saturation and fetal arterial blood oxygen content are not much lower than that of the adult. In utero the presence of high concentrations of HbF maintains higher affinity for oxygen and thus shifts the curve to left, and oxygen (which is bound more tightly to hemoglobin) is released more readily even with a small reduction in partial pressure of oxygen. (Fig. 15-3)

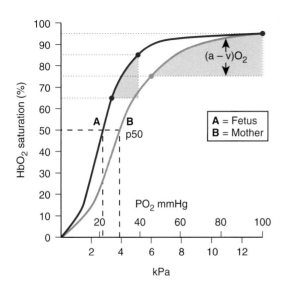

Figure 15-3 Oxyhemoglobin dissociation curve of fetus and mother. The partial pressure of oxygen is shown on the x-axis (PO_2) in mm of Hg, and the y-axis shows oxyhemoglobin saturation. The points A and B represent fetal and maternal P_{50} values respectively. The shaded area ((a-v) O_2) represents the oxygen unloading capacity between a given "arterial" and "venous" PO_2. (Adapted from Tin W, Wariyar U. Giving small babies oxygen: 50 years of uncertainty. Semin Neonatol 2002; 7:361 with permission from Elsevier.)

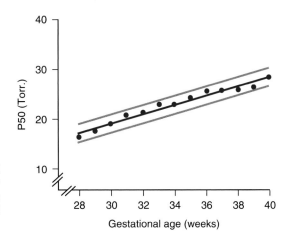

Figure 15-4 Relationship between gestational age and hemoglobin P_{50}. Each point represents mean value for age; outrider lines indicate +/− 2 SD. (Reproduced with permission from Polin RA, Fox WF. Fetal and Neonatal Physiology 2004, p. 885. Elsevier.)

In humans, fetal P_{50} is about 20 mmHg under standard conditions and there is a gradual decrease in blood oxygen affinity (increase in P_{50}) during the course of gestation (Fig. 15-4) (32). At the placental level, the high oxygen affinity of HbF favors oxygen uptake by the fetus and adequate oxygen transfer is achieved at relatively low PO_2. In the fetus, the umbilical venous blood has the highest PO_2, which usually does not go much above 30 mmHg. At that oxygen tension the saturation of fetal umbilical venous blood is 6–8% higher than saturation of maternal blood (33).

THE CRITICAL THRESHOLD OF FETAL OXYGENATION

Monitoring of fetal oxygen is technically difficult and conventional transmission oximeters are unsuitable for fetal use because of difficulty of access to fetal parts and the much lower pulse oxygen saturations (SpO_2) values observed in the fetus. With the advances in technology, fetal pulse oximetry is now available as a stand-alone or integrated with fetal monitoring but has its inherent limitations. The studies have been conducted during the first stage of labor and the mean fetal pulse oxygen saturation ($FSpO_2$) has been reported to be 49% (34). The establishment of a clinically useful value below which a fetus is considered to be at risk of hypoxia has been addressed in human studies (35). They have defined the lower limit of normal $FSpO_2$ (defined as mean − 2SD) to be approximately 30%. Goffinet et al. (36) reported a significant correlation between $FSpO_2$ less than 30% and poor neonatal condition defined as the presence of at least one of the following: 5 min Apgar score of less than 7, secondary respiratory distress, umbilical artery pH less than or equal to 7.15, transfer to neonatal intensive care unit or death. Based on animal and relevant human data, several groups (37, 38) have suggested that $FSpO_2$ values greater than or equal to 30% can be considered reassuring in the human fetus, and values less than 30% for greater than or equal to 10 min may require further assessment or intervention.

The fetal pulse oximetry has been compared with other monitoring techniques. The French multi-center study group (39) compared intrapartum $FSpO_2$ with fetal blood analysis (FBA) and reported similar sensitivity and specificity of FBA and $FSpO_2$ (threshold $FSpO_2$ of 30%) in predicting postpartum umbilical artery pH < 7.15. The German multicenter study group (37) used receiver operator characteristics (ROC) analysis and reported the best predictive range of $FSpO_2$ to be between 30 and 40% and a cut off at 30% for low scalp pH (< 7.20). They reported in this study a sensitivity of 81% and specificity of 100%. These intrapartum data of $FSpO_2$ illustrate that the fetus is capable of maintaining the metabolic function up to the critical $FSpO_2$ of 30%. However, there are no reported studies which correlate the optimal fetal saturation and clinical outcomes.

Near-infrared spectroscopy (NIRS) has also been used to assess oxygenation of blood and tissue in the fetus. The experimental studies conclude that the interpretation of NIRS data may be more relevant when used with other monitoring modalities such as fetal pulse oximetry rather than on its own. Studies with NIRS and color Doppler ultrasound have also shown that fetal hypoxemia (defined as $FSpO_2 < 30\%$) results in an increased cerebral volume and blood flow which is mediated by increased production of adrenal catecholamines (40).

OXYGENATION DURING FETAL TO NEONATAL TRANSITION

The birth of a fetus demands postnatal changes to meet the metabolic needs and to adapt to extrauterine life. This involves pulmonary, circulatory, temperature and metabolic adaptation. The high oxygen affinity of fetal blood has important disadvantages in postnatal life despite being optimally saturated. At the tissue level, the low P_{50} of fetal Hb decreases the driving potential for oxygen delivery and thus limits the rate at which oxygen can be unloaded. On the other hand the newborn needs more oxygen to adapt to postnatal life and this increase in oxygen consumption in most species is reported to be 100–150% (41). In addition, the stress of a cold environment and muscular activity further increase the metabolic demand for oxygen. Hence, a P_{50} adequate for tissue supply in the fetus may limit the rate of oxygen delivery in the newborn postnatally. This is compensated in babies born at term gestation by an increase in 2,3-DPG which shifts the dissociation curve to the right and thus helps in unloading the oxygen at tissue level.

The physiology of premature infants differs from that of term babies. They have higher fetal hemoglobin concentration, lower 2,3-DPG content and lower P_{50} levels. The functioning fractions of DPG are also significantly lower than those of term infants. They have less oxygen-unloading capacity initially as compared to term infants, and this persists during the first 3 months of life (42). This means that premature babies have even higher oxygen saturation (SaO_2) at any given level of arterial PO_2 (PaO_2), and also that the oxygen demands of most extremely premature infants can be met by maintaining PaO_2 levels just above 50 mmHg that will result in saturation levels above 88% (43).

Although the fetal hemoglobin levels remain high for the first few months and more so in premature infants, the compensatory rise in DPG levels from birth allows the newborn infant to meet the increased oxygen requirements. The low fetal saturations may not be appropriate at birth as the pulmonary, metabolic and circulatory adaptation takes place. This adaptation requires a drop in the pulmonary vascular resistance with a drop in pulmonary airway resistance after the first breaths and changes associated with the transition from fetal to adult circulation incorporating closure of fetal physiological shunts (ductus arteriosus, ductus venosus and foramen ovale). The effect of lung inflation and ventilation on the pulmonary blood flow was studied by Strang (44), who observed that if the lung is inflated from fetal state and ventilated with gas mixtures which do not change fetal composition of blood gases (i.e. pH 7.35, pCO_2 45 torr, PO_2 25 torr), an increase in pulmonary vascular conductance (decrease in resistance) and in blood flow can be achieved (Fig. 15-5). This increase in conductance was attributed to the expansion of collapsible pulmonary capillaries. In addition, when the blood gas composition was changed by the increase in PO_2 and decrease in PCO_2 similar to ventilation with air, further increases in vascular conductance and blood flow were achieved. These changes along with the increase in systemic vascular resistance contribute to circulatory adaptation at birth.

In addition to the reduction in pulmonary vascular resistance, another known important factor that facilitates the closure of the ductus arteriosus

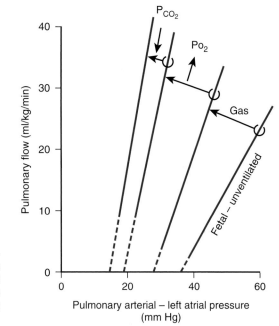

Figure 15-5 Pulmonary vascular conductance increases with the onset of ventilation. Separate curves depict the contributions of gaseous inflation, increased PO_2 and decreased PCO_2. (Reproduced with permission from Strang LB. The lungs at birth. Arch Dis Child 1965; 40:575.)

is "oxygen" (45). The high oxygen saturations would affect closure of physiological shunts in term babies without causing any adverse effects, but at present there is not enough evidence to suggest that babies born very premature and exposed to similar high saturations would have the physiological transition similar to term babies, particularly when the anatomical maturity is far from complete. The critical saturation in the fetus to prevent adverse metabolic effects has already been discussed. There is a growing interest in addressing the optimal saturations in the early postnatal period in the vulnerable premature babies to minimize the risk of potential oxygen toxicity whilst maintaining adequate tissue oxygenation during the desirable physiological transitional changes following birth.

Animal studies have shown that the rise in arterial oxygen tension is the main reason for ductal closure immediately after birth (46). It is also known that changes in arterial oxygen level have a profound effect on pulmonary vascular tone. The rise in partial pressure of oxygen is one of the three main factors triggering the fall in the pulmonary vascular tone (45) and the increase in the pulmonary blood flow seen in the period immediately after birth (the others being the mechanical ventilation of the lung and the $PaCO_2$ of blood perfusing the lung). The classic experiments of Cassin, Dawes et al. (47) in exteriorized fetal lambs have shown that increasing the oxygen tension in the pulmonary arterial blood from 16 to 34 mmHg caused an immediate fall in the pulmonary vascular tone. However, Dawes later cautioned that raising the PaO_2 from 50 to even as high as 150 mmHg had virtually no further effect on the pulmonary vascular tone. (48).

The effects of arterial oxygenation level on cardiac output, oxygen extraction and oxygen consumption in low birth weight infants receiving mechanical ventilation were studied by Schulze et al. (49). They adjusted the inspired oxygen concentration to achieve either low SpO2 (89–92%) or high SpO2 (93–96%) and concluded that there was no mismatch between systemic oxygen delivery and demand between the two groups. Furthermore, the mixed venous oxygen tension decreased with the simultaneous increase in oxygen extraction ratio in the low target range of oxygen saturation. There are limited data on the effects of oxygen on ductus arteriosus in premature fetuses or infants. Rasanen et al. (50) studied the effect of maternal hyperoxygenation on fetal physiology in 40 women, of whom half were between 20 and 26 weeks of gestation, and the other half between 31 and 36 weeks gestation. They randomized mothers to receive either 60% humidified oxygen or room air by face masks and measured various echocardiographic indices using Doppler ultrasound. They concluded that the reactivity of the human fetal pulmonary circulation increases with advancing gestation. There were no changes during maternal hyperoxygenation in fetuses between 20 and 26 week gestation, but in fetuses between 31 and 36 weeks gestation the impedance decreased with a corresponding reduction in the flow in the ductus arteriosus. However, the post-natal data comparing the effect of high and low saturations on ductus arteriosus in preterm babies at different gestation are rather limited.

One reason why the ductus arteriosus may remain patent in very preterm babies is that they are often not very well oxygenated in the period immediately after birth, and many clinicians are apprehensive that unnecessarily restricting arterial oxygen level in the period after birth for fear of the retinal consequences could result in more ductus arteriosus remaining patent. The only good experimental evidence relating to this is the study by Skinner et al. (51) on 18 oxygen-dependent preterm infants of gestational age between 27 and 36 weeks and with patent ductus arteriosus. These infants received varying concentrations of inspired oxygen to achieve the target arterial oxygen saturation range of 84–88%, 95–97% and 100%. The effect of these different SaO_2 levels on pulmonary and ductal blood flow was studied by echocardiography. The authors reported that a rise in SaO_2 can cause significant ductal constriction in this gestational age range of preterm babies, but the observation was based on a brief period of relative oxygen exposure. It is thus appropriate to say that oxygen does have an effect on closure of the ductus arteriosus after birth in more mature babies, but it remains uncertain whether the same holds true in extreme preterm babies, and the question of whether restricting oxygen levels impose any untoward effects on the ductus arteriosus remains debatable.

OXYGEN TOXICITY IN PRETERM INFANTS

Oxygen and Eye

Although the etiopathogenesis of ROP is considered multifactorial, it is primarily affected by the immaturity of the retina itself, and levels of retinal arterial oxygenation. The retina is avascular in early fetal life. With the advancement of gestational age, new retinal blood vessels grow outwards from the center around the optic nerve. Retinal vessel development begins at about 16 weeks gestation and is usually complete by 36 weeks during intrauterine life (52). In babies who are born extremely premature, the retina is incompletely vascularized and the peripheral part of the retina is most susceptible to injuries.

The role of oxygen in the pathogenesis of ROP has been explored by various studies. The chemical signaling by oxygen-regulated vascular endothelial growth factor (VEGF) and non-oxygen-regulated insulin-like growth factor-1 (IGF-1) contribute to the development of retinal vasculature. VEGF is up-regulated in a hypoxic environment and down regulated by hyperoxia (53), and low levels of IGF-1 prevent vascular growth (54). In utero, VEGF is found at the front end of growing vessels and the levels of IGF-1 are sufficient to allow vessel growth (55). Under "normal" physiological conditions, increased oxygen demand of the growing neural retina anterior to the vascularization creates localized hypoxia. This results in the expression of VEGF and growth of vessels toward this stimulus.

Following premature birth, the induction of ROP is characterized by the disruption of normal retinal vascularization process. The pathogenesis of ROP can be described in two "phases" (Fig. 15-6). The first phase of ROP is related to the exposure to excessive oxygen after premature birth when the normal retinal vascular

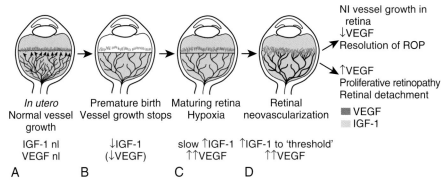

Figure 15-6 Schematic representation of IGF-1/VEGF control of blood vessel development in ROP. (A) In utero, VEGF is found at the growing front of vessels. IGF-1 is sufficient to allow vessel growth. (B) With premature birth, IGF-1 is not maintained at in utero levels, and vascular growth ceases, despite the presence of VEGF at the growing front of vessels. Both endothelial cell survival (AKT) and proliferation (MAPK) pathways are compromised. With low IGF-1 and cessation of vessel growth, a demarcation line forms at the vascular front. High oxygen exposure (as occurs in animal models and in some premature infants) may also suppress VEGF, further contributing to inhibition of vessel growth. (C) As the premature infant matures, the developing but non-vascularized retina becomes hypoxic. VEGF increases in retina and vitreous. With maturation, the IGF-1 level slowly increases. (D) When the IGF-1 level reaches a threshold at 34 weeks gestation, with high VEGF levels in the vitreous, endothelial cell survival and proliferation driven by VEGF may proceed. Neovascularization ensues at the demarcation line, growing into the vitreous. If VEGF vitreal levels fall, normal retinal vessel growth can proceed. With normal vascular growth and blood flow, oxygen suppresses VEGF expression, so it will no longer be overproduced. If hypoxia (and elevated levels of VEGF) persists, further neovascularization and fibrosis leading to retinal detachment can occur. (Reproduced from Smith LEH. Pathogenesis of retinopathy of prematurity. Semin Neonatol 2003; 8:469 with permission of the publisher, Elsevier.)

growth stops and regression of some already developed vessels ensues. In the relatively hyperoxic environment, vasoconstriction of retinal vessels occurs, and this leads on to arrest of the growth of blood vessels along the border between vascularized and avascular retina. Resolution of "normal" in utero hypoxic drive also suppresses VEGF mRNA expression (56); this in turn causes loss of the physiological wave of VEGF anterior to the growing vascular front. The low levels of IGF-1 due to loss of supply from placenta and amniotic fluid following birth also contribute to impairment of retinal vascular growth (55). In addition, vascular obliteration may also be caused by apoptosis of vascular endothelial cells.

In contrast, the second phase of ROP is characterized by retinal neovascularization, induced by hypoxia. It is similar to other proliferative retinopathies and occurs at about 32–34 weeks post-menstrual age. The magnitude of destruction in the second phase is determined by the extent of damage in the first phase (54). As the infant matures, the developing but non-vascularized retina becomes hypoxic. This stimulates and up-regulates the expression of VEGF in the retina and also in vitreous, a mechanism said to be the critical factor in ocular neovascularization. The levels of VEGF remain high throughout the progression of ROP during this phase. The IGF-1 is also critical to the development of ROP and the levels increase until ROP reaches the threshold stage. If hypoxia persists, the VEGF levels remain high and may lead to proliferative retinopathy, with or without further complication of retinal detachment.

Oxygen exposure, in terms of fluctuations and concentrations of inspired oxygen around different mean fractional concentration of inspired oxygen (FiO_2) levels, also seems to have an impact on development of ROP. It was observed in animal studies that variations around higher mean FiO_2 levels (mean 24% oxygen) had more severe vascular abnormalities compared to fluctuations around lower levels (mean 21% oxygen) (57), and also that breathing higher oxygen concentrations impaired retinal development to the extent of complete vessel ablation in 80% ambient oxygen (58). The effect of other biochemical mediators on ROP has also been studied. Carbon dioxide has been associated with development of ROP; although there have been conflicting reports (59–61). Hypercarbia in the presence of hyperoxia and variable oxygen levels is observed to increase the severity of ROP by causing vasodilatation, and resultant increase in blood flow and oxygenation to the retina. This leads on to down-regulation and decreased production of VEGF, and delay in the normal process of retinal vascularization (62). Blood transfusion and erythropoietin have also been postulated as risk factors for ROP (63, 64). This is explained by the effect on oxygen delivery to tissues and by increasing iron, a known oxidant.

Oxygen and Brain

The effects of high inspired and arterial oxygen concentrations on immature brain cells and their signaling cascades are not completely understood. It has been known for more than 30 years from an animal study that cerebral vasculature constricts in response to hyperoxia and this reduces cerebral blood flow (65). The effects of oxygen on the brain to some extent are similar to those on the retina as the latter is a specialized part of the central nervous system and thus may share the same pathophysiological processes, and it has been suggested that cerebral and retinal damage share a common vaso-reactive vascular origin (66).

Various factors and mechanisms that influence oxygen radical disease of the newborn have been described. These include antioxidants, and the metabolism of glutathione, iron and nitric oxide. In addition to lipid and protein oxidation, oxygen radicals may also induce neuronal damage by mitochondrial permeability transition and augmentation of the influx of calcium ion into mitochondria (67), thus leading to necrosis or apoptosis. The redoxins and peroxiredoxins are located in the inner mitochondrial membranes which scavenge reactive oxygen species and other free radicals and thus protect from oxidative stress injury. Glutathione is the most abundant antioxidant which can regenerate other antioxidants (68). It is also involved in regeneration of oxidized ascorbate and tocoferol, which have been linked with outcome in preterm infants (69). In preterm babies availability of glutathione and other antioxidants is limited, and thus they have a low capacity for detoxification. Nitric oxide (NO) in low concentrations is known to act as an antioxidant but its reaction with superoxide leads to production of peroxinitrite, which has potential for deleterious effects on immature cellular structures in the neonatal brain (70).

The effect of exposure to pure oxygen on the brain was described in an animal study as early as 1959 (71). Gyllensten found in this historic study that rearing mice in pure oxygen for 20–30 days had a marked deleterious effect on subsequent cortical vascularization and cellular differentiation, and a similar effect was observed on the growth of vessels into the frontal cortex in hamsters (72). Another animal study also showed that the brain of the newborn rat grew less well when the animal was reared in 70–80% oxygen for the first 9 days (73). In humans, development of an extensive form of periventricular leukomalacia (PVL) is found to have a strong correlation with sustained hyperoxia (74). More alarmingly, Ahdab-Barmada et al. described pontosubicular lesions in infants who had PaO_2 values of more than 150 mmHg in the first few weeks of life (75). More recently, Haynes et al. (76) described oxidative damage to premyelinating oligodendrocytes in cerebral white matter as a mechanism of development of PVL and, in a large clinical study of 1105 low birth weight infants by Collins et al. (77), the risk of disabling cerebral palsy was observed to be doubled in those exposed to hyperoxia. The adjusted odds for risk of cerebral palsy increased 8-fold in infants with the highest compared to the lowest quintiles of oxygen exposure. Even short exposures to non-physiologic oxygen levels were observed to trigger apoptotic neurodegeneration in the brain of infant rodents, and the vulnerability to oxygen neurotoxicity in the human was reported to extend from the sixth month of pregnancy to 3 years of age (78).

Oxygen and Lung

When bronchopulmonary dysplasia (BPD) was first described in preterm babies on mechanical respiratory support, it was widely felt that oxygen toxicity was a major contributory factor (79, 80). In early reports the condition was typically seen only in babies exposed to 80% oxygen or more for at least 6 days. Subsequent studies soon convinced most people that pressure damage or "barotrauma" from mechanical ventilation was another major factor (81, 82), and it was not long before clinicians had come to believe that this was the main cause.

The fact that oxygen, independently of mechanical ventilatory support, can cause lethal damage to the previously normal lung was shown by an elegant experiment involving 18-week-old lambs in 1969 (83). One group of lambs were allowed to breathe air, and another group breathed 100% oxygen. Half of each group were left to breathe spontaneously, and half were anesthetized and ventilated artificially. All the lambs breathing 100% oxygen died within 4 days, and respiratory support neither delayed nor speeded up their death. That oxygen in the inspired gas, rather than the oxygen levels in the blood is damaging to the lungs was addressed by another elegant study in 1970 which showed that cyanosis in dogs (created surgically by veno-arterial shunt) failed to protect the lung from the consequence of breathing 100% oxygen at normal barometric pressure for 48 h (84), thus implying that oxygen is a direct toxin on the bronchial and alveolar epithelium.

In preterm babies, the effect of high inspired oxygen concentration as an important cause of BPD is well documented (85, 86). The direct toxic effect of oxygen damages the bronchial and alveolar epithelium as well as capillary endothelium, leading to alveolar oedema, neutrophil infiltration, proliferation of alveolar cells and fibrosis (86). Even if the inspired oxygen concentration is not very high, oxidative stress (defined as imbalances between pro- and antioxidant forces) can still occur and impose lung tissue injury. Furthermore, high levels of biochemical markers of oxidative stress have been identified in the pulmonary lavage in the first few days of life in preterm babies who later develop BPD (87).

Newborn infants and especially premature babies are more prone to oxidative stress (87) as they have a higher risk of exposure to high oxygen concentrations, reduced antioxidant defense and more free iron leading to production of hydroxyl radicals. The "oxygen radical disease of neonatology" may affect different organs, but the presentations would depend on the organ which is most vulnerable (88). It is difficult to control all the pathophysiological processes underlying oxidative stress injury in preterm infants, but we do know that careful control of oxygen exposure may prevent the aforesaid complications in newborn infants.

"NORMAL" LEVELS OF OXYGENATION IN NEWBORNS

The fetus achieves normal growth in utero with arterial blood that is only about 70% saturated with oxygen (Fig. 15-3). Children with cyanotic heart disease make the transition to extra-uterine life without much difficulty with saturation levels similar to those of the fetus. Despite these facts, the practice in the neonatal units over the past three decades has generally been to attempt to keep oxygen levels in "all" newborns in line with those of term and non-compromised preterm infants. Several studies have documented what are often termed "normal" or reference values for arterial oxygen saturation and or PaO$_2$ levels for both term and well preterm infants (89–95). These studies demonstrate a relatively narrow range of normal baseline SpO$_2$ values during the regular breathing state of the newborn. For preterm and term infants in their neonatal period this is 93–100%, and for older term infants between 2 and 6 months age, 97–100%. These data correspond with the few existing studies of arterial partial pressures of oxygen, which have demonstrated mean PaO$_2$ of 70–76 mmHg in term infants on days 2–7 of life (96).

What is also known is that preterm infants, in particular those with prolonged dependency on supplemental oxygen, have lower baseline saturation levels (97), more frequent desaturation episodes (98), disturbed sleep patterns (99), greater risk of pulmonary hypertension (100, 101), and increased adverse pulmonary complications compared with preterm infants without chronic oxygen dependency or infants born at term (102). What is *not* known, however, is whether these associations are causal. It remains unclear whether attempts to ameliorate the states described above by oxygen administration, to reduce desaturation episodes, decrease PaO$_2$ variability, or improve sleep, actually make any material difference to long-term outcomes such as improving growth and development in infancy, or reducing serious adverse pulmonary complications or death.

OPTIMAL LEVELS OF OXYGENATION IN PRETERM INFANTS: NEONATAL PERIOD

There is no sufficient evidence to date to suggest what are the optimal oxygen saturation or PaO$_2$ values to aim for in preterm infants who receive supplemental oxygen therapy in order to avoid potential oxygen toxicity whilst ensuring adequate oxygen delivery to tissues.

Three trials published more than 50 years ago (1–3) clearly demonstrated the effect of unrestricted, high levels of ambient oxygen in causing severe eye disease in premature infants (Fig. 15-7). One randomized trial involving 79 infants with "respiratory distress syndrome" was carried out by Usher in Canada, comparing the "high" and "low" oxygen approaches as guided by oxygen tension. The high oxygen approach consisted in provision of supplemental oxygen during the first 72 h of life to maintain oxygen tension of 70–100 mmHg in arterial or 55–70 mmHg in capillary blood. Such infants often received 60–100% oxygen therapy. In contrast, infants randomized to the low oxygen approach received supplemental oxygen only when the arterial tension fell below 40 mmHg or capillary tension fell below 35 mmHg. Usher demonstrated in 1968 that a significantly higher proportion of infants randomized to "high approach" to oxygen therapy had radiological changes of marked pulmonary infiltrates on serial chest X-rays taken during the first 72 h (103). With the honorable exception of this trial, only published as an abstract, there has not been

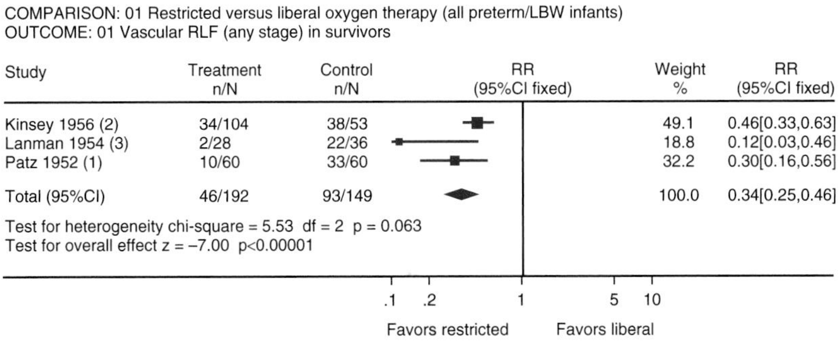

COMPARISON: 01 Restricted versus liberal oxygen therapy (all preterm/LBW infants)
OUTCOME: 01 Vascular RLF (any stage) in survivors

Study	Treatment n/N	Control n/N	RR (95%CI fixed)	Weight %	RR (95%CI fixed)
Kinsey 1956 (2)	34/104	38/53		49.1	0.46[0.33,0.63]
Lanman 1954 (3)	2/28	22/36		18.8	0.12[0.03,0.46]
Patz 1952 (1)	10/60	33/60		32.2	0.30[0.16,0.56]
Total (95%CI)	46/192	93/149		100.0	0.34[0.25,0.46]

Test for heterogeneity chi-square = 5.53 df = 2 p = 0.063
Test for overall effect z = −7.00 p<0.00001

.1 .2   1   5 10

Favors restricted   Favors liberal

Figure 15-7 Forest plot showing the meta-analysis of three trials included in the review: Askie L, Henderson-Smart DJ. Restricted versus liberal oxygen exposure for preventing morbidity and mortality in preterm or low birth weight infants. In: The Cochrane Library, Issue 3, 2003. Oxford: Update Software. (Reproduced with permission from J Wiley and Sons.)

any randomized trial to test the effect of restricting the level of oxygenation in preterm infants from or soon after birth since it became possible to monitor the oxygen tension or saturation continuously and non-invasively. Furthermore, there are no randomized trials looking at the effects of targeting a lower PaO$_2$ or SpO$_2$ range from the early neonatal period on important outcomes such as severe ROP, death or long-term growth and neurodevelopmental morbidity.

Recent evidence from several observational studies (104–107) has suggested that this hypothesis of "restrictive oxygen approach" is worth exploring (Table 15-1). A prospective observational study by Tin et al. (104), of every baby born alive before 28 weeks gestation to mothers resident in the north of England in 1990–94, came out with some fairly provocative findings in 2001. All the babies were born in or referred to one of five neonatal intensive care units, where the policy towards the monitoring of oxygen saturation varied, but several other care policies were fairly similar. Two of the five neonatal units shared the same oxygen saturation monitoring policy; hence there were four different practices of oxygen monitoring during the study period. Survival rates, and survivors without evidence of cerebral palsy at 18 months, were almost identical in the five units in the 294/568 babies of 23–27 weeks gestation (52%) still alive a year after birth (Table 15-2). In one unit, target fractional oxygen saturation was 80–90% (with the lower alarm limit set to operate only if saturation fell below 70%) once the baby was more than 2–3 h old. Such a policy was sustained for all babies thought to need supplemental oxygen until retinal vascularization was complete. In another unit, target functional oxygen saturation was 94–98% (with the lower alarm set to operate at 88%). The other three units had intermediate policies. Careful, uniform, ophthalmic review of all the survivors showed that retinopathy severe enough to merit treatment with cryotherapy occurred in 6.3% (95% CI 1.7–15.0%) of the babies in the first of these units, and 27.7% (95% CI 17.3–40.2%) in the latter. No child from the first unit but four from the latter unit became blind. The three units employing intermediate policies for target oxygen saturation had "threshold" retinopathy rates in the middle of this range (Fig. 15-8).

In the unit where target oxygen saturation was 80–90% half the 64 long-term survivors were managing without endotracheal intubation and mechanical ventilation by 7 days, and without supplemental oxygen by 30 days. In the unit where target oxygen saturation was 94–98%, these milestones were achieved by half the survivors in 21 and 72 days respectively. There was no evidence that targeting much lower oxygen saturation in these preterm babies had an adverse effect on growth between birth and at the time of their discharge. In fact growth was curtailed twice as much in the latter unit (possibly because nutritional intake was increased more cautiously in babies still requiring respiratory support). Neurodevelopmental outcome was similar at 18 months (no child having been lost to follow-up).

Sun and his colleagues (105) collated data from a subset of hospitals that participated in a national evidence-based quality improvement collaborative for neonatology (Vermont Oxford Network), and compared the survival, chronic lung disease and severe retinopathy of prematurity of 1544 extremely low birth weight babies (500–1000 g) who were cared for in units that aimed to keep oxygen saturation at or below 95% and those that intended to keep saturations above 95% whilst these babies were in supplemental oxygen. They reported significantly lower incidences of chronic lung disease (27% vs. 53%) as well as stage III/IV ROP (10% vs. 29%) amongst babies cared for with targeted saturations of 95% or less. Survival rate was marginally higher in the low saturation group, but not statistically significantly (83% vs. 76%). A study by Chow et al. (106) in 2004 showed that implementation of strict clinical practices of oxygen management and monitoring was associated with a significant decrease in the incidence of stage III/IV ROP (from 12% to 2.5%), and need for surgery (from 4.5% to 0%) in infants with

Table 15-1 Summary of Recent Observational Studies Showing the Potential Benefits of Lower SpO$_2$ Targeting

Reference	Study group	SpO$_2$ ranges compared	Survival	Chronic lung disease	ROP (stage 3-4)	ROP (treatment)
Tin, 2001 (104)	≤27 weeks	Low: 70–90% High: 88–98%	53% 52%	18% 46% $P < 0.01$		6% 27% $P < 0.01$
Sun, 2002 (105)	≤1500 g	Low: ≤95% High: > 95%	83% 76%	27% 53% $P < 0.01$	10% 29% $P < 0.01$	4% 12% $P < 0.01$
Anderson, 2004 (107)	≤1500 g, > 2 weeks old	Low: ≤92% High: > 92%			2.4% 5.5% $P < 0.01$	1.3% 3.3% $P < 0.01$
Chow, 2003 (106)	500–1500 g	Low: 85–93% High: 90–98%	88% 81%		2.5% 12.5% $P < 0.01$	0–1.3% 4.4% $P < 0.01$

Table 15-2 **Outcome at 1 year in all Babies of 23–27 Weeks Gestation born in 1990–1994 and its Relation to Minimum and Maximum Pulse Oximeter Alarm Settings (104)**

Oximeter alarm settings	Number of babies admitted	ONE YEAR SURVIVORS (NUMBER AND PERCENTAGE)			
		Number of survivors	Median number of days ventilated	Cerebral palsy	Threshold retinopathy
88–98%*	123	65 (52.8%)	21	11 (16.9%)	18 (27.7%)
85–95%	235	128 (54.5%)	16	20 (15.6%)	20 (15.6%)
84–94%	84	37 (44.0%)	15	6 (16.2%)	5 (13.5%)
70–90%	126	64 (50.7%)	7	10 (15.6%)	4 (6.3%)

Target saturation was in the upper half of the accepted range.
*Nellcor pulse oximeter measurements (functional saturation). Other measurements are fractional saturation.

birth weight of 500–1500 g. A national survey reported by Anderson et al. (107) in 2004 also showed significantly less stage III/IV ROP (2.4% vs. 5.5%) in babies of less than 1501 g at birth, and also significantly less retinal surgery (1.3% vs. 3.3%), in neonatal units where the upper alarm limit of pulse oxygen saturation in babies over 2 weeks old was ≤ 92% vs. > 92%.

In contrast to the report of these observational studies, Poets et al. (108) reported their observation on 891 babies of < 30 weeks gestation and admitted to two neonatal units, using different pulse oxygen saturation alarm limits (80–92% vs. 92–97%). Retrospective analysis of their data showed the incidence of ROP (more than stage 2) was significantly higher in the unit that used a lower alarm limit (13% vs. 6%) although no difference was seen in the incidence of ROP that required surgery. The difficulty with all these observational studies however, is that the association between target oxygen saturation and improved outcomes cannot be deemed causal and, as no randomized controlled trials exist to answer this question comprehensively, the uncertainty remains.

OPTIMAL LEVELS OF OXYGENATION IN PRETERM INFANTS: POST-NEONATAL PERIOD

Two randomized trials have recently been conducted to see whether it is better to keep arterial oxygen saturation high in very preterm babies when they are more

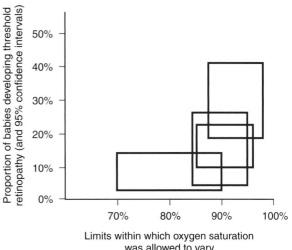

Figure 15-8 The relation between the limits within which oxygen saturation was allowed to vary and the proportion of 1-year survivors so nursed who later developed "threshold" ROP. A comparison of four policies. Staff aimed to keep saturation in the upper half of the allowed range. (Reproduced from Tin W, Milligan DWA, Pennefather P, et al. Pulse oximetry, severe retinopathy, and outcome at one year in babies of less than 28 weeks gestation. Arch Dis Child 2001; 84: F106 with permission of BMJ Publishing Group.)

than a few weeks old. The American STOP-ROP trial (109), which recruited 649 babies born between 1990 and 1994 with a mean birth gestation of 25.4 weeks and a mean postmenstrual age at trial entry of 35 weeks, showed that keeping fractional oxygen saturation above 95% slightly reduced the number of babies with pre-threshold retinopathy who went on to develop disease severe enough to require retinal surgery. However, benefit was only seen in those without evidence of "plus disease" (dilated and tortuous vessels in at least two quadrants of the posterior pole) at recruitment (32% vs. 46%). More unexpectedly, targeting the higher oxygen saturation significantly increased the number of infants who remained in hospital, in supplemental oxygen, and on diuretics at a postmenstrual age of 50 weeks. Significant pulmonary deterioration after recruitment (13.2% vs. 8.5%) was only seen in those with more than average evidence of chronic lung disease at trial entry. The higher oxygenation target did not improve growth or the eventual retinal outcome as assessed 3 months after the expected date of delivery.

The result of the Australian BOOST trial was published in 2004 (110). The aim of this randomized, double-blind study was to see whether maintaining higher oxygen saturations versus standard levels among oxygen-dependent preterm babies improved their growth and development. This study recruited 358 babies of less than 30 weeks gestation who remained in supplemental oxygen at 32 weeks post-menstrual age. Collaborating units had different policies with regard to optimum oxygenation in the period immediately after birth, but all monitored saturation using a pre-specified Nellcor N-3000® pulse oximeter after recruitment for as long as supplemental oxygen was deemed necessary. Trial oximeters were specially modified to keep targeted functional saturation in the range of either 91–94% or 95–98%, depending on allocation at entry, while displaying a targeted figure (masked) in the range 93–96%. This well-designed study showed no evidence that the growth and developmental outcome of the oxygen-dependent preterm infant was improved by keeping their functional oxygen saturation in the high range. This finding contradicts the substantial body of observational evidence that suggests higher oxygen targeting can improve growth (111, 112), ameliorate sleep pattern abnormalities (113) and reduce desaturation episodes (97). In keeping with the observation in the STOP-ROP study, the BOOST study also showed infants in the higher oxygen saturation range had greater use of postnatal steroids (58% vs. 50%) and diuretics (52% vs. 44%), more readmissions (54% vs. 48%) and more pulmonary-related deaths (6% vs. 1%). Although these were secondary outcomes in both trials and hence they lack the statistical power to assess these results reliably, the consistency of the direction of effect lends weight to the hypothesis that high concentrations of inspired oxygen in preterm infants in their post-neonatal life may result in more pulmonary damage.

APPROACHES TO OXYGEN THERAPY AND CLINICAL OUTCOMES

Neonatal Mortality and Morbidity Outcomes

The beneficial effect of restricting oxygen therapy on ROP was evident more than 50 years ago. Universal restriction of oxygen therapy, rather than restricting the level of oxygenation in response to this strong evidence, was felt to be responsible for excessive mortality and morbidity in preterm infants as a result of hypoxic respiratory failure (13,14). A time-series analysis of first-day infant mortality and still birth rates by Whyte (114), however, suggested that oxygen restriction could not have been the only reason for the observed increase in mortality during that historical era. Recent observational studies (104–107) already described have also suggested that the "restrictive" oxygen therapy compared to the "liberal" approach as guided by noninvasive, continuous pulse oxygen saturation monitoring shortly after birth was associated with significantly lower rates of severe ROP and BPD without the increase in mortality in preterm babies.

Impact of Neonatal Morbidities on Long-Term Outcomes

The prognostic impact of major neonatal morbidities, particularly severe ROP, BPD and brain injury, is additive, and was shown to be independently correlated to poor outcome at 18 months of age. Schmidt et al. reported that preterm babies who were free of these neonatal complications had 18% risk of death or severe neurosensory impairment at 18 months, compared to a risk of 42% for babies who developed one of these complications, and 62% for those with two. Babies with all three complications had a poor outcome rate as high as 88% (115).

The prognostic impact of defined "threshold" ROP on visual outcome should not be underestimated. The ophthalmological outcome at 10 years of children with birth weight of less than 1251 g who developed ROP, and randomized to the Multicenter Trial of Cryotherapy of Prematurity (CRYO-ROP), was reported in 2001 (116). Visual outcome was described as "unfavorable" based on functional outcome (near and distant visual acuity of 20/200 or worse) and structural outcome (posterior retinal folds or worse). Significantly fewer unfavorable outcomes were seen in "treated" compared to "control" eyes (44.4% vs. 62.1%) at 10 years of age, and the benefit of cryotherapy for treatment of threshold ROP for both structure and function was maintained till 15 years of age (117). It is, however, alarming to know that whilst cryotherapy lowers the risk of unfavorable outcome, more than 40% of infants had long-term visual disability. The results of these CRYO-ROP follow-up studies are likely to be applicable to the current practice of laser treatment for threshold ROP, considering that although a comparative study using historic controls showed that laser photocoagulation resulted in better structural outcome compared to trans-scleral cryotherapy (118), a small but well-designed prospective randomized trial did not show any significant difference in visual outcomes at 3 years of age (119).

Long-Term Outcomes at 18 Months and 10 Years

An observational study by Tin et al. (104) is the only published study that has provided data on neurodevelopmental outcome of "all" surviving children who received their early neonatal care under different oxygen-monitoring policies. Their findings from the initial follow-up that there was no difference in the rate of cerebral palsy (of any type or severity) amongst 294 survivors, though important, is still not entirely reassuring considering that the use of a "restrictive" oxygen therapy approach in early neonatal life may have a negative impact on cognitive and intellectual functions, adaptive skills and behavior; impairments which will not be apparent at about 18 months of age when these children are first assessed.

The second follow-up of the same cohort by Bradley, Tin and their colleagues (120), completed recently, involved a total of 124 surviving children who had early neonatal care under "restrictive" (target saturation 80–90%) and "liberal" (target saturation 94–98%) oxygen therapy approaches. Structured assessments were carried out on intellectual and cognitive function (Wechsler Intelligent Scale for Children, third edition) (121), literacy and numeracy skills (Wechsler Objective Reading and Numerical Dimensions) (122), adaptive functioning (Vineland Adaptive Behavior Scale) (123) and behavior (Child Behavior Check List) (124). In addition, information on health (including vision) and education status was also collected. Children were seen at about 10 years of age, and the follow-up rate in this cohort was 96%. The mean score for full-scale IQ of all the 119 children assessed was about one standard deviation below the population mean. More children cared for with the "liberal" approach were found to have cognitive disability compared to the "restrictive" approach (35% vs. 23%), and the mean full-scale IQ of children in the former group was eight points lower compared to the latter. The scores varied very widely and showed a skewed distribution, and the difference between the two mean IQ scores was not statistically significant. A similar trend was seen for literacy and numeracy skills. There was also a noticeable but non-significant excess of children with very low (less than 2nd centile) Vineland Adaptive Behavior Scale in the "liberal" approach group compared to the "restricted" group (34% vs. 20%). These results need to be treated with caution as they have not yet been subjected to rigorous scrutiny to see whether any perinatal factors (such as gestation at birth) or socio-economic factors might be responsible for these observed differences. However, these findings provide reassurance to clinicians that it is highly unlikely that restrictive oxygen therapy, with an aim of keeping functional oxygen saturations of between 80% and 90% in babies of less than 28 weeks gestation until they no longer need supplemental oxygen or their retinal vasculature is fully developed, is associated with any disadvantages in terms of intellectual skills, academic achievements, adaptive functioning and behavior amongst long-term surviving children.

Of 64 surviving children who had "liberal" oxygen therapy in the neonatal period, five were registered as blind at 10 years of age, but none of the 60 children in the "restrictive" oxygen therapy group had this degree of visual disability. Using the same definition as in the CRYO-ROP follow-up study (116), 12.7% of the eyes of children in the "liberal" group had unfavorable visual outcome compared to only 3% in the "restrictive" group, and this difference is highly significant. Despite cryotherapy, an unfavorable visual outcome was seen in 45% of the eyes that reached threshold ROP, highlighting once again the critical need for well-designed research to find out more effective ways of treating ROP (125), and more importantly preventing ROP in these preterm babies.

CONTROVERSIES ON OXYGEN THERAPY

The most historic and arguably the most important of all the questions and controversies on oxygen therapy and monitoring in preterm babies, a "restrictive" or a "liberal" approach, is the main subject of this chapter. There are some other questions and controversies related to maintenance of oxygenation in preterm infants. Commonly asked questions are discussed next.

Respiratory Support for Convalescent Preterm Infants: CPAP or Oxygen?

The dilemma of using continuous positive airway pressure (CPAP) as an alternative to oxygen therapy in a preterm baby who needs respiratory support is not easy to address, as positive airway pressure is also generated with the use of a high-flow nasal cannula (HFNC). Locke et al. (126) reported in 1993 that nasal cannulae can inadvertently generate a positive end-distending pressure, and that an air-oxygen mixture delivered through nasal cannulae at a flow of 2 L/min can generate a mean pressure of 9.8 cmH$_2$O. Sreenan et al. (127) demonstrated that flow rates between 1.0 and 2.5 L/min given through high-flow nasal cannulae can generate positive distending pressure (measured as end-expiratory esophageal pressure) in management of low birth weight infants with apnea of prematurity, comparable to pressures delivered by conventional CPAP devices at 6 cmH$_2$O. Walsh et al. (128)

recently reported a nested cohort study of 187 infants with birthweight < 1250 g, who were receiving oxygen via nasal cannulae. Fifty-two (27.8%) of the study infants were receiving minimal supplemental oxygen with an "effective FiO_2" of less than 23%. When subjected to room air challenge (129), 87 (46.5%) of study infants were weaned successfully to room air, and this success rate was as high as 72% for infants who were receiving an effective FiO_2 of < 0.23 prior to room air challenge. More interestingly, 7 out of 22 infants in this cohort who were receiving only room air with flow rates between 0.13 and 2.0 L/min failed the room air challenge, implying that resultant airway pressure due to the flow, rather than supplemental oxygen, may play an important part in contributing a clinical benefit in some infants perceived to be oxygen-dependent. The use of HFNC in excess of 1 L/min would demand further evaluation in the smallest infants to ascertain whether their natural airway orifices are capable of acting as intrinsic predictable blow-off valves to prevent the generation of excessive airway pressure (130). There is no comparative study to answer the question: Is it better to keep a preterm baby on CPAP with room air or off CPAP with supplemental oxygen? The knowledge of the relation between flow and airway pressure delivered by high-flow nasal cannulae, the concept of "effective FiO_2" (131) and the ability to calculate this in preterm infants should help the clinicians to rationalize the choice of respiratory support for convalescent preterm infants.

Continuous Non-Invasive Monitoring: Oxygen Saturation or Oxygen Tension?

The monitoring of oxygenation in the fetus or newborn demands a reliable way of estimating the oxygen content of blood. Although it is generally accepted that PaO_2 monitoring is the gold standard surrogate of tissue oxygenation in preterm infants, there is no clinical evidence to date to support this perception. Furthermore, PaO_2 monitoring has its inherent limitations, particularly of being invasive and the risk of iatrogenic complications. Although continuous PaO_2 monitoring is feasible through an indwelling catheter, this can only be used for a short term, and not throughout the period during which the preterm infant is vulnerable to oxygen toxicity as well as hypoxic damage. Moreover, PaO_2 monitoring only provides intermittent snapshots of oxygenation rather than providing a continuous trend in most clinical settings. Transcutaneous oxygen monitoring (TcO_2) did overcome these limitations, but its clinical use has declined over the past decade due to several reasons, including the regular need for calibration and local complications such as skin burns, particularly in extreme preterm babies. Studies have shown a good correlation between blood oxygen saturation and pulse oximeter saturation readings (132, 133). In newborns with high content of HbF, a small reduction of PaO_2 will be magnified into larger reductions in SaO_2 in the steep part of the oxygen-dissociation curve. Moreover, pulse oximeters are highly sensitive in detecting hyperoxia provided that type-specific alarm limits are set (based on whether the oximeter measures functional or fractional saturation) and a low specificity is accepted (134) (Box 15.1). However, pulse oximetry has its own technical limitations (e.g. motion artefacts, electromagnetic interference) and physiological limitations in clinical situations, including hypotension, hypoperfusion, severe anemia and dyshemoglobinemias (135). The flat parts of the sigmoid-shaped oxygen-hemoglobin dissociation curve also highlight the lack of accuracy in reflecting true arterial PO_2 when the saturations are very high or very low. Although there is no consensus on whether TcO_2 or SpO_2 is better as non-invasive monitoring, a questionnaire survey of 100 neonatal units in North America in the 1990s showed that 74% of the units were using pulse oximetry as the sole method of continuous monitoring (136), and it is very likely that this trend continues.

Optimum Oxygen Saturation in Preterm Infants: Does it Vary with Postnatal Age?

There is no clear defined range of oxygen saturation that is applicable to different postnatal ages of preterm infants. Perhaps it is more important to identify optimum saturation in the very early postnatal period, arguably from birth (and during resuscitation) so as to minimize the risk of oxidative stress and subsequent morbidities in preterm infants, and all clinicians would agree with this "preventive" approach. As already discussed, data available to date suggested the "low saturation targeting" approach may be preferable in the early neonatal period. Knowledge of the pathophysiology of ROP often raises the question as to whether targeting higher saturation is desirable in preterm infants who develop pre-threshold ROP. A well-designed randomized American STOP-ROP trial, though not conclusive, suggested "high saturation targeting" may benefit some infants with pre-threshold ROP.

Another question often raised by the clinicians is the effect of blood transfusion or reduction in the content of HbF with advancing postnatal age on optimum oxygen saturations. The effects of HbF and HbA on P_{50} have already been described. The change in P_{50} after blood transfusion in preterm infants has not been thoroughly investigated. However, in one small study (137) of preterm infants with a mean gestational age of 25.3 weeks, it was observed that the HbF content decreased from 92.9% to 43.5%, within 2.8 days after transfusion. This was associated with a parallel and significant increase in P_{50} from 18.1 to 21.0 mmHg. This knowledge of changes in P_{50} could be useful to predict the "optimum oxygen saturation range," but the clinical benefits of attempting to target this range at a different postnatal age or after blood transfusion remains debatable.

RESOLVING THE UNCERTAINTY: THE WAY FORWARD

The lack of knowledge and ongoing uncertainty for over 50 years on what is "normal" oxygenation for babies making the transition to extra-uterine life, particularly when they are born very prematurely, has led on to wide variation of acceptance as to what constitutes a safe minimum or maximum level of oxygenation for a small baby in the first few weeks of life. Figure 15-9 shows this variation in the UK (138) and policies in the USA vary just as much (136). Observational studies over the past 50 years have got us nowhere, and the only way to resolve the uncertainties and controversies of oxygen monitoring and therapy is to conduct large, well-designed randomized controlled trials (139–141).

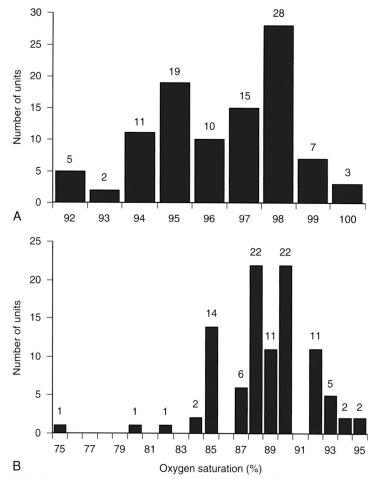

Figure 15-9 Oxygen saturation monitoring policies in the UK. Results from a telephone survey of 100 units with three or more intensive care cots caring for babies of less than 28 weeks gestation in 2001. High (A) and low (B) oximeter alarm settings. (Reproduced from Tin W, Wariyar U. Giving small babies oxygen: 50 years of uncertainty. Semin Neonatol 2002; 7:361 with permission of the publisher, Elsevier.)

The important features of an "ideal" randomized control trial to look at the effect of different approaches of oxygen monitoring and therapy include:

(1) Targeting a population that is at highest risk of neonatal morbidities as well as long-term mortality and adverse neurosensory outcome; in other words, preterm infants as defined by gestational age (since gestation rather than birth weight is the best predictor for both short- and long-term outcomes) (142).

(2) Early randomization and intervention based on assigned oxygen monitor soon after birth, ideally immediately from birth.

(3) Adequate sample size that will enable one to exclude the possibility that a reduction in important neonatal morbidities by the "restrictive" oxygen approach is not associated with a small but significant increase in death or serious neurosensory disability in survivors.

(4) Effective blinding of the assigned oxygen monitors using similar technology to that in the Australian BOOST trial (110), to minimize observers' bias and non-compliance.

(5) A system of continuous data monitoring on oxygen levels using similar technology to that in the American STOP-ROP trial (109), so as to detect

the variability of oxygen levels outside the target range, and also to minimize non-compliance.

(6) A model (practice within the trial) that would be likely to become "standard practice" in day-to-day clinical practice; a "pragmatic trial".

(7) A long-term composite of death or major neurosensory disability (predefined) being used as the "primary" outcome measure, along with several important neonatal morbidities as "secondary" outcomes. Arguably, even using "long-term" outcomes at 18 months or 2 years may not be satisfactory, and the cognitive outcome at school age may be a more meaningful outcome (143).

(8) Complete ascertainment of long-term follow-up information to minimize the distortion of the perceived outcome (144).

MULTICENTER RANDOMIZED CONTROLLED TRIALS – "THE OXYGEN SATURATION TRIALS"

In response to the growing demand to resolve the controversy on oxygen therapy in very preterm babies, an international collaborative effort has been mounted to conduct large multicenter randomized trials to address the main research question: Does varying the concentration of inspired oxygen to maintain a "low" oxygen saturation range of 85–89% versus a "high" range of 91–95% in babies of less than 28 weeks gestation from the day of birth till they are breathing air affect the incidence of: (1) death or severe neurosensory disability at corrected age of 2 years; (2) retinal surgery for ROP; (3) the need for supplemental oxygen therapy or respiratory support at 36 weeks post-menstrual age; (4) patent ductus arteriosus requiring treatment (medical or surgical), or necrotizing enterocolitis requiring surgery; (5) poor growth at 36 weeks post-menstrual age and at 2 years?

The trials have been designed as "double-blind" trials using central randomization. The strategy for blinding was shown to be successful in the first Australian BOOST trial (110), and this will help to minimize co-intervention bias and outcome ascertainment bias. The target oxygen saturation range of the study Masimo Radical Oximeters® (with the Signal Extraction Technology) is 88–92%, but these trial monitors will be adjusted to display the "offset" saturation that is either 3% higher or 3% lower than the actual oxygen saturation, thereby producing two study groups with two different ranges of saturation. The allocated oximeter will be used as long as oxygen saturation monitoring is required while the infant remains in hospital.

Infants of *< 28 weeks* gestation are eligible if they are *< 24 hours* of age. Recruitment is not appropriate if death is imminent, if there is a congenital anomaly affecting oxygenation or the likelihood of successful follow-up is low. *Primary outcome* of all the trials is the composite of death or major neurosensory disability at 2 years (corrected for prematurity). Uniformed definition of major disability constitutes: mental developmental index (MDI) using the Bayley Scales of Infant Development (BSID) (145) of less than 70 (< 2 SD below mean), severe visual loss, not walking unaided due to cerebral palsy and severe hearing loss requiring hearing aids. *Secondary outcomes* include: (i) retinal surgery; (ii) oxygen dependency at 36 weeks post-menstrual age; the need for supplemental oxygen will be assessed by physiological definition (130); (iii) duration of respiratory supports (endotracheal intubation, nasal CPAP, supplemental oxygen); (iv) patent ductus arteriosus; (v) necrotizing enterocolitis requiring surgery; (vi) growth parameters at discharge and at 2 years; (vii) hospital readmissions up to 2 years; (viii) cerebral palsy; (ix) visual impairment; (x) hearing loss; (xi) mean MDI on the BSID; and (xii) death after 4 weeks chronological age primarily due to pulmonary disease.

The Oxygen Saturation Trials across the continents include: BOOST 2 (Benefit Of Oxygen Saturation Targeting) Trial (Australia), BOOST 2 Trial (New Zealand), BOOST 2 Trial (United Kingdom), COT (Canadian Oxygen Trial), and the SUPPORT Trial (The Surfactant Positive Airway Pressure and Pulse Oximetry Trial in Extremely Low Birth Weight Infants) and POST-ROP (Pulse Oximetry Saturation Trial to prevent Retinopathy of Prematurity) in North America. There has already been a prospective agreement to combine the individual patient data from all the trials in order to increase the ability to detect much smaller differences of the primary outcome, and this controlled trial-strategy of *prospective meta-analysis* (146) is likely to be established for the first time in neonatal medicine from "the oxygen trials."

Collaboration across three continents helped Campbell to identify the cause of retinopathy in the preterm baby more than 50 years ago (10). The similar collaboration to mount the well-designed randomized trials and the strategy of prospective meta-analysis will provide important information to confirm or refute that the "restrictive" oxygen approach does more good than harm in preterm babies vulnerable to oxygen toxicity. However, clinicians should be aware that the current oxygen trials may not end the questions and controversies on "oxygen" – a powerful and most commonly used "drug" in neonatal medicine.

"The clinician must bear in mind that oxygen is a drug and must be used in accordance with well recognized pharmacologic principles; i.e., since it has certain toxic effects and is not completely harmless (as widely believed in clinical circles) it should be given only in the lowest dosage or concentration required by the particular patient."

—Julius Comroe (1945)

REFERENCES

1. Patz A, Hoeck LE, de la Cruz E. Studies on the effect of high oxygen administration in retrolental fibroplasia. 1. Nursery observations. Am J Ophthalmol 1952; 35:1248.
2. Kinsey VE, Jacobus JT, Hemphill F. Retrolental fibroplasia: cooperative study of retrolental fibroplasia and the use of oxygen. Arch Ophthalmol 1956; 56:481.
3. Lanman TJ, Guy LP, Dancis J. Retrolental fibroplasia and oxygen therapy. JAMA 1954; 155:223.
4. Priestley J, Experiments and observations on different kinds of air. London: J Johnson; 1775: 101.
5. Scheele KW. Chemische abhandlung von der luft und dem feuer. Upsala and Leipzig, 1777. (See also the English translation: Chemical observations and experiments on air and fire; with an introduction by Torbern Bergman. London: J Johnson; 1780.).
6. Lavoisier A-L. Experiences sur la respiration des animaux. Mém Soc Sci Paris 1777; 2:185 (actually published in 1780).
7. Tin W, Hey E. The medical use of oxygen: a century of research in animals and humans. Neo Reviews 2003; 4:e349.
8. Wilson JL, Long SB, Howard PJ. Respiration of premature infants: response to variations of oxygen and to increased carbon dioxide in inspired air. Am J Dis Child 1942; 63:1080.
9. Howard PJ, Bauer AR. Irregularities of breathing in the newborn period. Am J Dis Child 1949; 77:592.
10. Campbell K. Intensive oxygen therapy as a possible cause of retrolental fibroplasia: a clinical approach. Med J Austr 1951; ii:48.
11. Crosse VM, Evans PJ. Prevention of retrolental fibroplasia. Arch Ophthalmol 1952; 48:83.
12. Guy LP, Lanman TJ, Dancis J. The possibility of total elimination of retrolental fibroplasia by oxygen restriction. Pediatrics 1956; 17:247.
13. Avery ME, Oppenheimer EH. Recent increase in mortality in hyaline membrane disease. J Pediatr 1960; 57:553.
14. Cross KW. Cost of preventing retrolental fibroplasia? Lancet 1973; ii:954.
15. Bolton DPG, Cross KW. Further observations on the cost of preventing retrolental fibroplasia. Lancet 1974; i:445.
16. Duc G, Sinclair JC. Oxygen administration. In: Sinclair JC, Bracken MB, eds., Effective care of the newborn infant. Oxford: Oxford University Press; 1992: 178–199.
17. Mike V, Krauss AN, Ross GS. Doctors and the health industry: a case study of transcutaneous oxygen monitoring in neonatal intensive care. Social Sci Med 1996; 42:1247.
18. Yamanouchi I, Igarashi I, Ouchi E. Incidence and severity of retinopathy in low birth weight infants monitored by TCPO$_2$. Adv Exp Med Biol 1987; 220:105.

19. Grylack LJ. Transcutaneous oxygen monitoring and retinopathy of prematurity. Pediatrics 1987; 80:973.
20. Bancalari E, Flynn J, Goldberg RN, et al. Influence of transcutaneous oxygen monitoring on the incidence of retinopathy of prematurity. Pediatrics 1987; 79:663.
21. Flynn JT, Bancalari E, Snyder ES, et al. A cohort study of transcutaneous oxygen tension and the incidence and severity of retinopathy of prematurity. N Engl J Med 1992; 326:1050.
22. Hay W. The uses, benefits, and limitations of pulse oximetry in neonatal medicine: consensus on key issues. J Perinatol 1987; 7:347.
23. Walsh MC, Noble LM, Carlo WA, et al. Relationship of pulse oximetry to arterial oxygen tension in infants. Crit Care Med 1987; 15:1102.
24. Southall DP, Bignall S, Stebbens VA, et al. Pulse oximeter and transcutaneous arterial oxygen measurements in neonatal and paediatric intensive care. Arch Dis Child 1987; 62:882.
25. Bucher HU, Fanconi S, Baeckert P, et al. Hyperoxemia in newborn infants: detection by pulse oximetry. Pediatrics 1989; 84:226.
26. Poets CF, Wilken M, Seidenberg J, et al. Reliability of a pulse oximeter in the detection of hyperoxemia. J Pediatr 1993; 122:87.
27. Cochran DP, Shaw NJ. The use of pulse oximetry in the prevention of hyperoxaemia in preterm infants. Eur J Pediatr 1995; 154:222.
28. Brockway J, Hay WW. Prediction of arterial partial pressure of oxygen with pulse oxygen saturation measurements. J Pediatr 1998; 133:63.
29. Wasunna A, Whitelaw GL. Pulse oximetry in preterm infants. Arch Dis Child 1987; 62:957.
30. Blanchette V, Doyle J, Schmidt B, et al. Hematology. In: Avery GB, Fletcher MA, MacDonald MG, eds., Neonatology, pathophysiology and management of the newborn. Philadelphia: J.B. Lippincott; 1994: 972–973.
31. Hlastala MP, Woodson RD. Saturation dependency of the Bohr effect: interactions among H^+, CO_2 and DPG. J Appl Physiol 1975; 38:1126.
32. Barcroft J, Elsden SR. The oxygen consumption of the sheep fetus. J Physiol 1946; 105:25P.
33. Beer R, Doll E, Wenner J. Shift in oxygen dissociation curve of the blood of infants in the first month of life. Pflugers Arch 1958; 265(6):526.
34. East CE, Dunster KR, Colditz PB. Fetal oxygen saturation during maternal breathing down efforts in the second stage of labour. Am J Perinatol 1998; 15:121.
35. Chua S, Yeong SM, Razvi K, et al. Fetal oxygen saturation during labour. Br J Obstet Gynaecol 1997; 104:1080.
36. Goffinet F, Langer B, Carbonne B, et al. Multicenter study on the clinical value of fetal pulse oximetry: I. Methodologic evaluation. Am J Obstet Gynecol 1997; 177:1238.
37. Dildy GA, Clark SL, Garite TJ, et al. Current status of multicenter randomized clinical trial on fetal oxygen saturation monitoring in the United States. Eur J Obstet Gynaecol Reprod Biol 1997; 72:S43.
38. Sailing E. Fetal Pulse oximetry during labour: issues and recommendations for clinical use. J Perinat Med 1996; 24:467.
39. East CE, Colditz PB, Dunster KR, et al. Human fetal intrapartum oxygen saturation monitoring: agreement between readings from two sensors on the same fetus. Am J Obstet Gynaecol 1996; 174:1594.
40. Nijland R, Jongsma H, Nijhuis J, et al. Arterial oxygen saturation in relation to metabolic acidosis in fetal lambs. Am J Obstet Gynaecol 1995; 172:810.
41. Avery ME. The lung and its disorders. Philadelphia: WB Saunders; 1974.
42. Guyton AC. Regulation of cardiac output. Anesthesiology 1971; 29:235.
43. Dudell G, Cornish JD, Bartlett RH. What constitutes adequate oxygenation? Pediatrics 1990; 85:39.
44. Strang LB. The lungs at birth. Arch Dis Child 1965; 40:575.
45. Moss AJ, Emmanoulides GC, Adams FH, et al. Response of the ductus arteriosus and pulmonary and systemic arterial pressure to changes in oxygen environment in newborn infants. Pediatrics 1964; 33:937.
46. Born GV, Dawes GS, Mott JC. Oxygen lack and autonomic nervous control of the foetal circulation in the lamb. J Physiol 1956; 134(1):149.
47. Cassin S, Dawes GS, Ross BB. Pulmonary blood flow and vascular resistance in immature fetal lambs. J Physiol 1964; 171:80.
48. Dawes GS. Pulmonary circulation in the foetus and new-born. Br Med Bull 1966; 22(1):61.
49. Schulze A, Whyte RK, Way RC, et al. Effect of arterial oxygenation level on cardiac output, oxygen extraction, and oxygen consumption in low birth weight infants receiving mechanical ventilation. J Pediatr 1995; 126:777.
50. Rasanen J, Wood DC, Debbs RH, et al. Reactivity of the human fetal pulmonary circulation to maternal hyperoxygenation increases during the second half of pregnancy: a randomized study. Circulation 1998; 97:257.
51. Skinner JR, Hunter S, Poets CF, et al. Haemodynamic effects of altering arterial oxygen saturation in preterm infants with respiratory failure. Arch Dis Child 1999; 80:F81.
52. Roth AM. Retinal vascular development in premature infants. Am J Ophthalmol 1977; 84:636.
53. Shweiki D, Itin A, Soffer D, et al. Vascular endothelial growth factor induced by hypoxia may mediate hypoxia-initiated angiogenesis. Nature 1992; 359:843.
54. Hellstrom A, Perruzzi C, Ju M, et al. Low IGF-1 suppresses VEGF-survival signaling in retinal endothelial cells: direct correlation with clinical retinopathy of prematurity. Proc Natl Acad Sci USA 2001; 98:5804.

55. Smith LEH. Pathogenesis of retinopathy of prematurity. Semin Neonatol 2003; 8:469.
56. Pierce EA, Foley ED, Smith LE. Regulation of vascular endothelial growth factor by oxygen in a model of retinopathy of prematurity [see comments] [published erratum appears in Arch Ophthalmol 1997; 115:427]. Arch Ophthalmol 1996; 114:1219.
57. McColm JR, Cunningham S, Wade J, et al. Hypoxic oxygen fluctuations produce less severe retinopathy than hyperoxic fluctuations in a rat model of retinopathy of prematurity. Pediatr Res 2004; 55(1):107.
58. Phelps DL, Rosenbaum AL. Effects of marginal hypoxemia on recovery from oxygen induced retinopathy in the kitten model. Pediatrics 1984; 73(1):1.
59. Shohat M, Reisner SH, Krikler R, et al. Retinopathy of prematurity: incidence and risk factors. Pediatrics 1983; 72:159.
60. Tsuchiya S, Tsuyama K. Retinopathy of prematurity: birth weight, gestational age and maximum $PaCO_2$. Tokai J Exp Clin Med 1987; 12:39.
61. Brown DR, Milley JR, Ripepi UJ, et al. Retinopathy of prematurity. Risk factors in a five year cohort of critically ill premature neonates. Am J Dis Child 1987; 141:154.
62. Berkowitz BA. Adult and newborn rat inner retinal oxygenation during carbogen and 100% oxygen breathing. Invest Ophthalmol Vis Sci 1996; 37:2089.
63. Dani C, Reali MF, Bertini G, et al. The role of blood transfusions and iron intake on retinopathy of prematurity. Early Hum Dev 2001; 62:57.
64. Romagnoli C, Zecca E, Gallini F, et al. Do recombinant human erythropoietin and iron supplementation increase the risk of retinopathy of prematurity? Eur J Pediatr 2000; 159:627.
65. Kennedy C, Grave GD, Jehle JW. Effect of hyperoxia on the cerebral circulation of the newborn puppy. Pediatr Res 1971; 5:659.
66. Fledelius HC. Central nervous system damage and retinopathy of prematurity – an ophthalmic follow-up of prematures born in 1982–84. Acta Paediatr 1996; 85:1186.
67. Rybnikova E, Damdimopoulos AE, Gustafsson JA, et al. Expression of novel antioxidant thioredoxin-2 in the rat brain. Eur J Neurosci 2000; 12:1669.
68. Nangia S, Saili A, Dutta AK, et al. Free oxygen radicals – predictors of neonatal outcome following perinatal asphyxia. Indian J Pediatr 1998; 65:419.
69. Silvers KM, Gibson AT, Powers HJ. High plasma vitamin C levels at birth associated with low antioxidant status and poor outcome in premature babies. Arch Dis Child 1994; 71:F40.
70. Issa A, Lappalainen U, Kleinman M, et al. Inhaled nitric oxide decreases hyperoxia induced surfactant abnormality in preterm rabbits. Pediatr Res 1999; 45:247.
71. Gyllensten L. Influence of oxygen exposure on the differentiation of the cerebral cortex of growing mice. Acta Morphol Neerl Scand 1959; 2:311.
72. Hannah RS, Hannah KJ. Hyperoxia: effects on the vascularisation of the developing central nervous system. Acta Neuropathol 1980; 51:141.
73. Grave GD, Kennedy C, Sokoloff L. Impairment of growth and development of the rat brain by hyperoxia at atmospheric pressure. J Neurochem 1972; 19:187.
74. Grunnet ML. Periventricular leukomalacia complex. Arch Pathol Lab Med 1979; 103:6.
75. Ahdab-Barmada M, Moosy J, Painter M. Pontosubicular necrosis and hyperoxaemia. Pediatrics 1980; 65:840.
76. Haynes RL, Folkerth RD, Keefe RJ, et al. Nitrosative and oxidative injury to premyelinating oligodendrocytes in periventricular leukomalacia. J Neuropathol Exp Neurol 2003; 62:441.
77. Collins MP, Lorenz JM, Jetton JR, et al. Hypocapnia and other ventilation related risk factors for cerebral palsy in low birth weight infants. Pediatr Res 2001; 50:712.
78. Felderhoff MU, Bittigau P, Sifringer M, et al. Oxygen causes cell death in developing brain. Neurobiol Dis 2004; 17(2):273.
79. Northway WH, Rosan RC, Porter DY. Pulmonary disease following respirator therapy of hyaline membrane disease: bronchopulmonary dysplasia. N Engl J Med 1967; 267:357.
80. Anderson WR, Strickland MB, Tsai SH, et al. Light microscopic and ultrastructural study of the adverse effects of oxygen on the neonate lung. Am J Path 1973; 73:327.
81. Reynolds EOR, Taghizadeh A. Improved prognosis of infants mechanically ventilated for hyaline membrane disease. Arch Dis Child 1974; 49:505.
82. Taghizadeh A, Reynolds EOR. Pathogenesis of bronchopulmonary dysplasia following hyaline membrane disease. Am J Pathol 1976; 82:241.
83. deLemos R, Wolfsdorf J, Nachman R, et al. Lung injury from oxygen in lambs. The role of artificial ventilation. Anesthesiology 1969; 30:609.
84. Miller WM, Waldhausen JA, Rashkind WJ. Comparison of oxygen poisoning of the lung in cyanotic and acyanotic dogs. N Engl J Med 1970; 282:943.
85. Jobe AH, Bancalari E. Bronchopulmonary dysplasia. Am J Respir Crit Care Med 2001; 163:1723.
86. Weingerger B, Laskin DL, Heck DE, et al. Oxygen toxicity in premature infants. Toxicol Appl Pharmacol 2002; 181:60.
87. Saugstad OD. Bronchopulmonary dysplasia – oxidative stress and oxidants. Semin Neonatol 2003; 8:39.
88. Saugstad OD. Oxidative stress in newborn – a 30 year perspective. Biol Neonate 2005; 88:228.
89. Poets CF. When do infants need additional inspired oxygen? A review of the current literature. Pediatr Pulmonol 2001; 26:424.
90. Richard D, Poets CF, Neale S, et al. Arterial oxygen saturation in preterm neonates without respiratory failure. J Pediatr 1993; 123:963.
91. Poets CF, Stebbens VA, Alexander JR, et al. Arterial oxygen saturation in preterm infants at discharge from the hospital and six weeks later. J Pediatr 1992; 120:447.

92. Poets CF, Stebbens VA, Lang JA, et al. Arterial oxygen saturation in healthy term neonates. Eur J Pediatr 1996; 155(3):219.

93. Stebbens VA, Poets CF, Alexander JR, et al. Oxygen saturation and breathing patterns in infancy. 1. Full term infants in the second month of life. Arch Dis Child 1991; 66:569.

94. Poets CF, Stebbens VA, Alexander JR, et al. Oxygen saturation and breathing patterns in infancy. 2: Preterm infants at discharge from special care. Arch Dis Child 1991; 66:574.

95. Ng A, Subhedar N, Primhak RA, et al. Arterial oxygen saturation profiles in healthy preterm infants. Arch Dis Child 1998; 79:F64.

96. Koch G, Wendel H. Adjustment of arterial blood gases and acid base balance in the normal newborn infant during the first week of life. Biol Neonate 1968; 12:136.

97. Sekar K, Duke JC. Sleep apnoea and hypoxaemia in recently weaned premature infants with and without bronchopulmonary dysplasia. Pediatr Pulmonol 1991; 10:112.

98. Singer L. Oxygen desaturation complicates feeding in infants with bronchopulmonary dysplasia after discharge. Pediatrics 1992; 90:380.

99. Fitzgerald D, Van Asperen P, O'Leary P, et al. Sleep, respiratory rate, and growth hormone in chronic neonatal lung disease. Pediatr Pulmonol 1998; 26:241.

100. Fitzgerald D, Evans N, Van Asperen P, et al. Subclinical persisting pulmonary hypertension in chronic neonatal lung disease. Arch Dis Child 1994; 70:F118.

101. Subhedar NV, Shaw NJ. Changes in pulmonary arterial pressure in preterm infants with chronic lung disease. Arch Dis Child 2000; 82:F243.

102. Giacoia GP, Venkataraman PS, West-Wilson KI, et al. Follow-up of school-age children with bronchopulmonary dysplasia. J Pediatr 1997; 130:400.

103. Usher R. Treatment of respiratory distress. In: Winters RW, ed., Body fluids in pediatrics. Boston: Little Brown; 1973: 303–337.

104. Tin W, Milligan DWA, Pennefather P, et al. Pulse oximetry, severe retinopathy, and outcome at one year in babies of less than 28 weeks gestation. Arch Dis Child 2001; 84:F106.

105. Sun SC. Relation of target SpO_2 levels and clinical outcome in ELBW infants on supplemental oxygen. Pediatr Res 2002; 51:A350.

106. Chow L, Wright KW, Sola S. Can changes in clinical practice decrease the incidence of severe retinopathy in very low birth weight infants? Pediatrics 2003; 111:339.

107. Anderson CG, Benitz WE, Madan A. Retinopathy of prematurity and pulse oximetry: A national survey of recent practices. J Perinatol 2004; 24:164.

108. Poets C, Arand J, Hummler H, et al. Retinopathy of prematurity: a comparison between two centers aiming for different pulse oximetry saturation levels. Biol Neonate 2003; 84:267.

109. The STOP-ROP Multicenter Study Group. Supplemental Therapeutic Oxygen for Prethreshold Retinopathy Of Prematurity (STOP-ROP), a randomized, controlled trial. I. Primary outcomes. Pediatrics 2000; 105:295.

110. Askie LM, Henderson-Smart DJ, Irwig L, et al. Oxygen-saturation targets and outcomes in extremely preterm infants. N Engl J Med 2003; 349:953.

111. Groothuis JR, Rosenberg AA. Home oxygen promotes weight gain in infants with bronchopulmonary dysplasia. Am J Dis Child 1987; 141:992.

112. Hudak BB, Allen MC, Hudak ML, et al. Home oxygen therapy for chronic lung disease in extremely low-birthweight infants. Am J Dis Child 1989; 143:357.

113. Simakajornboon N, Beckerman RC, Mack C, et al. Effect of supplemental oxygen on sleep architecture and cardiorespiratory events in preterm infants. Pediatrics; 2002; 110:884.

114. Whyte RK. First day neonatal mortality since 1935: re-examination of Cross hypothesis. BMJ 1992; 304:343.

115. Schmidt B, Asztalos EV, Roberts RS, et al. Impact of bronchopulmonary dysplasia, brain injury, and severe retinopathy on the outcome of extremely low-birth-weight infants at 18 months: results from the trial of indomethacin prophylaxis in preterm. JAMA 2003; 289:1124.

116. Multicenter Trial of Cryotherapy for Retinopathy of Prematurity. Ophthalmological outcomes at 10 years. Cryotherapy for Retinopathy of Prematurity Cooperative Group. Arch Ophthalmol 2001; 119:1110.

117. 15 Year outcomes following threshold retinopathy of prematurity: final results from the Multicenter Trial of Cryotherapy for Retinopathy of Prematurity. Cryotherapy for Retinopathy of Prematurity Cooperative Group. Arch Ophthalmol 2005; 123:311.

118. Pearce IA, Pennie FC, Gannon LM, et al. Three year visual outcome for treated stage 3 retinopathy: cryotherapy versus laser. Br J Ophthalmol 1998; 82:1254.

119. White JE, Repka MX. Randomised comparison of diode laser photocoagulation versus cryotherapy for threshold retinopathy of prematurity: three year outcome. J Pediatr Ophthalmol Strabismus 1997; 34:83.

120. Bradley S, Anderson K, Tin W, et al. Early oxygen exposure and outcome at 10 years in babies of less than 28 weeks. Pediatr Res 2004; 55:A373.

121. Wechsler D. Intelligence Scale for Children. Texas: Psychological Corporation; 1991.

122. Wechsler D. Wechsler Objective Reading Dimension Test. Sidcup, UK: Psychological Corporation; 1993.

123. Sparrow SS, Balla DA, Cicchetti DV. Vineland adaptive behaviour scales: Interview Edition Survey Forms Manual. Circle Pines, MN: American Guidance Service; 1984.

124. Achenbach TM, Edelbrock C. Manual for the child behavior checklist and revised child behavior profile. Burlington, Vermont: Queen City Printers; 1983.

125. Early Treatment for Retinopathy of Prematurity Cooperative Group. Revised indications for the treatment of retinopathy of prematurity: results of the early treatment for retinopathy of prematurity randomized trial. Arch Ophthalmol 2003; 121:1684.

126. Locke RG, Wofson MR, Shaffer TH, et al. Inadvertent administration of positive end-distending pressure during nasal cannula flow. Pediatrics 1993; 91:135.

127. Sreenan C, Lemke RP, Hudson-Mason A, et al. High-flow nasal cannulae in the management of apnea of prematurity: a comparision with conventional nasal continuous positive airway pressure. Pediatrics 2001; 107:1081.

128. Walsh M, Engle W, Laptook A, et al. Oxygen delivery through nasal cannulae to preterm infants: can practice be improved? Pediatrics 2005; 116:857.

129. Walsh MC, Wilson-Costello D, Zadell A, et al. Safety, reliability, and validity of a physiologic definition of bronchopulmonary dysplasia. J Perinatol 2003; 23:451.

130. Finer NN. Nasal cannula use in the preterm infant: oxygen or pressure? Pediatrics 2005; 116:1216.

131. Benaron DA, Benitz WE. Maximizing the stability of oxygen delivered via nasal cannula. Arch Pediatr Adolesc Med 1994; 148(3):294.

132. Major D, Masson M. Estimation of PaO_2 using pulsatile oximetry and the HbO_2 dissociation curve in the premature infant. Union Med Can 1989; 118:21.

133. Walsh MC, Noble LM, Carlo WA, et al. Relationship of pulse oximetry to arterial oxygen tension in infants. Crit Care Med 1987; 15(12):1102.

134. Bucher H, Fanconi S, Baeckert P, et al. Hyperoxemia in newborn infants: detection by pulse oximetry. Pediatr 1989; 84(2):226.

135. Moyle JTB. Limitations. In: Hahn CEW, Adams AP, eds., Principles and practice series: pulse oximetry. Plymouth: BMJ; 1998:108.

136. Vijayakumar E, Ward GJ, Bullock CE, et al. Pulse oximetry in infants < 1500 gm at birth on supplemental oxygen: a national survey. J Perinatol 1997; 17:341.

137. Halleux V, De, Gagnon CG, Bard H. Decreasing oxygen saturation in very early preterm newborn infants after transfusion. Arch Dis Child 2003; 88:F163.

138. Tin W, Wariyar U. Giving small babies oxygen: 50 years of uncertainty. Semin Neonatol 2002; 7:361.

139. Tin W. Oxygen therapy: 50 years of uncertainty. Pediatrics 2002; 110:615.

140. Cole CH, Wright KW, Tarnow-Mordi W, et al. Resolving our uncertainty about oxygen therapy. Pediatrics 2003; 112:1415.

141. Silverman WA. A cautionary tale about supplemental oxygen: the albatross of neonatal medicine. Pediatrics 2004; 113:394.

142. Tin W, Wariyar U, Hey E. Changing prognosis for babies of less than 28 weeks gestation in the north of England between 1983 and 1994. BMJ 1997; 314:107.

143. Marlow N, Wolke D, Bracewell MA, et al. Neurologic and developmental disability at six years of age after extremely preterm birth. N Eng J Med 2005; 352:9.

144. Tin W, Fritz S, Wariyar U, et al. Outcome of very preterm birth: children reviewed with ease at two differ from those only traced and reviewed with difficulty. Arch Dis Child 1998; 79:83.

145. Bayley N. Manual for the Bayley scales of infant development. Texas: Psychological Corporation; 1993.

146. Simes RJ. Prospective meta-analysis of cholesterol-lowering studies: the Prospective Pravastatin Pooling (PPP) Project and the Cholesterol Treatment Trialists (CTT) Collaboration. Am J Cardiol 1995; 76:122C.

Chapter 16

Non-invasive Respiratory Support: An Alternative to Mechanical Ventilation in Preterm Infants

Peter G. Davis MD FRACP • Colin J. Morley MD FRACP FRCPCH

Physiological Principles

A Brief History of Invasive and Non-invasive Neonatal Ventilation

NCPAP for Post-Extubation Care

Augmenting NCPAP: Nasal Intermittent Positive Pressure Ventilation (NIPPV)

NCPAP for Babies with RDS or at Risk of Developing RDS

NCPAP Devices

High-Flow Nasal Cannulae for Respiratory Support

How Much Supporting Pressure Should be Used?

Complications of NCPAP

When has NCPAP Failed: i.e., When Should Infants be Intubated?

Weaning Continuous Positive Airway Pressure

Conclusions

When making choices about treatment, the primary concern of the clinician is whether one therapy leads to better outcomes than the alternatives. This chapter draws heavily on evidence from randomized trials found in the neonatal module of the Cochrane Library (http://www.nichd.nih.gov/cochrane/default.cfm). Consistent with presentation in the library, estimates of treatment effect are expressed as relative risk (RR) and the differences are statistically significant if the 95% confidence interval does not include one. Other levels of evidence, e.g. from observational studies, will be presented, particularly where no randomized trials exist. In some areas the highest level of available evidence is our own personal experience and we present this cautiously and with humility.

Before examining the available evidence, we believe that summarizing the physiological principles underpinning non-invasive respiratory support and the history of its application usefully informs clinicians and researchers in the field. Although other techniques exist, this chapter will focus on the mainstay of current non-invasive support, nasal continuous positive airway pressure (NCPAP).

MANAGEMENT OF RESPIRATORY FAILURE

PHYSIOLOGICAL PRINCIPLES

Why Do Preterm Infants Experience Respiratory Failure and How Can Non-invasive Support Help?

Respiratory Distress Syndrome (RDS)

RDS is a disease of newborn infants, increasing in prevalence with decreasing gestational age. It is characterized by immature lung development and inadequate surfactant production. The lungs of affected infants may not expand normally immediately after birth, do not easily maintain a residual volume and are at risk of atelectasis. Other factors also contribute to a loss of lung volume, including muscle hypotonia, a compliant chest wall and slow clearance of fetal lung liquid. Repeated lung expansion, followed by atelectasis during expiration, leads to shearing forces, which damage the alveolar epithelium and leakage of protein-rich fluid from the pulmonary capillaries, which in turn inhibits any endogenous surfactant present (1). Damage to the lungs is exacerbated by mechanical ventilation and high oxygen concentrations.

Apnea of Prematurity

The pharyngeal airway of the preterm newborn is very compliant. The cartilaginous components are more flexible and the fat-laden superficial fascia of the neck that stabilizes the upper airway of term infants is not well developed. The intrathoracic airways including trachea, bronchi and small airways are similarly compliant and prone to collapse.

The breathing patterns of very premature infants are frequently erratic and at times inadequate. Much time and effort is spent in neonatal intensive care units monitoring and treating apneic episodes. The causes of apnea of prematurity include hypoxia and reduced functional residual capacity (FRC), particularly in active sleep. Upper airway obstruction, alone or in combination with a central respiratory pause, accompanies most apneic events.

The Role of Nasal CPAP

NCPAP effectively supports the breathing of preterm infants through a number of mechanisms. It mechanically splints the upper airway thereby preventing obstruction and reducing apnea (2). Dilatation of the airways reduces resistance to air flow and so diminishes work of breathing (3). NCPAP aids lung expansion and so reduces ventilation perfusion mismatch and improves oxygenation. By preventing repeated alveolar collapse and re-expansion, NCPAP reduces protein leak and helps conserve surfactant.

Why Might Non-invasive Support Be Superior to Ventilation via an Endotracheal Tube?

Intermittent positive pressure ventilation via an endotracheal tube has been the mainstay of neonatal intensive care almost since its inception. Many lives have been saved by this technique but its adverse effects are well documented:

- complications of the endotracheal tube, including subglottic stenosis and tracheal lesions
- infections, both pulmonary and systemic
- acute and chronic lung damage due to large tidal volumes (volutrauma), excessive inflating pressure (barotrauma) and shear stress with each inflation.

362

By avoiding the local mechanical problems of an endotracheal tube as well as those of volutrauma, NCPAP has at least a theoretical advantage over invasive respiratory support.

A BRIEF HISTORY OF INVASIVE AND NON-INVASIVE NEONATAL VENTILATION

The first form of assisted ventilation for neonates was intermittent positive pressure ventilation provided via an endotracheal tube, which became widespread in the late 1960s and early 1970s. George Gregory was the first to describe the use of CPAP in neonates in 1971; a therapy he developed because of the high mortality observed in infants weighing less than 1500 g, particularly those requiring assisted ventilation in the first 24 h of life (4). The first series of 20 "severely ill" infants with RDS were treated with CPAP delivered predominantly via an endotracheal tube. In an attempt to avoid the complications of endotracheal intubation, other interfaces were developed, including a pressurized plastic bag (5) and a tight-fitting face mask (6). Two infants in Gregory's initial series were managed in a pressure chamber around the infant's head (4). In 1973, Ahlström et al. described the use of a face chamber providing pressures up to 15 cmH$_2$O (7). Rhodes and Hall conducted a controlled trial, based on alternate allocation of subjects to CPAP via a tight-fitting face mask or conventional therapy of warmed humidified oxygen (8). A trend towards increased survival was noted in the CPAP group, which was statistically significant in the subgroup of infants weighing more than 1500 g.

The local pressure effects of these devices, combined with the problems of accessibility, particularly for suctioning and feeding, led to the development of alternative interfaces for the delivery of CPAP. Novogroder et al. described a device composed of two Portex endotracheal tubes inserted through the nose and positioned under direct laryngoscopy in the posterior pharynx, joined by a Y-connector and attached to pressure source (9). Others described shorter bi-nasal devices which were simpler to manufacture and insert (10, 11). An even simpler single nasal prong, made by cutting down an endotracheal tube, became widely used (12). A recent development in the field is that of a variable-flow device which uses jet nozzles to assist inspiratory flow while diverting flow away from the patient in expiration (13). It is claimed that this design is superior to conventional CPAP in reducing work of breathing (14).

It should be noted that of all the above trials, only Rhodes and Hall used a control group (8). Novogroder et al. had plans to subject their device to a randomized trial but abandoned them when "the dramatic effect of CPAP (was) observed after a brief period of treatment in all patients" (9). It is likely that others were so convinced of the virtues of endotracheal intubation that trials of this therapy against CPAP were considered inappropriate. In an accompanying commentary to Rhodes et al.'s study (8), Chernick congratulated the authors on conducting a "daring controlled study" and suggested that while one or two such studies of nasal CPAP would be welcome, many more "would be foolish" (15). With some notable exceptions it seems researchers heeded his advice. The following sections present these exceptions.

NCPAP FOR POST-EXTUBATION CARE

It is generally accepted that early extubation of premature infants who have been managed with an endotracheal tube (ETT) is desirable. The perceived benefits of early extubation include reducing the risks of infection, local tissue damage and chronic lung disease. On the other hand, failed extubation and the need for reinsertion

COMPARISON: Nasal CPAP vs Headbox
OUTCOME: Failure of extubation

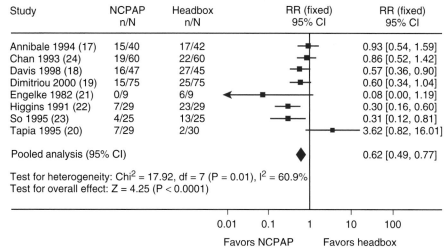

Study	NCPAP n/N	Headbox n/N	RR (fixed) 95% CI
Annibale 1994 (17)	15/40	17/42	0.93 [0.54, 1.59]
Chan 1993 (24)	19/60	22/60	0.86 [0.52, 1.42]
Davis 1998 (18)	16/47	27/45	0.57 [0.36, 0.90]
Dimitriou 2000 (19)	15/75	25/75	0.60 [0.34, 1.04]
Engelke 1982 (21)	0/9	6/9	0.08 [0.00, 1.19]
Higgins 1991 (22)	7/29	23/29	0.30 [0.16, 0.60]
So 1995 (23)	4/25	13/25	0.31 [0.12, 0.81]
Tapia 1995 (20)	7/29	2/30	3.62 [0.82, 16.01]
Pooled analysis (95% CI)			0.62 [0.49, 0.77]

Test for heterogeneity: Chi^2 = 17.92, df = 7 (P = 0.01), I^2 = 60.9%
Test for overall effect: Z = 4.25 (P < 0.0001)

Favors NCPAP   Favors headbox

Figure 16-1 NCPAP for extubation: failure.

of the ETT is associated with instability and the possibility of more local trauma. The Cochrane systematic review of the topic (16) identified eight randomized trials of varying methodological quality, using various levels of CPAP and devices (17–24). Pooled analysis showed that NCPAP reduced the rate of respiratory failure after extubation compared to management in an oxyhood (relative risk 0.62; 0.49–0.77) (Fig. 16-1). Four of the included studies allowed rescue NCPAP to be provided for babies failing oxyhood. As rescue treatment was frequently successful, there was no significant difference in rates of endotracheal intubation between the groups (RR 0.93 (0.72, 1.19)) (Fig. 16-2). A study that directly compared elective versus rescue NCPAP after extubation found no differences in reintubation rates (25). Therefore, it could reasonably be concluded that NCPAP should be used when an endotracheal tube is removed from a very premature infant to prevent the instability associated with possible subsequent respiratory failure and reintubation. However, if resources are

COMPARISON: Nasal CPAP vs Headbox
OUTCOME: Endotracheal reintubation

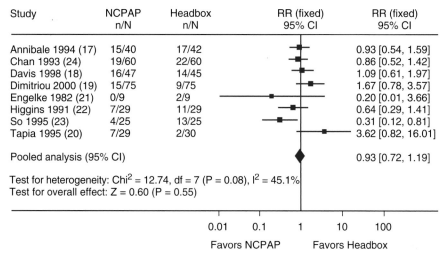

Study	NCPAP n/N	Headbox n/N	RR (fixed) 95% CI
Annibale 1994 (17)	15/40	17/42	0.93 [0.54, 1.59]
Chan 1993 (24)	19/60	22/60	0.86 [0.52, 1.42]
Davis 1998 (18)	16/47	14/45	1.09 [0.61, 1.97]
Dimitriou 2000 (19)	15/75	9/75	1.67 [0.78, 3.57]
Engelke 1982 (21)	0/9	2/9	0.20 [0.01, 3.66]
Higgins 1991 (22)	7/29	11/29	0.64 [0.29, 1.41]
So 1995 (23)	4/25	13/25	0.31 [0.12, 0.81]
Tapia 1995 (20)	7/29	2/30	3.62 [0.82, 16.01]
Pooled analysis (95% CI)			0.93 [0.72, 1.19]

Test for heterogeneity: Chi^2 = 12.74, df = 7 (P = 0.08), I^2 = 45.1%
Test for overall effect: Z = 0.60 (P = 0.55)

Favors NCPAP   Favors Headbox

Figure 16-2 NCPAP for extubation: reintubation.

limited, it appears that reserving the use of NCPAP for preterm infants who have developed symptoms of respiratory failure post-extubation does not lead to an increased rate of reintubation.

AUGMENTING NCPAP: NASAL INTERMITTENT POSITIVE PRESSURE VENTILATION (NIPPV)

Although NCPAP has proven to be an effective method of post-extubation support, researchers have sought to further improve the technique by adding positive pressure inflations to a background of nasal CPAP. The technique was widely used in the 1980s but became less popular when reports appeared linking its use to gastrointestinal perforation (26). The availability of ventilators that provided inflations synchronized with the infant's own efforts led to renewed interest in NIPPV. Systematic review identified three randomized trials (27–29) evaluating the technique for the post-extubation care of preterm infants (30). Pooled analysis showed that NIPPV significantly reduced the risk of respiratory failure compared with NCPAP (RR 0.21 (0.10, 0.45)) (Fig. 16-3). Two of the three studies allowed rescue therapy with NIPPV for infants failing NCPAP. The effect of NIPPV on rate of reintubation was therefore decreased, although still significant (RR 0.39 (0.18, 0.97)) (Fig. 16-4). Reassuringly, there was no significant difference in the rate of abdominal distension and no infant developed gastrointestinal perforation. All three trials in this systematic review used the Infant Star ventilator with a Graseby capsule to provide synchronized inflations to babies randomized to NIPPV. There is little to guide clinicians in determining the ventilator settings when using this technique. In the randomized trials the rate of ventilator breaths varied between 10 and 25/min and the peak pressures were set at or slightly above the peak inspiratory pressures used pre-extubation. Since publication, the ventilator used in these trials has ceased production. Anecdotally, many units have reverted to using non-synchronized NIPPV and the association with gastrointestinal perforations has not re-emerged.

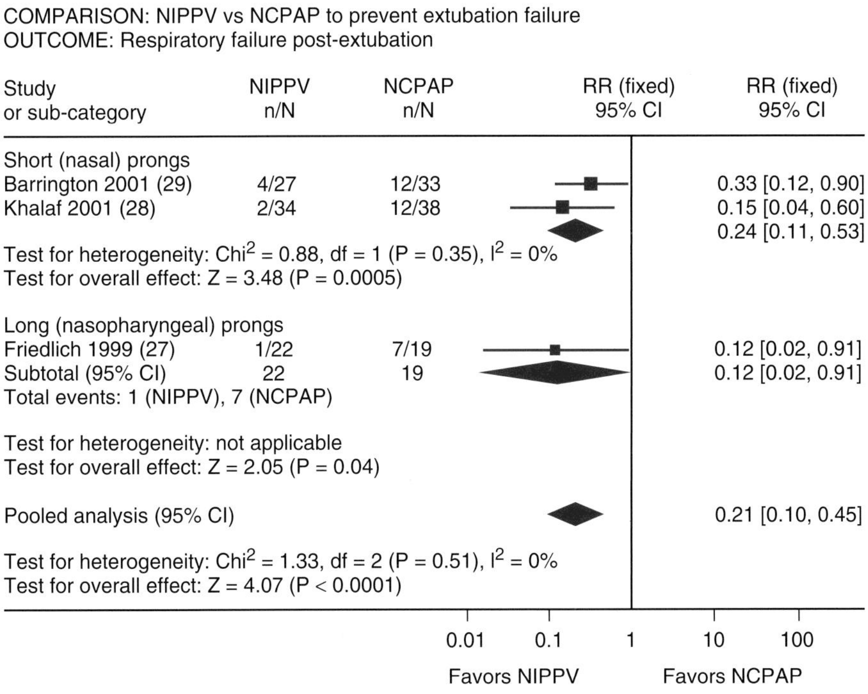

COMPARISON: NIPPV vs NCPAP to prevent extubation failure
OUTCOME: Respiratory failure post-extubation

Study or sub-category	NIPPV n/N	NCPAP n/N	RR (fixed) 95% CI	RR (fixed) 95% CI
Short (nasal) prongs				
Barrington 2001 (29)	4/27	12/33		0.33 [0.12, 0.90]
Khalaf 2001 (28)	2/34	12/38		0.15 [0.04, 0.60]
				0.24 [0.11, 0.53]

Test for heterogeneity: Chi^2 = 0.88, df = 1 (P = 0.35), I^2 = 0%
Test for overall effect: Z = 3.48 (P = 0.0005)

Long (nasopharyngeal) prongs				
Friedlich 1999 (27)	1/22	7/19		0.12 [0.02, 0.91]
Subtotal (95% CI)	22	19		0.12 [0.02, 0.91]

Total events: 1 (NIPPV), 7 (NCPAP)

Test for heterogeneity: not applicable
Test for overall effect: Z = 2.05 (P = 0.04)

Pooled analysis (95% CI)				0.21 [0.10, 0.45]

Test for heterogeneity: Chi^2 = 1.33, df = 2 (P = 0.51), I^2 = 0%
Test for overall effect: Z = 4.07 (P < 0.0001)

```
          0.01    0.1      1      10     100
          Favors NIPPV        Favors NCPAP
```

Figure 16-3 NIPPV for extubation: failure.

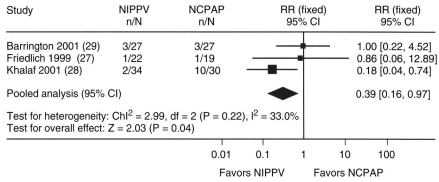

COMPARISON: NIPPV vs NCPAP to prevent extubation failure
OUTCOME: Endotracheal reintubation

Study	NIPPV n/N	NCPAP n/N	RR (fixed) 95% CI	RR (fixed) 95% CI
Barrington 2001 (29)	3/27	3/27		1.00 [0.22, 4.52]
Friedlich 1999 (27)	1/22	1/19		0.86 [0.06, 12.89]
Khalaf 2001 (28)	2/34	10/30		0.18 [0.04, 0.74]
Pooled analysis (95% CI)				0.39 [0.16, 0.97]

Test for heterogeneity: Chl^2 = 2.99, df = 2 (P = 0.22), I^2 = 33.0%
Test for overall effect: Z = 2.03 (P = 0.04)

0.01   0.1   1   10   100
Favors NIPPV   Favors NCPAP

Figure 16-4 NIPPV: reintubation.

NIPPV is used in other clinical situations. Systematic review of NIPPV for treating apnea of prematurity found only two studies, with a total of 54 infants (31, 32). The pooled analysis showed a modest benefit for NIPPV over NCPAP and no evidence of harm (33). It therefore seems reasonable to try NIPPV when infants are experiencing troublesome apnea while treated with NCPAP. Following its success in these situations, some have suggested NIPPV be used as an initial form of support for preterm infants with respiratory distress but this is not based on randomized trials. Observational studies suggest that this mode of support is worth testing in randomized trials either alone (34) or in conjunction with prior intubation and exogenous surfactant therapy (35).

NIPPV appears to be a useful method for augmenting the beneficial effects of NCPAP. Further studies of the best settings to use and the safety of the non-synchronized mode as well as its use as a primary method of support in RDS are required.

NCPAP FOR BABIES WITH RDS OR AT RISK OF DEVELOPING RDS

The focus of studies on this topic has changed over the decades. Questions will be dealt with in roughly historical order.

Is Prophylactic CPAP Better than No Assisted Ventilation for Very Preterm Infants?

The rationale for the use of NCPAP in this context is that it may assist the establishment and maintenance of an FRC and thereby alter the natural history of RDS. Observational studies comparing practices in different centers and in the same centers over time suggested that the early use of CPAP leads to a reduction in the need for IPPV and to a reduced rate of bronchopulmonary dysplasia (BPD) (36–38). Two randomized trials enrolling 312 preterm infants compared the use of NCPAP started in the first hours of life to headbox oxygen (oxyhood) (39, 40). Pooled analysis of these trials found no significant difference in rates of endotracheal intubation (Fig. 16-5), CLD, pneumothorax or mortality (41). However, these trials recruited relatively mature infants (up to 32 weeks) with a low incidence of adverse outcomes. More trials are required to answer this important question, particularly in very premature infants at greatest risk of death or CLD.

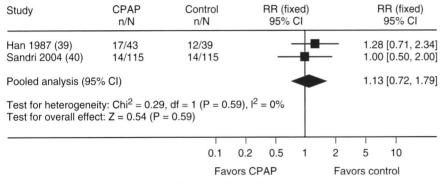

COMPARISON: Prophylactic CPAP vs control
OUTCOME: Endotracheal intubation

Study	CPAP n/N	Control n/N	RR (fixed) 95% CI	RR (fixed) 95% CI
Han 1987 (39)	17/43	12/39		1.28 [0.71, 2.34]
Sandri 2004 (40)	14/115	14/115		1.00 [0.50, 2.00]
Pooled analysis (95% CI)				1.13 [0.72, 1.79]

Test for heterogeneity: Chi^2 = 0.29, df = 1 (P = 0.59), I^2 = 0%
Test for overall effect: Z = 0.54 (P = 0.59)

0.1   0.2   0.5   1   2   5   10

Favors CPAP   Favors control

Figure 16-5 Prophylactic NCPAP: endotracheal intubation.

Is Continuous Distending Pressure (CDP) Better than No CDP for Treatment of RDS?

CDP includes any treatment where a continuous positive or negative pressure is applied to aid lung expansion. A review of this topic found five studies comparing continuous distending pressure with no assisted ventilation, four of which were undertaken in the 1970s (42). Two used negative pressure chambers (43, 44), two used face mask CPAP (8, 45) and one used negative pressure for less severe illness and endotracheal CPAP when more severe (46). Pooled analysis of these trials showed that CDP was associated with benefits in terms of reduced treatment failure (death or use of assisted ventilation) (RR 0.70 (0.55, 0.88)) and mortality (RR 0.53 (0.32, 0.87)) (Fig. 16-6). However, an increased rate of pneumothorax was noted in the CDP group (RR 2.36 (1.25, 5.54)) (Fig. 16-7).

These results are of limited relevance in the modern neonatal intensive care era because of the settings of the included studies and the techniques used. However, in developing countries where resources are limited, CPAP may be an inexpensive, effective technique for management of RDS.

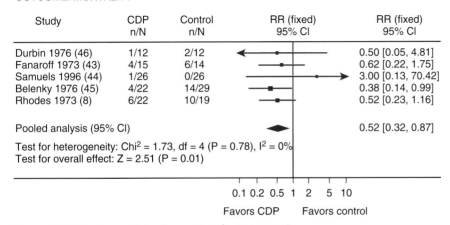

COMPARISON: CDP VS STANDARD CARE
OUTCOME: MORTALITY

Study	CDP n/N	Control n/N	RR (fixed) 95% CI	RR (fixed) 95% CI
Durbin 1976 (46)	1/12	2/12		0.50 [0.05, 4.81]
Fanaroff 1973 (43)	4/15	6/14		0.62 [0.22, 1.75]
Samuels 1996 (44)	1/26	0/26		3.00 [0.13, 70.42]
Belenky 1976 (45)	4/22	14/29		0.38 [0.14, 0.99]
Rhodes 1973 (8)	6/22	10/19		0.52 [0.23, 1.16]
Pooled analysis (95% CI)				0.52 [0.32, 0.87]

Test for heterogeneity: Chi^2 = 1.73, df = 4 (P = 0.78), I^2 = 0%
Test for overall effect: Z = 2.51 (P = 0.01)

0.1 0.2 0.5 1   2   5   10

Favors CDP   Favors control

Figure 16-6 Continuous distending pressure for RDS: mortality.

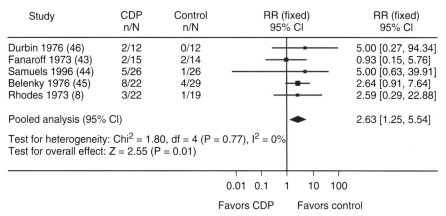

COMPARISON: CDP VS STANDARD CARE
OUTCOME: ANY PNEUMOTHORAX

Study	CDP n/N	Control n/N	RR (fixed) 95% CI	RR (fixed) 95% CI
Durbin 1976 (46)	2/12	0/12		5.00 [0.27, 94.34]
Fanaroff 1973 (43)	2/15	2/14		0.93 [0.15, 5.76]
Samuels 1996 (44)	5/26	1/26		5.00 [0.63, 39.91]
Belenky 1976 (45)	8/22	4/29		2.64 [0.91, 7.64]
Rhodes 1973 (8)	3/22	1/19		2.59 [0.29, 22.88]
Pooled analysis (95% CI)				2.63 [1.25, 5.54]

Test for heterogeneity: Chi^2 = 1.80, df = 4 (P = 0.77), I^2 = 0%
Test for overall effect: Z = 2.55 (P = 0.01)

0.01 0.1 1 10 100

Favors CDP   Favors control

Figure 16-7 Continuous distending pressure for RDS: pneumothorax.

CPAP in the "Surfactant Era"

Two questions have emerged. Is CPAP with early intubation for surfactant and brief ventilation better than CPAP and selective intubation, surfactant and continued ventilation? Is CPAP better than endotracheal intubation at birth?

Surfactant is the most comprehensively evaluated treatment in neonatology. Whether given to ventilated babies prophylactically or as treatment, it reduces mortality and the combined outcome of death or chronic lung disease (47, 48). It appears that surfactant is more beneficial when given early in the course of RDS (49). Although other methods of administration have been tried (50), surfactant is given via an endotracheal tube. It has become common practice for very preterm infants to be intubated in the delivery room for the purpose of surfactant administration as well as the perceived stability that endotracheal intubation ensures. However, the process of intubation is destabilizing for the infant (51) and pediatric trainees often struggle to achieve satisfactory performance in this area (52). A systematic review was conducted of studies addressing the question of whether early, brief intubation for surfactant administration followed by extubation to NCPAP was better than NCPAP and selective intubation, surfactant and continued ventilation (53). Meta-analysis of included studies showed no significant difference in mortality or the combined outcome death or BPD. There was a reduction in the subsequent need for ventilation (RR 0.79 (0.59. 0.85)) but an increased use of surfactant (0.51 doses (0.36, 0.65)) in the early intubation group. Further trials are required to determine whether the instability associated with intubation is outweighed by the benefits of surfactant therapy.

The second question is whether premature infants at high risk of RDS should be intubated and ventilated in the delivery room, given surfactant and have continuing ventilation in the NICU or be managed with NCPAP and only be intubated if they develop respiratory failure. Several groups have reported their experience over time as they have changed policy from intubation to NCPAP in the delivery room (54, 55). They describe lower mortality and morbidity in the group treated with NCPAP.

The design of these trials does not allow therapeutic recommendations to be made but provided the stimulus for a randomized trial currently in progress designed to answer the question of whether NCPAP or endotracheal intubation in the delivery room is better (56).

NCPAP DEVICES

Since the introduction of NCPAP, several interfaces have been developed to transmit pressure to the infant. The nasal prongs may be short, lying 1–2 cm inside the nose or long, with the tip in the nasopharynx (Fig. 16-8). They may be single or binasal. An important determinant of effectiveness of CPAP devices is their ability to transmit the pressure set by the clinician to the infant. This depends on the resistance to flow of the device, which in turn depends on the length and diameter of the prongs. Not surprisingly, in an in vitro comparison of popular devices, short binasal prongs with the largest internal diameters had the lowest resistance (57).

Since its description by Moa et al. in 1988 (13), the variable-flow NCPAP device (known as the Aladdin, EME infant flow Nasal CPAP or Infant Flow Driver) has become widely used around the world. In vitro studies using models of neonatal ventilation have demonstrated less pressure variation and work of breathing with the variable flow device (58). Pandit et al. have measured work of breathing (WOB) in preterm infants using respiratory inductance plethysmography and esophageal pressure monitoring (59). They demonstrated a reduction in WOB with variable-flow CPAP compared to constant-flow CPAP. The same group showed, in a crossover study, that the variable-flow device led to better lung recruitment than either nasal cannulae or continuous flow CPAP (60).

While understanding the properties of different devices is useful, for clinicians the primary question regarding NCPAP devices is whether one is better than the others at reducing the severity of the respiratory problems and the incidence of endotracheal intubation. Head to head comparisons of different devices are few. Pooled analysis of the two trials (61, 62) comparing single and double nasal prongs after extubation of preterm infants confirms that double prongs are better for preventing extubation failure (RR 0.59 (CI: 0.42, 0.85)) (Fig. 16-9) (63). Two trials have compared different binasal devices. Stefanescu et al. compared the Infant Flow system to Inca prongs and found no difference in rates of extubation failure, death or BPD (64). Sun et al., however, reported a lower rate of reintubation using the Infant Flow system than Medicorp short binasal prongs (65).

Mazzella et al. compared the Infant Flow Driver with a single long nasopharyngeal tube for the treatment of preterm infants with respiratory distress (66). Although infants randomized to the Infant Flow Driver had lower oxygen requirements and

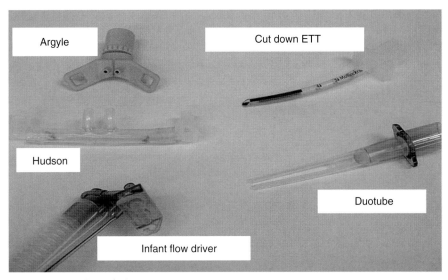

Figure 16-8 NCPAP devices.

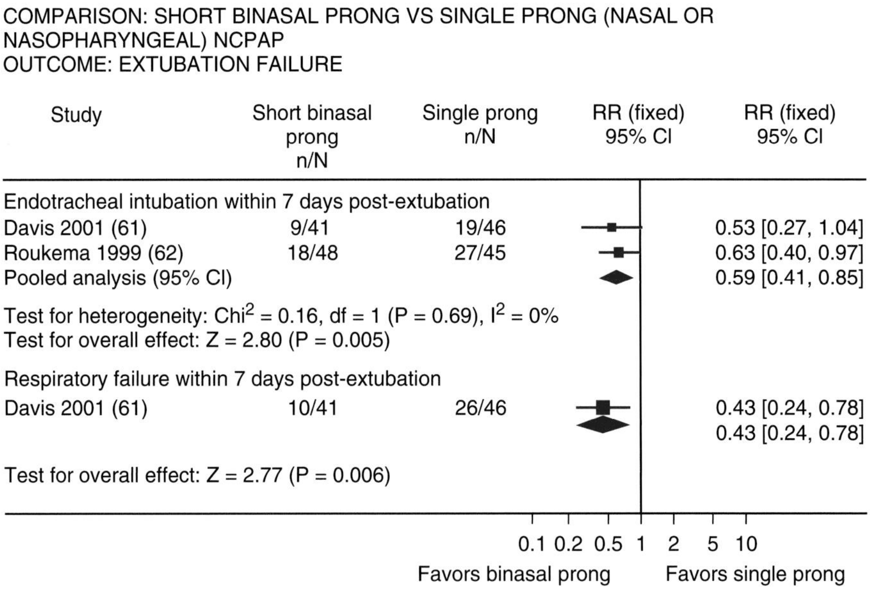

COMPARISON: SHORT BINASAL PRONG VS SINGLE PRONG (NASAL OR
NASOPHARYNGEAL) NCPAP
OUTCOME: EXTUBATION FAILURE

Study	Short binasal prong n/N	Single prong n/N	RR (fixed) 95% CI	RR (fixed) 95% CI
Endotracheal intubation within 7 days post-extubation				
Davis 2001 (61)	9/41	19/46		0.53 [0.27, 1.04]
Roukema 1999 (62)	18/48	27/45		0.63 [0.40, 0.97]
Pooled analysis (95% CI)				0.59 [0.41, 0.85]

Test for heterogeneity: Chi^2 = 0.16, df = 1 (P = 0.69), I^2 = 0%
Test for overall effect: Z = 2.80 (P = 0.005)

Respiratory failure within 7 days post-extubation				
Davis 2001 (61)	10/41	26/46		0.43 [0.24, 0.78]
				0.43 [0.24, 0.78]

Test for overall effect: Z = 2.77 (P = 0.006)

```
        0.1 0.2 0.5  1   2   5  10
     Favors binasal prong   Favors single prong
```

Figure 16-9 Single vs. double prong NCPAP.

respiratory rates there were no significant differences in the need for mechanical ventilation or the duration of CPAP treatment.

The lower resistance offered by binasal prongs appears to translate to a clinical advantage for these devices over short or long single nasal prongs. Further research is required to determine whether the features of the Infant Flow system lead to clinically important benefits over less expensive binasal systems.

HIGH-FLOW NASAL CANNULAE FOR RESPIRATORY SUPPORT

Nasal cannulae delivering high flows of oxygen or air have become a popular form of respiratory support without the intensive scrutiny applied to other modes of assisted ventilation (67). In preterm infants, Locke et al. showed that a flow of 2 L/min through 0.3 cm diameter nasal prongs produced a mean positive end distending pressure of 9.8 cm H_2O as measured by differences in esophageal pressure (68). While noting that some of the infants studied experienced improved respiratory parameters, the group warned, "it is inherently unsafe to use nasal cannulae for the purpose of generating positive end-distending pressure." They cautioned against the indiscriminate use of nasal cannulae in preterm infants. Sreenan et al. undertook a crossover study comparing high-flow nasal cannulae with conventional NCPAP via Argyle prongs (69). They studied 40 premature infants with an average postconceptual age of 30 weeks being treated for apnea with NCPAP for two consecutive 6-h periods. Using esophageal probes to measure end expiratory pressure, they titrated nasal cannula flow to achieve an esophageal pressure equal to that measured when the infant was on NCPAP. They found no significant difference in rate of apneic and bradycardic events between NCPAP and nasal cannula periods and no evidence of nasal trauma or drying during the 6 h of the study. They concluded that high-flow nasal cannulae were simpler to use and as effective as NCPAP in the management of apnea of prematurity. Problems have been noted with nasal cannulae. In a retrospective cohort study, Kopelman and Holbert compared infants supported with oxygen cannulae to a group managed with oxyhoods (70). They found cannula usage was associated with nasal mucosal injury and a trend towards increased infection with coagulase-negative staphylococcal sepsis. The availability of heated and humidified delivery systems has reduced anxiety about these adverse effects.

Uncertainty about the efficacy and safety of high-flow nasal oxygen means that this technique should be regarded as promising and warranting further evaluation rather than considered ready for widespread application.

HOW MUCH SUPPORTING PRESSURE SHOULD BE USED?

The purpose of nasal CPAP is to deliver a supporting pressure to the upper airways and lungs. If this is achieved consistently, it may not matter which device is used. A pressure of 5 cm H_2O is a traditional starting point. Some NICUs hardly vary this and claim good results (71). There is some evidence from the Cochrane NCPAP for extubation review that pressures below 5 cm H_2O are ineffective in this setting (Fig. 16-10) (16). In their landmark publication on CPAP Gregory et al. used pressures up to 15 mmHg (4). A study of infants with mild RDS showed the highest end expiratory lung volume, tidal volume and lowest respiratory rate and thoraco-abdominal asynchrony at a pressure of 8 cmH_2O, compared with 0, 2, 4, and 6 cm H_2O (72).

A baby with RDS, relatively stiff lungs, a high FiO_2 and a chest X-ray showing opaque lungs may need a higher pressure to support lung volume than a baby with a low FiO_2 treated for apneic episodes. If CPAP is to be effective, the pressure may occasionally need to be increased to 10 cm H_2O (73). High pressures, if used inappropriately in a baby with compliant lungs, can compromise cardiopulmonary function, interfere with blood flow through the lungs and cause over-distension leading to carbon dioxide retention. Judging which pressure is needed remains an art. If an infant shows evidence of lung disease with increasing oxygen requirements and a more opaque chest X-ray, we would increase the pressure in increments of 1 cm H_2O and observe the effect.

The optimal CPAP pressure is not known and may depend on the condition treated. Future research should be directed towards evaluating strategies of titrating CPAP pressures to an infant's requirements. In the absence of evidence-based

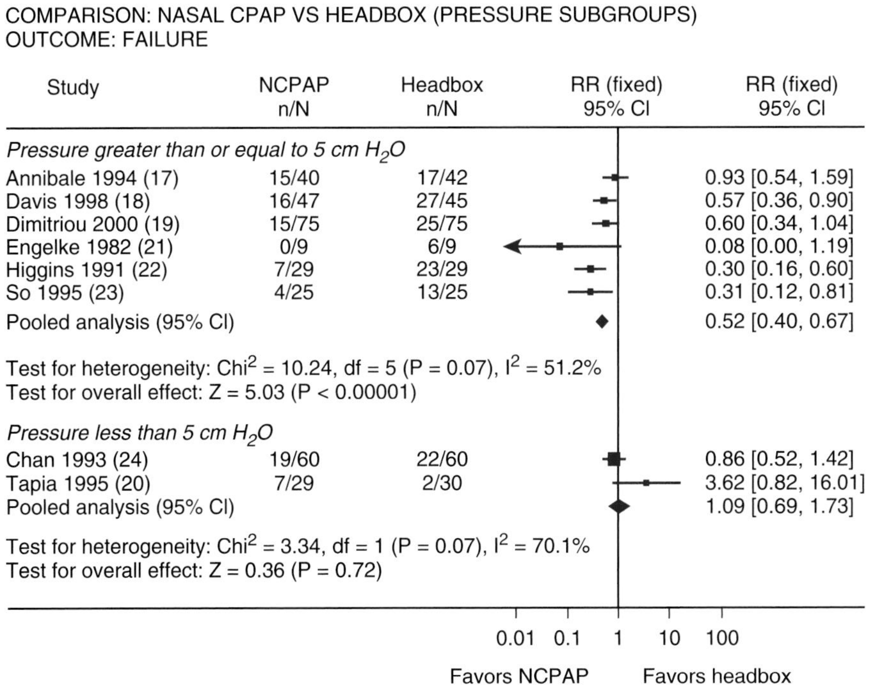

COMPARISON: NASAL CPAP VS HEADBOX (PRESSURE SUBGROUPS)
OUTCOME: FAILURE

Study	NCPAP n/N	Headbox n/N	RR (fixed) 95% CI	RR (fixed) 95% CI
Pressure greater than or equal to 5 cm H_2O				
Annibale 1994 (17)	15/40	17/42		0.93 [0.54, 1.59]
Davis 1998 (18)	16/47	27/45		0.57 [0.36, 0.90]
Dimitriou 2000 (19)	15/75	25/75		0.60 [0.34, 1.04]
Engelke 1982 (21)	0/9	6/9		0.08 [0.00, 1.19]
Higgins 1991 (22)	7/29	23/29		0.30 [0.16, 0.60]
So 1995 (23)	4/25	13/25		0.31 [0.12, 0.81]
Pooled analysis (95% CI)				0.52 [0.40, 0.67]

Test for heterogeneity: Chi^2 = 10.24, df = 5 (P = 0.07), I^2 = 51.2%
Test for overall effect: Z = 5.03 (P < 0.00001)

Pressure less than 5 cm H_2O				
Chan 1993 (24)	19/60	22/60		0.86 [0.52, 1.42]
Tapia 1995 (20)	7/29	2/30		3.62 [0.82, 16.01]
Pooled analysis (95% CI)				1.09 [0.69, 1.73]

Test for heterogeneity: Chi^2 = 3.34, df = 1 (P = 0.07), I^2 = 70.1%
Test for overall effect: Z = 0.36 (P = 0.72)

```
          0.01  0.1   1   10  100
```

Favors NCPAP   Favors headbox

Figure 16-10 NCPAP for extubation – subgroup analysis by pressure used.

guidelines, we use CPAP pressures in the range 5–10 cm H_2O, adjusting these on the basis of oxygen requirements and clinical assessment of work of breathing.

COMPLICATIONS OF NCPAP

NCPAP is a comparatively simple form of respiratory support, yet it is not without complications. The major problems of the early days of CPAP, intracerebellar hemorrhages (74) and hydrocephalus (75), were solved by alterations in delivery technique. However, nasal trauma may occur with the use of prongs and ranges in severity from redness and excoriation of the nasal passages to necrosis of the columella and nasal septum requiring surgery. Observational studies suggest that all CPAP devices may cause trauma and that neither Hudson prongs, single naso-pharyngeal tubes or Infant Flow systems are particularly better or worse than the others (76). Robertson et al. described a complication rate of 20% in a series of very low birthweight babies managed on the Infant Flow Driver. Techniques to prevent nasal trauma are entirely anecdotal. We try to select a prong of sufficient diameter to snugly fit the infant's nostril (avoiding excessive leak around the device) but which does not cause blanching of the nostril wall. Positioning of binasal prongs so that there is no pressure on the columella is sometimes difficult to achieve but critical. We have observed that, within our unit, supervision by skilled nurses experienced in the technique of securing CPAP prongs has led to a low rate of nasal trauma.

WHEN HAS NCPAP FAILED: I.E., WHEN SHOULD INFANTS BE INTUBATED?

There is no universally accepted definition of CPAP failure. Polin et al. suggested that "an infant with ventilation that is not improving or inadequate oxygenation with $FiO_2 > 0.6$" should be intubated and given surfactant (77). Others recommend intubation when oxygen requirements exceed 0.35–0.40 (78). We set the following failure criteria for infants randomized to NCPAP in the COIN trial (56): $FiO_2 > 0.6$ or pH < 7.25 with a $pCO_2 > 60$ mmHg or more than 1 apneic episode per hour requiring stimulation. Whatever threshold is applied, it is important that remediable causes of failure are looked for and treated before intubation. These include airway obstruction with secretions and inappropriate (too small) prong size. Treating a large mouth leak and increasing applied pressure may be useful strategies before accepting that CPAP has failed.

WEANING CONTINUOUS POSITIVE AIRWAY PRESSURE

There are many ways of weaning babies from NCPAP and the optimal method remains uncertain. A survey of neonatal units in the northern region of England showed that while most units wanted formal weaning procedures only 6% had a protocol (79). The majority of units weaned by gradually increasing the time off NCPAP. Robertson and Hamilton randomized 58 premature babies to either a "weaning" or a "rescue" strategy of NCPAP after extubation (80). The weaning strategy gradually increased the time spent off CPAP. In the rescue arm, babies were extubated to headbox oxygen and NCAP was only commenced if predefined failure criteria were reached: NCPAP was discontinued after 12 h and recommenced only if the same failure criteria were met. They found no significant difference in the total number of ventilator days or days on NCPAP. A randomized trial comparing a strategy of weaning pressure with one of increasing time off NCPAP showed a significantly shorter duration of weaning with the "pressure" strategy (81).

In the absence of good evidence, our practice is to wean infants to a CPAP of 5 cm H_2O, discontinue when the infant is stable with an $FiO_2<0.30$ and recommence if oxygen requirements or frequency of apneas increase.

CONCLUSIONS

For Clinicians

On the basis of randomized trials and systematic reviews:

- NCPAP reduces respiratory instability and the need for extra support after extubation
- NCPAP reduces the rate of apnea
- NIPPV is a useful method for augmenting the benefits of NCPAP
- Binasal prongs are superior to single nasal prongs for the delivery of CPAP
- It is *possible* to manage very preterm infants on NCPAP from delivery – whether this approach is better than early endotracheal intubation and surfactant therapy will be clarified by trials currently in progress.

For Researchers

Opportunities to advance knowledge in the field of non-invasive ventilation include studies of:

- Alternative techniques of surfactant administration that do not require endotracheal intubation
- Methods available at the bedside to judge optimal levels of CPAP
- High-flow nasal cannulae to establish safety and efficacy of this technique
- NIPPV to determine the best settings in terms of pressures, rates and synchronization as well as testing its role in the initial management of RDS.

Acknowledgments

PGD is supported by an Australian National Health and Medical Research Council Fellowship.

REFERENCES

1. Ikegami M, Jacobs H, Jobe A. Surfactant function in respiratory distress syndrome. J Pediatr 1983; 102:443–447.
2. Alex CG, Aronson RM, Onal E, Lopata M. Effects of continuous positive airway pressure on upper airway and respiratory muscle activity. J Appl Physiol 1987; 62:2026–2030.
3. Saunders RA, Milner AD, Hopkin IE. The effects of continuous positive airway pressure on lung mechanics and lung volumes in the neonate. Biol Neonate 1976; 29:178–186.
4. Gregory GA, Kitterman JA, Phibbs RH, et al. Treatment of the idiopathic respiratory-distress syndrome with continuous positive airway pressure. N Engl J Med 1971; 284:1333–1340.
5. Barrie H. Simple method of applying continuous positive airway pressure in respiratory-distress syndrome. Lancet 1972; 1:776–777.
6. Ackerman BD, Stein MP, Sommer JS, Schumacher M. Continuous positive airway pressure applied by means of a tight-fitting face-mask. J Pediatr 1974; 85:408–411.
7. Ahlström H, Jonson B, Svenningsen NW. Continuous postive airways pressure treatment by a face chamber in idiopathic respiratory distress syndrome. Arch Dis Child 1976; 51:13–21.
8. Rhodes PG, Hall RT. Continuous positive airway pressure delivered by face mask in infants with the idiopathic respiratory distress syndrome: a controlled study. Pediatrics 1973; 52:1–5.

9. Novogroder M, MacKuanying N, Eidelman AI, Gartner LM. Nasopharyngeal ventilation in respiratory distress syndrome. A simple and efficient method of delivering continuous positive airway pressure. J Pediatr 1973; 82:1059–1062.

10. Wung JT, Driscoll JM Jr, Epstein RA, Hyman AI. A new device for CPAP by nasal route. Crit Care Med 1975; 3:76–78.

11. Caliumi-Pellegrini G, Agostino R, et al. Twin nasal cannula for administration of continuous positive airway pressure to newborn infants. Arch Dis Child 1974; 49:228–230.

12. Field D, Vyas H, Milner AD, Hopkin IE. Continuous positive airway pressure via a single nasal catheter in preterm infants. Early Hum Dev 1985; 11:275–280.

13. Moa G, Nilson K, Zetterstrom H, Jonsson LO. A new device for administration of nasal continuous positive airway pressure in the newborn: an experimental study. Crit Care Med 1988; 16:1238–1242.

14. Courtney SE, Aghai ZH, Saslow JG, et al. Changes in lung volume and work of breathing: a comparison of two variable-flow nasal continuous positive airway pressure devices in very low birth weight infants. Pediatr Pulmonol 2003; 36:248–252.

15. Chernick V. Continuous distending pressure in hyaline membrane disease: of devices, disadvantages, and a daring study. Pediatrics 1973; 52:114–115.

16. Davis PG, Henderson-Smart DJ. Nasal continuous positive airways pressure immediately after extubation for preventing morbidity in preterm infants. Cochrane Database Syst Rev 2003; CD000143.

17. Annibale DJ, Hulsey TC, Engstrom PC, et al. Randomized, controlled trial of nasopharyngeal continuous positive airway pressure in the extubation of very low birth weight infants. J Pediatr 1994; 124:455–460.

18. Davis P, Jankov R, Doyle L, Henschke P. Randomised, controlled trial of nasal continuous positive airway pressure in the extubation of infants weighing 600 to 1250 g. Arch Dis Child Fetal Neonatal Ed 1998; 79:F54–F57.

19. Dimitriou G, Greenough A, Kavvadia V, et al. Elective use of nasal continuous positive airways pressure following extubation of preterm infants [In Process Citation]. Eur J Pediatr 2000; 159:434–439.

20. Tapia JL, Bancalari A, Gonzalez A, Mercado ME. Does continuous positive airway pressure (CPAP) during weaning from intermittent mandatory ventilation in very low birth weight infants have risks or benefits? A controlled trial. Pediatr Pulmonol 1995; 19:269–274.

21. Engelke SC, Roloff DW, Kuhns LR. Postextubation nasal continuous positive airway pressure. a prospective controlled study. Am J Dis Child 1982; 136:359–361.

22. Higgins RD, Richter SE, Davis JM. Nasal continuous positive airway pressure facilitates extubation of very low birth weight neonates. Pediatrics 1991; 88:999–1003.

23. So BH, Tamura M, Mishina J, et al. Application of nasal continuous positive airway pressure to early extubation in very low birthweight infants. Arch Dis Child Fetal Neonatal Ed 1995; 72:F191–F193.

24. Chan V, Greenough A. Randomised trial of methods of extubation in acute and chronic respiratory distress. Arch Dis Child 1993; 68:570–572.

25. Robertson NJ, Hamilton PA. Randomised trial of elective continuous positive airway pressure (CPAP) compared with rescue CPAP after extubation. Arch Dis Child Fetal Neonatal Ed 1998; 79:F58–F60.

26. Garland JS, Nelson DB, Rice T, Neu J. Increased risk of gastrointestinal perforations in neonates mechanically ventilated with either face mask or nasal prongs. Pediatrics 1985; 76:406–410.

27. Friedlich P, Lecart C, Posen R, et al. A randomized trial of nasopharyngeal-synchronized intermittent mandatory ventilation versus nasopharyngeal continuous positive airway pressure in very low birth weight infants after extubation. J Perinatol 1999; 19:413–418.

28. Khalaf MN, Brodsky N, Hurley J, Bhandari V. A prospective randomized, controlled trial comparing synchronized nasal intermittent positive pressure ventilation versus nasal continuous positive airway pressure as modes of extubation. Pediatrics 2001; 108:13–17.

29. Barrington KJ, Bull D, Finer NN. Randomized trial of nasal synchronized intermittent mandatory ventilation compared with continuous positive airway pressure after extubation of very low birth weight infants. Pediatrics 2001; 107:638–641.

30. Davis PG, Lemyre B, De Paoli AG. Nasal intermittent positive pressure ventilation (NIPPV) versus nasal continuous positive airway pressure (NCPAP) for preterm neonates after extubation. Cochrane Database Syst Rev, 2001; CD003212.

31. Ryan CA, Finer NN, Peters KL. Nasal intermittent positive-pressure ventilation offers no advantages over nasal continuous positive airway pressure in apnea of prematurity. Am J Dis Child 1989; 143:1196–1198.

32. Lin CH, Wang ST, Lin YJ, Yeh TF. Efficacy of nasal intermittent positive pressure ventilation in treating apnea of prematurity. Pediatr Pulmonol 1998; 26:349–353.

33. Lemyre B, Davis PG, De Paoli AG. Nasal intermittent positive pressure ventilation (NIPPV) versus nasal continuous positive airway pressure (NCPAP) for apnea of prematurity. Cochrane Database Syst Rev, 2002; CD002272.

34. Manzar S, Nair AK, Pai MG, Paul J, Manikoth P, George M, et al. Use of nasal intermittent positive pressure ventilation to avoid intubation in neonates. Saudi Med J 2004; 25:1464–1467.

35. Santin R, Brodsky N, Bhandari V. A prospective observational pilot study of synchronized nasal intermittent positive pressure ventilation (SNIPPV) as a primary mode of ventilation in infants > or = 28 weeks with respiratory distress syndrome (RDS). J Perinatol 2004; 24:487–493.

36. Avery ME, Tooley WH, Keller JB, et al. Is chronic lung disease in low birthweight infants preventable? A survey of 8 centres. Pediatrics 1987; 79:26–30.

37. Jacobsen T, Gronvall J, Petersen S, Andersen GE. "Minitouch" treatment of very low-birth-weight infants. Acta Paediatr 1993; 82:934–938.

38. Gittermann MK, Fusch C, Gittermann AR, et al. Early nasal continuous positive airway pressure treatment reduces the need for intubation in very low birth weight infants [see comments]. Eur J Pediatr 1997; 156:384–388.

39. Han VK, Beverley DW, Clarson C, et al. Randomized controlled trial of very early continuous distending pressure in the management of preterm infants. Early Hum Dev 1987; 15:21–32.

40. Sandri F, Ancora G, Lanzoni A, et al. Prophylactic nasal continuous positive airways pressure in newborns of 28–31 weeks gestation: multicentre randomised controlled clinical trial. Arch Dis Child Fetal Neonatal Ed 2004; 89:F394–F398.

41. Subramaniam P, Henderson-Smart D, Davis P. Prophylactic nasal continuous positive airways pressure for preventing morbidity and mortality in very preterm infants. Cochrane Database Syst Rev 2005; CD001243.

42. Ho JJ, Subramaniam P, Henderson-Smart DJ, Davis PG. Continuous distending pressure for respiratory distress syndrome in preterm infants. Cochrane Database Syst Rev, 2002; CD002271.

43. Fanaroff AA, Cha CC, Sosa R, et al. Controlled trial of continuous negative external pressure in the treatment of severe respiratory distress syndrome. J Pediatr 1973; 82:921–928.

44. Samuels MP, Raine J, Wright T, et al. Continuous negative extrathoracic pressure in neonatal respiratory failure. Pediatrics 1996; 98:1154–1160.

45. Belenky DA, Orr RJ, Woodrum DE, Hodson WA. Is continuous transpulmonary pressure better than conventional respiratory management of hyaline membrane disease? A controlled study. Pediatrics 1976; 58:800–808.

46. Durbin GM, Hunter NJ, McIntosh N, et al. Controlled trial of continuous inflating pressure for hyaline membrane disease. Arch Dis Child 1976; 51:163–169.

47. Soll RF. Synthetic surfactant for respiratory distress syndrome in preterm infants. Cochrane Database Syst Rev 2000; CD001149.

48. Soll RF. Prophylactic natural surfactant extract for preventing morbidity and mortality in preterm infants. Cochrane Database Syst Rev 2000; CD000511.

49. Yost CC, Soll RF. Early versus delayed selective surfactant treatment for neonatal respiratory distress syndrome. Cochrane Database Syst Rev 2000; CD001456.

50. Kattwinkel J, Robinson M, Bloom BT, et al. Technique for intrapartum administration of surfactant without requirement for an endotracheal tube. J Perinatol 2004; 24:360–365.

51. O'Donnell CP, Kamlin CO, Davis PG, Morley CJ. Endotracheal intubation attempts during neonatal resuscitation: success rates, duration, and adverse effects. Pediatrics 2006; 117:e16–e21.

52. Leone TA, Rich W, Finer NN. Neonatal intubation: success of pediatric trainees. J Pediatr 2005; 146:638–641.

53. Stevens TP, Blennow M, Soll RF. Early surfactant administration with brief ventilation vs selective surfactant and continued mechanical ventilation for preterm infants with or at risk for RDS. Cochrane Database Syst Rev 2002; CD003063.

54. Lindner W, Vossbeck S, Hummler H, Pohlandt F. Delivery room management of extremely low birth weight infants: spontaneous breathing or intubation. Pediatrics 1999; 103:961–967.

55. Aly H, Massaro AN, Patel K, El Mohandes AA. Is it safer to intubate premature infants in the delivery room? Pediatrics 2005; 115:1660–1665.

56. Morley CJ, Davis P, Doyle L. Continuous positive airway pressure: randomized, controlled trial in Australia. Pediatrics 2001; 108:1383.

57. De Paoli AG, Morley CJ, Davis PG, et al. In vitro comparison of nasal continuous positive airway pressure devices for neonates. Arch Dis Child Fetal Neonatal Ed 2002; 87:F42–F45.

58. Klausner JF, Lee AY, Hutchison AA. Decreased imposed work with a new nasal continuous positive airway pressure device. Pediatr Pulmonol 1996; 22:188–194.

59. Pandit PB, Courtney SE, Pyon KH, et al. Work of breathing during constant- and variable-flow nasal continuous positive airway pressure in preterm neonates. Pediatrics 2001; 108:682–685.

60. Courtney SEM. Lung recruitment and breathing pattern during variable versus continuous flow nasal continuous positive airway pressure in premature infants: an evaluation of three devices [Article]. Pediatrics 2001; 107:304–308.

61. Davis P, Davies M, Faber B. A randomised controlled trial of two methods of delivering nasal continuous positive airway pressure after extubation to infants weighing less than 1000 g: binasal (Hudson) versus single nasal prongs. Arch Dis Child Fetal Neonatal Ed 2000; 85:F82–85.

62. Roukema H, O'Brine K, Nesbitt K, Zaw W. A randomized controlled trial of Infant Flow continuous positive airway pressure (CPAP) versus nasopharyngeal CPAP in the extubation of babies ≤1250 g (abstract). Pediatr Res 1999; 45:318A.

63. De Paoli AG, Davis PG, Faber B, Morley CJ. Devices and pressure sources for administration of nasal continuous positive airway pressure (NCPAP) in preterm neonates. Cochrane Database Syst Rev 2002; CD002977.

64. Stefanescu BM, Murphy WP, Hansell BJ, et al. A randomized, controlled trial comparing two different continuous positive airway pressure systems for the successful extubation of extremely low birth weight infants. Pediatrics 2003; 112:1031–1038.

65. Sun SC, Tien HC. Randomized controlled trial of two methods of nasal CPAP (NCPAP): Flow Driver vs conventional NCPAP (abstract). Ped Res 1999; 45:322A.

66. Mazzella M, Bellini C, Calevo MG, et al. A randomised control study comparing the Infant Flow Driver with nasal continuous positive airway pressure in preterm infants. Arch Dis Child Fetal Neonatal Ed 2001; 85:F86–F90.

67. Walsh M, Engle W, Laptook A, et al. Oxygen delivery through nasal cannulae to preterm infants: can practice be improved? Pediatrics 2005; 116:857–861.

68. Locke RG, Wolfson MR, Shaffer TH, et al. Inadvertent administration of positive end-distending pressure during nasal cannula flow. Pediatrics 1993; 91:135–138.

69. Sreenan C, Lemke RP, Hudson-Mason A, Osiovich H. High-flow nasal cannulae in the management of apnea of prematurity: a comparison with conventional nasal continuous positive airway pressure. Pediatrics 2001; 107:1081–1083.

70. Kopelman AE, Holbert D. Use of oxygen cannulas in extremely low birthweight infants is associated with mucosal trauma and bleeding, and possibly with coagulase-negative staphylococcal sepsis. J Perinatol 2003; 23:94–97.

71. De Klerk AM, De Klerk RK. Nasal continuous positive airway pressure and outcomes of preterm infants. J Paediatr Child Health 2001; 37:161–167.

72. Elgellab A, Riou Y, Abbazine A, et al. Effects of nasal continuous positive airway pressure (NCPAP) on breathing pattern in spontaneously breathing premature newborn infants. Intensive Care Med 2001; 27:1782–1787.

73. Kamper J, Wulff K, Larsen C, Lindequist S. Early treatment with nasal continuous positive airway pressure in very low-birth-weight infants. Acta Paediatr 1993; 82:193–197.

74. Pape KE, Armstrong DL, Fitzhardinge PM. Central nervous system pathology associated with mask ventilation in the very low birthweight infant: a new etiology for intracerebellar hemorrhages. Pediatrics 1976; 58:473–483.

75. Vert P, Andre M, Sibout M. Continuous positive airway pressure and hydrocephalus. Lancet 1973; 2:319.

76. Buettiker V, Hug MI, Baenziger O, et al. Advantages and disadvantages of different nasal CPAP systems in newborns. Intensive Care Med 2004; 30:926–930.

77. Polin RA, Sahni R. Newer experience with CPAP. Semin Neonatol 2002; 7:379–389.

78. Goldbart AD, Gozal D. Non-invasive ventilation in preterm infants. Pediatr Pulmonol Suppl 2004; 26:158–161.

79. Bowe L, Clarke P. Current use of nasal continuous positive airways pressure in neonates. Arch Dis Child Fetal Neonatal Ed 2005; 90:F92–F93.

80. Robertson NJ, Hamilton PA. Randomised trial of elective continuous positive airway pressure (CPAP) compared with rescue CPAP after extubation. Arch Dis Child Fetal Neonatal Ed 1998; 79:F58–F60.

81. Bowe L, Smith J, Clarker P, et al. Nasal CPAP weaning of VLBW Infants: is decreasing CPAP pressure or increasing time off the better strategy – results of a randomised controlled trial. Pediatric Academic Society Meeting, San Francisco (Abstract) 2006.

Chapter 17

High-Frequency Ventilation in Neonatal Respiratory Failure

Ulrich H. Thome MD • Waldemar A. Carlo MD

Gas Exchange During High-Frequency Ventilation

Classification of High-Frequency Ventilators

Clinical Applications of HFV

Conclusion

Advances in neonatal respiratory and general care have improved survival of preterm infants. However, the rate of bronchopulmonary dysplasia (BPD) has not decreased and may be increasing (1). While the high rate of BPD is in part due to survival of very immature infants, it is possible that improved ventilatory strategies, tailored to avoid volutrauma, may reduce BPD rates and severity. Although conventional ventilation at very high respiratory rates may reduce air leaks and even mortality (2), clinical data on effective strategies to reduce lung injury in neonates is scarce. Extensive research in animal models of neonatal lung disease suggests that high-frequency ventilation (HFV) may reduce lung injury. Small tidal volumes that reduce volutrauma, volume recruitment, and mechanisms of enhanced gas exchange that improve blood gases may explain why HFV can reduce lung injury. While some investigators have shown markedly improved clinical outcomes with HFV, an overall assessment of the clinical studies and trials of HFV is hampered by heterogeneity in the ventilation strategies and observed clinical effects. This chapter will address basic and clinical data on HFV, focused on the heterogeneity in the results of clinical trials.

GAS EXCHANGE DURING HIGH-FREQUENCY VENTILATION

During normal breathing CO_2 elimination is proportional to alveolar ventilation. Alveolar ventilation is dependent on the product of frequency times tidal volume minus dead space and can be calculated with the following equation:

$$V_A = f(V_T - V_D)$$

Where V_A is alveolar ventilation, f is frequency, V_T is tidal volume, and V_D is dead-space volume. As V_T approaches V_D, alveolar ventilation will be decreased, limiting CO_2 elimination. HFV is capable of overcoming this limitation, as normal CO_2 elimination and normocapnia can be maintained with tidal volumes less than dead-space during both high-frequency oscillatory ventilation (HFOV) (3) and high-frequency jet ventilation (HFJV) (4, 5). Several mechanisms have been proposed to contribute to gas transport during HFV (6). Although the relative importance of these mechanisms for each type of HFV is not known, all proposed mechanisms together convincingly explain why HFV has such a high capacity to eliminate CO_2, sometimes at the risk of causing hypocapnia.

Mechanisms of Enhanced Gas Exchange during HFV

All gas transport occurs by convection (i.e., bulk-gas flow) and diffusion. Convection is the predominant mechanism for gas transport in the trachea and large airways, while diffusion is the most important in the small airways and alveoli.

ENTRAINMENT

Gas entrainment (the addition of gas from areas surrounding the jet injector cannula to that intrinsically delivered by the jet ventilator) is an important characteristic of jet ventilators. Entrainment occurs because of viscous shearing forces between moving and static layers of gas causing the nonmoving gas to be dragged into the moving stream (7). It is also possible that entrainment occurs when areas of relative negative pressure develop near the injector as gas with a high flow rate is delivered to the patient (8). Whether entrainment actually occurs during HFJV depends on gas dynamics (9).

NON-UNIFORMITY OF GAS EXCHANGE

Non-uniformity of gas exchange is due to preferential ventilation of some parts of the lungs and can occur during HFV just as it occurs during conventional ventilation and spontaneous breathing. At high frequencies and low tidal volumes, ventilation of the pulmonary apex is favored over the base. The opposite occurs at low frequencies and high tidal volumes, favoring ventilation of the base (10). Central regions of the lungs are ventilated better than peripheral ones at high frequencies (11).

CONVECTIVE STREAMING AND ASYMMETRICAL VELOCITY PROFILES

When a pressure gradient is generated at the airway opening, a bolus of gas moves into the airways. This bolus has a parabolic profile with gas in the center moving faster than gas near the walls of the airway. During exhalation, there is a flat velocity profile. The combined effect is a net movement of the gas particles from the center of the airway into the lungs and a net movement out of the lungs for gas particles near the wall (Fig. 17-1). With many ventilator cycles, the gas is advanced progressively into the lungs in a streaming fashion even with small tidal volumes. Furthermore, gas transport is about an order of magnitude greater because the multiple airway bifurcations and the higher velocity near the outer wall of the daughter airways make the velocity profiles asymmetric.

DIRECT ALVEOLAR VENTILATION

Some direct ventilation of the alveoli occurs even when tidal volumes are less than dead space because of the length between the airway opening and alveoli varies. Therefore, alveoli with shorter path lengths may receive fresh gas during ventilation even with tidal volumes smaller than dead space.

AUGMENTED DIFFUSION

The diffusion of one gas into another is caused by the continuous random motion of gas molecules. The rate of diffusion is largely dependent on concentration gradients, molecular mass, and temperature (5). Because of the high velocity profile during HFV, gas particles diffuse better (radial diffusion), which enhances gas transport. However, augmented diffusion appears to be of minor importance in explaining the enhanced gas transport during HFV, although this remains controversial (5, 6).

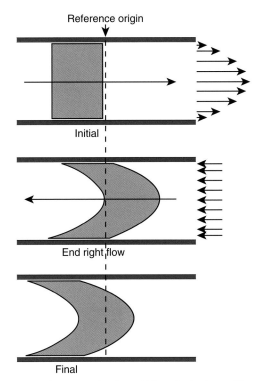

Figure 17-1 Convective-exchange mechanism within a single airway. The position and shape of a plug of gas are shown at three times in an oscillatory cycle: initially, at the end of flow to the right, and at the end of flow to the left. At the end of the cycle, the net axial flow is zero, with 25% of the particles displaced to the right and 25% displaced to the left. Reproduced from Haselton FR, Scherer PW. Bronchial bifurcations and respiratory mass transport. Science 1980; 208:69–71, with permission.

Pendelluft

Pendelluft is the transport of gas between parallel lung units and is due to differences in the time constant of the units or due to asymmetrical bifurcations. Pendelluft has been observed during HFV at frequencies above 5 Hz (12).

CO₂ Elimination

One of the most consistent observations about gas exchange during HFV is that CO_2 elimination is more effective than during conventional ventilation. This is, in part, due to the increased minute ventilation that HFV allows and the mechanisms of enhanced gas exchange. The results of these mechanisms of enhanced gas exchange is that physiological dead space can be decreased with HFV and that tidal volumes smaller than dead space can maintain normal CO_2 elimination during HFJV (4) and HFOV (3). CO_2 elimination during both HFJV and HFOV is more dependent on tidal volume than on frequency. Since it is difficult to measure tidal volume during HFV, practically, it is better to relate CO_2 elimination to the chest vibration or oscillation which is determined by the difference between peak inspiratory (PIP) and positive end-expiratory pressure (PEEP) or the pressure amplitude (Fig. 17-2). PaCO₂ in arterial blood decreases with increases in the airway pressure gradient. During HFV the effective diffusion coefficient, and thus CO_2 elimination, is proportional to approximately $V_T^2 \times f$ (3, 4, 13), in contrast to conventional mechanical ventilation (CMV) and spontaneous breathing, for which the CO_2 elimination is proportional to $V_T \times f$.

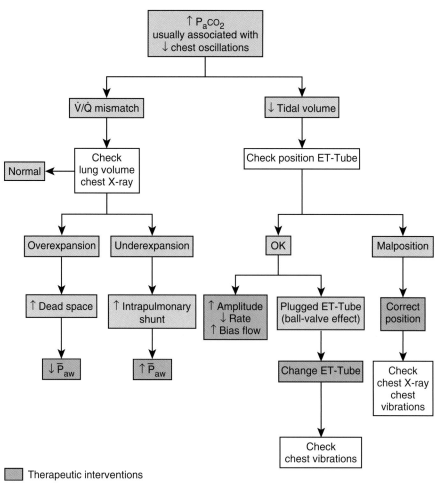

Figure 17-2 Algorithm for correction of hypercapnia during HFOV. For HFJV, mean airway pressure (P_{aw} or MAP) can be changed by varying PEEP, PIP or I:E ratio/frequencies. For example, if there is overexpansion, mean airway pressure can be lowered by decreasing PEEP, decreasing PIP, or decreasing the frequency while increasing the expiratory time. If there is decreased chest vibration during HFJV, PIP should be increased.

However, as tidal volumes and ventilator frequencies are increased, HFV may lead to an inadvertent increase in functional residual capacity, sometimes identified clinically as inadvertent positive end-expiratory pressure or gas trapping, which can result in ventilation perfusion mismatch (Fig. 17-2). The increase in functional residual capacity leads to an increase in functional dead space and subsequent impairment of CO_2 elimination (4). A decrease in ventilator frequency or I:E ratio (14, 15) can reduce gas trapping. A decrease in mean airway pressure can also be effective in reducing gas trapping. On the other hand, underexpansion of the lungs can also lead to a ventilation perfusion mismatch and hypercapnia (Fig. 17-2).

Oxygenation during HFV

In contrast to the tidal volume and frequency dependence of CO_2 elimination, oxygenation during HFV is dependent on lung volume (14). When lung volume is decreased, HFV can be very effective in volume recruitment through an increase in mean airway pressure (16) or the use of periodic sustained inflation (17, 18). Therapeutic interventions to manage hypoxemia during HFV are depicted in Fig. 17-3. If hypoxemia is due to atelectasis or low lung volume, an increase in mean airway pressure (P_{aw} or MAP) or sustained inflations with increases in MAP of up

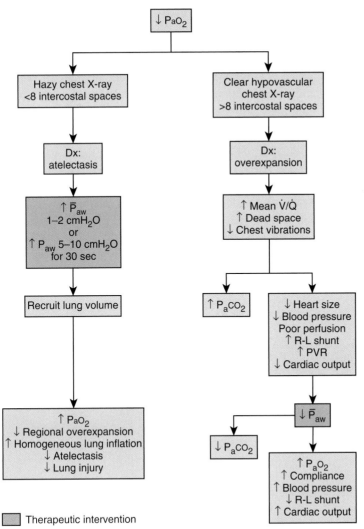

Figure 17-3 Algorithm for correction of hypoxemia during HFOV. For HFJV, the therapeutic interventions for atelectasis are to increase positive end-expiratory pressure (PEEP) by 1–2 cmH$_2$O, increase peak inspiratory pressure (PIP) by 1–2 cmH$_2$O, or increase back-up rate on the conventional ventilator by 5–10 breaths per min. For overexpansion during HFJV, the interventions are to decrease PEEP, decrease rate, or increase expiratory time.

to 5–10 cmH$_2$O for as long as 30 s have been recommended (19). The lung volume prior to initiation of HFV correlates inversely with the increase in mean airway pressure necessary to optimize oxygenation (20) but there can be marked dissociation between improvement in oxygenation and lung function during HFV (21). Thus, implementation of the volume recruitment strategy may be difficult in the clinical setting. If functional residual capacity is normal, increasing it further with an elevated mean airway pressure will not improve oxygenation (22). It is important to note that the improvement in oxygenation is dependent on the increase of lung volume and not a direct effect of mean airway pressure. However, hypoxemia with overexpansion would require a decrease in MAP (Fig. 17-3). Clinically it is often difficult to make an assessment of lung volume, which may explain why air leaks may occur more frequently during HFV (see later).

The mechanism behind improved oxygenation during HFV appears to be a reduction in intrapulmonary shunting (5). In addition, volume recruitment can improve pulmonary mechanics (18) and reduce lung injury (16). However, care should be exercised when volume recruitment is attempted. Cardiac output can decrease if the high mean airway pressure is transmitted to the central veins or the heart, particularly in association with improving lung compliance (23–25). Using measurements of superior vena cava flow to estimate cardiac output indicated that HFOV resulted in a higher proportion of infants with low superior vena cava flow (48% vs. 20%) and receiving intravenous volume expanders and inotropes (61% vs. 40%) when compared to conventional ventilation, although the effects were not significant (26). Reducing mean airway pressure during HFJV resulted in improved cardiac output (27).

CLASSIFICATION OF HIGH-FREQUENCY VENTILATORS

Various ventilators capable of delivering small tidal volumes at high frequencies have been developed. These ventilators differ largely in the method used to generate the tidal volume. Circuits and delivery-system designs also vary, and these may have major impact on the functioning of a high-frequency ventilator. Furthermore, the strategies employed with a high-frequency ventilator may also affect its functioning. Considerable overlap also exists between the various high-frequency ventilators currently in use. We have classified and characterized the principal techniques presently employed to deliver HFV (Table 17-1).

High-Frequency Positive-Pressure Ventilation

High-frequency positive-pressure ventilation (HFPPV) is the term used for conventional ventilation at rates above 60/min and up to 150–180/min. HFPPV employs ventilators with low-compliance tubing and connectors so that an adequate tidal volume may be delivered despite very short inspiratory times. The tidal volume delivered is smaller than during CMV but larger than dead space. As with CMV, expiration is passive. The pressure wave-form may be square if pressure-limited ventilation or inspiratory hold is used but will tend to become triangular, particularly at higher frequencies. Ventilator and circuit design as well as pulmonary mechanics of the patient may limit the range in which the ventilator can be used safely. As the frequency is increased, tidal-volume delivery may become compromised because of an incomplete inspiration or expiration with gas trapping. Because of this, minute ventilation can decrease at higher frequencies (28). This technique was developed by Sjöstrand and co-workers (29) in an effort to reduce cardiac side-effects from assisted ventilation but was found to be effective in achieving normal blood gases at reduced airway pressures.

High-Frequency Jet Ventilation

With HFJV, a high-pressure source is allowed to deliver a volume of gas through a small-bore injector cannula. Delivered tidal volumes may be large, but volumes

Table 17–1 Techniques for High-Frequency Ventilation

	Tidal volume	Expiration	Airway pressure wave form	Usual frequency
HFPPV	> Dead space	Passive	Variable	60–150/min
Jet ventilation	> or < dead space	Passive	Triangular	240–600/min
Flow interruption	> or < dead space	Passive	Triangular	300–900/min
Oscillation	> or < dead space	Active	Sine wave*	300–900/min

*Can vary depending on I:E ratio.

smaller than dead space can maintain normal CO_2 elimination (4). Gas entrainment may occur during HFJV as discussed earlier. However, gas entrainment may only occur at ventilator settings, circuit, and patient characteristics that allow addition of gas from the bias flow circuit to the jet flow without additional pressures (8, 30). During jet ventilation, humidification of gases is particularly difficult, and inadequate humidification may cause tracheal lesions. Thus, humidification of bias-flow gases alone is not sufficient during HFJV, and jet ventilation should not depend exclusively on the bias flow to provide humidity to the jet gas. Most jet ventilators provide bias flow like a constant-flow time-cycled ventilator, and the pressure waveform typically is triangular. Expiration during HFJV is completely passive. Frequencies used vary widely and have ranged from about 240 to 600/min.

High-Frequency Flow Interruption

Similar to jet ventilation, high-frequency flow interruption (HFFI) employs small volumes delivered at high frequencies by interrupting a flow or high-pressure source (31). However, in contrast to jet ventilation, there is no injector cannula or gas entrainment. As with jet ventilation, tidal volumes may be smaller or larger than dead space; expiration is passive unless an additional venturi system generating negative pressure swings is added. The pressure waveform is also triangular and frequencies used are in the range 300–900/min. There is limited experimental or clinical experience using HFFI. Different nomenclatures (including HFV and HFOV) have been used to describe this technique in some publications.

High-Frequency Oscillatory Ventilation

HFOV, also called high-frequency oscillation (HFO), is a unique form of high-frequency ventilation because, in contrast to all other techniques, expiration is active. There is abundant literature of successful application of HFOV in experimental and clinical studies. There are more neonatal trials with HFOV than with any other type of HFV. These trials are discussed later.

Few reports of comparisons of the various types of high-frequency ventilators are available. Evaluation of eight commercially manufactured neonatal high-frequency ventilators, including HFJV, HFFI, and HFOV using a test lung, revealed that, independent of the ventilator type, delivered tidal volume decreased with increasing ventilatory frequencies or decreasing endotracheal tube size. However, tidal volume delivery was relatively insensitive to lung compliance (32).

CLINICAL APPLICATIONS OF HFV

Preterm Infants with Respiratory Distress Syndrome

Multiple trials of HFV have been performed in preterm neonates with respiratory distress syndrome. The trials differ in the ventilatory strategies, time between birth and randomization, the ventilator technology, patient population, the study end points, and, in later studies, the use of antenatal steroids and exogenous surfactant. These differences limit the comparison of the trials and limit the confirmatory power of meta-analyses. Furthermore, new trends such as the use of higher ventilation rates during CMV (33–35) and permissive hypercapnia (36–38) may have benefited the control groups in some trials and thereby diminished the possible advantage of HFV. The most extensively discussed reasons for conflicting results included the ventilation strategies used for HFV (39) and CMV (40, 41), the age when HFV was started (42), and the ventilator technology and devices used. Meta-analyses of available trials comparing elective HFV and CMV have summarized the available data (43–45).

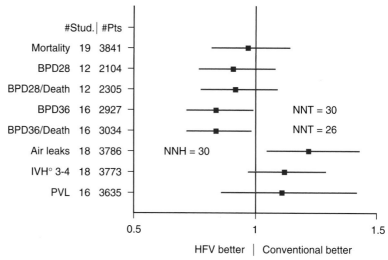

	#Stud.	#Pts	
Mortality	19	3841	
BPD28	12	2104	
BPD28/Death	12	2305	
BPD36	16	2927	NNT = 30
BPD36/Death	16	3034	NNT = 26
Air leaks	18	3786	NNH = 30
IVH° 3-4	18	3773	
PVL	16	3635	

HFV better │ Conventional better

Figure 17-4 Overall results showing odds ratios and 95% confidence intervals, calculated according to a fixed effect model for the analyzed outcome parameters. The significant differences in the incidence of BPD36, BPD36/death, and air leaks remained significant in a random effects model. BPD28, bronchopulmonary dysplasia, defined as oxygen or ventilator dependency at 28 days postnatal age; BPD28/D, BPD28 or death; BPD36, bronchopulmonary dysplasia, defined as oxygen or ventilator dependency at 36 weeks post-menstrual age; BPD36/D, BPD36 or death; air leaks, pneumothorax, pneumomediastinum, or pulmonary interstitial emphysema; NNT, number needed to treat; NNH, number needed to harm.

Figure 17-4 shows the results of an updated meta-analysis from our previous publication (45) including the most recent trials. As not all outcome parameters were available from all studies, the analysis of some outcomes had to be based on fewer trials. Most importantly, bronchopulmonary dysplasia at 36 weeks post-menstrual age (BPD36) was not reported in the HIFI trial (46), which reduced the sample size for this outcome. There was no statistically significant difference regarding mortality, BPD at 28 days (BPD28), BPD28 combined with mortality, severe intraventricular hemorrhages grades 3–4 (IVH3–4) or periventricular leukomalacia (PVL) by either fixed or random effects models. Trends favoring HFV were observed for BPD36 and the combined outcome BPD36 or death achieved marginal statistical significance according to a fixed effects statistical model but not in the more appropriate random effects model, which includes adjustments for heterogeneity between trials. In contrast to expectations, there was a statistically significant increase in the incidence of air leaks with HFV in both the fixed and random effects models.

For brevity, subgroup meta-analyses are only shown for BPD36 or death, air leaks, IVH3–4 and PVL (Fig. 17-5 and Fig. 17-6). After limiting the analysis to trials using a high lung volume strategy (HLVS) or to trials using the SensorMedics 3100A for HFV, the reductions of BPD or death and air leaks were marginally significant. However, an analysis limited to studies which optimized also their CMV groups by using a low-pressure or tidal-volume strategy (LPVS) did no longer demonstrate a significant difference in either outcome, even though all studies in this subgroup used an HLVS for HFV. In trials using a high-rate low-tidal-volume strategy for CMV (HRCMV), there is even a trend in the opposite direction for BPD36 or death, favoring HRCMV over HFV. A trend towards more IVH3–4 with HFV in the overall analysis disappears when the analysis is limited to trials using an HLVS, which is reassuring as it indicates that appropriately applied HFV may not predispose to more IVH. For this reason, and because of the significant reduction of BPD36 or death, the HLVS is recommended when HFOV is used. The results of individual trials for the combined BPD36 or death outcome are shown in Figure 17-7.

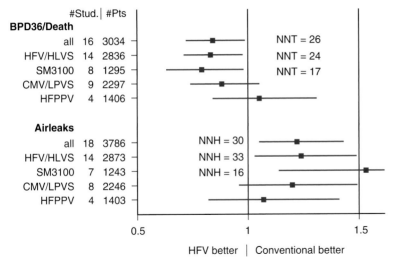

Figure 17-5 Results of subgroup analyses for the incidence of bronchopulmonary dysplasia, defined as oxygen or ventilator dependency at 36 weeks postmenstrual age or death (BPD36/D) and air leaks in a fixed effects model. The differences in the HFV/HLVS and SM3100 subgroups remained significant in a random effects model. All, all available studies included; HFV/HLVS, only studies using a high lung volume strategy for HFV; SM3100, only studies using the Sensor Medics 3100A for HFV; CMV/LPVS, only studies using a low pressure and tidal volume strategy for CMV; HRCMV, only studies using a high-rate low pressure and tidal volume strategy for CMV; NNT, number needed to treat; NNH, number needed to harm.

Only trials using an HLVS for HFV while limiting CMV to lower rates than 60/min yielded significant results favoring HFV. Further analysis of survival without BPD36 against birthweight indicates that studies which show a benefit of HFV over CMV (47–53) had CMV results below the regression line indicating the average outcome whereas their HFV results were not better than the CMV results of several other studies, therefore showing no advantage of HFV (40, 54–57) (Fig. 17-8).

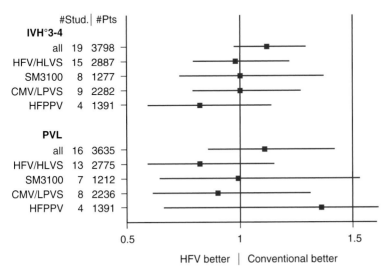

Figure 17-6 Results of subgroup analyses for the incidence of intraventricular hemorrhage grade 3 to 4 according to Papile et al. (58) (IVH°3–4) and periventricular leukomalacia (PVL) in a fixed effects model. There were no significant differences in any of the subgroups in a random effects model. HFV/HLVS, only studies using a high lung volume strategy for HFV; SM3100, only studies using the Sensor Medics 3100A for HFV; CMV/LPVS, only studies using a low pressure and tidal volume strategy for CMV; HRCMV, only studies using a high-rate low pressure and tidal volume strategy for CMV.

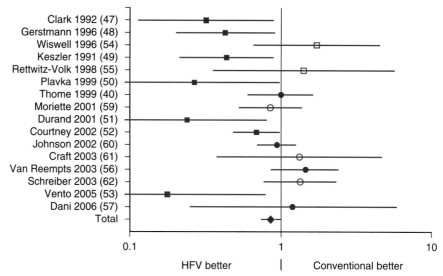

Figure 17-7 Individual study results for the incidence of bronchopulmonary dysplasia, defined as oxygen or ventilator dependency at 36 weeks post-menstrual age, or death (BPD36/D). Trials are ordered by the publication year and identified by the first author names. ■, Trials using HFV with an HLVS and CMV with a low rate; □, trials without clear definition of ventilatory strategies; ●, trials using HFV with an HLVS and CMV with a high starting rate of at least 60/min; ○, trials using HFV with an HLVS and unclear CMV strategy; ◆, overall result according to a fixed effect model.

Recursive cumulative meta-analyses showed how the advantage associated with HFV decreased as more and more evidence was added (45). Cumulative meta-analyses with trials ordered by the time elapsed before randomization and commencement of the randomized ventilation mode or by the $PaCO_2$ limits did

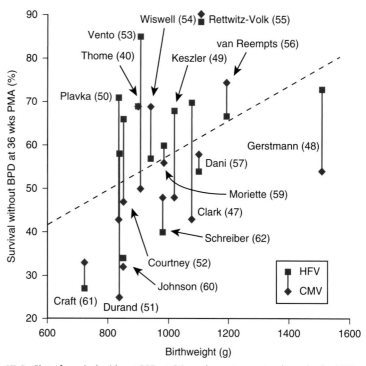

Figure 17-8 Plot of survival without BPD at 36 weeks post-menstrual age in the HFV and CMV randomization groups by mean birthweight of all studies reporting that outcome. Trials are identified by the first author names. The dotted line is the overall linear regression line.

not show clear patterns (45), indicating that the time to randomization or the use of permissive hypercapnia did not impact on trials results (45).

Follow-up of infants treated with HFV during the newborn period usually report no long-term advantage in pulmonary function (63–65) in the negative trials but at least one trial with short-term positive results reported also improved long-term pulmonary outcomes (46).

In conclusion, heterogeneity among trials of elective HFV in comparison to CMV in preterm infants appears to arise mainly from differences in ventilatory strategies. The time lag before enrollment and the use of permissive hypercapnia do not appear to influence study outcomes. Optimizing both modes, HFV by using an HLVS and CMV by using a high rate and minimal tidal volumes, appears to lead to comparable outcomes. Therefore, meticulous attention to the ventilator settings seems to be more important than the choice of a particular mode or machine.

Other Potential Clinical Uses of HFV

BRONCHOPLEURAL FISTULA/PNEUMOTHORAX

Pneumothorax is a frequent occurrence in neonatal ventilatory therapy. HFJV was used in six infants who had severe pulmonary disease and persistent air leaks via thoracotomy tubes placed for pneumothoraces (66). When infants were treated with HFJV, the flow through the bronchopleural fistula decreased. Simultaneously, peak and mean airway pressures were decreased during HFJV while adequate gas exchange was maintained. This study confirmed previous case reports describing similar observations in animals and adult patients. It is likely that the reduction of bronchopleural fistula was due to a reduction in the mean airway pressure (67) rather than the HFJV itself. However, HFV does not prevent the development of air leaks. To the contrary, HFOV was associated with increased air leaks in randomized trials of preterm infants (Fig. 17-4).

PULMONARY HYPERTENSION

A randomized trial which enrolled term infants with pulmonary hypertension or meconium aspiration who fulfilled ECMO (extracorporeal membrane oxygenation) criteria demonstrated decreased need for ECMO in infants randomized to HFOV versus CMV (68). In another study which enrolled similar patients HFOV was as effective as CMV with inhaled nitric oxide (iNO) (69). HFOV combined with iNO had the highest rate of responders. However, a third trial of term infants with severe respiratory failure did not demonstrate any benefits of HFOV over CMV (70). The reasons for this discrepancy may be differences in study protocols and the specific strategies used during application of the ventilation modes. Some evidence suggest that HFOV may be a valuable treatment alternative for infants with congenital diaphragmatic hernia (71). These infants have hypoplastic lungs which can be damaged by normal tidal volumes, so HFOV with its small tidal volumes may be the best alternative to protect the lungs from volutrauma in patients failing CMV, especially as these infants frequently have severe pulmonary hypertension.

IMPAIRED CARDIAC FUNCTION

Although several authors have reported worsening cardiac hemodynamics during HFV, the increased mean airway pressure employed in those studies may have accounted for the adverse cardiac effects. Animal studies in which mean airway pressure was comparable during HFV and CV have shown no change in cardiac output. HFOV used with a mean airway pressure 2 cm H_2O higher than CMV did not impair cardiac output (72). However, HFOV can result in decreased cardiac output and increased need of fluid volume intake and inotropes (26).

Following cardiac surgery in infants and children, cardiac output either improved or remained unchanged during periods of either HFFI (73) or HFJV (27). Interestingly, cardiac output improved during HFJV in those infants who initially had poor cardiac output during CV. Regardless of the ventilatory mode, cardiac output was dependent on mean airway pressure (27). Thus, the lower mean airway pressure used during HFJV may reduce the cardiovascular side-effects of positive airway pressure and HFOV may be used safely at slightly higher mean airway pressure without adversely affecting cardiac output.

BRONCHOSCOPY AND AIRWAY AND THORACIC SURGERY

Because HFV allows adequate gas exchange with small tidal volumes, it reduces airway and thoracic structure movement and thus may facilitate surgical procedures. We devised a system using a combination of jet ventilation and constant air suction, both of which deliver gas through a single interface valve providing active inspiration and expiration through the suction channel of a bronchoscope (74). When tested in vitro and in rabbits with normal lungs, baseline functional residual capacity remained constant. This system also improved ventilation when used during bronchoscopy. High-frequency ventilation may also facilitate airway and thoracic surgery as excursions during ventilation are decreased (75). When delivered transtracheally, HFJV may be an alternative mode of ventilation during cardiopulmonary resuscitation (76).

OTHER USES

Rescue HFV in neonates failing CMV is commonly performed. A large non-randomized but controlled study documented the rapid improvement in gas exchange when infants were switched from CMV to HFV (77).

Nasal HFV has been employed in neonates with moderate respiratory failure resulting in a significant decrease in PCO_2 (78).

CONCLUSION

HFV is a technique that enhances gas exchange and can be used to improve blood gases in many critically ill neonates. However, clinicians should pay meticulous attention to indications and ventilatory strategies that optimize the use of these ventilators. Excellent results can be obtained with CMV but selected patients may benefit from HFV.

REFERENCES

1. St. John EB, Carlo WA. Respiratory distress syndrome in VLBW infants: changes in management and outcomes observed by the NICHD Neonatal Research Network. Semin Perinatol 2003; 27:288–292.
2. Greenough A, Milner AD, Dimitriou G. Synchronized mechanical ventilation for respiratory support in newborn infants. Cochrane Database Systematic Review (Abstract); 2004.
3. Boynton BR, Hammond MD, Fredberg JJ, et al. Gas exchange in healthy rabbits during high-frequency oscillatory ventilation. J Appl Physiol 1989; 66:1343–1351.
4. Korvenranta H, Carlo WA, Goldthwait DA, et al. Carbon dioxide elimination during high-frequency jet ventilation. J Pediatr 1987; 111:107–113.
5. Boynton B, Carlo WA. Pulmonary gas exchange during high frequency ventilation. In: Boynton B, Carlo WA, Jobe A, eds. New therapies for neonatal respiratory failure: a physiologic approach. Cambridge, England: Cambridge University Press; 1994: 202–217.
6. Chang HK. General concepts of molecular diffusion. In: Engel LA, Paiva M, eds. Gas mixing and distribution in the lung. New York: Marcel Dekker; 1985: 1–22.
7. Scacci R. Air entrainment masks: jet mixing is how they work; the Bernoulli and Venturi principles are how they don't. Respir Care 1979; 24:928.
8. Hamilton LH, Londino JM, Linehan JH, et al. Pediatric endotracheal tube designed for high-frequency ventilation. Crit Care Med 1984; 12:988–993.
9. Weisberger SA, Carlo WA, Chatburn R, et al. Effect of varying inspiratory and expiratory times during high-frequency jet ventilation. J Pediatr 1986; 108:596–600.

10. Allen J, Frantz ID, Fredberg JJ. Regional alveolar pressure during periodic flow: dual manifestation of gas inertia. J Clin Invest 1985; 76:620–629.

11. Fernandez P, Hernaiz MI, Houtz P, et al. Relation between esophageal and costal pleural pressures during high frequency ventilation in rabbits. FASEB J 1992; 6:A1480.

12. Lehr J, Butler JP, Westerman PA, et al. Photographic measurement of pleural surface motion during lung oscillation. J Appl Physiol 1985; 59:623–633.

13. Kamm RK, Slutsky AS, Drazen JM. High frequency ventilation. CRC Crit Rev Biomech Engin 1984; 9:347–379.

14. Thome U, Pohlandt F. Effect of the TI/TE ratio on mean intratracheal pressure in high-frequency oscillatory ventilation. J Appl Physiol 1998; 84:1520–1527.

15. Pillow JJ, Wilkinson MH, Ramsden CA. Effect of I/E ratio on mean alveolar pressure during high-frequency oscillatory ventilation. J Appl Physiol 1999; 87:407–414.

16. McCulloch PR, Forkert PG, Froese AB. Lung volume maintenance prevents lung injury during high frequency oscillatory ventilation in surfactant-deficient rabbits. Am Rev Respir Dis 1988; 137:1185–1192.

17. Byford LJ, Finkler JH, Froese AB. Lung volume recruitment during high frequency ventilation in surfactant-deficient rabbits. Fed Proc 1985; 44:1557.

18. Walsh MC, Carlo WA. Sustained inflation during HFOV improves pulmonary mechanics and oxygenation. J Appl Physiol 1988; 65:368–372.

19. Fernándex-Martorell P, Boyton BR. High-frequency oscillatory ventilation and high-frequency flow interruption. In: Boynton B, Carlo WA, Jobe A, eds. New therapies for neonatal respiratory failure: a physiologic approach. Cambridge, England: Cambridge University Press; 1994: 218–259.

20. Dimitriou G, Cheesman P, Greenough A. Lung volume and the response to high volume strategy, high frequency oscillation. Acta Paediatr 2004; 93:613–617.

21. Kalenga M, Battisti O, Francois A, et al. High-frequency oscillatory ventilation in neonatal RDS: initial volume optimization and respiratory mechanics. J Appl Physiol 1998; 84:1174–1177.

22. Boynton BR, Villanueva D, Hammond MD, et al. The effect of mean airway pressure on gas exchange during high frequency oscillatory ventilation. J Appl Physiol 1991; 70:701–707.

23. Traverse JH, Korvenranta H, Adams EM, et al. Impairment of hemodynamics with increasing airway pressure during high-frequency oscillatory ventilation. Pediatr Res 1988; 23:628–631.

24. Laubscher B, van Melle G, Fawer CL, et al. Haemodynamic changes during high frequency oscillation for respiratory distress syndrome. Arch Dis Child 1996; 74:F172–F176.

25. Burkhard S, Fritz M, Fink C, et al. Conventional ventilation versus high-frequency oscillation: hemodynamic effects in newborn infants. Crit Care Med 2000; 28:227–231.

26. Osborn DA, Evans E. Randomized trial of high-frequency oscillatory ventilation versus conventional ventilation: effect on systemic blood flow in very preterm infants. J Pediatr 2003; 143:192–198.

27. Weiner JH, Chatburn RL, Carlo WA. Ventilatory and hemodynamic effects of high-frequency jet ventilation following cardiac surgery. Respir Care 1987; 32:332–338.

28. Boros SJ, Bing DR, Mammel MC, et al. Using conventional infant ventilators at unconventional rates. Pediatrics 1984; 74:487–492.

29. Sjöstrand U. High-frequency positive-pressure ventilation (HFPPV): a review. Crit Care Med 1980; 8:345–364.

30. Weisberger SA, Carlo WA, Fouke JM, et al. Determination of tidal volume and gas entrainment during high frequency jet ventilation. Am Rev Resp Dis 1985; 131:A253.

31. Frantz ID III, Werthammer J, Stark AR. High-frequency ventilation in premature infants with lung disease: adequate gas exchange at low tracheal pressures. Pediatrics 1983; 71:483–488.

32. Fredberg JJ, Glass GM, Boynton BR, et al. Factors influencing mechanical performance of neonatal high-frequency ventilators. J Appl Physiol 1987; 62:2485–2490.

33. Heicher DA, Kasting DS, Harrod JR. Prospective clinical comparison of two methods for mechanical ventilation of neonates: rapid rate and short inspiratory time versus slow rate and long inspiratory time. J Pediatr 1981; 98:957–961.

34. Oxford Region controlled trial of artificial ventilation (OCTAVE) study group. Multicenter randomized controlled trial of high against low frequency positive pressure ventilation. Arch Dis Child 1991; 66:770–775.

35. Pohlandt F, Saule H, Schröder H, et al. Decreased incidence of extra-alveolar air leakage of death prior to air leakage in high versus low rate positive pressure ventilation: results of a randomised seven-center trial in preterm infants. Eur J Pediatr 1992; 151:904–909.

36. Mariani G, Cifuentes J, Carlo WA. Randomized trial of permissive hypercapnia in preterm infants. Pediatrics 1999; 104:1082–1088.

37. Carlo WA, Stark AR, Wright LL, et al. Minimal ventilation to prevent bronchopulmonary dysplasia in extremely-low-birth-weight infants. J Pediatr 2002; 141:370–374.

38. Thome UH, Carroll W, Wu TJ, et al. Outcome of extremely preterm infants randomized at birth to different PaCO$_2$ targets during the first seven days of life. Biol Neonate 2006; 90:218–225.

39. Bryan AC, Froese AB. Reflections on the HIFI trial. Pediatrics 1991; 87:565–567.

40. Thome U, Kössel H, Lipowsky G, et al. Randomized comparison of high-frequency ventilation with high rate intermittent positive pressure ventilation in preterm infants with respiratory failure. J Pediatr 1999; 135:39–46.

41. Thome UH, Carlo WA. High-frequency ventilation in neonates. Am J Perinatol 2000; 17:1–9.

42. Rimensberger PC, Beghetti M, Hanquinet S, et al. First intention high-frequency oscillation with early lung volume optimization improves pulmonary outcome in very low birth weight infants with respiratory distress syndrome. Pediatrics 2000; 105:1202–1208.

43. Henderson-Smart DJ, Bhuta T, Cools F, et al. Elective high frequency oscillatory ventilation versus conventional ventilation for acute pulmonary dysfunction in preterm infants (Cochrane Review). Cochrane Database of Systematic Reviews (Abstract); 2004.

44. Bhuta T, Henderson-Smart DJ. Elective high frequency jet ventilation versus conventional ventilation for respiratory distress syndrome in preterm infants (Cochrane Review). Cochrane Database of Systematic Reviews (Abstract); 2004.

45. Thome WH, Carlo WA, Pohlandt F. Ventilation strategies and outcome in randomised trials of high frequency ventilation. Arch Dis Child Fetal Neonatal Ed 2005; 90:466–473.

46. HIFI Study Group. High-frequency oscillatory ventilation compared with conventional mechanical ventilation in the treatment of respiratory failure in preterm infants. N Engl J Med 1989; 320:88–93.

47. Clark RH, Gerstmann DR, Null DM, et al. Prospective randomized comparison of high-frequency oscillatory and conventional ventilation in respiratory distress syndrome. Pediatrics 1992; 89:5–12.

48. Gerstmann DR, Minton SD, Stoddard RA, et al. The Provo multicenter early high-frequency oscillatory ventilation trial: improved pulmonary and clinical outcome in respiratory distress syndrome. Pediatrics 1996; 98:1044–1057.

49. Keszler M, Donn SM, Bucciarelli RL, et al. Multicenter controlled trial comparing high-frequency jet ventilation and conventional mechanical ventilation in newborn infants with pulmonary interstitial emphysema. J Pediatr 1991; 119:85–93.

50. Plavka R, Kopecky P, Sebron V, et al. A prospective randomized comparison of conventional mechanical ventilation and very early high frequency oscillatory ventilation in extremely premature newborns with respiratory distress syndrome. Intens Care Med 1999; 25:68–75.

51. Durand DJ, Asselin JM, Hudak ML, et al. Early high-frequency oscillatory ventilation versus synchronized intermittent mandatory ventilation in very low birth weight infants: a pilot study of two ventilation protocols. J Perinatol 2001; 21:221–229.

52. Courtney SE, Durand DJ, Asselin JM, et al. High-frequency oscillatory ventilation versus conventional mechanical ventilation for very-low-birth-weight infants. N Engl J Med 2002; 347:643–652.

53. Vento G, Matassa PG, Ameglio F, et al. HFOV in premature neonates: effects on pulmonary mechanics and epithelial lining fluid cytokines. A randomized controlled trial. Intens Care Med 2005; 31:463–470.

54. Wiswell TE, Graziani LJ, Kornhauser MS, et al. High-frequency jet ventilation in the early management of respiratory distress syndrome is associated with a greater risk for adverse outcomes. Pediatrics 1996; 98:1035–1043.

55. Rettwitz-Volk W, Veldman A, Roth B, et al. A prospective, randomized, multicenter trial of high-frequency oscillatory ventilation compared with conventional ventilation in preterm infants with respiratory distress syndrome receiving surfactant. J Pediatr 1998; 132:249–254.

56. Van Reempts P, Borstlap C, Laroche S, et al. Early use of high frequency ventilation in the premature neonate. Eur J Pediatr 2003; 162:219–226.

57. Dani C, Bertini G, Pezzati M, et al. Effects of pressure support ventilation plus volume guarantee vs. high-frequency oscillatory ventilation on lung inflammation in preterm infants. Pediatr Pulmonol 2006; 41:242–249.

58. Papile LA, Burstein J, Burstein R, et al. Incidence and evolution of subependymal and intraventricular hemorrhage: a study of infants with birth weights less than 1,500 gm. Pediatrics 1978; 92:529–534.

59. Moriette G, Paris-Llado J, Walti H, et al. Prospective randomized multicenter comparison of high-frequency oscillatory ventilation and conventional ventilation in preterm infants of less than 30 weeks with respiratory distress syndrome. Pediatrics 2001; 107:363–372.

60. Johnson AH, Peacock JL, Greenough A, et al. High-frequency oscillatory ventilation for the prevention of chronic lung disease of prematurity. N Engl J Med 2002; 347:633–642.

61. Craft AP, Bhandari V, Finer NN. The sy-fi study: a randomized prospective trial of synchronized intermittent mandatory ventilation versus a high-frequency flow interrupter in infants less than 1000 g. J Perinatol 2003; 23:14–19.

62. Schreiber MD, Gin-Mestan K, Marks JD, et al. Inhaled nitric oxide in premature infants with the respiratory distress syndrome. N Engl J Med 2003; 349:2099–2107.

63. Gerhardt T, Reifenberg L, Goldberg RN, et al. Pulmonary function in preterm infants whose lungs were ventilated conventionally or by high-frequency oscillation. J Pediatr 1989; 115:121–126.

64. HIFI Study Group High-frequency oscillatory ventilation compared with conventional mechanical ventilation in the treatment of respiratory failure in preterm infants: assessment of pulmonary function at 9 months of corrected age. J Pediatr 1990; 116:933–941.

65. Thomas MR, Rafferty GF, Limb ES, et al. Pulmonary function at follow-up of very preterm infants from the United Kingdom oscillation study. Am J Respir Crit Care Med 2004; 169:868–872.

66. Gonzales F, Harris T, Black P, et al. Decreased gas flow through pneumothoraces in neonates receiving high-frequency jet versus conventional ventilation. J Pediatr 1987; 110:464–466.

67. Walsh MC, Carlo WA. Determinants of gas flow through a bronchopleural fistula. J Appl Physiol 1989; 67:1591–1598.

68. Clark RH, Yoder BA, Snell MS. Prospective, randomized comparison of high-frequency oscillation and conventional ventilation in candidates for extracorporeal membrane oxygenation. J Pediatr 1994; 124:447–454.

69. Kinsella JP, Truog WE, Walsh WF, et al. Randomized, multicenter trial of inhaled nitric oxide and high-frequency oscillatory ventilation in severe, persistent pulmonary hypertension of the newborn. J Pediatr 1997; 131:55–62.

70. Rojas MA, Lozano JM, Rojas MX, et al. Randomized, multicenter trial of conventional ventilation versus high-frequency oscillatory ventilation for the early management of respiratory failure in term or near-term infants in Colombia. J Perinatol 2005; 11:720–724.

71. Desfrere L, Jarreau PH, Dommergues M, et al. Impact of delayed repair and elective high-frequency oscillatory ventilation on survival of antenatally diagnosed congenital diaphragmatic hernia: first application of these strategies in more "severe" subgroup of antenatally diagnosed newborns. Intensive Care Med 2000; 26:934–941.

72. Cambonie G, Guillaumont S, Luc F, et al. Haemodynamic features during high-frequency oscillatory ventilation in preterms. Acta Paediatr 2003; 92:1068–1073.

73. Vincent RN, Stark AR, Lang P, et al. Hemodynamic response to high-frequency ventilation in infants following cardiac surgery. Pediatrics 1984; 73:426–430.

74. Nutman J, Carlo WA, Chatburn RL. Low frequency oscillatory ventilation through the suction channel of a pediatric bronchoscope. Ann Otol Rhinol Laryngol 1989; 98:251–255.

75. Greenspan JS, Davis DA, Russo P, et al. High frequency jet ventilation: intraoperative application in infants. Pediatr Pulmonol 1994; 17:155–160.

76. Klain M, Keszler H, Brader E. High frequency jet ventilation in CPR. Crit Care Med 1981; 9:421–422.

77. Morcillo F, Gutierrez A, Izquierdo I, et al. High-frequency oscillatory ventilation as salvage strategy in the newborn infant. An Esp Pediatr 1999; 50:269–274.

78. Van der Hoeven M, Brouwer E, Blanco CE. Nasal high frequency ventilation in neonates with moderate respiratory insufficiency. Arch Dis Child Fetal Neonatal Ed 1998; 79:F61–F63.

Chapter 18

New Modalities of Mechanical Ventilation in the Newborn

Nelson Claure MSc PhD • Eduardo Bancalari MD

Conventional Mechanical Ventilation

New Modalities of Mechanical Ventilation

Noninvasive Ventilation of the Newborn

Experimental Modalities of Neonatal Mechanical Ventilation

Summary and Future Directions

Initial reports of assisted neonatal ventilation in the 19th century describe simple devices for resuscitation and brief ventilation. In 1881 Alexander G. Bell designed a metal jacket to produce breathing by vacuum after his son's death from respiratory problems, a design that is believed to be the precursor of the iron lung (1). Later on various reports describe the use of intubation tools and mechanical devices for positive and negative pressure ventilation in children (2–7). In the 1960s pioneering reports on the use of intermittent positive pressure ventilation (IPPV) in neonates with respiratory failure were published (8–10). These were followed by introduction of continuous distending airway pressure to maintain lung volume in the management of infants with RDS by Gregory et al. in the 1970s (11, 12).

Earlier IPPV devices initiated every tidal breath and did not adapt to spontaneous breathing. This produced inspiratory loading, rebreathing and patient discomfort. Adaptation of the Ayre's T used in anesthesia to IPPV devices facilitated spontaneous breathing from a continuous flow of gas (13). This method became the mainstay of adult and neonatal ventilation.

The introduction of modern mechanical ventilation for the newborn in respiratory failure as a rescue therapy in the 1960s was subsequently extended to premature infants with RDS and resulted along with other interventions in a dramatic increase in survival of critically ill preterm newborns. However, this was accompanied by the appearance of a new complication described as bronchopulmonary dysplasia (BPD) (14).

Some of the most striking advances in perinatal medicine over the last decades resulted from introduction of therapies such as antenatal corticosteroids and exogenous surfactants that produced a marked increase in survival of extremely premature infants. In spite of this, an important fraction of the newborn population develop severe respiratory failure and mechanical ventilation plays a significant role in their survival. Preterm infants represent the vast majority of all ventilated neonates. More than 90% of infants born at 25–26 weeks of gestation and 60–70% of infants born between 29–30 weeks of gestation require mechanical ventilation (15).

The severe forms of lung injury described by Northway et al. attributed to aggressive mechanical ventilation, and exposure to high concentrations of oxygen are less frequent today. This is in part due to the increased awareness of the deleterious effects of aggressive respiratory support (16–18). Although BPD is milder, its incidence remains high (19) and its relevance on long-term pulmonary (20) and neurodevelopmental outcome is important (21).

Newer modalities of mechanical ventilation have been developed with the introduction of microprocessor and sensing technology for control and monitoring of respiratory parameters. In spite of this and the widespread use of mechanical ventilation in the newborn since the 1960s, there is no clear evidence of an optimal ventilatory strategy for the preterm infant across different gestational ages and types of pulmonary disease.

CONVENTIONAL MECHANICAL VENTILATION

Neonatal ventilators adapted the Ayre's T to IPPV devices to maintain a continuous flow of gas in the breathing circuit (13). Intermittent partial closure of a valve at the expiratory end increases the airway pressure until the set peak inspiratory pressure (PIP) is reached and produces tidal inflation during a fixed inspiratory time (Ti). A continuous distending pressure for maintenance of end-expiratory lung volume is provided by the positive end-expiratory pressure (PEEP). This method, termed time-cycled pressure-limited (TCPL) ventilation, was also coined as intermittent mandatory ventilation (IMV) (13) and became the mainstay of neonatal ventilation. Since then, both terms have been used interchangeably in the literature. IMV is often referred to as conventional or controlled mandatory ventilation (both abbreviated as CMV) with the latter referring to high ventilator rates that override the spontaneous respiratory drive.

Limitations of Conventional Mechanical Ventilation

Patient-ventilator asynchrony occurs frequently during IMV since mechanical breaths of a fixed duration delivered at fixed intervals interact in various ways with the infant's spontaneous breathing and reflex activity. The effects vary depending on the timing and volume of the spontaneous inspiration or positive pressure (22–24). Respiratory reflexes influence the infant's spontaneous respiratory rhythm. Activation of the Hering-Breuer vagal inhibitory reflex by lung inflation can shorten neural inspiration whereas its activation by lung inflation during neural expiration will prolong its duration. Also active in the newborn, the head's paradoxical reflex can be activated by lung inflation and elicit a greater inspiratory effort.

Inspiratory asynchrony occurs when the mechanical breath is delivered towards the end of the spontaneous inspiration and extends beyond the end of inspiration. The resulting additional lung inflation or inspiratory hold can limit the spontaneous respiratory rate and may increase the risk of volutrauma. Expiratory asynchrony occurring when the mechanical breath is delivered during exhalation prolongs the spontaneous expiratory phase and it can elicit active exhalation against an elevated pressure at the airway, producing a rise in intrathoracic pressure.

Asynchrony can adversely affect gas exchange and it has been associated with the occurrence of air leaks (25, 26). Concerns also exist regarding its effects on brain blood flow and the possible increased risk of intraventricular hemorrhage (IVH) (27). Earlier reports of elimination of asynchrony by neuromuscular paralysis suggested a reduction in IVH and air leaks (28, 29). Manipulation of the IMV settings can decrease asynchrony (30, 31) but this requires experienced and continuous fine tuning of inspiratory time and rate. The use of high ventilator rates was suggested to prevent asynchrony and avoid the need for paralysis (32). This may not be desirable for the preterm infant in whom hypocapnia has been associated with increased CNS and lung injury.

Lack of ventilation monitoring was common in the earlier IMV devices. Monitoring was limited to visual assessment of chest expansion and breathing rate, thus lacking the ability to accurately detect inadequate or excessive lung inflation, hypoventilation, gas trapping and impaired lung mechanics. Total ventilation in preterm infants varies as the underlying lung disease evolves and also as a result of changes in lung function and spontaneous respiratory drive. The support during IMV is fixed and, without ventilation monitoring, periods of excessive or insufficient ventilation may go undetected.

NEW MODALITIES OF MECHANICAL VENTILATION

Advances in the neonatal ventilators were accelerated in the 1990s with the use of microprocessor and sensing technology for control and monitoring the ventilator. An increased number of ventilatory techniques were developed for use in neonates or were adapted from adult ventilation. Their classification as conventional or new is mostly for historical and illustrative purposes as some of the new modalities have been used for many years.

Synchronized Mechanical Ventilation

The modality resulting from the synchronization of positive pressure ventilation with the infant's every spontaneous inspiration was coined patient triggered ventilation (PTV) (33). This modality also became known as synchronized IPPV (SIPPV) and assist/control ventilation (A/C). Initial PTV devices provided a low IMV backup in the absence of spontaneous breathing. Later it was noted that the preterm infant's inconsistent respiratory drive required having a backup (or controlled) rate set by the caregiver. Thus, the term A/C indicates more appropriately the manner in which this modality is currently applied. A new modality, synchronized IMV (SIMV), was also introduced. SIMV maintained the features of IMV with the added synchrony and was rapidly adopted in many centers.

The ability to synchronize the mechanical breath with the onset of spontaneous inspiration was expanded to terminate the mechanical breath when inflation had stopped or at the end of spontaneous inspiration. The additional breath-termination feature became available in A/C and SIMV and also led to the introduction of pressure support ventilation (PSV).

Synchronization Methods

Synchronization of the ventilator breath with the spontaneous inspiration was successfully attained using signals obtained from measurements of respiratory activity. Their efficacy and reliability on reducing asynchrony in the neonate have been assessed by many investigators.

ABDOMINAL WALL MOTION

Outward motion of the abdomen during inspiration is noticeable in the newborn and even more in preterm infants with lung disease and compliant chest wall (34). This outward motion is used for ventilator triggering with signals obtained from the Graseby pressure capsule, Hall-effect magnetic field sensors, magnetic induction and strain gauge transduction (35–38). These signals are not entirely specific to inspiration and there is a risk of autocycling during patient activity.

ESOPHAGEAL PRESSURE

The negative deflection in esophageal pressure during inspiration measured with an air-filled thin latex balloon was used experimentally to trigger a ventilator.

This led to an improved V_T and gas exchange with an apparent minimal interference from peristaltic waves (39).

Thoracic Impedance

This method was used by the synchronized assisted ventilation in infants (SAVI) module to trigger a ventilator during the upward deflection of the signal and to terminate the breath with a downward slope (40). This required careful electrode placement to avoid cardiogenic artifact. Later measurements indicated delayed triggering due to chest wall distortion and inward motion in early inspiration (35, 41).

Airway Pressure

Changes in airway pressure produced by spontaneous inspiration are used for triggering (42, 43). Initial data indicated similar sensitivity and trigger delay to other methods (35, 43). However, more recent data in preterm infants recovering from RDS indicate lower sensitivity and delays (44–46). Due to their respiratory disease and anatomy, preterm infants may not consistently produce the required pressure changes at the airway.

Air Flow

Flow sensors in neonatal ventilators provide synchrony and monitoring of V_T and ventilation. These sensors are mainstream or built into the ventilator. Triggering occurs when the inspiratory flow (or volume) exceeds a set threshold. The small flows required for triggering make this method appealing for use in the sicker more immature infants in whom flow triggering is comparable or superior to other methods (35, 36, 41, 45). Initial reports described its feasibility in preterm infants (47–51), but some with limited success (47–49). This may have resulted from an insufficient backup rate in A/C, device-specific refractory periods, or increased trigger delay in volume triggering (37). The time to reach a small volume may be prolonged in small infants.

Although mainstream flow sensors are usually small they increase the instrumental dead space and reduce CO_2 elimination (52). This appears to be more relevant in the smaller infants (53). In some ventilators internal sensors are used in lieu of mainstream sensors. It is unknown whether these differ in synchrony, but there are concerns about their accuracy in small infants as their V_T and flows are many times smaller than the circuit volume and background flows (54, 55). Autocycling can occur due to water condensation in the circuit and due to gas leaks around the ETT at the PEEP level (56). These leaks are common among infants who remain ventilated for long periods as they outgrow the ETT size.

Ventilatory Modalities

Assist/Control Ventilation (A/C)

In this modality every spontaneous inspiratory effort is assisted with a mechanical breath. A/C is also referred as SIPPV. If the infant stops breathing a "controlled" rate is initiated shortly after to provide backup ventilation. In A/C, all mechanical breaths have the same PIP, which is gradually reduced during weaning. The backup rate is usually maintained below the assist frequency to prevent a takeover if the controlled rate provides all the required minute ventilation.

Synchronized Intermittent Mandatory Ventilation (SIMV)

This modality represents a modification of conventional IMV. In IMV and SIMV the number of delivered breaths in every minute is the same while the interval between mechanical breaths, which is constant in IMV, is variable in SIMV. In SIMV, with some variance between manufacturers, time windows of duration equal to the IMV breath-to-breath interval are consecutively opened and a mechanical breath is triggered by the first spontaneous inspiration. A "backup" mechanical breath is delivered at the end of the time window if no spontaneous inspiration is detected. Synchronous and backup breaths have the same PIP.

PRESSURE SUPPORT VENTILATION (PSV)

This is a flow-cycled modality where, similarly to A/C, every breath is assisted and the positive pressure is terminated at the end of inspiration. It is believed that the infant has a greater control of the frequency and duration of inspiration. The synchronous "support" pressure is aimed at compensating for the disease and instrumental increased mechanical loads, i.e. increased airway resistance, reduced compliance, and narrow ETT (59, 60).

Similarly to A/C, a consistent respiratory drive is needed to ensure maintenance of ventilation in PSV. If apnea occurs, ventilators offer a backup ventilation level consisting of IMV. In some ventilators PSV can be combined with SIMV and most spontaneous breaths are pressure-supported. Since the aim of PSV is mainly to boost the spontaneous effort, the pressure-supported breaths are usually assisted with lower peak airway pressures and result in smaller volumes than those breaths assisted with SIMV.

Advantages and Limitations of Synchronized Ventilation

The main advantage offered by synchronized ventilation is the avoidance of asynchrony between infant and ventilator. This may be more relevant today as ventilatory management has changed from mandatory ventilation to a more gentle assistance of the spontaneous effort and preservation of the infant's breathing rhythm.

Physiologic studies have reported important potential benefits of synchronized ventilation for preterm infants compared to conventional ventilation. These include improved gas exchange and ventilation with more consistent V_T (42, 47, 50, 51, 60–65). Although one would expect that patient triggering would limit excessive ventilation, the incidence of hypocarbia in the acute phase of RDS was not affected by synchronized ventilation (69).

Synchronous ventilation was also shown to reduce the stress response (66) and fluctuations in blood pressure (61, 64, 67) in preterm infants. A recent report indicates fewer spontaneous fluctuations in oxygenation during SIMV vs. IMV (70). Synchronized ventilation has also been shown to reduce breathing effort and work of breathing (64, 65) but it is not clear whether synchrony reduces the metabolic demands of respiration (68).

Limitations attributed to synchronized ventilation are often related to inadequate function of the synchronization mechanism that leads to delayed triggering, autocycling or lack of triggering. These can result from differences between ventilators and their triggering methods but it is likely that greater variability exists during routine clinical practice depending on the infant population, the underlying lung disease and the trigger sensitivity setting.

Delayed triggering can result in an increased breathing effort (71) and produce a prolonged inspiratory hold. The latter can have effects similar to those of long Ti such as limiting the breathing frequency (57) and disrupting the breathing pattern (58). Although purposely delaying the synchronous breath did not affect ventilation or gas exchange during SIMV (72), the effects of delayed triggering may be more relevant with A/C ventilation. Asynchronous or delayed triggering is usually due to a low trigger-sensitivity setting. Trigger failure occurs due to trigger malfunction or a low trigger sensitivity. As a result, the infant is being supported as in IMV.

Autocycling is more serious in A/C than in SIMV due to the potential for hyperventilation, hypocapnia and gas trapping. If the autocycling persists, it is likely to blunt the spontaneous respiratory drive due to hyperventilation.

End-inspiratory asynchrony can occur due to delayed triggering or ventilator breaths with long Ti. This produces a prolonged plateau in the volume signal similar to an inspiratory hold and can result in active exhalation against the positive pressure. In addition to synchronization with the onset of inspiration, the mechanical breath can be synchronized to terminate at the end of inflation or the spontaneous inspiration which is often based on the inspired flow. This is aimed at avoiding prolonged positive pressure breaths as they can limit breathing frequency (57) and disrupt the neural breathing pattern (58). This may be quite relevant as reports indicate that in preterm infants most mechanical breaths extend beyond the end of spontaneous inspiration (46).

Clinical Evidence with Synchronized Ventilation

Evidence obtained in short-term studies using specific physiologic parameters indicated potential beneficial effects of various modalities of synchronized ventilation. Most of these studies preceded the randomized trials that prospectively compared synchronized against conventional ventilation. To date, six randomized controlled trials and one quasi-randomized trial have compared A/C or SIMV to conventional IMV (38, 40, 73–77).

The individual or combined results of the randomized trials did not indicate significant beneficial effects of synchronization compared to conventional mechanical ventilation on survival or IVH. Synchronization appears to have accelerated the weaning process, leading to a shorter course of mechanical ventilation, but it did not consistently reduce the rate of acute respiratory complications such as air leak or the incidence of BPD. The lack of clear beneficial effects of synchronized ventilation is disappointing given the possible benefits suggested in acute physiologic studies.

There were important differences between the clinical trials. Some of the studied populations included infants of a wide range of gestational age (or birth weight). The sample size of these also varied greatly between studies, ranging from 30 to over 800 infants. These variations limit the ability to generalize the findings of these studies to multifactorial outcomes that are closely related to prematurity. This is especially relevant to respiratory outcomes such as BPD. The largest trial (78) has been criticized because of a large rate of crossover and for ventilating most of the infants with a lower-performance airway pressure triggered ventilator. Many studies had an insufficient sample to assess the effects on BPD (73–75) or their design was aimed at assessing the effects of synchronized ventilation only on weaning with a brief exposure to the control or intervention modalities. In one of these studies the age of study entry varied from a few hours to several days (73). These aspects limit interpretation of the data with regard to BPD since exposure to the therapy may be insignificant or many infants could have lung injury before study entry.

An important but often ignored difference between studies that test similar interventions is given by the incidence of the negative outcome measure in the control population. It is possible that the effects of reducing asynchrony may be greater in populations where this plays a greater role on outcome. The relative effect of synchronized ventilation on respiratory outcome referenced to the existing risk in the base population (the CMV group) is illustrated in Figure 18-1. Data abstracted from the surviving infants in studies that enrolled at least 100 infants in the birth weight (BW) ≤ 2 kg strata indicate a greater risk reduction in studies with a higher rate of BPD in the control groups, suggesting a baseline population-dependent difference in the effect.

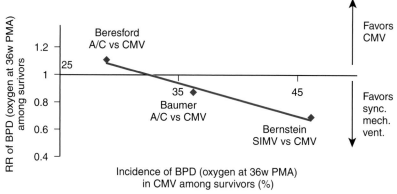

Figure 18-1 Data on surviving infants abstracted from studies that enrolled at least 100 infants in the BW ≤ 2000 g strata.Data from the study by Bernstein et al. abstracted from the BW 500–2000 g infants (reproduced from Claure N., Bancalari E., Arch. Dis. Child. Fetal Neonatal Ed., 2007 online, doi: 10,136/adc, 2006108852).

Today, most of the BPD cases and other morbidities are observed among those infants born with BW < 1000 g or <28 weeks GA. However, no study has focused on this population exclusively and only one consistently stratified the enrollment and reported the effects within strata (38). In that study, synchronization reduced BPD among survivors in the BW < 1000 g strata.

Based on the reported findings there is no consensus on the effects of synchronized ventilation on outcome. However, based on the apparent effects on duration of ventilation, the reported physiologic effects and the observations mentioned above, it is probably safe to conclude that with an adequate setup, judicious management and proper monitoring there may be benefits to the use of synchronized ventilation.

Clinical and Physiological Differences between Synchronized Modalities

Synchronized ventilation for the preterm infant is mostly used in A/C (PTV, SIPPV) or SIMV. The management of these two modalities differs and there is no consensus on the superiority of one over the other. Proponents of A/C point out as beneficial the assistance of every inspiration to prevent fatigue and a better V_T to dead space (V_D) ratio than unassisted spontaneous breaths. On the other hand, benefits indicated by proponents of SIMV include exposure to fewer positive pressure breaths, a potentially increased diaphragmatic fitness and a greater control of the contribution of the ventilator to total ventilation.

Although SIMV and A/C seem to be conceptually different, there are in practice a number of conditions where these modalities have striking similarities. This is evident in the acute phase of respiratory failure, where an SIMV rate ranging between 40 and 60 b/min is likely to assist every inspiration, yielding a similar support to that of A/C. Although such a range can be exceeded in A/C, it is uncommon, as the resulting V_T reduces the need for a high spontaneous breathing rate. A study indicated similarities in ventilator frequency and gas exchange between A/C and SIMV with tightly regulated PIP following surfactant administration (79).

Ventilatory management in A/C and SIMV is primarily driven at limiting PIP in order to avoid excessive V_T. As lung disease improves, weaning of PIP in A/C continues, whereas in SIMV weaning of PIP is often accompanied by a reduction in ventilator rate. Weaning the PIP in A/C increases the role of the inspiratory effort in the generation of V_T of the synchronous breath, whereas weaning of the ventilator rate and PIP in SIMV leads to a greater contribution of the spontaneous breathing effort to minute ventilation and to V_T generation of the synchronized breath.

This explains the lower spontaneous inspiratory effort in A/C compared to SIMV (64, 80) and the attenuation in intrathoracic pressure swings that resulted in smaller beat-to-beat blood pressure fluctuations (64). Reports indicate a lower metabolic cost of respiration in A/C compared to SIMV (68) among infants ventilated for over 3 weeks who had a high metabolic cost of breathing (81). This difference did not exist during the first week, suggesting that the metabolic effects of assisting every breath may be greater in more chronically ventilated infants.

Two randomized controlled studies compared the efficacy of weaning with A/C and SIMV in the recovery phase of RDS (82, 83). These studies suggested a more rapid weaning with A/C. However, many infants were ventilated for an extended length of time prior to study entry and therefore it is unclear whether the preferential use of one of these modalities throughout the entire course of mechanical ventilation could be responsible for the improved respiratory outcome.

As described above, A/C breaths can be terminated in synchrony with the end of the spontaneous inspiration (as in PSV). Physiologic studies showed that, compared to A/C ventilation with a fixed Ti, synchronous termination of the breath allowed an increase in the respiratory rate without affecting V_T (46). Compared to intermittent mandatory ventilation, PSV reduces the breathing effort and the respiratory rate to levels similar to those with A/C (81, 84). This, according to animal studies, occurs in proportion to the support pressure used (85). PSV has also been shown to enhance spontaneous ventilation and reduce thoracoabdominal asynchrony in neonates with congenital heart disease and decrease breathing effort in children following cardiac surgery (85, 86, 87).

Today, the acute phase of RDS is relatively short in most preterm infants, but many of them go on to require ventilatory support for several days or weeks. In those cases, low levels of support in A/C or SIMV can have some limitations. Many of these infants have an inconsistent respiratory drive and during apnea the controlled (backup) rate delivers breaths with the same PIP. The missing inspiratory effort also results in a lower V_T and the infant can develop hypoventilation if the controlled rate is not sufficient. At low SIMV rates, further weaning of PIP is slower because a minimal V_T may be required to avoid hypoventilation during apnea. Data on the effects of different ventilator rates in SIMV or as backup in A/C are lacking.

Limitations of the different modalities of synchronized ventilation may be overcome by the use of hybrid or combined modalities. These include the combined use of PSV and SIMV to provide a background ventilator rate or an apnea backup ventilator rate. Combining PSV and SIMV in preterm infants follows the rationale of providing some support level to all the spontaneous breaths with the aim of reducing the reliance on the larger SIMV breaths (Fig. 18-2). PSV prevented an increase in breathing effort and maintained ventilation and gas exchange in preterm infants who were acutely challenged with a reduction in SIMV frequency (88).

A recent randomized trial indicated that the combined use of PSV and SIMV during the first 4 weeks after birth facilitated weaning in infants of BW ≤ 1000 g (89). The benefits of this strategy appear to be greater in the BW 700–1000 g strata, as indicated by a shorter need for supplemental oxygen. This combined modality may be helpful in preterm infants in whom early weaning and reduced exposure to SIMV may lower the risk of lung injury. These data also suggest a dependency on the maturation of the respiratory center to benefit from a modality such as PSV that depends on a consistent respiratory drive.

Volume-Targeted Ventilation

Structural and functional characteristics of the lung in preterm infants make them susceptible to mechanical injury. Evidence indicates the lung is damaged by

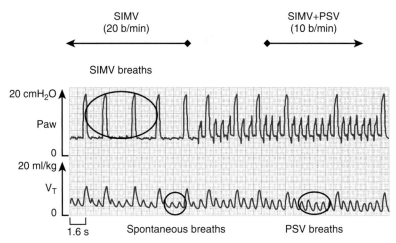

Figure 18-2 Recordings of airway pressure and V_T during a transition from SIMV at a rate of 20 b/min to SIMV at 10 b/m combined with PSV. V_T in spontaneous breaths assisted with PSV increases compared to non-assisted spontaneous breaths.

excessive lung inflation and by ventilation with insufficient lung volume rather than high positive pressure alone (17, 18, 90). It is likely that inadvertent exposure to excessive inflation due to high pressures or alveolar volume loss due to insufficient end-expiratory pressure or ventilation with small V_T plays a role in the development of lung injury in the preterm infant.

Resolution or aggravation of conditions such as inadequate surfactant function or excessive lung fluid can influence lung mechanics. Changes in lung volume, compliance and airway resistance are common in preterm infants and lead to changes in V_T and ventilation during mechanical ventilation with a constant PIP. During synchronized ventilation the inspiratory effort contributes to the generation of V_T but the preterm infant's respiratory drive is inconsistent and this further increases the variability in V_T and minute ventilation. These conditions make an adaptive modality appealing. The proposed beneficial effects of volume-targeted ventilation are based on avoidance of excessive lung inflation and maintenance of a stable lung volume by preventing alveolar de-recruitment due to insufficient V_T.

There are several modalities of volume-targeted ventilation that aim at delivering a target mechanical V_T by adjustments to the pressure or inspiratory duration. These modalities vary with regard to the controlled volume parameter, whether this is the volume delivered by the ventilator or the actual patient V_T (inspired or exhaled). In some of these modalities the adjustments occur as the volume is delivered, while in others they occur from breath to breath.

VOLUME-CONTROLLED (VC)

In this ventilatory modality the ventilator delivers on each cycle a constant volume of gas that is partitioned into the volume compressed in the circuit and V_T. VC breaths can be delivered in A/C, SIMV or IMV. In preterm infants V_T is a small fraction of the volume delivered by the ventilator in a VC breath. This limits the effectiveness of VC in preserving V_T during a decrease in C_L that would require a proportionally greater increase in the set ventilator volume. Also, leaks around the ETT during inspiration, which are common in preterm infants, can result in early termination of the VC breath.

VOLUME-ASSURED PRESSURE SUPPORT (VAPS)

This is a hybrid ventilatory modality that combines pressure support and VC within the same breath. If the measured volume during a pressure-supported breath is smaller than the set volume the breath will transition to a VC breath and continue until the set volume is delivered or the set inspiratory duration elapses.

Pressure-Regulated Volume-Controlled (PRVC)

In this modality PIP is automatically regulated to deliver a set volume in the A/C mode. A diagnostic VC breath is used to calculate respiratory compliance. Subsequently PIP is adjusted stepwise based on volume measurements obtained by internal flow sensors during the inspiratory phase of prior breaths. In preterm infants PRVC may be limited by the accuracy of internally measured volumes (54, 55). Although circuit compliance compensation methods appear to be effective these have not been tested in small preterm infants. Also, measurements of inspired volume may overestimate V_T in the presence of leaks around the ETT.

Volume Guarantee (VG)

This modality consists of automatic adjustments to PIP aimed at maintaining the measured exhaled V_T at a target level to compensate for changes in lung mechanics and spontaneous breathing effort. The PIP for the next breath is adjusted based on the difference between the target and measured exhaled V_T from previous breaths. Proximal measurements of exhaled V_T help in circumventing the effects of inspiratory leaks and gas compression in the circuit.

Physiologic and Clinical Evidence on Volume-Targeted Ventilation

The possible beneficial effects of volume-targeted ventilation include the prevention of volutrauma, avoidance of insufficient V_T, and more stable blood gases from a tighter control of V_T compared to constant peak pressure modes of ventilation in preterm infants. However, most of volume-targeted modalities were not designed specifically for the neonate but were adopted from adults and their physiologic effects were not examined prior to their use in clinical trials.

The understanding of volume-targeted ventilation in the preterm infant was increased with examination of VG in physiologic studies. The use of VG for automatic PIP weaning in SIMV in the recovery phase of RDS revealed a dependency on the target V_T. A minimal reduction in PIP was observed when the target V_T was similar to the mean V_T of pressure-limited SIMV (95, 96). Weaning of PIP was achieved only when the target V_T was set below such level, but this led to an increase in spontaneous breathing effort and a tendency towards a higher CO_2 (96).

Avoidance of excessive V_T was expected to stabilize gas exchange. A lower incidence of hypocapnia and a lower number of breaths with excessive V_T were reported when VG was used in A/C in infants with RDS (97) and a low incidence of abnormal CO_2 during clinical use of VG (98). When used in combination with A/C or PSV in stable infants with RDS, VG reduced V_T variability compared to pressure-limited ventilation (94, 95). On the other hand, VG in combination with PSV increased mean airway pressure and ventilation without improving gas exchange compared to pressure-limited SIMV in the early and weaning phases of RDS (99–101).

Under some conditions the variability in V_T can increase in VG with respect to pressure-limited ventilation. This could occur with a low target V_T because the infant contribution to V_T is greater (and often more variable). Conversely, the variability could decrease with a high target V_T because the spontaneous effort decreases when the ventilator provides most of the ventilation. Interaction with reflex activity may also lead to unexpected variability in PIP or V_T. In preterm infants, synchronized breaths can trigger an augmented spontaneous inspiration (72) or elicit a form of expiratory braking that interrupts exhalation (92).

In a randomized trial in infants with RDS there was a lower incidence of IVH in PRVC compared to IMV (101). The duration of ventilation did not differ in the entire group, but it was shorter with PRVC in the BW < 1000 g strata. It is unclear whether this was due to PRVC alone or to synchronized assistance of every breath. In a more recent trial PRVC was compared to SIMV in infants with RDS (103). In this trial, PRVC did not influence the duration of ventilation or respiratory outcome, but lowered the proportion of infants with severe respiratory deterioration.

VC was compared to pressure-limited among infants of BW ≥ 1200 g (102). This study was limited to larger preterm infants due to device limitations for delivery of small volumes. VC resulted in a more rapid weaning and shorter duration of ventilation but the sample size was insufficient to detect effects on BPD. Following the availability of delivering smaller volumes, VC was compared to pressure-limited ventilation in infants of BW 600–1500 g with RDS (104). This trial indicated that VC led to a faster weaning particularly among the BW < 1000 g infants, but the overall duration of ventilation and other outcomes did not differ.

A proposed benefit of volume-targeted ventilation is avoidance of excessive V_T believed to contribute to lung injury by promoting an inflammatory cascade. Analysis of tracheoalveolar fluid from preterm infants with RDS showed lower levels of proinflammatory cytokines among infants ventilated with PSV+VG compared to PSV during the first week (105). In spite of this and probably due to an insufficient sample size, ventilator or oxygen dependency did not differ.

The limited effects on respiratory outcome in the above-mentioned trials may be in part due to an improved management of pressure-limited ventilation. Although these modes do not have the benefit of the rapid and automatic adjustments to PIP, most of the devices used in the trials have volume-monitoring capabilities and therefore the clinician can adjust the PIP to avoid excessive volumes.

Although there is clear consensus regarding the benefits of avoiding excessive or insufficient V_T, there is a paucity of data on the optimal V_T. A comparison of 3 and 5 mL/kg as V_T targets in PSV+VG in preterm infants with RDS showed increased levels of proinflammatory cytokines in the small V_T group (106). Although radiographic markers of atelectasis were not evident, inadvertent changes in lung volume with cycling between collapse and recruitment could occur when insufficient V_T is targeted. A low target V_T could be attained by the infants, resulting in periods of reduced peak pressure or even endotracheal CPAP, which could lead to losses in lung volume. These infants are not likely to maintain a consistent effort and particularly if the loss in lung volume worsens lung mechanics. A decrease in V_T when the breathing effort is insufficient or absent will be followed by a rise in peak pressure. The resulting interaction between the target V_T and the spontaneous effort needs to be further explored.

Preterm infants often present with rapid and acute changes in C_L that lead to hypoventilation and episodes of hypoxemia (107, 108). The efficacy of an automatic rise in PIP by VG in attenuating these episodes was evaluated in a group of preterm infants. The episodes were not reduced by VG in SIMV mode when the target V_T was similar to the V_T of SIMV alone, but a higher target V_T reduced the number of breaths with small V_T and shortened the episodes of hypoxemia (109). A delayed response when VG is used in SIMV may have limited its efficacy. Alternatively, VG in A/C led to a shorter hypoventilation and faster recovery compared to pressure-limited A/C (110). Instantaneous adjustments to the pressure as V_T is delivered were expected to avert these episodes due to a faster response, but the effects were not striking (91).

Current evidence regarding the use of volume-targeted ventilation points towards beneficial effects in the preterm neonate. It is possible that the institution of gentler ventilatory strategies may have minimized the potential advantages over pressure-limited ventilation. The optimal V_T for different stages of lung disease or the different ventilatory modalities is still to be determined.

NONINVASIVE VENTILATION OF THE NEWBORN

The respiratory care provided to the premature newborn has shifted towards gentler and less invasive forms of support in an effort to avert adverse pulmonary outcome. For this, avoidance of intubation and reduction in the exposure to mechanical ventilation are among the proposed strategies. The use of nasal continuous positive airway pressure (NCPAP) is known to alleviate many of the conditions leading to the need for invasive ventilation. These conditions include apnea, upper airway obstruction, lung volume instability, and thoraco-abdominal asynchrony among others. In an effort to further alleviate these conditions in the preterm infant, the use of noninvasive positive pressure ventilation has been proposed and tested.

From the instrumental standpoint, there is little difference between invasive and noninvasive ventilation with a nasal interface in lieu of the ETT. In fact, noninvasive ventilation was one of the initial forms of respiratory support for preterm infants with RDS (111). Reports of individual center experiences with noninvasive ventilation indicated beneficial effects (112, 113) while others reported a higher risk of gastrointestinal perforation (114). Initially, noninvasive ventilation of the newborn was done using conventional ventilators in IMV (N-IMV). Abdominal and flow triggering synchronization techniques were extended into noninvasive neonatal ventilation and enabled delivery of nasal A/C (N-A/C) or PSV and nasal SIMV (N-SIMV). A proposed benefit of the addition of synchrony to noninvasive ventilation is the avoidance of gastric distension.

Apnea is a common indication for invasive ventilation in preterm infants. In addition to the increased ventilation, ventilator cycling may stimulate the respiratory center or induce reflex activity. In crossover and randomized comparisons N-IMV reduced apnea and bradycardia compared to NCPAP in preterm infants (115, 116), with an observed pattern of sighs and resumption of breathing following cycling of the ventilator.

Preterm infants have a compliant chest wall that often caves in during inspiration, partially dissipating the spontaneous effort. N-SIMV reduced thoraco-abdominal asynchrony in preterm infants immediately after extubation in comparison to NCPAP (117), while a crossover study showed that assisting every inspiration with flow-triggered N-A/C reduced breathing effort and improved ventilation (118). Interestingly, noninvasive high-frequency ventilation (HFV) improved $PaCO_2$ in a group of term and preterm infants with moderate respiratory insufficiency (119).

Clinical Evidence

The desire to reduce the use of invasive ventilation in preterm infants increased the interest in noninvasive ventilation, resulting in the execution of three randomized trials. A randomized comparison of NCPAP and N-SIMV via binasal nasopharyngeal prongs in preterm infants after extubation showed a better respiratory evolution in the SIMV group (120). Most infants who failed NCPAP were later managed with N-SIMV. A subsequent comparison of NCPAP and N-SIMV via short nasal prongs in preterm infants showed that extubation failure in N-SIMV was one-third of that in the NCPAP group (121). The frequency of apnea was lower in the N-SIMV group and apnea itself was the most common cause of failure in both groups but more so in NCPAP. In another trial a similar improvement in the rate of successful extubation was observed with N-SIMV versus NCPAP (122). In that trial, infants with worse lung mechanics on NCPAP were more likely to fail extubation, whereas N-SIMV sustained all infants similarly regardless of their lung function.

This suggests that N-SIMV may be particularly beneficial for infants with limitations in their respiratory pump.

These studies, although individually small, present convincing evidence of a better respiratory course following extubation to low-rate N-SIMV. There were some tendencies towards shorter oxygen dependency and lower rates of BPD among infants extubated to N-SIMV but these were less consistent. These studies report no or minimal gastrointestinal complications with the use of N-SIMV, which is reassuring in view of earlier concerns. These data have been examined in systematic reviews and analysis of the pooled data confirms individual study observations. In spite of this, noninvasive ventilation is not as widely used as would be expected and there are few devices available. There is a need for further investigation with the use of noninvasive ventilation early in the respiratory course.

Respiratory stimulants were widely used in the above-mentioned trials but, nonetheless, apnea and hypoxemia were the most common causes of failure, followed by increased CO_2. This may be due to low N-SIMV rates or the lung function status at extubation. The use of noninvasive ventilation in modalities such as PSV or apnea backup ventilation may be beneficial. There is a possible association between extubation failure and the documented vulnerability of respiratory control and increased hypoxemia in preterm infants in the supine position (123, 124), which may be overcome by improved patient interfaces that facilitate positioning.

Noninvasive ventilation is, similarly to NCPAP, dependent on the proper airway interface and its maintenance. A common concern is the risk of nasal injury in all forms of noninvasive support. There is a critical need to develop better interfaces for the tiniest infants. Many interfaces are too rigid and heavy for the smallest infants (those who could benefit most), which can produce injurious torque forces or lead to excessive tightening. It is also common to find dislodged interfaces rendering the support ineffective. This may be addressed by smarter monitoring in noninvasive devices.

EXPERIMENTAL MODALITIES OF NEONATAL MECHANICAL VENTILATION

Classifying neonatal ventilatory modalities as conventional, new or experimental is not straightforward as these terms have become less specific. Some modalities are no longer considered experimental simply because they are available commercially and have received approval for use clinically although knowledge on their short- and long-term physiologic and therapeutic benefits or drawbacks is limited. The experimental modalities described below differ, but they share the common aim of optimizing the interaction with the patient, providing gentler forms of support and ameliorating the still-prevalent pulmonary sequelae.

Proportional Assist Ventilation (PAV)

The respiratory pump of the ventilated preterm infant has to overcome mechanical impediments for generation of an adequate V_T. These loads are induced by obstructive or restrictive conditions due to the underlying lung disease and narrow ETT. PAV is designed to compensate for these impediments. In PAV, the ventilator pressure increases instantaneously in proportion to the volume, flow or both generated by the respiratory pump. Thus, it enhances the infant's volume- or flow-generating ability and results in a perceived reduction in the impediments to breathe. PAV is intrinsically different from synchronized pressure or volume modalities and its management is quite different. In PAV, the user determines the degree of mechanical unloading by setting the elastic (volume-proportional) and resistive (flow-proportional) gains in pressure. These gains must be suited to each infant and require estimation of the respiratory mechanics. An elastic gain that exceeds the elastic recoil of the lungs can lead to a runaway increase in pressure, whereas a resistive gain that unloads beyond the total airway resistance leads to pressure oscillations.

Physiologic Effects and Clinical Evidence

The acute physiologic and short-term clinical effects of PAV in preterm infants have been assessed. PAV reduced breathing effort and chest wall asynchrony in preterm infants during the weaning phase of RDS in whom the effects were proportional to the degree of elastic unloading (125). This is a beneficial effect of PAV since part of the diaphragmatic force is dissipated in distorting the chest wall (34). Also in the weaning phase of RDS in preterm infants, a crossover comparison showed improved ventilation and oxygenation accompanied by a reduction in peak pressures with PAV compared to A/C and IMV. The better coupling of the ventilator to the patient effort throughout inspiration led to lower transpulmonary pressures (67). Prior reports indicated a decrease in beat-to-beat blood pressure variability in A/C compared to IMV (61, 64). In this study, these fluctuations were also reduced compared not only to IMV but also to A/C.

In a subsequent crossover study, PAV was compared to SIMV in a group of preterm infants recovering from RDS or in the evolving phases of lung disease. In these infants PAV reduced peak and mean airway pressures in comparison to SIMV and maintained similar gas exchange (126). A backup IMV rate was needed during PAV to ensure ventilation during variations in respiratory drive. The improved synchrony in PAV was expected to reduce the "fighting" of the ventilator. In spite of this, episodes of hypoxemia were longer during PAV. These episodes are often associated with increased patient activity (107, 108, 127) and are frequent among infants with lung disease (128, 129). Further research is needed to identify the population or lung disease stage that could benefit most from PAV and to determine its role in improving long-term pulmonary outcome.

Targeted Minute Ventilation

Preterm infants often require mechanical ventilation beyond the initial respiratory failure because of inconsistent respiratory effort and residual lung damage. Although most infants require low levels of support, the prolonged duration of ventilation increases the risk of lung injury. Currently used modalities do not adapt to the changing needs of these infants. During SIMV and A/C both infant and ventilator contribute to total ventilation, and reduction in breathing effort impairs ventilation to different degrees depending on the ventilator rate or backup rate, respectively. The apparent constant ventilation with a fixed ventilator rate can also decline if lung mechanics worsen. A high ventilator rate in SIMV or backup rate in A/C can prevent hypoventilation, but it may also inhibit the spontaneous drive and unduly increase the risk of lung injury, whereas an insufficient ventilator rate can increase the risk of hypoventilation.

Targeted minute ventilation is based on the rationale that adjustment of the ventilator rate to supply (or remove) the required ventilatory deficit (or excess) with respect to a target minute ventilation would maintain a more stable gas exchange and, if the spontaneous minute ventilation is consistent, lead to a lower ventilatory support. Automated regulation of the ventilator rate based on measured exhaled minute ventilation (V_E) was developed with the aim of adapting to the varying needs of the preterm infant. This experimental modality reduced the ventilator rate to almost half without impairing gas exchange compared to SIMV in a group of preterm infants recovering from RDS (130). These infants maintained their ventilation for considerable periods, requiring only transient increases in

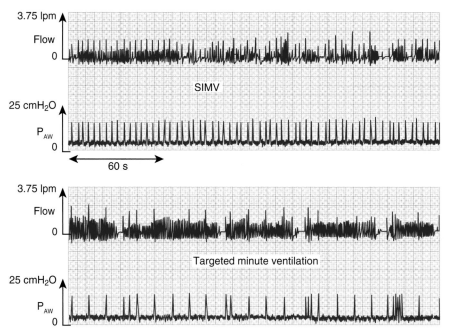

Figure 18-3 These recordings illustrate how compared to SIMV, targeted minute ventilation markedly weaned the ventilator rate with a few brief periods of increased ventilator rate and a more consistent spontaneous ventilation.

ventilator rate (Fig. 18-3). This suggests that maintenance of ventilation and gentle support do not depend on the number of ventilator breaths alone but also on their distribution over time.

MANDATORY MINUTE VENTILATION (MMV)

This is an adult weaning modality (131, 132) that has recently become available for neonates (133). In MMV, spontaneous breaths are non-assisted or assisted by pressure support and, if minute ventilation falls below a preset level, volume-controlled breaths are delivered at a constant rate. MMV combined with PSV led to automatic weaning of rate and mean airway pressure compared to SIMV in a group of near-term infants without parenchymal disease (134). MMV has not been studied in small preterm infants but, when combined with PSV, it may lead to effects similar to those of SIMV+PSV (88, 89).

APNEA BACKUP VENTILATION AND AUTOMODE

These modalities are alternative forms of targeted ventilation that have become available for neonatal ventilation. In these, spontaneous breaths can be non-assisted or assisted, while mandatory breaths in the absence of spontaneous breathing can be volume- or pressure-controlled breaths. There are no reports of these modalities in preterm infants.

ADAPTIVE MECHANICAL BACKUP VENTILATION

This hybrid modality combines PAV with a backup ventilator rate for periods of apnea. This mode has been expanded to initiate or maintain the backup rate on the occurrence of hypoxemia. The SpO_2-sensitive backup mode was compared to backup ventilation in response to apnea alone in preterm infants recovering from RDS (135). The SpO_2-sensitive backup reduced the incidence and duration of hypoxemia, suggesting a role for hybrid ventilatory strategies that promote weaning and gentle ventilation while maintaining a stable gas exchange.

Neurally Adjusted Ventilatory Assist (NAVA)

Different sensing methods have been used to synchronize the spontaneous inspiratory effort and the ventilator. Some of these methods have been used not only for synchronization but also for regulation of pressure and volume. Depending on specific infant characteristics and disease conditions, these methods may be limited by inadequate coupling of the force generated by the respiratory muscles and the components of the respiratory system. This can lead to a delayed or inadequate reflection of the timing and magnitude of the respiratory center's neural output. In 1970 Huszczuk described a ventilator controlled by phrenic nerve activity but the invasive nature of the technique restricted its use to animal studies on control of breathing (136).

NAVA is a modality consisting of adjustments to the ventilator pressure in proportion to the electrical activity of the crural diaphragm measured by esophageal electrodes (137). NAVA was shown effective in unloading the respiratory muscles without inactivation of the neural afferent signal in healthy adults (138) and in a pediatric animal model of lung injury with non-invasive ventilation (139). NAVA has not been evaluated in neonates, but it may become useful in both invasive and non-invasive ventilation of the newborn.

Dead-Space Reduction Techniques

Preserving lung volume and ventilation with the lowest possible pressures to maintain V_T and $PaCO_2$ within acceptable ranges is one of the main goals of neonatal ventilation. This, however, is not always easily attained. Preterm infants have a relatively large anatomical dead space that reduces the fraction of V_T that contributes to alveolar ventilation (140). Elimination of alveolar CO_2 is further impaired by instrumental setups including long endotracheal tubes and mainstream flow sensors (52). The limited alveolar ventilation produced by spontaneous and ventilator breaths can delay weaning or require higher ventilator settings. Dead-space reduction methods aim at reducing the ventilatory demands and mechanical support by enhancing alveolar ventilation.

CONTINUOUS TRACHEAL GAS INSUFFLATION (CTGI)

This technique is used in addition to the standard ventilator setup. In CTGI a small flow of gas drawn from the inspiratory limb of the circuit is pumped through small capillaries built in the wall of a specially designed ET tube to its distal end. The insufflated gas produces a washout of the internal lumen of the ET tube and flow sensor. In a crossover study in small preterm infants CTGI reduced $PaCO_2$ under constant ventilator settings or maintained a constant $PaCO_2$ when settings were lowered (141). In an RCT preterm infants assisted by CTGI were weaned off ventilatory support sooner (142). There were indications of a better respiratory outcome but the sample size was insufficient to yield conclusive evidence.

In CTGI safety in the event of a proximal ET tube obstruction is ensured by proper monitoring. A multi-lumen ET tube has a smaller internal diameter than a conventional ET tube of comparable external diameter, but newer designs have apparently overcome this limitation (143).

INTRATRACHEAL VENTILATION, ASPIRATION OF DEAD SPACE, AND DISTAL BIAS FLOW

These techniques have also explored the reduction of dead space. These techniques consist of flushing fresh gas at or aspirating gases from the distal end of the ETT. Experimental data indicate their effectiveness in reducing arterial CO_2 or mechanical support (144–149).

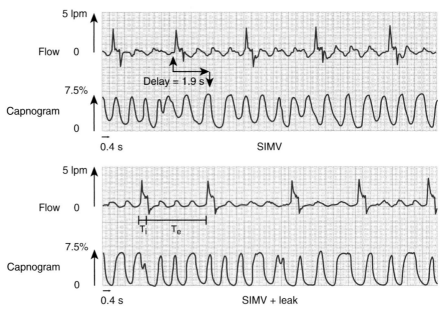

Figure 18-4 These recordings during SIMV (with the mainstream flow sensor) show the reduction in CO_2 concentration at end-inspiration and end-expiration by a continuous wash out of the sensor while synchrony is maintained (from Claure N, D'Ugard C, Bancalari E. Elimination of ventilator dead space during synchronized ventilation in premature infants. J Pediatr, 2003; 143:315-320, with permission).

CONTINUOUS WASHOUT OF THE FLOW SENSOR

Mainstream flow sensors are used in neonatal ventilation for synchronization and volume monitoring. Their apparent negligible dead-space volume can increase the V_D/V_T ratio, reducing ventilation efficiency and leading to higher CO_2 (52). These effects are more striking in small preterm infants ventilated at low SIMV rates in spite of higher spontaneous ventilation (53). Continuous washout of the flow sensor with a proximal side-stream gas leak is a simple technique that clears the sensor from exhaled CO_2, maintaining the ability to synchronize, as shown in Figure 18-4. Similar concerns about the side-effects of mainstream flow sensors led to new flow sensor designs (150–152).

Other components of the ventilator setup, including long endotracheal tubes, large Y connectors, closed suction devices, heat-moisture exchangers, and aerosol reservoir devices, could also impair alveolar ventilation in small infants (153–155). Low circulating bias flows in the ventilator circuit could also impair at least theoretically the removal of exhaled gases. The individual or combined effects of these factors in preterm infants remain to be investigated.

Automated Adjustment of the Inspired Oxygen in the Preterm Infant

Supplemental oxygen is the therapy with the most striking effect on blood oxygen content and is used in the preterm infant to avoid the effects of hypoxia on the CNS and other organs. Structural and functional immaturity of the lungs, anti-oxidant system and retina predisposes the preterm infant on supplemental oxygen to oxidative stress, development of lung injury and retinopathy of prematurity (ROP) (14, 16, 156–160). The management of the fraction of inspired oxygen (FiO2) tries to balance adequate oxygenation against oxygen toxicity. However, this is very difficult because most preterm infants present with frequent and wide fluctuations in oxygenation. These occur gradually when associated with respiratory deterioration or improvement, while other fluctuations are characterized by rapid and frequent changes in blood oxygen (107, 108, 127–129).

Center policies guide the adjustment of the basal FiO_2 to maintain oxygenation within a desired range. However, there are no clear guidelines on the handling of episodes of hypoxemia. Caregivers respond to these events to primarily resolve the hypoxemia, which is usually done by an increase in FiO_2 followed by a timely weaning of FiO_2 when normoxemia is restored. Under routine conditions, the timeliness of the response is affected by personnel workload and delays expose the infants to periods of insufficient oxygenation or unnecessary oxygen exposure. The rationale for automated FiO_2 regulation in the preterm infant is based on avoidance of the above-mentioned conditions by timely adjustments. An automated system can execute this repetitive and time-demanding task that cannot be achieved without additional workload.

Clinical Experience with Automated FiO₂ Regulation

Reports of experiences with methods of automated FiO_2 regulation vary in terms of the control method, oxygenation parameter and the studied population. They all showed the feasibility of this approach and advantages over conventional routine or dedicated care in infants (161–167). Automated FiO_2 adjustments at 1 min intervals based on PaO_2 readings from an indwelling electrode prolonged the time within a target range compared to routine care in preterm infants with RDS while on a ventilator, NCPAP or on an oxygen-hood (161, 162).

Later reports describe automated regulation of FiO_2 based on noninvasive measurements of arterial oxygen saturation by pulse oximetry (SpO_2). These measurements are quite appealing in this population due to the prolonged need for supplemental oxygen and monitoring. In BPD infants breathing on a hood, automated control extended the time around a target SpO_2 compared to manual adjustments every 2–3 min and even more compared to adjustments made every 20–30 min (163). Similar findings of increased stability around a target SpO_2 level were observed with automated or semi-automated FiO_2 control in ventilated preterm infants (164, 165).

Although these reports indicated increased stability within a desired range or around a target SpO_2 level with automated FiO_2 regulation, it is apparent that in some of these studies the infants did not present with frequent or acute episodes of hypoxemia (161) or, when these episodes occurred, the response of the automated regulation was dampened (162, 164) or consisted of a user alert (161). A recently described automated method, which according to the authors was not designed to respond to acute episodes of hypoxemia, increased the time within a target range of SpO_2 compared to dedicated and even more compared to routine manual control in a group of preterm infants on nasal CPAP (166). The need for manual adjustments was sharply reduced during automated control but it was not completely eliminated.

An automated FiO_2 method was recently developed with the parallel goals of maintaining SpO_2 within a desired range, assisting during acute episodes of hypoxemia and minimizing FiO_2. In order to evaluate this method under the most challenging conditions and quantify the effort required for tight control, it was compared to a fully dedicated nurse in a group of ventilated preterm infants with frequent episodes of hypoxemia (167). Automated FiO_2 control increased the time within the desired range, while the nurse adjusted the FiO_2 a mean of 29 times per hour, suggesting the need for dedicated attention at the onset and throughout the episode of hypoxemia, as shown in Figure 18-5 (168).

Fluctuations in oxygenation have been linked to the development of ROP (169–172). Also, many infants undergoing chronic lung changes present with

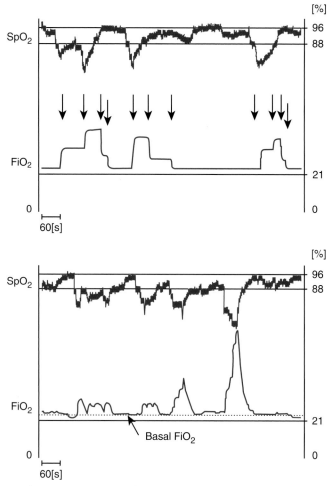

Figure 18-5 Adjustments to FiO$_2$ at the onset and throughout the episodes of hypoxemia (arrows) by a fully dedicated nurse at bedside (top) and during automated FiO$_2$ regulation (bottom), (from Claure N, Bancalari E. Automatic adjustment of the inspired oxygen during hypoxemic episodes in ventilated preterm infants. Ital J Pediatr 2003; 29:187–193 with permission).

episodes of hypoxemia (128, 129) and BPD is often associated with poor neurological outcome (173, 174). Other data indicate negative effects of repeated hypoxemia on the airway, lung vasculature and other organs (175–178). Only further investigation will determine the role of this strategy in obtaining the best balance between pulmonary, ophthalmic and neurological outcome in preterm infants.

Today, there is no consensus on the most appropriate range of oxygenation for preterm infants. Difficulties in maintaining oxygenation within a certain range has limited research in this area. This type of automation will facilitate this area of research.

Liquid Ventilation

Neonates in respiratory failure present with unstable lung volume and insufficient surfactant function. Liquid ventilation (LV) with perfluorocarbon (PFC) is aimed at ameliorating such conditions by reducing the surface tension of gas-fluid interfaces and recruiting collapsed areas. PFC liquids are inert, water-insoluble fluorinated hydrocarbons of high gas solubility and low surface tension. The viscosity of PFC increases the resistance to flow. Initial experiments with submersion of animals in PFC showed survival and laborious breathing (179).

Total Liquid Ventilation (TLV)

In this technique the lungs are filled with PFC to FRC and gas exchange is achieved by ventilation with oxygenated PFC. PFC exchange is assisted by gravity or liquid ventilators where rate and volume determine CO_2 removal and O_2 content in PFC determines oxygenation (180–182). TLV improved surface forces, C_L, lung volume, and gas exchange in surfactant-deficient preterm and term animals (183–187) and in chemical lung injury models (188–190).

Partial Liquid Ventilation (PLV)

In this technique the lungs are also filled with PFC to FRC but gas exchange is achieved by conventional gas ventilation. In PLV, PFC recruits collapsed alveoli and reduces surface tension. Compared to gas ventilation, PLV improved C_L and gas exchange in animal models of RDS even at low doses of PFC (191–193), meconium aspiration (190, 194), and lung hypoplasia (195). Avoidance of high settings in gas ventilation may be an important benefit of PLV, as suggested by reduced lung inflammation in preterm animals with RDS (191) and in surfactant-deficient term animals (196).

Clinical Evidence of Liquid Ventilation in the Newborn

The initial use of LV in neonates was mostly as a rescue therapy in very sick infants in whom conventional therapies were failing (197, 198). LV was provided by intermittent instillation of PFC to FRC assisted by gravity alternating with gas ventilation. Lung compliance and oxygenation improved but, due to their severity, none of these infants survived. PLV was subsequently used in 13 preterm infants with severe RDS (199). Three infants had a prior need of HFV for hypercapnia and were returned to HFV after a brief PLV course as hypercapnia persisted. Ten infants received PLV for up to 76 h with improved oxygenation and lung mechanics, with eight of them eventually surviving.

PLV was used with the rationale of optimizing extra-corporeal life support (ECLS) in sick infants with acute RDS or CDH by recruiting gas-exchanging spaces (200). C_L improved gradually within 2 days. Both infants with CDH died and two of four infants with acute RDS died due to non-pulmonary reasons. Case reports of PLV in acute respiratory failure requiring ECMO or HFV, persistent interstitial emphysema and alveolar proteinosis also indicate acute improvement in lung function but without striking effects on survival (201–204).

As observed in the animal data, the mechanism of LV action in infants with RDS appears to be related to recruitment of collapsed air spaces and reduced surface tension. In more mature infants with RDS, the improvement with LV seems to be slower. This more gradual response appears to be related to recruitment and clearance of areas with debris and exudate.

There is interest in the possibility of inducing lung growth in CDH by TLV. Thirteen infants on ECLS for CDH were randomized to TLV and gas ventilation to assess the effects on lung growth (205). Infants on TLV had a slightly shorter ECLS and ventilator course. Eventually, six infants on TLV survived, compared to two on gas ventilation. The effects on lung growth remain to be determined, as the few deaths in the study did not allow for reporting on this outcome.

Although extensive animal data support LV and in spite of the relatively encouraging findings in the most severe cases, LV has not left the experimental stage. The introduction of alternative techniques, including ECMO, inhaled nitric oxide and HFV, may have addressed individually or combined some of the conditions LV was intended to improve.

SUMMARY AND FUTURE DIRECTIONS

From its initial use as a rescue therapy, improvements in the methods and management of neonatal respiratory support have contributed to the survival of thousands of newborn infants in respiratory failure. The improved survival of the most premature infants, a population with a high risk of poor respiratory and neurologic outcome, increased the need for gentler yet effective ventilatory strategies.

The emergent availability of technology led to the development of new ventilatory modalities, but not all modern technology has impacted patient care. There is a further need to improve their performance and understand their effects across different stages of lung disease in the preterm infant. This is even more relevant with ventilatory strategies adapted from other populations.

There is a need to further improve both invasive and noninvasive ventilatory support in the preterm infant and tailor the support to their often variable needs. It is hoped that new modalities could alleviate some of the shortcomings of existing care and result in better outcomes. New developments should be carefully evaluated for evidence of their short- and long-term physiologic and clinical effects before adopting them as routine in the care of the preterm infant.

Parallel advances in neonatal care have perhaps masked the effects of some advances in respiratory support. This is likely to continue as most outcomes are multifactorial. Newer strategies introduced in practice are not likely to change an outcome alone but they could contribute to improving it. Clearly, there is much to learn and improve in the respiratory care of the newborn and the potential benefits are priceless to the infants and their families.

REFERENCES

1. Library of Congress. Alexander Graham Bell Family Papers. 2000.
2. O'Dwyer J. Intubation of the larynx. New York Med J 1885.
3. O'Dwyer J. Fifty cases of croup in private practice treated by intubations of the larynx with a description of the method and of the danger incident thereto. Med Res 1887; 32:557.
4. Doe OW. Apparatus for resuscitating asphyxiated children. Boston Med Surg 1889; 9:122.
5. Green CM. Reports of Societies. Boston Med Surg J 1889; 120–1.
6. Bloxsom A. Resuscitation of the newborn infant. Use of the positive pressure oxygen-air lock. J Pediatr 1950; 37:311–319.
7. Donald I. Augmented respiration: an emergency positive-pressure patient-cycled respirator. Lancet 1954; 1:895–899.
8. Benson F, Celander O. Respirator treatment of pulmonary insufficiency in the newborn. Acta Paediatr 1959; 48:49–50.
9. Heese H, Wittman W, Malan A. The management of the respiratory distress of the newborn with positive pressure respiration. S Afr Med Jour 1963; 37:123.
10. Delivoria-Papadopooulos M, Swyier P. Assisted ventilation in terminal hyaline membrane disease. Arch Dis Child 1964; 39:481–484.
11. Gregory GA, Kitterman JA, Phibbs RH, et al. Treatment of the idiopathic respiratory-distress syndrome with continuous positive airway pressure. N Engl J Med 1971; 284:1333–1340.
12. Kattwinkel J, Fleming D, Cha CC, et al. A device for administration of continuous positive airway pressure by the nasal route. Pediatrics 1973; 52:131–134.
13. Kirby R, Robison E, Schulz J, et al. Continuous-flow ventilation as an alternative to assisted or controlled ventilation in infants. Anesth Analg 1972; 51:871–875.
14. Northway WH Jr, Rosan RC, Porter DY. Pulmonary disease following respirator therapy of hyaline-membrane disease. Bronchopulmonary dysplasia. N Engl J Med 1967; 276:357–368.
15. St John EB, Carlo WA. Respiratory distress syndrome in VLBW infants: changes in management and outcomes observed by the NICHD Neonatal Research Network. Semin Perinatol 2003; 27:288–292.
16. Taghizadeh A, Reynolds EO. Pathogenesis of bronchopulmonary dysplasia following hyaline membrane disease. Am J Pathol 1976; 82:241–264.
17. Dreyfuss D, Basset G, Soler P, et al. Intermittent positive-pressure hyperventilation with high inflation pressures produces pulmonary microvascular injury in rats. Am Rev Respir Dis 1985; 132:880–884.
18. Dreyfuss D, Soler P, Basset G, et al. High inflation pressure pulmonary edema. Respective effects of high airway pressure, high tidal volume, and positive end-expiratory pressure. Am Rev Respir Dis 1988; 137:1159–1164.

19. Fanaroff AA, Hack M, Walsh MC. The NICHD neonatal research network: changes in practice and outcomes during the first 15 years. Semin Perinatol 2003; 27:281–287.

20. Ehrenkranz RA, Walsh MC, Vohr BR, et al. Validation of the National Institutes of Health consensus definition of bronchopulmonary dysplasia. Pediatrics 2005; 116:1353–1360.

21. Walsh MC, Morris BH, Wrage LA, et al. Extremely low birthweight neonates with protracted ventilation: mortality and 18-month neurodevelopmental outcomes. J Pediatr 2005; 146:798–804.

22. Greenough A, Morley C, Davis J. Interaction of spontaneous respiration with artificial ventilation in preterm babies. J Pediatr 1983; 103:769–773.

23. Greenough A, Morley CJ, Davis JA. Respiratory reflexes in ventilated premature babies. Early Human Dev 1983; 8:65–75.

24. Greenough A, Morley CJ, Davis JA. Provoked augmented inspirations in ventilated premature babies. Early Human Dev 1984; 9:111–117.

25. Stark AR, Bascom R, Frantz ID 3rd. Muscle relaxation in mechanically ventilated infants. J Pediatr 1979; 94:439–443.

26. Greenough A, Morley CJ. Pneumothorax in infants who fight ventilators. Lancet 1984; 1:689.

27. Perlman JM, McMenamin JB, Volpe JJ. Fluctuating cerebral blood-flow velocity in respiratory-distress syndrome. Relation to the development of intraventricular hemorrhage. N Engl J Med 1983; 309:204–209.

28. Perlman JM, Goodman S, Kreusser KL, et al. Reduction in intraventricular hemorrhage by elimination of fluctuating cerebral blood-flow velocity in preterm infants with respiratory distress syndrome. N Engl J Med 1985; 312:1353–1357.

29. Greenough A, Wood S, Morley CJ, et al. Pancuronium prevents pneumothoraces in ventilated premature babies who actively expire against positive pressure inflation. Lancet 1984; 1:1–3.

30. Field D, Milner AD, Hopkin IE. Manipulation of ventilator settings to prevent active expiration against positive pressure inflation. Arch Dis Child 1985; 60:1036–1040.

31. South M, Morley CJ. Synchronous mechanical ventilation of the neonate. Arch Dis Child 1986; 61:1190–1195.

32. Greenough A, Morley CJ, Pool J. Fighting the ventilator – are fast rates an effective alternative to paralysis? Early Human Dev 1986; 13:189–194.

33. Mehta A, Wright BM, Callan K, et al. Patient - triggered ventilation in the newborn. Lancet 1986; 2:17–19.

34. Heldt GP, McIlroy MB. Distortion of the chest wall and work of diaphragm in preterm infants. J Appl Physiol 1987; 62:164–169.

35. John J, Bjorklund LJ, Svenningsen NW, et al. Airway and body surface sensors for triggering in neonatal ventilation. Acta Paediatr 1994; 83:903–909.

36. Nikishin W, Gerhardt T, Everett R, et al. Patient-triggered ventilation: a comparison of tidal volume and chestwall and abdominal motion as trigger signals. Pediatr Pulmonol 1996; 22:28–34.

37. Bernstein G, Cleary JP, Heldt GP, et al. Response time and reliability of three neonatal patient-triggered ventilators. Am Rev Respir Dis 1993; 148:358–364.

38. Bernstein G, Mannino FL, Heldt GP, et al. Randomized multicenter trial comparing synchronized and conventional intermittent mandatory ventilation in neonates. J Pediatr 1996; 128:453–463.

39. Greenough A, Greenall F. Patient triggered ventilation in premature neonates. Arch Dis Child 1988; 63:77–78.

40. Visveshwara N, Freeman B, Peck M, et al. Patient-triggered synchronized assisted ventilation of newborns. Report of a preliminary study and three years' experience. J Perinatol 1991; 11:347–354.

41. Hummler H, Gerhardt T, Gonzalez A, et al. Patient triggered ventilation in neonates: comparison of a flow/volume and an impedance-triggered system. Am J Resp Crit Care Med 1996; 145:1049–1054.

42. Greenough A, Hird MF, Chan V. Airway pressure triggered ventilation for preterm neonates. J Perinat Med 1991; 19:471–476.

43. Hird MF, Greenough A. Comparison of triggering systems for neonatal patient triggered ventilation. Arch Dis Child 1991; 66:426–428.

44. Laubscher B, Greenough A, Kavadia V. Comparison of body surface and airway triggered ventilation in extremely premature infants. Acta Paediatr 1997; 86:102–104.

45. Dimitriou G, Greenough A, Cherian S. Comparison of airway pressure and airflow triggering systems using a single type of neonatal ventilator. Acta Paediatr 2001; 90:445–447.

46. Dimitriou G, Greenough A, Laubscher B, et al. Comparison of airway pressure-triggered and airflow-triggered ventilation in very immature infants. Acta Paediatr 1998; 87:1256–1260.

47. Greenough A, Pool J. Neonatal patient triggered ventilation. Arch Dis Child 1988; 63:394–397.

48. Mitchell A, Greenough A, Hird M. Limitations of patient triggered ventilation in neonates. Arch Dis Child 1989; 64:924–929.

49. Hird MF, Greenough A. Gestational age: an important influence on the success of patient triggered ventilation. Clin Phys Physiol Meas 1990; 11:307–312.

50. Hird MF, Greenough A. Patient triggered ventilation using a flow triggered system. Arch Dis Child 1991; 66:1140–1142.

51. Servant GM, Nicks JJ, Donn SM, et al. Feasibility of applying flow-synchronized ventilation to very low birthweight infants. Respir Care 1992; 37:249–253.

52. Figueras J, Rodriguez-Miguelez JM, Botet F, et al. Changes in $TcPCO_2$ regarding pulmonary mechanics due to pneumotachometer dead space in ventilated newborns. J Perinat Med 1997; 25:333–339.

53. Claure N, D'Ugard C, Bancalari E. Elimination of ventilator dead space during synchronized ventilation in premature infants. J Pediatr 2003; 143:315–320.

54. Cannon ML, Cornell J, Tripp-Hammel DS, et al. Tidal volumes for ventilated infants should be determined with a pneumotachometer placed at the endotracheal tube. Am J Respir Crit Care Med 2000; 162:2109–2112.

55. Chow LC, Vanderhal A, Raber J, et al. Are tidal volume measurements in neonatal pressure-controlled ventilation accurate? Pediatr Pulmonol 2002; 34:196–202.

56. Bernstein G, Knodel E, Heldt GP. Airway leak size in neonates and autocycling of three flow-triggered ventilators. Crit Care Med 1995; 23:1739–1744.

57. Upton CJ, Milner AD, Stokes GM. The effect of changes in inspiratory time on neonatal triggered ventilation. Eur J Pediatr 1990; 149:648–650.

58. Beck J, Tucci M, Emeriaud G, et al. Prolonged neural expiratory time induced by mechanical ventilation in infants. Pediatr Res 2004; 55:747–754.

59. Brochard L, Harf A, Lorino H, Lemaire F. Inspiratory pressure support prevents diaphragmatic fatigue during weaning from mechanical ventilation. Am Rev Respir Dis 1989; 139:513–521.

60. Brochard L, Rua F, Lorina H, et al. Inspiratory pressure support compensates for the additional work of breathing caused by the endotracheal tube. Anesthesiology 1991; 75:739–745.

61. Amitay M, Etches PC, Finer NN, et al. Synchronous mechanical ventilation of the neonate with respiratory disease. Crit Care Med 1993; 21:118–124.

62. Bernstein G, Heldt GP, Mannino FL. Increased and more consistent tidal volumes during synchronized intermittent mandatory ventilation in newborn infants. Am J Respir Crit Care Med 1994; 150:1444–1448.

63. Cleary JP, Bernstein G, Mannino FL, et al. Improved oxygenation during synchronized intermittent mandatory ventilation in neonates with respiratory distress syndrome: a randomized, crossover study. J Pediatr 1995; 126:407–411.

64. Hummler H, Gerhardt T, Gonzalez A, et al. Influence of different methods of synchronized mechanical ventilation on ventilation, gas exchange, patient effort and blood pressure fluctuations in premature neonates. Pediatr Pulmonol 1996; 22:305–313.

65. Jarreau PH, Moriette G, Mussat P, et al. Patient-triggered ventilation decreases the work of breathing in neonates. Am J Respir Crit Care Med 1996; 153:1176–1181.

66. Quinn MW, de Boer RC, Ansari N, et al. Stress response and mode of ventilation in preterm infants. Arch Dis Child Fetal Neonatal Ed 1998; 78:F195–198.

67. Schulze A, Gerhardt T, Musante G, et al. Proportional assist ventilation in low birth weight infants with acute respiratory disease: a comparison to assist/control and conventional mechanical ventilation. J Pediatr 1999; 135:339–344.

68. Roze JC, Liet JM, Gournay V, et al. Oxygen cost of breathing and weaning process in newborn infants. Eur Respir J 1997; 10:2583–2585.

69. Luyt K, Wright D, Baumer JH. Randomised study comparing extent of hypocarbia in preterm infants during conventional and patient triggered ventilation. Arch Dis Child Fetal Neonatal Ed 2001; 84:F14–17.

70. Firme SR, McEvoy CT, Alconcel C, et al. Episodes of hypoxemia during synchronized intermittent mandatory ventilation in ventilator-dependent very low birth weight infants. Pediatr Pulmonol 2005; 40:9–14.

71. Lorino H, Moriette G, Mariette C, et al. Inspiratory work of breathing in ventilated preterm infants. Pediatr Pulmonol 1996; 21:323–327.

72. Hummler H, Gerhardt T, Gonzalez A, et al. Increased incidence of sighs (augmented inspiratory efforts) during synchronized intermittent mandatory ventilation (SIMV) in preterm neonates. Pediatr Pulmonol 1997; 24:195–203.

73. Chan V, Greenough A. Randomised controlled trial of weaning by patient triggered ventilation or conventional ventilation. Eur J Pediatr 1993; 152:51–54.

74. Donn SM, Nicks JJ, Becker MA. Flow-synchronized ventilation of preterm infants with respiratory distress syndrome. J Perinatol 1994; 14:90–94.

75. Chen J-Y, Ling U-P, Chen J-H. Comparison of synchronized and conventional intermittent mandatory ventilation in neonates. Acta Paediatr Japonica 1997; 39:578–583.

76. Baumer JH. International randomised controlled trial of patient triggered ventilation in neonatal respiratory distress syndrome. Arch Disease Child 2000; 82:F5–10.

77. Beresford MW, Shaw NJ, Manning D. Randomised controlled trial of patient triggered and conventional fast rate ventilation in neonatal respiratory distress syndrome. Arch Dis Child 2000; 82:F14–18.

78. Letters to the editor. Arch Dis Child Fetal Neonatal Ed 2000; 83:F224–226.

79. Mrozek JD, Bendel-Stenzel EM, Meyers PA, et al. Randomized controlled trial of volume-targeted synchronized ventilation and conventional intermittent mandatory ventilation following initial exogenous surfactant therapy. Pediatr Pulmonol 2000; 29:11–18.

80. Kapasi M, Fujino Y, Kirmse M, et al. Effort and work of breathing in neonates during assisted patient-triggered ventilation. Pediatr Crit Care Med 2001; 2:9–16.

81. Ilizarov AM, Toubas PL, Weedon J, et al. Assist controlled versus synchronized intermittent mandatory ventilation: oxygen consumption, metabolic energy expenditure and minute ventilation. Neonatal Int Care 2004; 16:27–9.

82. Chan V, Greenough A. Comparison of weaning by patient triggered ventilation or synchronous mandatory intermittent ventilation. Acta Paediatr 1994; 83:335–337.

83. Dimitriou G, Greenough A, Giffin FJ, et al. Synchronous intermittent mandatory ventilation modes versus patient triggered ventilation during weaning. Arch Dis Child 1995; 72:F188–190.

84. Migliori C, Cavazza A, Motta M, et al. Effect on respiratory function of pressure support ventilation versus synchronised intermittent mandatory ventilation in preterm infants. Pediatr Pulmonol 2003; 35:364–367.

85. Uchiyama A, Imanaka H, Taenaka N, et al. Comparative evaluation of diaphragmatic activity during pressure support ventilation and intermittent mandatory ventilation in animal model. Am J Respir Crit Care Med 1994; 150:1564–1568.

86. Tokioka H, Nagano O, Ohta Y, et al. Pressure support ventilation augments spontaneous breathing with improved thoracoabdominal synchrony in neonates with congenital heart disease. Anesth Analg 1997; 85:789–793.

87. Tokioka H, Kinjo M, Hirakawa M. The effectiveness of pressure support ventilation for mechanical ventilatory support in children. Anesthesiology 1993; 78:880–884.

88. Osorio W, Claure N, D'Ugard C, et al. Effects of pressure support during an acute reduction of synchronized intermittent mandatory ventilation in preterm infants. J Perinatol 2005; 25:412–416.

89. Reyes Z, Claure N, Tauscher M, et al. Randomized Controlled Trial Comparing Synchronized Intermittent Mandatory Ventilation (SIMV) and SIMV plus Pressure Support (SIMV+PS) in Preterm Infants. Pediatrics 2006; 118:1409–1417.

90. Muscedere JG, Mullen JBM, Gan K, et al. Tidal ventilation at low airway pressures can augment lung injury. Am J Respir Crit Care Med 1994; 149:1327–1334.

91. Hummler H, Engelmann A, Pohlandt F, et al. Volume-controlled intermittent mandatory ventilation in preterm infants with hypoxemic episodes. Int Care Med 2006; 32:577–584.

92. McCallion N, Lau R, Dargaville PA, et al. Volume guarantee ventilation, interrupted expiration, and expiratory braking. Arch Dis Child 2005; 90:865–870.

93. Abubakar KM, Keszler M. Patient-ventilator interactions in new modes of patient-triggered ventilation. Pediatr Pulmonol 2001; 32:71–75.

94. Cheema IU, Ahluwalia JS. Feasibility of tidal volume-guided ventilation in newborn infants: a randomized, crossover trial using the volume guarantee modality. Pediatrics 2001; 107:1323–1328.

95. Herrera CM, Gerhardt T, Claure N, et al. Effects of volume-guaranteed synchronized intermittent mandatory ventilation in preterm infants recovering from respiratory failure. Pediatrics 2002; 110:529–533.

96. Keszler M, Abubakar K. Volume guarantee: stability of tidal volume and incidence of hypocarbia. Pediatr Pulmonol 2004; 38:240–245.

97. Dawson C, Davies MW. Volume-targeted ventilation and arterial carbon dioxide in neonates. J Paediatr Child Health 2005; 41:518–521.

98. Olsen SL, Thibeault DW, Truog WE. Crossover trial comparing pressure support with synchronized intermittent mandatory ventilation. J Perinatol 2002; 22:461–466.

99. Nafday SM, Green RS, Lin J, et al. Is there an advantage of using pressure support ventilation with volume guarantee in the initial management of premature infants with respiratory distress syndrome? A pilot study. J Perinatol 2005; 25:193–197.

100. Abd El-Moneim ES, Fuerste HO, Krueger M, et al. Pressure support ventilation combined with volume guarantee versus synchronized intermittent mandatory ventilation: a pilot crossover trial in premature infants in their weaning phase. Pediatr Crit Care Med 2005; 6:286–292.

101. Piotrowski A, Sobala W, Kawczynski P. Patient-initiated, pressure-regulated, volume-controlled ventilation compared with intermittent mandatory ventilation in neonates: a prospective, randomised study. Intensive Care Med 1997; 23:975–981.

102. Sinha SK, Donn SM, Gavey J, et al. Randomised trial of volume controlled versus time cycled, pressure limited ventilation in preterm infants with respiratory distress syndrome. Arch Dis Child Fetal Neonatal Ed 1997; 77:F202–205.

103. D'Angio CT, Chess PR, Kovacs SJ, et al. Pressure-regulated volume control ventilation vs synchronized intermittent mandatory ventilation for very low-birth-weight infants: a randomized controlled trial. Arch Pediatr Adolesc Med 2005; 159:868–875.

104. Singh J, Sinha SK, Donn SM, et al. Mechanical ventilation of very low birth weight infants: is volume or pressure a better target variable? J Pediatr 2006; 149:308–313.

105. Lista G, Colnaghi M, Castoldi F, et al. Impact of targeted-volume ventilation on lung inflammatory response in preterm infants with respiratory distress syndrome (RDS). Pediatr Pulmonol 2004; 37:510–514.

106. Lista G, Castoldi F, Fontana P, et al. Lung inflammation in preterm infants with respiratory distress syndrome: effects of ventilation with different tidal volumes. Pediatr Pulmonol 2006; 41:357–363.

107. Bolivar JM, Gerhardt T, Gonzalez A, et al. Mechanisms for episodes of hypoxemia in preterm infants undergoing mechanical ventilation. J Pediatr 1995; 127:767–773.

108. Dimaguila MA, DiFiore JA, Martin R, et al. Characteristics of hypoxemic episodes in very low birth weight infants on ventilatory support. J Pediatr 1997; 130:577–583.

109. Polimeni V, Claure N, D'Ugard C, et al. Effects of volume-targeted synchronized intermittent mandatory ventilation on spontaneous episodes of hypoxemia in preterm infants. Biol Neonate 2006; 89:50–55.

110. Keszler M, Abubakar KM. Volume guarantee accelerates recovery from forced exhalation episodes. PAS 2004; 3092.

111. Llewellyn MA, Tilak KS, Swyer PR. A controlled trial of assisted ventilation using an oro-nasal mask. Arch Dis Child 1970; 45:453–459.

112. Allen LP, Blake AM, Durbin GM, et al. Continuous positive airway pressure and mechanical ventilation by facemask in newborn infants. Br Med J 1975; 4:137–139.

113. Moretti C, Marzetti G, Agostino R, et al. Prolonged intermittent positive pressure ventilation by nasal prongs in intractable apnea of prematurity. Acta Paediatr Scand 1981; 70:211–216.

114. Garland JS, Nelson DB, Rice T, et al. Increased risk of gastrointestinal perforations in neonates mechanically ventilated with either face mask or nasal prongs. Pediatrics 1985; 76:406–410.

115. Ryan CA, Finer NN, Peters KL. Nasal intermittent positive-pressure ventilation offers no advantages over nasal continuous positive airway pressure in apnea of prematurity. Am J Dis Child 1989; 143:1196–1198.

116. Lin CH, Wang ST, Lin YJ, et al. Efficacy of nasal intermittent positive pressure ventilation in treating apnea of prematurity. Pediatr Pulmonol 1998; 26:349–353.

117. Kiciman NM, Andreasson B, Bernstein G, et al. Thoracoabdominal motion in newborns during ventilation delivered by endotracheal tube or nasal prongs. Pediatr Pulmonol 1998; 25:175–181.

118. Moretti C, Gizzi C, Papoff P, et al. Comparing the effects of nasal synchronized intermittent positive pressure ventilation (nSIPPV) and nasal continuous positive airway pressure (nCPAP) after extubation in very low birth weight infants. Early Hum Dev 1999; 56:167–177.

119. van der Hoeven M, Brouwer E, Blanco CE. Nasal high frequency ventilation in neonates with moderate respiratory insufficiency. Arch Dis Child Fetal Neonatal Ed 1998; 79:F61–63.

120. Friedlich P, Lecart C, Posen R, et al. A randomized trial of nasopharyngeal-synchronized intermittent mandatory ventilation versus nasopharyngeal continuous positive airway pressure in very low birth weight infants after extubation. J Perinatol 1999; 19:413–418.

121. Barrington KJ, Bull D, Finer NN. Randomized trial of nasal synchronized intermittent mandatory ventilation compared with continuous positive airway pressure after extubation of very low birth weight infants. Pediatrics 2001; 107:638–641.

122. Khalaf MN, Brodsky N, Hurley J, et al. A prospective randomized, controlled trial comparing synchronized nasal intermittent positive pressure ventilation versus nasal continuous positive airway pressure as modes of extubation. Pediatrics 2001; 108:13–17.

123. Martin RJ, DiFione JM, Korenke CB, et al. Vulnerability of respiratory control in healthy preterm infants placed supine. J Pediatr 1995; 127:609–614.

124. McEvoy C, Mendoza ME, Bowling S, et al. Prone positioning decreases episodes of hypoxemia in extremely low birth weight infants (1000 grams or less) with chronic lung disease. J Pediatr 1997; 130:305–309.

125. Musante G, Schulze A, Gerhardt T, et al. Proportional assist ventilation decreases thoracoabdominal asynchrony and chest wall distortion in preterm infants. Pediatr Res 2001; 49:175–180.

126. Schulze A, Rieger-Fackeldey E, Gerhardt T, et al. Randomized crossover comparison of proportional assist ventilation and patient triggered ventilation in extremely low birth weight infants with evolving chronic lung disease. Neonatology 2007; 92:1–7.

127. Lehtonen L, Johnson MW, Bakdash T, et al. Relation of sleep state to hypoxemic episodes in ventilated extremely-low-birth-weight infants. J Pediatr 2002; 141:363–369.

128. Garg M, Kurzner SI, Bautista DB, et al. Clinically unsuspected hypoxia during sleep and feeding in infants with bronchopulmonary dysplasia. Pediatrics 1988; 81:635–642.

129. Durand M, McEvoy C, MacDonald K. Spontaneous desaturations in intubated very low birth weight infants with acute and chronic lung disease. Pediat Pulmonol 1992; 13:136–142.

130. Claure N, Gerhardt T, Hummler H, et al. Computer controlled minute ventilation in preterm infants undergoing mechanical ventilation. J Pediatr 1997; 131:910–913.

131. Hewlett AM, Platt AS, Terry VG. Mandatory minute volume. A new concept in weaning from mechanical ventilation. Anaesthesia 1977; 32:163–169.

132. Davis S, Potgieter PD, Linton DM. Mandatory minute volume weaning in patients with pulmonary pathology. Anaesth Intensive Care 1989; 17:170–174.

133. Donn SM, Becker MA. Mandatory minute ventilation: A neonatal mode of the future. Neonatal Intensive Care 1998; 11:22–24.

134. Guthrie SO, Lynn C, Lafleur BJ, et al. A crossover analysis of mandatory minute ventilation compared to synchronized intermittent mandatory ventilation in neonates. J Perinatol 2005; 25:643–646.

135. Herber-Jonat S, Rieger-Fackeldey E, Hummler H, et al. Adaptive mechanical backup ventilation for preterm intents on respiratory assist modes – a pilot study. Int Care Med 2006; 32:302–308.

136. Huszczuk A. A respiratory pump controlled by phrenic nerve activity. J Physiol (Lond) 1970; 210:183P–184P.

137. Sinderby C, Navalesi P, Beck J, et al. Neural control of mechanical ventilation in respiratory failure. Nat Med 1999; 5:1433–1436.

138. Beck J, Spahija J, DeMarchie M, et al. Unloading during neurally adjusted ventilatory assist (NAVA). Eur Respir J 2002; 20:(Suppl. 38):627s.

139. Beck J, Campoccia F, Allo JC, et al. Improved synchrony and respiratory unloading by neurally adjusted ventilatory assist (NAVA) in lung-injured rabbits. Pediatr Res 2007; 61:289–294.

140. Numa AH, Newth CJ. Anatomic dead space in infants and children. J Appl Physiol 1996; 80:1485–1489.

141. Danan C, Dassieu G, Janaud JC, et al. Efficacy of dead-space washout in mechanically ventilated premature newborns. Am J Respir Crit Care Med 1996; 153:1571–1576.

142. Dassieu G, Brochard L, Agudze E, et al. Continuous tracheal gas insufflation enables a volume reduction strategy in hyaline membrane disease: technical aspects and clinical results. Intens Care Med 1998; 24:1076–1082.

143. Kolobow T, Berra L, DeMarchi L, et al. Ultrathin-wall, two-stage, twin endotracheal tube: a tracheal tube with minimal resistance and minimal dead space for use in newborn and infant patients. Pediatr Crit Care Med 2004; 5:379–383.

144. Bancalari A, Bancalari E, Hehre D, et al. Effect of distal endotracheal bias flow on $PaCO_2$ during high frequency oscillatory ventilation. Biol Neonate 1988; 53:61–67.

145. Muller EE, Kolobow T, Mandava S, et al. How to ventilate lungs as small as 12.5% of normal: the new technique of intratracheal pulmonary ventilation. Pediatr Res 1993; 34:606–610.

146. Kolobow T, Powers T, Mandava S, et al. Intratracheal pulmonary ventilation (ITPV): control of positive end-expiratory pressure at the level of the carina through the use of a novel ITPV catheter design. Anesth Analg 1994; 78:455–461.

147. Makhoul IR, Kugelman A, Garg M, et al. Intratracheal pulmonary ventilation versus conventional mechanical ventilation in a rabbit model of surfactant deficiency. Pediatr Res 1995; 38:878–885.

148. Handman H, Rais-Bahrani K, Rivera O, et al. Use of intratracheal pulmonary ventilation versus conventional ventilation in meconium aspiration syndrome in a newborn pig model. Crit Care Med 1997; 25:2025–2030.

149. De Robertis E, Sigurdsson SE, Drefeldt B, et al. Aspiration of airway dead space. A new method to enhance CO_2 elimination. Am J Resp Crit Care Med 1999; 159:728–732.

150. Foitzik B, Schaller P, Schmidt M, et al. Accuracy of deadspace free ventilatory measurements for lung function testing in ventilated newborns: a simulation study. J Clin Monit Comput 2000; 16:563–573.

151. Foitzik B, Schmidt M, Proquitte H, et al. Deadspace free ventilatory measurements in newborns during mechanical ventilation. Crit Care Med 2001; 29:413–419.

152. Wald M, Kalous P, Lawrenz K, et al. Dead-space washout by split-flow ventilation. A new method to reduce ventilation needs in premature infants. Intensive Care Med 2005; 31:674–679.

153. Wald M, Jeitler V, Lawrenz K, et al. Effect of the Y-piece of the ventilation circuit on ventilation requirements in extremely low birth weight infants. Intensive Care Med 2005; 31:1095–1100.

154. Briassoulis G, Paraschou D, Hatzis T. Hypercapnia due to a heat and moisture exchanger. Intensive Care Med 2000; 26:147.

155. Lugo RA, Keenan J, Salyer JW. Accumulation of CO_2 in reservoir devices during simulated neonatal mechanical ventilation. Pediatr Pulmonol 2000; 30:470–475.

156. Palta M, Gabbert D, Weinstein MR, et al. Multivariate assessment of traditional risk factors for chronic lung disease in very low birth weight neonates. J Pediatr 1991; 119:285–292.

157. Saugstad OD. Chronic lung disease: the role of oxidative stress. Biol Neonatol 1998; 87:819–824.

158. Saugstad OD. Free radical disease in neonatology. Semin Neonatol 1998; 3:22–38.

159. Frank L, Sosenko IRS. Failure of premature rabbits to increase antioxidant enzymes during hyperoxic exposure: increased susceptibility to pulmonary oxygen toxicity compared with term rabbits. Pediatr Res 1991; 29:292–296.

160. Avery G, Glass P. Retinopathy of prematurity: what causes it? Clin Perinatol 1988; 15:917–928.

161. Beddis JR, Collins P, Levy NM, et al. New technique for servo-control of arterial oxygen tension in preterm infants. Arch Dis Child 1979; 54:278–280.

162. Dugdale RE, Cameron RG, Lealman GT. Closed-loop control of the partial pressure of arterial oxygen in neonates. Clin Physics Physiol Meas 1988; 9:291–305.

163. Bhutani VK, Taube JC, Antunes MJ, Delivoria-Papadopoulos M. Adaptive control of the inspired oxygen delivery to the neonate. Pediatr Pulmonol 1992; 14:110–117.

164. Morozoff PE, Evans RW. Closed-loop control of SaO_2 in the neonate. Biomed Instrum Technol 1992; 26:117–123.

165. Sun Y, Kohane IS, Start AR. Computer-assisted adjustment of inspired oxygen concentration improves control of oxygen saturation in newborn infants requiring mechanical ventilation. J Pediatr 1997; 131:754–756.

166. Claure N, Gerhardt T, Everett R, et al. Closed-loop controlled inspired oxygen concentration for mechanically ventilated very low birth weight infants with frequent episodes of hypoxemia. Pediatrics 2001; 107:1120–1124.

167. Claure N, Bancalari E. Automatic adjustment of the inspired oxygen during hypoxemic episodes in ventilated preterm infants. Ital J Pediatr 2003; 29:187–193.

168. Urschitz MS, Horn W, Seyfang A, et al. Automatic control of the inspired oxygen fraction in preterm infants: a randomized crossover trial. Am J Respir Crit Care Med 2004; 170:1095–1100.

169. Penn JS, Henry MM, Tolman BL. Exposure to alternating hypoxia and hyperoxia causes severe proliferative retinopathy in the newborn rat. Pediatr Res 1994; 36:724–731.

170. Saito Y, Omoto T, Cho Y, et al. The progression of retinopathy of prematurity and fluctuation in blood gas tension. Graefes Arch Ophthal 1993; 231:151–156.

171. Reynaud X, Dorey CK. Extraretinal neovascularization induced by hypoxic episodes in the neonatal rat. Invest Ophthalmol Vis Sci 1994; 35:3169–3177.

172. Phelps DL, Rosenbaum A. Effects of marginal hypoxemia on recovery from oxygen-induced retinopathy in the kitten model. Pediatrics 1984; 73:1–6.

173. Lifschitz MH, Seilheimer DK, Wilson GS, et al. Neurodevelopmental status of low birth weight infants with bronchopulmonary dysplasia requiring prolonged oxygen supplementation. J Perinatol 1987; 7:127–132.

174. Schmidt B, Asztalos EV, Roberts RS, et al. Impact of bronchopulmonary dysplasia, brain injury, and severe retinopathy on the outcome of extremely low-birth-weight infants at 18 months: results from the trial of indomethacin prophylaxis in preterms. JAMA 2003; 289:1124–1129.

175. Tay-Uyboco JS, Kwiatkowski K, Cates DB, et al. Hypoxic airway constriction in infants of very low birth weight recovering from moderate to severe bronchopulmonary dysplasia. J Pediatr 1989; 115:456–459.

176. Unger M, Atkins M, Briscoe WA, et al. Potentiation of pulmonary vasoconstrictor response with repeated intermittent hypoxia. J Appl Physiol 1977; 43:662–667.

177. Custer JR, Hales CA. Influence of alveolar oxygen on pulmonary vasoconstriction in newborn lambs versus sheep. Am Rev Respir Dis 1985; 132:326–331.

178. Barlow B, Santulli T. Importance of multiple episodes of hypoxia or cold stress on the development of enterocolitis in an animal model. Surgery 1975; 77:687–690.

179. Clark LC Jr, Gollan F. Survival of mammals breathing organic liquids equilibrated with oxygen at atmospheric pressure. Science 1966; 152:1755–1756.

180. Moskowitz GD, Dubin S, Shaffer TH. Technical report: demand regulated control of a liquid breathing system. J Assoc Adv Med Instrum 1971; 5:273–278.

181. Shaffer TH, Moskowitz GD. Demand-controlled liquid ventilation of the lungs. J Appl Physiol 1974; 36:208–213.

182. Moskowitz GD, Shaffer TH, Dubin SE. Liquid breathing trials and animal studies with a demand-regulated liquid breathing system. Med Instrum 1975; 9:28–33.

183. Shaffer TH, Rubenstein D, Moskowitz D, et al. Gaseous exchange and acid-base balance in premature lambs during liquid ventilation since birth. Pediatr Res 1976; 10:227–231.

184. Shaffer TH, Tran N, Bhutani VK, et al. Cardiopulmonary function in very preterm lambs during liquid ventilation. Pediatr Res 1983; 17:680–684.

185. Shaffer TH, Douglas PR, Lowe CA, et al. The effects of liquid ventilation on cardiopulmonary function in preterm lambs. Pediatr Res 1983; 17:303–306.

186. Wolfson MR, Tran N, Bhutani VK, et al. A new experimental approach for the study of cardio-pulmonary physiology during early development. J Appl Physiol 1988; 65:1436–1443.

187. Tarczy-Hornoch P, Hildebrandt J, Mates EA, et al. Effects of exogenous surfactant on lung pressure-volume characteristics during liquid ventilation. J Appl Physiol 1996; 80:1764–1771.

188. Shaffer TH, Lowe CA, Bhutani VK, et al. Liquid ventilation: effects on pulmonary function in distressed meconium-stained lambs. Pediatr Res 1984; 18:47–52.

189. Richman PS, Wolfson MR, Shaffer TH. Lung lavage with oxygenated perfluorochemical liquid in acute lung injury. Crit Care Med 1993; 21:768–774.

190. Foust R 3rd, Tran NN, Cox C, et al. Liquid assisted ventilation: an alternative ventilatory strategy for acute meconium aspiration injury. Pediatr Pulmonol 1996; 21:316–322.

191. Kinsella JP, Parker TA, Galan H, et al. Independent and combined effects of inhaled nitric oxide, liquid perfluorochemical, and high-frequency oscillatory ventilation in premature lambs with respiratory distress syndrome. Am J Respir Crit Care Med 1999; 159:1220–1227.

192. Thome UH, Schulze A, Schnabel R, et al. Partial liquid ventilation in severely surfactant-depleted, spontaneously breathing rabbits supported by proportional assist ventilation. Crit Care Med 2001; 29:1175–1180.

193. Nakamura T, Tamura M. Partial liquid ventilation with low dose of perflubron and a low stretch ventilation strategy improves oxygenation in a rabbit model of surfactant depletion. Biol Neonate 2002; 82:66–69.

194. Hummler HD, Thome U, Schulze A, et al. Spontaneous breathing during partial liquid ventilation in animals with meconium aspiration. Pediatr Res 2001; 49:572–580.

195. Wilcox DT, Glick PL, Karamanoukian HL, et al. Perfluorocarbon-associated gas exchange improves pulmonary mechanics, oxygenation, ventilation, and allows nitric oxide delivery in the hypoplastic lung congenital diaphragmatic hernia lamb model. Crit Care Med 1995; 23:1858–1863.

196. von der Hardt K, Schoof E, Kandler MA, et al. Aerosolized perfluorocarbon suppresses early pulmonary inflammatory response in a surfactant-depleted piglet model. Pediatr Res 2002; 51:177–182.

197. Greenspan JS, Wolfson MR, Rubenstein SD, et al. Liquid ventilation of preterm baby. Lancet 1989; 2:1095.

198. Greenspan JS, Wolfson MR, Rubenstein SD, et al. Liquid ventilation of human preterm neonates. J Pediatr 1990; 117:106–111.

199. Leach CL, Greenspan JS, Rubenstein SD, et al. Partial liquid ventilation with perflubron in premature infants with severe respiratory distress syndrome. The LiquiVent Study Group. N Engl J Med 1996; 335:761–767.

200. Greenspan JS, Fox WW, Rubenstein SD, et al. Partial liquid ventilation in critically ill infants receiving extracorporeal life support. Philadelphia Liquid Ventilation Consortium. Pediatrics 1997; 99:E2.

201. Gross GW, Greenspan JS, Fox WW, et al. Use of liquid ventilation with perflubron during extracorporeal membrane oxygenation: chest radiographic appearances. Radiology 1995; 194:717–720.

202. Migliori C, Bottino R, Angeli A, et al. High-frequency partial liquid ventilation in two infants. J Perinat 2004; 24:118–120.

203. Dani C, Reali MF, Bertini G, et al. Liquid ventilation in an infant with persistent interstitial pulmonary emphysema. J Perinat Med 2001; 29:158–162.

204. Tsai WC, Lewis D, Nasr SZ, et al. Liquid ventilation in an infant with pulmonary alveolar proteinosis. Pediatr Pulmonol 1998; 26:283–286.

205. Hirschl RB, Philip WF, Glick L, et al. A prospective, randomized pilot trial of perfluorocarbon-induced lung growth in newborns with congenital diaphragmatic hernia. J Pediatr Surg 2003; 38:283–289.

Chapter 19

Role of Pulmonary Function Testing in the Management of Neonates on Mechanical Ventilation

Tilo Gerhardt MD • Nelson Claure MSc PhD • Eduardo Bancalari MD

Limitations to the Measurement of Pulmonary Mechanics in the Clinical Setting

Ventilator Graphics in Neonatal Ventilation

Summary and Future Implications

Lung mechanics were first measured in infants and neonates in the 1950s and 1960s by pioneers in the areas of neonatology and pediatric pulmonology (1–5). The equipment used for these measurements was not commercially available and had to be custom-made and miniaturized from equipment used in larger subjects. Mechanical and electronic components of the equipment were not always compatible so that the frequency response was insufficient and phase shifts between the signals affected the results. Calculation of compliance and resistance from the recordings of flow, volume and pressure was time-consuming and required a thorough understanding of pulmonary physiology and of the assumptions made in the models on which these calculations were based. In addition, experience was required to identify sections of the recordings that were distorted by artifacts and therefore would not yield accurate results. Often only a few breaths were chosen for analysis from recordings obtained over long periods.

Investigators realized that not only technical problems but, more importantly, patient-related problems contributed to the variability of the measurements and were a frequent source of error in the results. Prone or supine position, neck flexion or extension, status before or after feeding, sleep state, and reliability of pleural pressure transmission through an esophageal catheter could all affect the recordings and needed to be standardized. The results could also be influenced by the infant's variable breathing pattern due to changes in frequency, tidal volume (V_T), functional residual capacity, and expiratory grunting. These experiences and recommendations for standardization of measurements are summarized in detail elsewhere (6–12).

Initially the measurements of lung mechanics were mainly for investigational purposes. Measurements were obtained in groups of infants before and after therapy, or as part of randomized studies to test new modalities of mechanical ventilation. The information obtained from these studies contributed to the understanding of pulmonary changes occurring in disease and recovery, and during lung growth and maturation. This understanding was also important in the development of effective neonatal ventilators. It was shown that measurements of compliance correlate with the risk of mortality and development of bronchopulmonary dysplasia (BPD) (13–15). Potential benefits of medications such as diuretics, bronchodilators, steroids, and surfactant were evaluated using pulmonary function testing (16–20). Similarly, pulmonary function testing was used to assess newer modalities of ventilatory support (21–24).

In the 1980s with the development of microprocessors, computerized pulmonary function systems were introduced for clinical use. These systems had largely overcome the technical limitations of the earlier equipment, could record a large number of breaths and provided computer-aided analysis. Still the investigator needed the skill to attach the sensors to the infant's airway or nose without causing obstruction or irritability, and had to standardize the measuring conditions and recognize artifact or disorganized breathing on the recordings.

Because the measurements of pulmonary mechanics were an important research tool, it was hoped that their clinical use would help in the management of individual patients and improve their outcome. However, these expectations were never convincingly documented and there is no clear evidence that these measurements are useful diagnostic or prognostic tools. Some of the limitations to the usefulness of lung mechanics measurements will be discussed in the first part of this chapter.

In contrast to measurements of compliance and resistance in spontaneously breathing infants, graphic display of flow, V_T and airway pressure traces in mechanically ventilated infants are more reproducible and can be useful in fine tuning of the ventilator to identify the optimal respiratory support for individual infants. The use of graphic display of the respiratory signals allows the clinician to tailor the ventilatory support specifically to the condition of each individual infant. This fine tuning may help in reducing the risk of lung injury and, in consequence, improve outcome. Furthermore, pulmonary graphics can be used to identify problems with patient-ventilator interaction and to assist in detecting asynchrony between the infant's breathing effort and ventilator, and to identify ventilator autocycling. These potential benefits are discussed in the second part of this chapter.

LIMITATIONS TO THE MEASUREMENT OF PULMONARY MECHANICS IN THE CLINICAL SETTING

Methodological Problems

Inspiratory and expiratory flow, V_T and pressure need to be measured for the calculation of compliance and resistance. In non-intubated infants a flow sensor is attached to the airway through nasal prongs or a face mask. Skill is needed to get the infant used to the device, to prevent irritation and agitation and to avoid airway obstruction, as may occur by angling the prongs or pushing the mandible backwards while applying pressure to the face mask to avoid leaks. Leaks between patient and sensor are a frequent source of error. In intubated infants the attachment of the flow sensor is easier and without the risk of airway obstruction. V_T is obtained by electronic integration of the flow signal.

Esophageal pressure that reflects pleural pressure in spontaneously breathing infants is obtained through an esophageal tube. Esophageal manometry introduces additional variability and potential errors. Water-filled tubes with multiple end-holes are used in small infants, while esophageal balloons are utilized in larger infants. The difficulties with esophageal manometry have been described in detail elsewhere (9, 27). In short, positioning of the tube or balloon in the lower part of the esophagus is critical but difficult in small preterm infants. If the tube is too high, cardiac activity will be superimposed on the pressure signal. When the tube is too low, reaching into the stomach, the signal will be dampened. Gagging and esophageal peristalsis can interfere with pressure transmission, and an inappropriate amount of air in a balloon or gas bubbles forming in a water-filled tube will dampen the signal. With experience most of these problems can be avoided, but esophageal manometry requires constant vigilance and assessment of proper measurement.

In intubated ventilated infants spontaneous breathing effort in general is weaker and the main driving force responsible for inflation of the lungs is the positive airway pressure. Airway pressure can be recorded easily and more reliably than esophageal pressure. Measurements of compliance and resistance in infants whose breathing is controlled by a ventilator are therefore more reproducible than in spontaneously breathing infants (28–30).

The calculation of compliance and resistance by the method of Mead and Wittenberger or by utilizing the equation of motion assumes a single-compartment lung model and a linear relationship between volume and pressure and also between flow and pressure (31, 32). Both of these assumptions may not be valid in small infants with a low FRC and are definitely inappropriate in infants with lung disease, where the compliance decreases with increasing V_T and different time constants exist in different areas of the lung (33, 34). Measurements of compliance and resistance in infants with respiratory failure are, therefore, more variable than measurements in infants with normal lung function.

Recordings should be obtained only during quiet and regular breathing, ideally during quiet sleep. During REM-sleep the breathing pattern is more variable. Measurements obtained during periods of movement or agitation are unreliable and should not be analyzed (7, 8, 10, 11).

In intubated ventilated infants recordings should be done on the same PEEP level and with the same peak inspiratory pressure (PIP) to make the measurements comparable with previously obtained measurements. Using a different PEEP or PIP will result in the V_T being measured over different sections of the pressure/volume (P/V) curve, which in infants with lung pathology can significantly affect the measurements (35, 36).

Intrapatient Variability of Measurements

The above-mentioned problems contribute to the variability of measurements when repeated in the same infant (intrapatient). With experience and a strict control of measurement conditions this variability can be reduced. However, changes in the breathing strategy of spontaneously breathing infants cannot be controlled, and they are a major source of the observed intrapatient variability. The infant may breathe at a high frequency in order to stabilize the FRC (37, 38) and this can make the compliance measurements frequency-dependent. The same infant may take deep and slow breaths starting from the lower FRC level and reaching into the flat portion of the P/V curve at the end of inspiration. In this case, compliance measurements are likely to be different from those obtained previously.

The infant may have episodes of "grunting respiration" to increase expiratory resistance and stabilize FRC (37, 38). Because of the interdependence between compliance and resistance measurements, this can also affect the measurements of compliance. The FRC is highly variable in spontaneously breathing infants. After a forceful expiration (e.g. crying, Valsalva maneuver) the FRC can decrease to the closing volume. In this case, the following breaths show a marked reduction in compliance and an increase in resistance (39). Similar observations of a decrease in FRC and change in lung mechanics have been described after episodes of apnea, while compliance frequently increases after sighs and alveolar recruitment maneuvers (40, 41).

In spontaneously breathing infants the intrapatient variability for compliance measurements has been found to be 10–20% and for resistance 30–50% (30). This large variability limits the usefulness of these measurements in evaluating the response to therapy (diuretics, bronchodilators, and surfactant) in individual infants, because small improvements may be masked by the large variability. In contrast, when groups of infants are compared, this variability becomes less of a problem because statistical analysis allows the estimation of means and the probability for these means to be different from each other.

Lack of Normal Reference Values

For the same reasons that there is large intrapatient variability in these measurements, there is an even larger interpatient variability. Because of the lack of standardization in the measurement techniques and the variability in the measurements, there are no reference values for preterm and term infants that may be used for comparison of individual measurements. Several studies have compared compliance measurements from preterm infants with and without BPD to term infants to determine their diagnostic or prognostic value. However, there was a large overlap between the groups, with the majority of infants with BPD having compliance measurements within the 95% confidence interval of the control group (42–45). Because of this overlap, measurements in individual infants are of limited value as a diagnostic or prognostic tool for BPD. Furthermore, after the introduction of surfactant it became evident that the majority of infants developing BPD later on have a benign clinical course initially, requiring low peak pressures and low FiO_2 during the first week after birth, suggesting relatively normal lung function at that time (46). This observation suggests that factors other than low compliance and severity of initial respiratory failure play an important role in the risk of developing BPD, factors that cannot be identified with lung function measurements (47–49).

Lack of Correlation between Compliance Measurements and Gas Exchange

Based on experience from the adult it was expected that manipulation of PEEP and PIP on the ventilator could define a "best compliance" when ventilation avoids the extremes of low lung volume with alveolar collapse or high lung volume with alveolar overdistension. This "best compliance" would correlate with optimal gas exchange (50). However, respiratory failure in neonates is characterized more by abnormalities in ventilation/perfusion matching and right to left shunting through fetal channels than by abnormal lung mechanics.

The use of PEEP in infants with HMD improves their oxygenation and reduces the risk of lung injury (51–55). However, this improvement is generally not accompanied by an increase in compliance but by a decrease (36, 56). In contrast, a lowering of PEEP may result in a higher compliance because alveoli that were kept open with the higher PEEP are now closing and reopening with every breath, thus increasing the tidal volume. At the same time oxygenation worsens because ventilation/perfusion matching at the end of expiration is impaired.

Similarly, surfactant administration results in rapid improvement in gas exchange, but the improvement in compliance may lag behind for many hours or days (57–60). The lack of correlation between compliance and oxygenation is even more pronounced in infants with persistent pulmonary hypertension. Pulmonary hypertension with right to left shunting through the ductus arteriosus or the foramen ovale results in severe hypoxemia and can occur among infants free of lung pathology with essentially normal pulmonary mechanics but also among infants with markedly abnormal pulmonary mechanics caused by severe lung disease such as HMD, MAS or pneumonia (61, 62). In infants with PFC, therefore, compliance measurements are highly variable, do not correlate with oxygenation and are not useful in deciding when to start therapies such as NO or ECMO.

Limitations of Pulmonary Function Measurements in Setting Ventilator Parameters

As mentioned before, a better compliance rarely correlates with optimal gas exchange. For this reason it is difficult to decide how to adjust PEEP or PIP in response to an abnormal compliance measurement. Other clinical information, such as level of the diaphragm, signs of gas trapping or interstitial emphysema on the radiographs, presence of retractions and degree of tachypnea, and most importantly blood gas measurements, is more useful in optimizing ventilator settings than measurements of pulmonary mechanics.

Ventilator induced lung injury can occur rapidly in preterm infants with diseased lungs, the main cause being pulmonary overdistension (63–65). Therefore, the optimal ventilatory strategy may not be to maximize oxygenation and CO_2 elimination, which can easily be done by increasing PIP and ventilator rate, but to aim for a gas exchange just sufficient to prevent tissue hypoxia with the lowest possible ventilatory support (66–69). To achieve this goal monitoring of V_T, SaO_2, PCO_2 and pH, blood pressure and capillary perfusion as a reflection of cardiac output is more helpful than measurements of pulmonary compliance and resistance. The limitations and pitfalls of pulmonary function testing are discussed in detail elsewhere (70).

VENTILATOR GRAPHICS IN NEONATAL VENTILATION

The traces of flow, V_T and airway pressure are depicted on the screen of newer ventilators which use a flow sensor to synchronize the patient's breathing with ventilatory support. The shapes of these waveforms are displayed, providing a wealth of information for the clinician. However, this information is frequently ignored because of lack of familiarity with the tracings and difficulties in their interpretation. The following pages are intended to familiarize the clinician with pulmonary graphics and facilitate their interpretation to improve ventilatory support.

In contrast to the traditional measurement of lung mechanics in spontaneously breathing infants, measurements in intubated infants do not require attachment of the sensors to the nose or mouth. The signals are obtained from sensors that are part of the ventilator and are used for synchronized ventilation. The reproducibility of flow and airway pressure measurements in mechanically ventilated infants is adequate (28–30). Most graphic modules in neonatal ventilators calculate dynamic lung compliance and airway resistance. However, the accuracy and the validity of the methods employed have not been thoroughly examined.

The information obtained from scalar traces is not very useful for prognostic or diagnostic purposes, but it may be used to optimize the ventilatory support and reduce the risks of baro-volutrauma in individual patients.

Graphic Display of Flow, Volume and Pressure During Mechanical Ventilation

The following traces illustrating how graphics can be interpreted and used to the benefit of patients were obtained from a mechanically ventilated lung model.

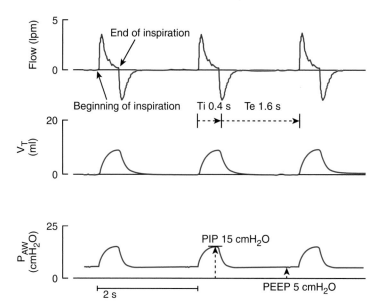

Figure 19-1 Normal trace of flow, V_T, and airway pressure (P_{AW}) in a patient on time-cycled pressure-limited (TCPL) ventilation.

Figure 19-1 shows a representative recording of flow, V_T and airway pressure in the time-cycled pressure-limited ventilation (TCPL) mode. By definition positive flow (above zero line) is inspiration and negative flow (below zero line) indicates expiration. The points where the flow trace crosses the zero line mark the beginning and end of inspiration and expiration. From these points inspiratory time (Ti) and expiratory time (Te) can be calculated. The volume trace that mimics the shape of the pressure wave form rises from baseline, reaches a plateau towards the end of inspiration and falls back to baseline during expiration. The rise is slower and the duration of the plateau is shorter than in the pressure wave. Under normal conditions (no change in FRC, no leak around the ET tube) inspired and exhaled volumes are equal and reflect the tidal volume of the breath. In this trace, airway pressure (P_{AW}) rises steeply, reaches a plateau at a peak inspiratory pressure (PIP) of 15 cmH$_2$O, and returns to the baseline pressure which is not zero but a PEEP of 5 cmH$_2$O.

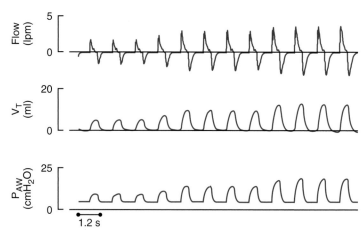

Figure 19-2 Effect of airway pressure (P_{AW}) on V_T in a lung model with linear relationship between volume and pressure.

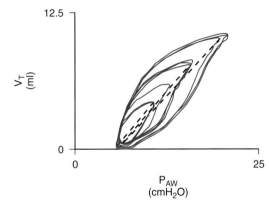

Figure 19-3 P/V loops of the breaths shown in Figure 19-2. The slopes of the dotted lines indicate the compliance of the system.

Effect of Pressure on Tidal Volume

Figure 19-2 shows the normal relationship between pressure and volume. As airway pressure (P_{AW}) is increased stepwise from 5 to 10 and then to 15 cmH_2O above the PEEP level of 4 cmH_2O, V_T increases in proportion from 5 to 10, and then to 15 mL. The ratio between V_T and change in P_{AW} is the compliance, which in this trace remains unchanged at 1.0 mL/cmH_2O.

The pressure generated by the ventilator has to overcome the elastic forces of the lung and chest wall. The compliance calculated from V_T and P_{AW}, therefore, is the compliance of the respiratory system and includes lung and chest wall compliance. Because compliance of the chest wall is very high in preterm infants, 80–90% of the pressure applied is necessary to overcome the elastic forces of the lungs and only 10–20% is needed to counteract the elastic forces of the chest wall. The compliance of the lung and total respiratory system, therefore, are quite similar in preterm infants (71).

The linear portion of the P/V curve in preterm infants is short and does not stretch far beyond the normal tidal volume range. When a peak pressure of 15–20 cmH_2O is reached, the lung becomes stiffer because of overdistension, and compliance drops. It has been documented that overdistension (volutrauma) damages the alveolar epithelium and the capillary integrity, leading to pulmonary edema. Overdistension is the main mechanism for ventilator-induced lung injury (63–65). In preterm infants with a reduced number of alveoli or no alveoli at all, the linear part of the P/V curve is short or non-existent. In addition, their lungs are frequently already injured before mechanical ventilation begins, secondary to lack of surfactant and/or inflammatory changes that begin in utero or as the result of unskilled and traumatic resuscitation in the delivery room. The preexisting injury makes the lungs more susceptible to further injury and therefore avoidance of overdistension is essential (69, 72, 73).

Figure 19-3 shows the P/V loops of the breaths shown in Figure 19-2. The breaths start at the PEEP level of 4 cmH_2O and a volume of zero. The right side of the loops shows the inspiratory phase. During inspiration P_{AW} increases faster than volume because the airway pressure has to overcome not only the elastic forces of chest and lungs but also the resistance of the respiratory system. Inspiration ends where volume and pressure reach their maximum. At this point flow has stopped and motion of lung and chest wall has come to a rest, so that pressure measured at this point reflects the pressure necessary to overcome only the elastic forces of the respiratory system. The slope of the line drawn from beginning to end of inspiration, therefore, reflects the compliance of the respiratory system, V_T/P_{AW}. It is evident from the loops that with increasing P_{AW}, volume increases proportionally. The lines drawn from beginning to end of the breaths have nearly identical slopes.

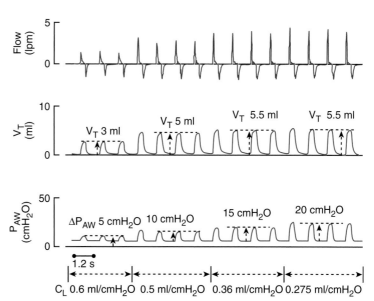

Figure 19-4 Effect of airway pressure on V_T in lung disease. Volume does not increase in proportion to pressure indicating pulmonary overdistension.

Evidence of Pulmonary Overdistension

Figure 19-4 provides an example of pulmonary overdistension. The change in airway pressure (delta P_{AW}) is gradually increased from 5 to 10, 15, and finally 20 cmH$_2$O above PEEP. Initially V_T increases in proportion to the pressure change from 2.5 to 5.0 mL but then the increments in V_T become progressively smaller. Pressure changes from 15 to 20 cmH$_2$O result in only minimal increments in V_T. The compliance of the initial breaths is 0.6 mL/cmH$_2$O, while that of the last breath

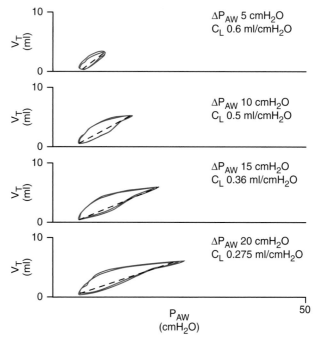

Figure 19-5 P/V loops of the breaths in Figure 19-4. The slope of the dotted line indicates a decreasing compliance with increasing pressure. The loops form a "beak."

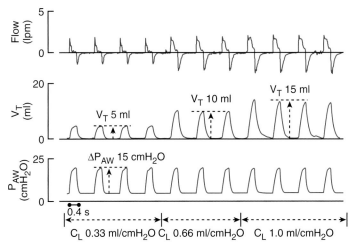

Figure 19-6 Improvement in compliance. V_T increases while pressure remains unchanged.

only 0.275 mL/cmH$_2$O. It is evident from this observation that the lung has exceeded the limits of its distensibility and has become overstretched.

Figure 19-5: the presence of pulmonary overdistension can be better appreciated from the P/V loops of the previous breaths (from Fig. 19-4). It is clear from the loops that as pressure increases, the slope of the dotted line drawn between the beginning and end of inspiration decreases, and the elliptical shape of the loops is lost. The loops become bent, shaped like a banana. The loops become pointed into the pressure direction and they resemble the beak of a bird. These distortions of the normal P/V loop are secondary to increases in pressure not being accompanied by proportional increases in volume. Therefore a banana shape and, even more so, a beak shape in a P/V loop indicate pulmonary overdistension (74). When this is observed in an infant, the airway pressure should be reduced until the beak or the banana shape disappears. If, as a result, oxygenation drops, a higher FiO$_2$ or a higher PEEP can be applied. If hypercapnia is a concern, a higher ventilator rate can be attempted or the higher CO$_2$ may be accepted as in permissive hypercapnia. These alternatives are not risk-free, but they are less damaging than pulmonary overdistension resulting in volutrauma (66–68, 75).

Changes in Compliance

Figure 19-6 shows a trace where the airway pressure remains unchanged at 15 cmH$_2$O over 4 cmH$_2$O of PEEP. However, the V_T increases over time from 5 to 10, to 15 mL. This indicates an improvement in compliance, as can be observed more gradually, occurring over hours not seconds, when atelectatic areas in the lung open up or surface tension decreases after the administration of surfactant. High airway pressures that were necessary earlier now become excessive and may produce lung overdistension. In preterm infants the V_T of spontaneous breaths ranges between 3.0 and 5.0 mL/kg. A V_T in this range should be aimed for during mechanical ventilation. Because of the short linear portion of the P/V curve in preterm infants, a larger V_T that could reach into the flat portion of the P/V curve, where the risk of lung injury secondary to overdistension is high, should be avoided (24, 73).

Effects of PEEP

Figure 19-7: PEEP plays an important part in the ventilatory management of infants. After tracheal intubation infants lose control over their larynx, which plays an essential role in stabilizing their FRC (laryngeal braking, grunting) (37, 38).

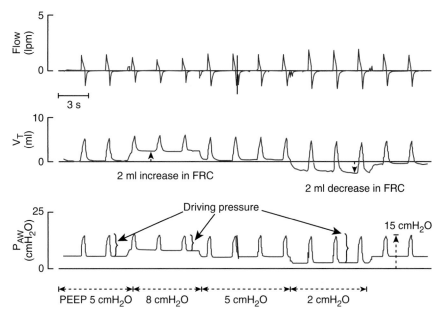

Figure 19-7 Effect of PEEP on V_T and FRC when peak pressure is kept constant.

Furthermore, there is an increased risk of lung injury not only due to high but also secondary to low lung volumes. The low volume injury occurs with surfactant deficiency when the closing pressure of the alveoli is high, or when the chest wall is very soft and does not provide enough outward recoil to maintain a normal resting lung volume. In this situation small airways and alveoli may collapse at end-expiration and then undergo cycles of reopening and closing during inspiration and expiration. The shear forces generated during these cycles gradually injure the respiratory epithelium, denuding the cells from their basal membrane and making the barrier leaky. This allows the development of hyaline membranes and further compromises lung function by inactivating surfactant (65, 73, 76–78).

It is important to avoid this cycle of collapse and recruitment. Application of PEEP or CPAP is an effective way to prevent alveolar collapse. All intubated preterm infants should be on a minimal PEEP of 4 cmH$_2$O. A higher PEEP of 6 or 8 cmH$_2$O may be necessary in cases of surfactant deficiency, recurrent atelectasis or pulmonary hemorrhage. However, PEEP has unwanted side-effects. In Figure 19-7 PEEP is increased after the first two breaths from 5 to 8 cmH$_2$O while peak inspiratory pressure (PIP) remains at 15 cmH$_2$O. It is evident from this trace that as PEEP increases, the driving pressure ($\Delta P = PIP - PEEP$) decreases by the amount of the increase in PEEP. This leads to a proportionately smaller V_T. At the same time FRC increases by the same amount that V_T has become smaller. When PEEP returns to 5 cmH$_2$O the increase in FRC is lost and V_T also returns to its initial size. When PEEP is reduced from 5 to 2 cmH$_2$O, FRC decreases and V_T increases by the same amount. PEEP prevents a complete exhalation to resting FRC, thus increasing lung volume but decreasing the size of V_T. The risks of applying PEEP are hypoventilation and hypercapnia.

Figure 19-8: in order to prevent the drop in V_T occurring with the application of PEEP the driving pressure needs to be maintained at its initial value. This is done by increasing PIP by the same amount of PEEP. In this figure PEEP is increased from zero to 4 and further to 8 cmH$_2$O. PIP increases from 15 to 19 and then to 23 cmH$_2$O, keeping the driving pressure constant at 15 cmH$_2$O. FRC increases by 4, then by 8 mL; however, V_T decreases steeply when PEEP of 8 cmH$_2$O is applied

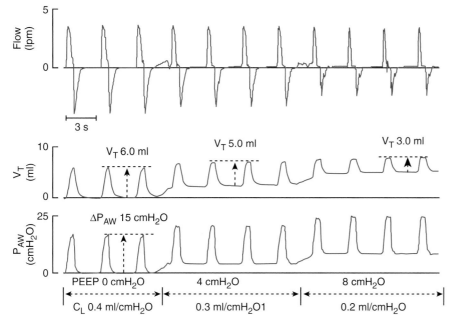

Figure 19-8 Effect of PEEP on V_T when driving pressure is kept constant.

despite a constant driving pressure. The reason for this observation is that the higher PEEP moves V_T up into the flatter part of the P/V curve where the lung becomes overdistended and stiffer.

Figure 19-9: the decrease in compliance after the application of PEEP is reflected in the P/V loops. On top is the loop without PEEP. The breath starts at a volume and pressure of zero. With an airway pressure change of 15 cmH_2O a volume change of 6.0 mL is achieved. After application of PEEP 8 cmH_2O the breath starts at higher volume and the same pressure change of 15 cmH_2O results in a V_T of only 3.0 mL. Compliance, which is reflected by the slope of the line drawn from the beginning of inspiration to its end, decreased to nearly one-half of the breath without PEEP. Application of a PEEP of 4 cmH_2O also shows a decrease in compliance but to lesser degree than with a PEEP of 8 cmH_2O.

In summary, PEEP stabilizes the FRC and prevents alveolar collapse, thus reducing lung injury. But PEEP also reduces compliance and V_T by shifting ventilation to the flat upper portion of the P/V curve. To prevent ventilation in this range where overdistension is a risk the peak pressure should be kept as low as possible, preferably below 20 cmH_2O. Adjustment of PIP should be done with an eye on V_T aiming for the lower values of the normal range of 3–5 mL/kg. In addition, the resulting $PaCO_2$ needs to be followed. If hypercapnia develops and appears unacceptable, an increase in ventilator rate may be less damaging than the higher PIP.

Circuit Flow

Figure 19-10 shows the influence of circuit or bias flow on inspiratory flow, V_T, and the pressure wave form. Inspiratory duration remains unchanged at 0.4 s. Bias flow is decreased from 9 to 6, and then to 3 L/min. With a decrease in bias flow, airway pressure rises more slowly, and in consequence inspiratory flow also decreases. With a bias flow of 9 L/min the pressure rises rapidly, allowing for a well defined plateau

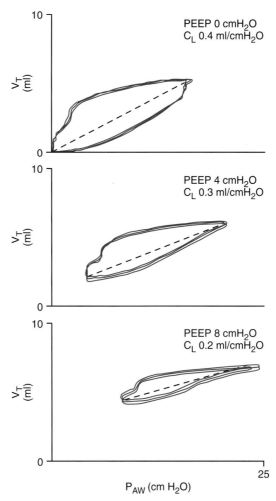

Figure 19-9 P/V loops with PEEP 0, 4, and 8 cmH$_2$O while keeping driving pressure constant. With increasing PEEP the slopes of the dotted lines, indicating compliance, decrease.

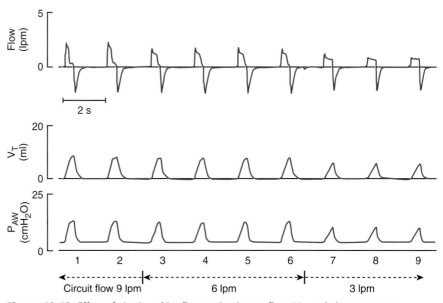

Figure 19-10 Effect of circuit or bias flow on inspiratory flow, V$_T$, and airway pressure.

time, a high inspiratory flow is reached and V_T shows a leveling off toward a plateau. With 6 L/min bias flow the pressure rise is slower so that the plateau becomes much shorter, inspiratory flow is lower and V_T barely reaches a plateau. With a bias flow of only 3 L/min inspiratory flow has become so low that the lung cannot fill within the preset time. The pressure wave becomes triangular because pressure rises so slowly that after 0.4 s the set pressure limit has not been reached and in consequence V_T drops. The trace illustrates the point that a minimal bias flow is needed to reach peak pressure and volume equilibration within the preset Ti, otherwise peak pressure and V_T decrease. The larger the patient, the larger V_T is, the higher this necessary minimal flow has to be set, otherwise peak pressure and tidal volume will decrease. In preterm infants a flow of 6–8 L/min is generally sufficient. In term infants approximately 12 L/min are needed, whereas in older air-hungry infants higher circuit flows are necessary.

The bias flow can be varied with the intent to alter the pressure wave form. High flows result in a square wave pattern, a low flow in a triangular pattern. No studies exist in neonates describing advantages of one pattern over the other. The square wave pattern is believed to reduce work of breathing at the beginning of inspiration, when flow acceleration is needed. On the other hand, a rapid inflation that exceeds normal physiologic rates may be injurious. The advantages or shortcomings of these patterns have not been assessed in neonates.

Duration of Inspiration

Figure 19-11 shows the influence of inspiratory time on the waveforms of flow, V_T, and airway pressure. Ti is decreased from 0.5 s to 0.4, and then to 0.3 s. The bias flow remains at 10 L/min. With the shortening of Ti the slopes of the flow, V_T, and pressure waves do not change. Their rise is only determined by the bias flow and the mechanical properties of the respiratory system but is not influenced by the duration of inspiration. However, the flow needs to be maintained for a minimum amount of time to deliver a desired V_T or to reach a certain pressure plateau. If not enough time is available, inspiration is cut short before it is completed and the desired pressure limit and tidal volume may not be reached (breaths 5 and 6). If too

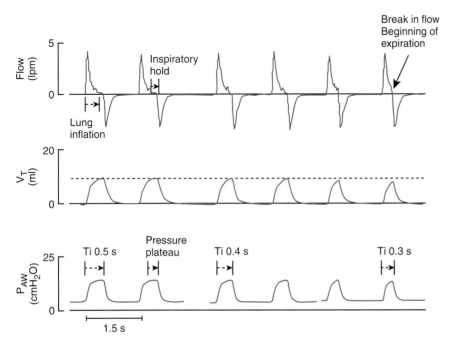

Figure 19-11 Effect of inspiratory time (Ti) on inspiratory flow, V_T, and airway pressure.

much time is allotted, inspiration will be completed before the ventilator cycles off and the respiratory system is held inflated at the end inspiratory level (breaths 1 and 2). Proper timing for inspiration is shown in breaths 3 and 4. This trace illustrates that the proper combination of bias flow and Ti is needed to reach the intended peak pressure and to produce the desired V_T.

Theoretically, a longer inspiratory duration could compensate for a low bias flow and vice versa. However, inspiratory duration should not depend on bias flow and rise time of the pressure wave, but it should be close to what is dictated by the time constant of the respiratory system or similar to what the infant's breathing strategy determines. The time constant is equal to the product of compliance and resistance of the respiratory system. It is short in preterm infants with stiff lungs and longer in term infants with airway obstruction. Therefore preterm infants in general need a shorter Ti set on the ventilator than term neonates. For clinical purposes the time constant does not need to be measured. Analysis of the flow trace indicates the time required for inspiration, provided that circuit flow is sufficient to generate a rapid rise in airway pressure to a plateau.

The first two breaths in Figure 19-11 show an inspiratory flow that peaks and then decreases towards the zero flow line. It remains at zero for some time before expiration starts. This is an example of an inspiratory hold. Inspiration has been completed as is evident from the cessation of inspiratory flow and the volume reaching a plateau at the end of inspiration. Expiration does not begin even after inspiration is complete because inspiratory time is fixed and peak airway pressure is maintained until the allotted inspiratory time elapses.

An inspiratory hold should be avoided since it does not contribute to a further increase in V_T. It increases the risk of pneumothorax and interstitial emphysema, and it makes the patient uncomfortable. An infant usually attempts to exhale as soon as V_T has been delivered and may start with an active expiration against the ventilator's inspiratory pressure. This leads to fighting the ventilator, asynchrony, inefficient ventilation, increased intrathoracic pressure and a higher risk of lung rupture and hypoxemia (79–81).

The inspiratory time, therefore, should be shortened until the period of near-zero flow at the end of inspiration disappears. Such an ideal inspiratory duration is shown in the next two breaths. It is evident from the recordings that this shortening of inspiration does not affect V_T. The main change in the V_T is the loss of the inspiratory plateau. Further shortening of Ti, as illustrated in the next two breaths, results in the loss of a pressure plateau and a decrease in V_T. An insufficient inspiratory time can be best determined from the inspiratory flow pattern. In breaths 5 and 6 inspiratory flow does not return back to zero gradually as seen in breaths 3 and 4, but the flow drops steeply to zero towards the end of inspiration and continues at the same steep angle into expiration because the airway pressure plateau ends before inspiration is completed. The example shown in breaths 5 and 6 will not have an adverse effect on ventilation because inspiration is terminated at a point where it has nearly been completed. That the breath is close to completion is reflected by the inspiratory flow having decreased to approximately 20% of its peak when expiration starts. However, any further shortening of inspiratory duration would result in a further decrease in V_T, and may leave the infant air-hungry, trying to prolong his/her inspiration beyond what the machine is set to deliver. During synchronized ventilation too short a Ti may lead to double trigger and therefore increase asynchrony.

In summary, a proper duration of inspiration is important for avoidance of harmful ventilatory patterns and improvement of synchrony between patient and ventilator. Recognition of insufficient or prolonged Ti is based on the analysis of the flow trace. Adjustments of Ti observing the flow trace can be made until a pattern similar to the one shown in breaths 3 and 4 is achieved.

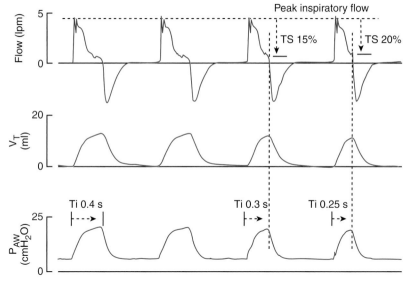

Figure 19-12 Effect of automatic termination of inspiration on duration of inspiration (Ti). Termination sensitivity of 15 and 20% of peak flow is applied.

Automatic Termination of Inspiration

Newer ventilators have an automatic inspiratory termination feature that provides the appropriate inspiratory duration. This algorithm relies on measurements of inspiratory flow, and inspiration is terminated when flow has decreased to a preset percentage of peak flow towards the end of inspiration. Usually 10, 15 or 20% of peak flow is chosen for the termination of inspiration. This feature avoids an inspiratory hold because the minimal flow at the end of inspiration characteristic of a prolonged inspiration will be below the selected percentage of peak flow, and inspiration is terminated before such a low flow is reached. The automatic termination of inspiration thus overrides the set Ti.

The effect of automatic inspiratory termination is shown in Figure 19-12. The first breath shows a fixed Ti of 0.4 s. The inspiratory hold can be recognized from the inspiratory plateau of airway pressure and V_T, and from the minimal flow at end of inspiration. An inspiratory termination of 15 and 20% of peak flow progressively shortens inspiration from 0.4 to 0.3 and further to 0.25 s. The minimal flow at end of inspiration disappears, and pressure and V_T plateaus become shorter; however, inspiration is not shortened to the degree that V_T drops or the intended pressure limit is not reached. As explained later, automatic inspiratory termination should be used in all infants on A/C or high IMV/SIMV rate, to avoid asynchrony and gas trapping.

Increased Pulmonary Resistance

Attention to the proper duration of inspiration is even more important in infants with upper (vascular ring) or lower (BPD, bronchial hyperreactivity) airway obstruction. Figure 19–13 simulates airway obstruction. As airway resistance is increased, peak inspiratory flow drops although airway pressure remains unchanged. The previous V_T is no longer reached during the set inspiratory time of 0.4 s. When the ventilator cycles off to expiration, inspiratory flow has barely dropped from its peak, indicating that inspiration is far from completed. As shown in the next breath, a longer inspiratory duration of 0.8 s is required to complete inspiration. It takes 0.8 s from the start of inspiration for the flow to decrease slowly towards zero and for V_T to reach its previous level. This example illustrates that not

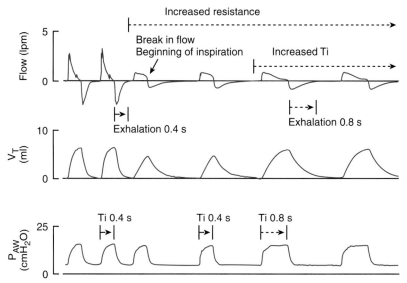

Figure 19-13 Effect of high airway resistance on flow, V_T. Necessary adjustments in duration of inspiration and expiration (Ti, Te).

only is there a minimal time needed for the airway pressure to reach its plateau, but additional time is needed for equilibration of pressures between airway and alveoli, which is considerable in infants with airway obstruction. It should be noted that expiration is a mirror image of inspiration. Airway pressure drops rapidly; however, flow and V_T continue to decrease for another 0.8 s. In cases of increased airway resistance adjustments in the ventilator rate need to be made to allow for an appropriate length of expiratory duration and prevent gas trapping. The complete cycle in this example takes 1.6 s and therefore the ventilator rate should not exceed 37 breaths per minute.

In the presence of airway obstruction a normal inspiratory time will lead to a decreased tidal volume, as will a high ventilatory rate. Because of a relative increase in dead-space ventilation in the presence of smaller V_T, alveolar ventilation may actually decrease at higher frequencies. In infants with airway obstruction, therefore, a higher ventilatory rate may not result in improved CO_2 elimination. After adjusting inspiratory and expiratory duration as described above, the only effective way to increase ventilation is increasing V_T by using higher airway pressures.

An increased airway resistance can be recognized from the low inspiratory and expiratory flows and the prolonged duration of inspiration and expiration. As shown in Figure 19-14 the problem is also reflected in the P/V loop. On top is a normal, elliptical P/V loop of breath 1 for comparison. Increased airway resistance makes the loops much wider. They now appear like squares because the high airway resistance leads to a rapid rise in airway pressure at the beginning of inspiration accompanied by only a very slow rise in V_T. During expiration the opposite occurs. Airway pressure drops rapidly to baseline while volume decreases slowly thereafter. The width of the loop is an indicator of airway resistance.

Duration of Expiration and Gas Trapping

In the description of Figure 19-13 it was mentioned that the factors (resistance and compliance) that determine the time necessary for inspiration are the same that affect the time needed for expiration. Normally the expiratory resistance is higher than the inspiratory resistance, resulting in a longer time constant during expiration than during inspiration. In this case expiratory time needs to be proportionately longer than the inspiration.

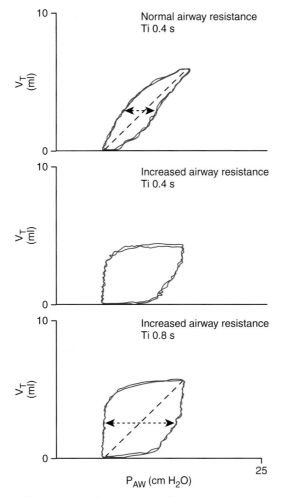

Figure 19-14 Typical presentation of P/V loops with increased resistance.

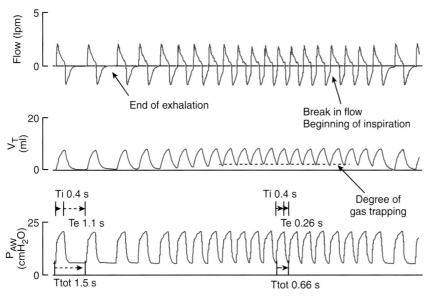

Figure 19-15 Effect of shortened expiratory duration (high rate) on expiratory flow, V_T and degree of gas trapping.

Even in infants with normal airway resistance a decrease in V_T and gas trapping may occur when a high frequency is used, as shown in Figure 19-15. The inspiratory time is kept fixed at 0.4 s. It can be seen on the flow trace that this is the time necessary to complete inspiration (it takes 0.4 s from the beginning of inspiration until the inspiratory flow has decreased again to the zero line). Therefore, at least 0.4 s should also be available for expiration. As the expiratory time is progressively shortened by increasing the IMV rate (increasing the rate does not affect Ti but only Te) V_T remains unchanged for the first five breaths until Ti and Te have become equal. When Te becomes shorter than Ti, the time available for a full expiration is insufficient and as a result the expiratory V_T is smaller than the inspiratory V_T. The volume trace does not return back to zero where the breath started, but finds a new base above the zero line. This upward shift reflects the degree of gas trapping. It can also be seen that V_T becomes smaller. The increase in rate above what was reached in breath number 5 (75 bpm), therefore, may not result in a further increase in alveolar ventilation. Indeed, alveolar ventilation may even decrease at higher frequencies because of smaller V_T and increased dead-space ventilation. Looking at the expiratory flow pattern, a pattern similar to that during too short an inspiration can be appreciated. If enough time is available for expiration (breaths 1 to 5), expiratory flow returns to zero before the next inspiration starts. If expiratory time is too short (following breaths) a break in expiratory flow with a fast return to zero and continuation at the same steep slope in flow into the inspiratory phase are noted. This happens because the rise in airway pressure of the next breath cuts expiration short before it is completed. If a flow pattern like this indicating gas trapping is detected, the ventilator rate should be lowered until expiratory flow returns to zero before the next inspiration begins.

Leaks Around the Endotracheal Tube

A frequent problem seen in intubated neonates is a leak around the ET tube. The maximal leak occurs at end of inspiration, when airway pressure is at its maximum. The pressure dilates the trachea, which is quite compliant in preterm infants, and thus increases the risk of a leak. An example of ET tube leak during inspiration is shown in Figure 19-16. The trace is characterized by an inspiratory V_T

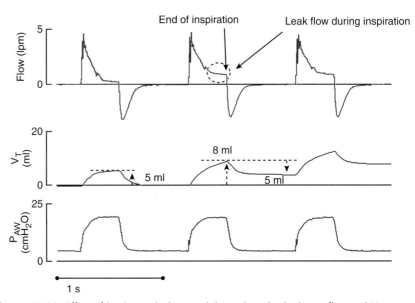

Figure 19-16 Effect of inspiratory leak around the endotracheal tube on flow and V_T.

being consistently larger than the expiratory V_T, resulting in the upward shift in the trace. Inspiratory V_T is larger because the volume entering the lungs plus the leak volume are measured during inspiration. During expiration, however, only the volume returning from the lungs is measured. The difference between inspiratory and expiratory V_T reflects the percentage of leak.

Because the leak flow is driven by the airway pressure, it continues as long as this pressure is applied, i.e. for the duration of the set inspiratory time. Even if Ti is prolonged, there is no plateau in tidal volume and no return of inspiratory flow to zero as in breaths without leaks (Fig. 19-16). After pressure equilibration between circuit and alveoli has occurred, inspiratory flow continues through the leak. At this point it becomes constant and equal to the leak flow. End of lung inflation can be determined as the point where the flow becomes flat and constant.

The inspiratory leak creates a small drop in pressure along the ET tube so that at the end of inspiration alveolar pressure will be slightly lower than the pressure measured at the airway opening. Generally this does not interfere with effective ventilation. However, if the leak is too large reintubation with a larger tube may be necessary. The inspiratory leak may interfere with automatic termination of inspiration because inspiratory flow may never fall below 10% or 20% of the measured peak flow. As a result, inspiration may not be terminated automatically. As shown in Figure 19-17, application of automatic inspiratory termination at 25% of peak flow reduces inspiratory time effectively from 0.4 to 0.3 s (breaths 3, 4) in the absence of any leak. However, when an inspiratory leak occurs automatic termination becomes ineffective. Similarly the automatic termination of inspiration during the Pressure Support mode will not work as intended. Inspiration may last longer than needed and will only be terminated when the set Ti has elapsed or the infant actively exhales. In case of inspiratory leaks, therefore, the automatic termination of inspiration needs to be set at a percentage of peak flow which is above leak flow. If the automatic termination cannot be achieved, the most appropriate inspiratory time should be determined from the flow trace.

Leakage around the ET tube during the expiratory phase is less common since the leak is driven by the PEEP. Because PEEP is considerably lower than PIP, the leak during expiration is generally smaller. Figure 19-18 shows the characteristics of a leak during inspiration as described before. In addition it can be noticed that after

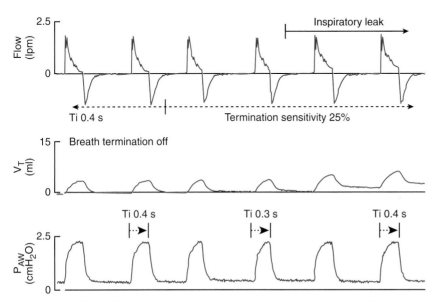

Figure 19-17 Effect of inspiratory leak around the endotracheal tube on automatic termination of inspiration.

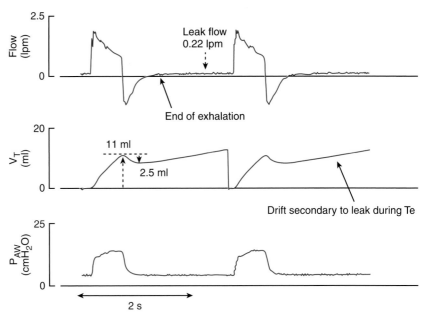

Figure 19-18 Effect of leak around the endotracheal tube during the expiratory phase on flow and V_T.

expiration has been completed, the flow is not zero but slightly above zero. This is leak flow during the expiratory phase caused by the PEEP pressure. This leak flow is responsible for the rising slope in the volume trace, an upward drift, occurring during the expiratory phase.

The leak flow during expiration is directed from the circuit into the patient and may be interpreted by the ventilator's algorithm as the next inspiration. In consequence autocycling may result in flow-triggered ventilators. Autocycling should be suspected if the ventilator cycles at a relatively high and constant frequency (Fig. 19-19). Autocycling should be avoided because it exposes the infant to

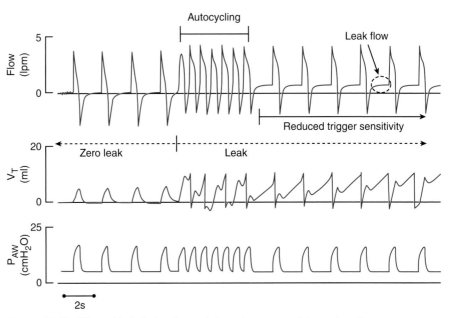

Figure 19-19 Effect of leak during the expiratory phase on ventilator autocycling.

an unnecessary high rate and mean airway pressure. In addition, it can produce hypocapnia and depress the patient's respiratory drive (82).

Autocycling due to expiratory leaks can be detected by reducing PEEP to decrease the expiratory leak, revealing the infants' true breathing rate. Alternatively, an increase in the flow trigger threshold above the leak flow should also stop autocycling and unveil the infants' own breathing rate. However, after periods of autocycling, the infants could become apneic due to hyperventilation. The latter maneuver will display the expiratory leak flow and allow its measurement. Thereafter, trigger sensitivity should be set 0.2 or 0.3 L/min above the measured leak flow to prevent autocycling.

Asynchrony between Infant and Ventilator

The following recordings were obtained from simulations of spontaneous breathing during mechanical ventilation and depict problems in ventilator/infant interaction or lack of synchrony between the infant and the mechanical breaths.

The first part of Figure 19-20 shows IMV breaths superimposed upon more rapid spontaneous breathing. Small spontaneous tidal volumes can be seen alternating with larger breaths of longer duration associated with the cycling of the ventilator. Only occasionally do spontaneous and mechanical breaths coincide. The mechanical cycle falls into the end of inspiration or the very beginning of expiration. The resulting ventilatory pattern is erratic and disorganized. It is clear from this trace that the infant's breathing strategy is disrupted with every mechanical breath, that part of his respiratory effort is wasted and not producing a volume change, indicating a compromised minute ventilation. This can result in episodes of hypoxemia and agitation (83, 84).

These unwanted effects can be avoided by SIMV. The dramatic change in the flow and volume pattern can be appreciated in the second part of the recording. The small spontaneous V_T and the larger V_T from synchronized breaths are clearly separated without overlap or disruption. The breathing pattern is regular and organized, illustrating an ideal pattern of synchronized ventilation (85, 86).

Figure 19-21 provides another example of poor synchrony between patient and ventilator. The ventilator mode is A/C, so each spontaneous breath should trigger a mechanical cycle. Inspiratory flow coincides with a rise in airway pressure, indicating that the ventilator is triggered reliably. However, the infant tries to breathe at a much faster rate and the ventilator cannot follow. The reason for this is a too long inspiratory time (0.4 s) for the infant's rapid spontaneous breathing. The patient tries to exhale and breathe in again while the inspiratory pressure is still maintained.

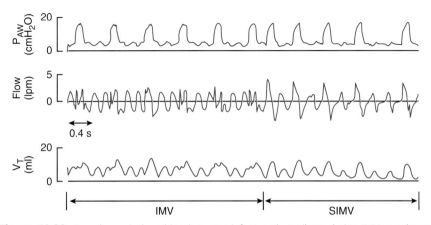

Figure 19-20 Asynchrony in breathing between infant and ventilator during IMV, synchrony during SIMV.

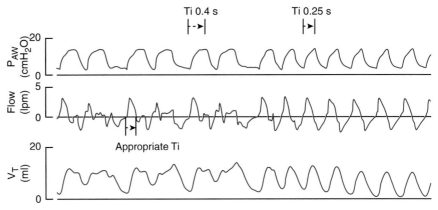

Figure 19-21 Inappropriate inspiratory duration can cause asynchronous breathing during assist/control ventilation.

This, however, is a futile effort and no significant volume change is achieved against the high airway pressure. The combination of high spontaneous rate and a relatively long Ti of the mechanical breaths can cause asynchrony, inspiratory hold, and a decrease in ventilation even when a synchronizing ventilatory mode is used. Again the flow pattern is erratic and the volumes are distorted and show a prolonged inspiratory phase. The Ti needed for this infant, approximately 0.25 s, can be measured from the duration of inspiratory flow after a breath was triggered. In the second half of the trace, a decrease in Ti from 0.4 to 0.25 s results in the ventilator cycling off at the time when inspiration is complete and the patient begins to exhale. In addition, the ventilator is now able to follow the infant's high rate. Minute ventilation and comfort are clearly improved. The flow and volume patterns have become organized and regular.

Another approach to improve synchrony during A/C or high-rate SIMV is the use of the automatic termination of inspiration. As explained in the description of Figure 19-12 this algorithm ends inspiration as soon as the inspiratory flow approaches a certain percentage of peak flow at the end of the inspiratory phase. This technique prevents periods of asynchronous breathing when the infant actively exhales against a prolonged positive airway pressure, or when the physiologic duration of inspiration is shorter than the set Ti. As in Figure 19-21, the first part of Figure 19-22 shows the ventilation pattern with an excessive Ti of 0.4 s.

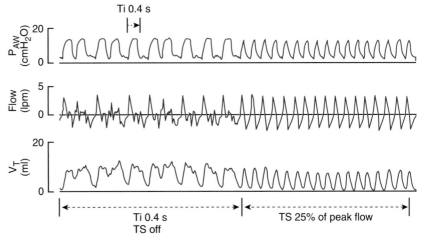

Figure 19-22 Use of automatic termination of inspiration during assist/control ventilation to improve synchrony of breathing.

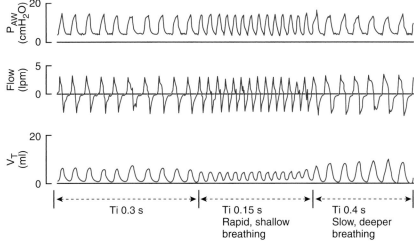

Figure 19-23 Variability of inspiratory duration (Ti) with use of automatic termination of inspiration.

In the second half of the trace an inspiratory termination at 25% of peak flow was applied, and ventilation becomes regular and synchronous. Inspiratory duration becomes very short and inspiratory pressure is applied only for the time that the infant breathes in and drops as soon as the infant breathes out. As explained in Figure 19-17, a large leak around the ET tube can render this automatic termination of inspiration unreliable.

An advantage of using the automatic termination of inspiration over a shortened but fixed Ti is that the automatic termination offers a variable Ti. The variability in Ti when using the automatic termination of inspiration is shown in Figure 19-23. As the patient's breathing strategy changes over time, including periods of rapid shallow and slow deep breathing, Ti changes accordingly from 0.15 to 0.4 s. This variable Ti gives the infant the ability to determine the inspiratory duration that best fits his/her spontaneous breathing strategy.

Clinical Relevance of Pulmonary Function Data During Neonatal Ventilation

The traces shown in Figures 19-1 to 19-23 illustrate the points made in the introduction. Ventilator graphics provide a wealth of information about an infant's respiratory status and whether his/her specific type of respiratory failure is being supported optimally.

Furthermore, the interplay between ventilator and patient is reflected continuously by these graphics, so that any failure of the automatic features of the ventilator in providing synchrony can be detected in time. Especially during sudden deterioration of an infant's condition, ventilator graphics can provide clues regarding the function of the ventilator, problems arising from the infant or their interaction.

In preterm infants undergoing mechanical ventilation, changes in ventilation and lung mechanics can occur in a gradual manner (e.g. onset or resolution of lung disease) or acutely (e.g. lung collapse or pneumothorax). In addition, many of the changes in ventilation and lung mechanics can occur inadvertently due to inappropriate adjustments of the ventilator settings or result from inappropriate infant/ventilator interaction. Ventilator graphics can be useful in detecting and correcting these conditions. In addition, ventilator graphics can be quite useful in assessing the contribution of the spontaneous breathing effort to ventilation and evaluating the consistency of the infant's respiratory drive.

In practice, fine tuning the ventilatory support may not always lead to improved arterial blood gases. Perhaps for this reason ventilator graphics are not widely used in the management of preterm infants. In view of this, it should be mentioned that a number of ventilator adjustments when using ventilator graphics are intended to make the support provided to the preterm infant gentler and thus avoid the risk of lung injury. The benefits of this may not be evident immediately but in the long term.

There are limited data in the literature assessing the effects of utilizing ventilator graphics and pulmonary mechanics in ventilated preterm infants. A retrospective observation in ventilated preterm infants indicated a lower incidence of air leaks and IVH among infants in whom pulmonary mechanics were measured and their V_T was kept within limits compared to the non-monitored infants (25). In a randomized comparison of monitoring of lung mechanics versus no monitoring, lung mechanics data did not reduce the duration of ventilation or oxygen therapy, but led to a shorter duration of ventilation among survivors (26). Interestingly, in the monitored group, lung mechanics data given to the clinicians did not include information on tidal volume.

SUMMARY AND FUTURE IMPLICATIONS

Although there is no clear evidence that the use of pulmonary function testing or graphic display of respiratory signals improves short- or long-term outcome in ventilated infants, the use of ventilator graphics does not entail risks and in well-trained hands is a valuable tool in the management of the ventilated preterm infant. Also, its use helps in the understanding and demonstration of the effects of different interventions and infant-ventilator interaction. Although it still remains to be proven, if used consistently it may contribute to improving the outcome of this fragile population.

REFERENCES

1. Cook CD, Sutherland JM, Segal S, et al. Studies of respiratory physiology in the newborn infant: III. Measurements of mechanics of respiration. J Clin Invest 1957; 37:440.
2. Karlberg P, Cherry RB, Escardo F, et al. Respiratory studies in newborn infants. I. Apparatus and methods for studies of pulmonary ventilation and the mechanics of breathing. Principle of analysis in mechanics of breathing. Acta Paediatr Scand 1960; 49:345.
3. Nelson NM. Neonatal pulmonary function. Pediatr Clin North Am 1966; 13:769.
4. Swyer PR, Reiman RC, Wright JJ. Ventilation and ventilatory mechanics in the newborn: methods and results in 15 resting infants. J Pediatr 1960; 56:612.
5. Polgar G. Opposing forces to breathing in newborn infants. Biol Neonat 1967; 11:1.
6. England SJ. Current techniques for assessing pulmonary function in the newborn and infant: advantages and limitations. Pediatr Pulmonol 1988; 4:48.
7. Gerhardt T, Bancalari E. Measurement and monitoring of pulmonary function. Clin Perinatol 1991; 18:581.
8. American Thoracic Society/European Respiratory Society. Respiratory mechanics in infants: physiologic evaluation in health and disease. Am Rev Respir Dis 1993; 147:474.
9. Coates AL, Stocks J. Esophageal pressure manometry in human infants. Pediatr Pulmonol 1991; 11:350.
10. Stocks JC, Beardsmore C, Helms P. Infant lung function: measurement conditions and equipment. Eur Respir J 1989; 2:123.
11. American Thoracic Society/European Respiratory Society. Respiratory function measurements in infants: measurement conditions. Am J Respir Crit Care Med 1995; 151:2058.
12. Stocks J, Sly PD, Tepper RS, et al., editors. Infant respiratory function testing. New York: Wiley-Liss; 1996.
13. Graff MA, Novo RP, Diaz M, et al. Compliance measurement in respiratory distress syndrome: the prediction of outcome. Pediatr Pulmonol 1986; 2:332.
14. Simbruner G, Coradello H, Cubec G, et al. Respiratory compliance of newborns after birth and its prognostic value for the course and outcome of respiratory disease. Respiration 1982; 43:414.

15. Gerhardt T, Hehre D, Feller R, et al. Serial determination of pulmonary function in infants with chronic lung disease. J Pediatr 1987; 110:448.

16. Engelhardt B, Elliott S, Hazinski TA. Short and long-term effects of furosemide on lung function in neonates with increased pulmonary resistance. Pediatr Pulmonol 1986; 2:287.

17. Gomez del Rio M, Gerhardt T, Hehre D, et al. Effect of a beta-agonist nebulization on lung function in neonates with increased pulmonary resistance. Pediatr Pulmonol 1986; 2:287.

18. Avery GB, Fletcher AB, Kaplan M, et al. Controlled trial of dexamethasone in respirator dependent infants with bronchopulmonary dysplasia. Pediatrics 1985; 75:106.

19. Goldsmith LS, Greenspan JS, Rubenstein SD, et al. Immediate improvement in lung volume after exogenous surfactant: alveolar recruitment versus increased distention. J Pediatr 1991; 119:424.

20. Bhutani VK, Abbasi S, Long WA, et al. Pulmonary mechanics in premature infants one month after treatment with synthetic surfactant. J Pediatr 1992; 120:S18.

21. Hummler H, Gerhardt T, Gonzalez A, et al. Influence of different methods of synchronized mechanical ventilation on ventilation, gas exchange, patient effort, and blood pressure fluctuations in premature neonates. Pediatr Pulmonol 1996; 22:305–313.

22. Claure N, Gerhardt T, Hummler H, et al. Computer-controlled minute ventilation in preterm infants undergoing mechanical ventilation. J Pediatr 1997; 131:910–913.

23. Schulze A, Gerhardt T, Musante G, et al. Proportional assist ventilation in low birth weight infants with acute respiratory disease: A comparison to assist/control and conventional mechanical ventilation. J Pediatr 1999; 135:339–344.

24. Herrera CM, Gerhardt T, Claure N, et al. Effects of volume-guaranteed synchronized intermittent mandatory ventilation in preterm infants recovering from respiratory failure. Pediatrics 2002; 110:529–533.

25. Rosen WC, Mammal MC, Fisher JB, et al. The effects of bedside pulmonary mechanics testing during infant mechanical ventilation. Pediatr Pulmonol 1993; 16:147–152.

26. Stenson BJ, Glover RM, Wilkie RA, et al. Randomized controlled trial of respiratory system compliance measurements in mechanically ventilated neonates. Arch Dis Child Fetal Neonatal Ed 1998; 78:F15–F19.

27. Silva Neto G, Gerhardt T, Claure N, et al. Influence of chestwall distortion and esophageal catheter position on esophageal manometry in preterm infants. Pediatr Res 1995; 36:617.

28. Gupta SK, Wagener JS, Erenberg A. Pulmonary mechanics in healthy term neonates: variability in measurements obtained with a computerized system. J Pediatr 1990; 117:603.

29. Ratjen FA, Wiesemann HG. Variability of dynamic compliance measurements in spontaneously breathing and ventilated newborn infants. Pediatr Pulmonol 1992; 12:73.

30. Gonzalez A, Tortorolo L, Gerhardt T, et al. Intrasubject variability of repeated pulmonary function measurements in preterm ventilated infants. Pediatr Pulmonol 1996; 21:35–41.

31. Mead J, Whittenberger JL. Physical properties of human lungs measured during spontaneous respiration. J Appl Physiol 1953; 5:779.

32. Bhutani VK, Sivieri EM, Abbasi S. Evaluation of neonatal pulmonary mechanics and energetics: a two factor least mean square analysis. Pediatr Pulmonol 1988; 4:150.

33. Silva Neto G, Gerhardt TO, Silberberg A, et al. Nonlinear pressure/volume relationship and measurements of lung mechanics in infants. Pediatr Pulmonol 1992; 12:146.

34. Kano S, Lanteri CJ, Duncan AW, et al. Influence of nonlinearities on estimates of respiratory mechanics using multilinear regression analysis. J Appl Physiol 1994; 77:1185.

35. Spoelstra AJG, Srikasibhandha S. Dynamic pressure volume relationship of the lung and position in healthy neonates. Acta Paediatr Scand 1973; 62:176.

36. Shaffer TH, Koen PA, Moskowitz GD, et al. Positive end expiratory pressure: effects on lung mechanics of premature lambs. Biol Neonate 1978; 34:1.

37. Kosch PC, Stark AR. Dynamic maintenance of end-expiratory lung volume in full-term infants. J Appl Physiol 1984; 57:1126.

38. Stark AR, Cohlan BA, Waggener TB, et al. Regulation of end-expiratory lung volume during sleep in premature infants. J Appl Physiol 1987; 62:117.

39. Bolivar JM, Gerhardt T, Gonzalez A, et al. Mechanisms for episodes of hypoxemia in preterm infants undergoing mechanical ventilation. J Pediatr 1995; 127:767.

40. Davis GM, Moscato J. Changes in lung mechanics following sighs in premature newborns without lung disease. Pediatr Pulmonol 1994; 17:26.

41. Smaldone GC, Mitzner W, Itoh H. Role of alveolar recruitment in lung inflation: influence of pressure-volume hysteresis. J Appl Physiol 1983; 55:1321.

42. Gerhardt T, Hehre D, Feller R, et al. Serial determination of pulmonary function in infants with chronic lung disease. J Pediatr 1987; 110(3):448–456.

43. Freezer NJ, Sly PD. Predictive value of measurements of respiratory mechanics in preterm infants with HMD. Pediatr Pulmonol 1993; 16:116–123.

44. Merth IT, de Winter JP, Zonderland HM, et al. Pulmonary function in infants with neonatal chronic lung disease with or without hyaline membrane disease at birth. Eur Respir J 1997; 10:1606–1613.

45. Baraldi E, Filippone M, Trevisanuto D, et al. Pulmonary function until two years of life in infants with bronchopulmonary dysplasia. Am J Respir Crit Care Med 1997; 155:149–155.

46. Rojas MA, Gonzalez A, Bancalari E, et al. Changing trends in the epidemiology and pathogenesis of neonatal chronic lung disease. J Pediatr 1995; 126:605.

47. Van Marter LJ, Pagano M, Allred E, et al. Rate of bronchopulmonary dysplasia as a function of neonatal intensive care practices. J Pediatr 1992; 120:938–946.

48. Jobe A, Bancalari E. Bronchopulmonary dysplasia. Am J Respir Crit Care Med 2001; 163:1723–1729.

49. Bancalari E. Changes in the pathogenesis and prevention of chronic lung disease of prematurity. Am J Perinatol 2001; 18(1):1–9.

50. Suter PM, Fairley HB, Isenberg MD, et al. Optimum end-expiratory airway pressure in patients with acute pulmonary failure. N Engl J Med 1975; 292:284–289.

51. Gregory GA, Kitterman JA, Phibbs RH. Treatment of the idiopathic respiratory distress syndrome with continuous positive airway pressure. N Engl J Med 1971; 284:133.

52. Chernick V. Hyaline membrane diseases: therapy with constant lung distending pressure. N Engl J Med 1973; 298:302.

53. Froese AB, McCulloch PR, et al. Optimizing alveolar expansion prolongs the effectiveness of exogenous surfactant therapy in the adult rabbit. Am Rev Respir Dis 1993; 148:569–577.

54. Tremblay LN, Slutsky AS. Ventilator-induced injury: from barotrauma to biotrauma. Proc Assoc Am Physicians 1998; 110:482–488.

55. Naik AS, Kallapur SG, Bachurski CJ, et al. Effects of ventilation with different positive end-expiratory pressures on cytokine expression in the preterm lamb lung. Am J Respir Crit Care Med 2001; 164:494–498.

56. Yu VYH, Rolfe P. Effect of continuous positive airway pressure breathing on cardiorespiratory function in infants with respiratory distress syndrome. Acta Paediatr Scand 1977; 66:59.

57. Couser RJ, Ferrara TB, Ebert J, et al. Effects of exogenous surfactant therapy on dynamic compliance during mechanical breathing in preterm infants with hyaline membrane disease. J Pediatr 1990; 116:119–124.

58. Edberg KE, Ekstrom-Jodal B, Hallman M, et al. Immediate effects on lung function of instilled human surfactant in mechanically ventilated newborn infants with IRDS. Acta Paediatr Scand 1990; 79:750.

59. Armsby DH, Bellon G, Carlisle K, et al. Delayed compliance increase in infants with respiratory distress syndrome following synthetic surfactant. Pediatr Pulmonol 1992; 14:206–213.

60. Cotton RB. A model of the effect of surfactant treatment on gas exchange in hyaline membrane disease. Semin Perinatol 1994; 18:19–22.

61. Morin FC III, Stenmark KR, et al. Persistent pulmonary hypertension of the newborn. Am J Respir Crit Care Med 1995; 151:2010–2032.

62. Walsh MC, Stork EK. Persistent pulmonary hypertension of the newborn: rational therapy based on pathophysiology. Clin Perinatol 2001; 28(3):609–627.

63. Dreyfuss D, Soler P, Bassett G, et al. High inflation pressure pulmonary edema: respective effects of high airway pressure, high tidal volume, and positive end-expiratory pressure. Am Rev Respir Dis 1988; 137:1159–1164.

64. Dreyfuss D, Saumon G. Role of tidal volume, FRC and end-inspiratory volume in the development of pulmonary edema following mechanical ventilation. Am Rev Respir Dis 1993; 148:1194–1203.

65. Dreyfuss D, Saumon G. Ventilator-induced lung injury lessons from experimental studies. Am J Respir Crit Care Med 1998; 157:294–323.

66. Hudson LD. Protective ventilation for patients with acute respiratory distress syndrome. N Eng J Med 1998; 338:385–387.

67. Clark RH, et al. Lung protective strategies of ventilation in the neonate: what are they? Pediatrics 2000; 105(1):112–114.

68. Clark RH, Gerstmann DR, Jobe AH, et al. Lung injury in neonates: causes, strategies for prevention, and long-term consequences. J Pediatr 2001; 139:478–486.

69. Frank JA, Gutierrez JA, Jones KD, et al. Low tidal volume reduces epithelial and endothelial injury in acid-injured rat lungs. Am J Respir Crit Care Med 2002; 165:242–249.

70. Gerhardt T. Limitations and pitfalls of pulmonary function testing and pulmonary graphics in the clinical setting. In: Donn SM, ed. Neonatal and pediatric pulmonary graphics: principles and clinical applications. New York: Futura Publishing; 1998.

71. Gerhardt T, Bancalari E. Chestwall compliance in full-term and premature infants. Acta Paediatr Scand 1980; 69:359.

72. Bjorklund LJ, Ingimarsson J, Curstedt T, et al. Manual ventilation with a few large breaths at birth compromises the therapeutic effect of subsequent surfactant replacement in immature lambs. Pediatr Res 1997; 42:348–355.

73. Jobe AH, Ikegami M. Mechanisms initiating lung injury in the preterm. Early Human Dev 1998; 53:81–94.

74. Fisher JB, Mammel MC, Coleman JM, et al. Identifying lung overdistention during mechanical ventilation by using volume-pressure loops. Pediatr Pulmonol 1988; 5:10.

75. Carlo WA, Stark AR, Wright LL, et al. Minimal ventilation to prevent bronchopulmonary dysplasia in extremely-low-birth-weight infants. J Pediatr 2002; 141:370–375.

76. Muscedere JG, Mullen JBM, Gan K, et al. Tidal ventilation at low airway pressures can augment lung injury. Am J Respir Crit Care Med 1994; 149:1327–1334.

77. Michna J, Jobe AH, Ikegami M. Positive end-expiratory pressure preserves surfactant function in preterm lambs. Am J Respir Crit Care Med 1999; 160:634–639.

78. Verder H, Albertsen P, Ebbesen F, et al. Nasal continuous positive airway pressure and early surfactant therapy for respiratory distress syndrome in newborns of less than 30 weeks' gestation. Pediatrics 1999; 103:491.

79. Boros SJ, Campbell K. A comparison of the effects of high frequency–low tidal volume and low frequency–high tidal volume mechanical ventilation. J Pediatr 1980; 97:108–112.
80. Pohlandt F, Saule H, Schroder H, et al. Decreased incidence of extra-alveolar air leakage or death prior to air leakage in high versus low rate positive pressure ventilation: results of a randomised seven-centre trial in preterm infants. Eur J Pediatr 1992; 151:904–909.
81. Casetti AV, Bartlett RH, Hirschl RB. Increasing inspiratory time exacerbates ventilator-induced lung injury during high-pressure/high-volume mechanical ventilation. Crit Care Med 2002; 30:2295.
82. Bernstein G, Knodel E, Heldt GP. Airway leak size in neonates and autocycling of three flow-triggered ventilators. Crit Care Med 1995; 23:1739.
83. Quinn MW, de Boer RC, Ansari N, et al. Stress response and mode of ventilation in preterm infants. Arch Dis Child Fetal Neonatal Ed 1998; 78:F195–F198.
84. Cleary JP, Bernstein G, Mannino FL, et al. Improved oxygenation during synchronized intermittent mandatory ventilation in neonates with respiratory distress syndrome: a randomized, crossover study. J Pediatr 1995; 126:407–411.
85. Bernstein G, Heldt GP, Mannino FL. Increased and more consistent tidal volumes during synchronized intermittent mandatory ventilation in newborn infants. Am J Respir Crit Care Med 1994; 150:1444–1448.
86. Jarreau PH, Moriette G, Mussat P, et al. Patient-triggered ventilation decreases the work of breathing in neonates. Am J Respir Crit Care Med 1996; 153:1176–1181.

Section IV

Respiratory Control and Apnea of Prematurity

Chapter 20

Neonatal Respiratory Control and Apnea of Prematurity

Oded Mesner MD • Juliann M. Di Fiore BSEE
• Richard J. Martin MBBS FRACP

Physiologic Considerations

Diagnostic Dilemmas

Management Options, Questions and Controversies

Resolution and Outcome

The field of developmental respiratory neurobiology has made great advances in recent years by employing molecular and histochemical techniques to integrate new knowledge in physiology and neuroanatomy. Despite such new scientific insight, therapeutic strategies for neonatal apnea have barely changed in three decades. This review will initially focus on new physiologic insights during the transition from fetal to neonatal life, and characterize the interrelationship among apnea, bradycardia, and desaturation in preterm infants. We will then attempt to translate this body of knowledge into a rationale for established and proposed therapeutic interventions, and consider the risk/benefit of such interventions during early postnatal life.

PHYSIOLOGIC CONSIDERATIONS

Fetal Breathing Movements

Since the placenta is the site of gas exchange in utero, the function of fetal breathing movements may not be immediately clear. There is strong evidence, however, that fetal respiratory muscle activity is important for fetal lung growth and development. Increasing or decreasing the frequency of fetal breathing has a direct correlation with accelerating or inhibiting lung growth, respectively. Phasic and tonic contraction of airway smooth muscle also has been reported in utero, and presumably serves to aid the propulsion of lung fluid. Therefore, the irregular fetal diaphragmatic contraction that characterizes gestation serves a prominent developmental role. In the third trimester of gestation fetal breathing becomes limited to REM sleep and there is total cessation of breathing during NREM sleep, even in the presence of hypercapnia. The mechanism behind the absence of fetal breathing during NREM sleep seems to originate from the predominance of descending inhibitory pathways to the medullary rhythm-generating center (1). The periodic nature of fetal breathing changes into a continuous pattern after birth in order to allow for the survival of the newborn. Several factors associated with the fetal transition to extrauterine life have been shown to induce continuous breathing in the fetus, although the precise relative roles of cord occlusion, lung inflation, circulatory changes, sensory stimulation, and biochemical factors in this process remain unclear.

Postnatal Respiratory Patterns

Preterm infants exhibit pronounced immaturity of respiratory control, the net result of which is a high incidence of apnea and periodic breathing. There seems to be an overriding inhibitory influence of central origin in the control of breathing in the neonate that persists from the fetal state. This is manifested by a decrease in breathing in response to CO_2, a paradoxical response to hypoxia, an enhanced reflex apnea elicited by laryngeal stimulation and irregularities in breathing pattern. Apneic episodes are almost universal in extremely low birth weight infants, and extremely common in all preterm infants, depending on precise definitions, as discussed later. The incidence of apnea of prematurity decreases with advancing postnatal age, such that by 43–44 weeks postmenstrual or postconceptional age the incidence is comparable to that of a term infant (2). This observation has been extremely reassuring for the monitoring and management of such infants. As is the case for apnea, the short cyclic respiratory pauses that constitute periodic breathing may be accompanied by bradycardia and/or desaturation, with the resolution of periodic breathing following a similar trajectory to longer apneic events. Greater dependence on peripheral (vs. central) chemoreceptors associated with fluctuations in arterial oxygen tension has been proposed to underlie periodic breathing in neonates. This is consistent with the observation in preterm infants that greater peripheral chemoreceptor responses to hypoxia may be associated with more frequent apnea (3).

Ventilatory Responses to Hypercapnia

The diminished ventilatory response to CO_2 of preterm infants, especially those with apnea, is thought to be a primary mechanism underlying apnea of prematurity (4). CO_2 is sensed primarily centrally at or underlying the ventrolateral medulla of the brainstem, although peripheral chemoreceptors, e.g., the carotid body, do contribute (5). Central chemoreceptors, originally thought to be confined to the ventrolateral medulla, have been found to be widely spread in the brainstem. It is unclear at this point whether there is developmental maturation in location of central chemoreceptors, since most studies have been done in adult animals; hence the biologic basis for the immature hypercapnic response remains to be explored.

A likely explanation for decreased CO_2 responses is that during early postnatal life there is up-regulation of inhibitory neurotransmitters or neuromodulators, and their receptors at respiratory-related neurons or interneurons in the brainstem. Gamma-aminobutyric acid (GABA), adenosine and endorphins are likely candidates, although the effects of adenosine may be excitatory as well as inhibitory, depending on the adenosine receptor subtype activated. As xanthines are non-specific adenosine receptor subtype inhibitors, their use may have widespread effects on neurotransmitter functions (see Ch. 21). Of interest is the observation that the respiratory inhibition induced by simulated sepsis in a rat pup model may be reversed by indomethacin, implicating release of endogenous prostaglandins as a potential mechanism in sepsis-induced apnea (6). This is consistent with the widely observed respiratory inhibition in preterm infants exposed to prostaglandin therapy.

Ventilatory Responses to Hypoxia

The hypoxic ventilatory response has been well characterized in newborn, especially preterm, infants. Unlike adults, who express a relatively sustained response to

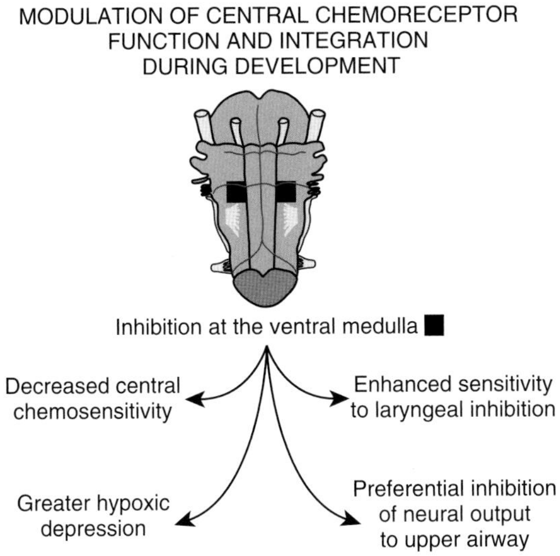

MODULATION OF CENTRAL CHEMORECEPTOR
FUNCTION AND INTEGRATION
DURING DEVELOPMENT

Inhibition at the ventral medulla ■

Decreased central
chemosensitivity

Enhanced sensitivity
to laryngeal inhibition

Greater hypoxic
depression

Preferential inhibition
of neural output
to upper airway

Figure 20-1 Experimental inhibition at the ventral medulla, where central chemosensitivity is processed (squares), has been shown to simulate many of the physiological characteristics of apnea in early postnatal life.

hypoxia, neonates have an initial increase in ventilation that lasts 1–2 min, followed by a decline in breathing to below baseline ventilation. This late decline has been traditionally termed hypoxic ventilatory depression. The initial increase in ventilation is secondary to stimulation of peripheral chemoreceptors primarily in the carotid body. This biphasic ventilatory response to hypoxia has been shown to persist in convalescing preterm neonates at 4–6 weeks of age (7). The same inhibitory neurotransmitters in the brainstem (most notably GABA) that diminish hypercapnic responses have been implicated in neonatal hypoxic respiratory depression. This phenomenon may contribute to inhibition of fetal breathing in the relatively hypoxemic intrauterine environment, but enhance respiratory instability when it persists postnatally. Of interest is the observation that experimental inhibition at the ventral medulla in animal models can inhibit central chemosensitivity, enhance hypoxic depression, and simulate other pathophysiologic features of neonatal apnea (Fig. 20-1).

In neonatal care there is still considerable controversy surrounding the use of supplemental oxygen and what constitutes optimal oxygenation of preterm infants (see Chs 14 and 15). This has implications for respiratory control in this population. Neonatal resuscitation with 100% oxygen has been shown to significantly delay onset of spontaneous respiratory efforts when compared to 21% oxygen (8). This appears to be an example of peripheral chemoreceptor inhibition and resultant respiratory depression during acute hyperoxic exposure (9). It has been recently observed in rat pups that even mild hyperoxia, as occurs during resuscitation with 40% oxygen, has a comparable depressant effect on spontaneous respiratory efforts as occurs with 100% oxygen (10). Although there is considerable interest in optimizing the oxygenation of preterm infants exposed to prolonged periods of supplemental oxygen, the potential effect of baseline oxygen saturation on incidence of apneic episodes is unclear. In addition, based on animal models, there is real interest in the potential for long-lasting effects of repetitive hypoxia on respiratory control (11).

Therefore, it should be apparent that a rational approach to diagnosis and management of apneic episodes in preterm infants necessitates a clear understanding of underlying physiologic mechanisms and their relevance to gas exchange in early postnatal life. Unfortunately, there are significant pitfalls in our diagnostic techniques for this population, and the risk/benefit ratio for any intervention must be carefully considered, especially considering that this problem is almost universal and appears to resolve over time.

DIAGNOSTIC DILEMMAS

Current clinical practice requires a cardiorespiratory event-free period before hospital discharge, although the specific length of time varies among institutions (12). Adequate detection of such events can only be accomplished through accurate measurements of respiration, oxygenation and heart rate. Discrepancies in event recognition can occur between cardiorespiratory monitoring systems, as the type and number of events detected are dependent on the form of respiratory monitoring, alarm settings and inclusion of continuous pulse oximetry. Keeping this in mind, the ideal monitoring system should be non-invasive, insensitive to motion artifact, and capable of detecting and storing all events of interest with a rapid response time.

Respiratory Monitoring

Measurements of respiration can be accomplished through a variety of strategies where a compromise must be made between accurate detection of respiration and invasiveness. As a result devices are divided into two basic categories; flow detectors applied to the nose and/or mouth and sensors that detect chest wall excursions, i.e. impedance or respiratory inductance plethysmography. Respiratory inductance plethysmography (RIP) entails two bands placed around the chest and abdomen. With the addition of a software algorithm to calibrate the rib cage and abdominal waveforms a semi-quantitative volume waveform can be acquired. Although RIP requires two additional bands placed around the infant, it has the advantage of detecting obstructive apnea by identifying periods of absent ventilation on the volume waveform in conjunction with asynchronous chest wall and abdominal excursions. In contrast, measurements of respiration via impedance utilize ECG electrodes with no additional leads needed on the infant. Although impedance is more conducive for patient care, obstructive efforts cannot be readily distinguished from normal respiration and the addition of a nasal and/or oral flow sensor would be required to identify obstructive or mixed apnea.

The mask pneumotachograph is the gold standard for measuring airflow in infants. However, the need for a complete seal around the nose and/or mouth for accurate measurements of flow and volume make it unrealistic in the clinical setting. For qualitative measurements of flow the pneumotach has been replaced in the sleep lab setting by the thermistor or end tidal CO_2 monitoring. As these devices have a poor correlation to measured flow and volume (13) they should only be used to detect the presence or total absence of flow, keeping in mind that comparisons between the various modes of apnea identification may lead to conflicting results (14). Clearly measurement of flow with devices placed on the infant's nose or mouth can be quite cumbersome and interfere with patient care outside of the sleep lab environment. Therefore, there continues to be general acceptance of impedance monitoring in clinical practice for detection of central apnea, and sacrifice of the ability to distinguish obstructive apnea from normal respiration. Under these conditions, an obstructive event may only be detected if accompanied by a desaturation and/or bradycardic episode.

Oxygen Saturation

Measurement of blood gas values is the ideal mode for estimating oxygen levels in infants. However, this procedure is invasive and can only provide information on an intermittent basis. Pulse oximetry has gained widespread acceptance for continuous long-term measurements of oxygen saturation. Oximeters are easy to use, require no calibration or heating of the skin (in contrast to transcutaneous PO_2), and provide immediate information regarding oxygenation and heart rate. Accurate interpretation of pulse oximetry employs the relationship between oxygen saturation and oxygen tension as described by the oxygen dissociation curve. Although this curve presents data in the total range of oxygen saturation levels, it is generally accepted that accuracy of pulse oximetry decreases at saturation levels less than 70–80%. Interpretation of high levels of oxygen saturation must also be done with extreme caution. Blood is almost completely saturated at a PaO_2 of 90–100 mmHg and it becomes increasingly difficult to estimate oxygen tension above 60–70 mmHg as the dissociation curve begins to plateau. As baseline levels in healthy preterm infants in room air may occur in this plateau range with oxygen saturations ranging from 97 to 99%, these same levels may result in hyperoxic exposure in infants receiving supplemental oxygen. The ideal saturation range in preterm infants has yet to be determined. However, the reduction of the upper alarm limit to 95% has been proposed to have sufficient sensitivity to detect episodes of hyperoxemia (15).

Body motion has been a previous problem with false alarms or loss of signal and a major obstacle in utilizing this technology to its fullest potential. Recent advances in software algorithms with new-generation monitors have resulted in a decrease in the incidence of false alarms. This improvement in SaO_2 software has been offset by an increased incidence of missed events of both bradycardia and hypoxemia when compared to conventional monitors, with the incidence of false alarms and missed events varying by manufacturer (16). Further discrepancies between manufacturers may be due to variations in types of hemoglobin (fractional versus functional), averaging rates and motion artifact filtering.

Additional features of the new-generation pulse oximeters include data storage over extended periods that can be downloaded for more extensive data analysis. Summary reports, including amount of time at a range of saturation levels, can be provided over varying periods to assist in patient care. These options are becoming increasingly popular in both clinical practice and as a research tool.

Heart Rate

Instantaneous measurements of heart rate can be detected by placement of ECG electrodes on the infant, with the conventional arrangement being right arm, left arm and left leg or abdomen. This method of heart rate monitoring uses impedance technology including R-wave detector algorithms from the QRS portion of the ECG waveform for calculation of heart rates. Alternatively, heart rate can be monitored via pulse oximetry, resulting in less equipment on the patient but with an increased potential for motion artifact when compared to standard ECG electrodes.

Definition of Events

Unfortunately there is inconsistency in standard definitions of apnea, bradycardia and desaturation. This has been problematic as publications have used a multitude of thresholds and descriptions to describe cardiorespiratory events.

Apnea has been defined in the literature as a respiratory pause ranging from 10 to 20 s. The current American Academy of Pediatrics Guidelines employ the original 1986 NIH Consensus Statement defining a respiratory pause of 20 s in duration as the minimum criterion for a clinically relevant apnea, or a shorter duration if accompanied by bradycardia or cyanosis (17). Once identified, apnea can be stratified into three types: a central pause with no respiratory effort (central apnea), an obstructed event with chest wall motion but no corresponding flow (obstructive apnea), or a combination of both (mixed apnea). Detection and distinction of apnea type may aid in determining the mode of clinical intervention.

There are no current standard thresholds for bradycardia in terms of threshold or duration. Lower limits have ranged from 70 to 100 beats/min, with data suggesting possible detrimental hypoxic ischemic effects of apnea with bradycardia <80 beats/min in the most vulnerable preterm infants (18). The inclusion or omission of duration in defining bradycardia is driven by both individual preferences and monitor capabilities as the option for duration is manufacturer-specific.

Levels ranging from 80 to 85% are commonly considered thresholds for defining oxygen desaturation. Although prolonged periods of hypoxemia can occur in preterm infants episodic desaturation is usually associated with apnea or short respiratory pauses (i.e., periodic breathing). In very low birth weight infants these events can occur during both spontaneous respiration and mechanical ventilation, and have been shown to progressively increase during the first month of life (19).

MANAGEMENT OPTIONS, QUESTIONS AND CONTROVERSIES

The management of apnea of prematurity is largely influenced by the existence and the nature of any underlying conditions causing the apneic episodes. A thorough consideration of possible causes is always warranted, especially when there is an unexpected increase in the frequency of episodes of apnea and/or bradycardia. Episodes of apnea with an underlying cause (generally referred to as secondary apnea) may be eliminated by treating such a cause, including infection, patent ductus arteriosus, seizures, maternal or neonatal medication exposure, and possibly gastro-esophageal reflux, as discussed later. Treatment of symptomatic idiopathic apnea generally involves pharmacologic and nonpharmacologic approaches. The risks and benefits of any therapeutic option in the premature infant must be carefully weighed before any such intervention is made. Some management options have been demonstrated as beneficial, while others require further study (Table 20-1).

TABLE 20–1 Therapeutic Interventions for Apnea of Prematurity	
Interventions with proven benefit	**Interventions requiring further study**
Positive airway pressure: – Nasal CPAP – NIPPV – High-flow nasal cannula* – Mechanical ventilation* Methylxanthines: – Caffeine – Aminophylline	Body positioning Sensory stimulation: – Kinesthetic – Skin-to-skin – Olfactory Improved oxygen-carrying capacity: – Oxygen supplementation – Red blood cell transfusion Control of hyperbilirubinemia Inspired CO_2 supplementation Nutritional supplementation – L–Carnitine – Creatine Doxapram* Anti-reflux medication

*Benefit should be carefully weighed against risk.

Therapeutic Interventions with Proven Benefit

Continuous Positive Airway Pressure

Apnea of prematurity is frequently managed with nasal continuous positive airway pressure (NCPAP). NCPAP appears to both splint and stabilize the upper airway with positive pressure and increase functional residual capacity. The result is a decrease in the risk of pharyngeal or laryngeal obstruction and improved oxygenation status. This in turn may prolong the time from cessation of breathing to resultant desaturation and bradycardia. While CPAP in premature infants has been found to markedly decrease the incidence of both mixed and obstructive apnea episodes, the effect on central apneas is less clear.

Nasal intermittent positive pressure ventilation (NIPPV) is a mode of respiratory support in which intermittent ventilator-derived inflations are superimposed on NCPAP. A review of randomized controlled trials of NIPPV versus CPAP for the prevention of apnea of prematurity has found NIPPV to be a useful method of augmenting the beneficial effects of NCPAP in preterm infants with apnea that is frequent or severe (20). There is considerable current interest in identifying the optimal mode of delivery for the various CPAP systems with or without ventilatory support.

There are, however, a number of problems associated with NCPAP use. Pressure effects can occur, which may lead to local tissue necrosis with resulting nasal stenosis and deformity (21). The prongs are irritating to the nares and can increase nasal secretions and potentially lead to an increased risk of nasal and systemic infection. In addition, infants frequently become agitated to such a degree that sedation may be required to maintain the prongs in the nares. This has led to considerable interest in alternate modes of CPAP delivery.

Nasal cannulae were originally designed to deliver oxygen at low flow without intentionally creating continuous positive airway pressure. However, cannulae can deliver significant positive distending pressure to premature neonates if the flow is increased to 1–2 L/min. The pressure generated is generally proportional to the gas flow rate, but it is dependent on a number of factors, including the structure of the cannula and the anatomy of the infant's airway. The common practice of using high-flow nasal cannula to deliver an effective fraction of inspired oxygen was reported and discussed in a recent multi-center study (22). This technique has been demonstrated to be an effective means to deliver a positive distending pressure of approximately 6 cmH_2O, which is comparable to NCPAP in the management of apnea of prematurity (23). Delivery of higher flow rates through nasal cannula devices may generate dangerously high airway distending pressures in premature infants. Moreover, due to a variable leak around the cannula the resultant airway pressure produced with a given flow in a given infant is not reliably predictable. Adequate humidification of the air flowing through a nasal cannula is also problematic. Currently, the use of nasal cannulae to deliver end-expiratory pressure or gas flow to reduce the frequency of apnea and desaturation remains to be adequately tested and cannot be routinely recommended, despite its common use.

For severe or refractory episodes of apnea and bradycardia endotracheal intubation and mechanical ventilation may be needed. Minimal ventilator settings should be used to allow for spontaneous ventilatory efforts and to minimize lung injury.

Methylxanthines

Methylxanthines have been the mainstay of pharmacological treatment of apnea for more than three decades. Considerable data exist about their mechanism of action and their beneficial and adverse effects. This topic is discussed elsewhere in this book (see Ch. 21 by Schmidt and Bassler).

Therapeutic Interventions Requiring Further Study

Body Positioning

Body position has a potential to influence lung function and breathing pattern. The supine position facilitates application of CPAP devices but infants nursed in the prone position have been shown, in some studies, to have less apnea, both central (24) and mixed (25). In contrast, Keene et al. found no significant differences in the incidence of clinically significant apnea, bradycardia, or desaturation between supine and prone positions (26). The optimal body position for the prevention of apnea is probably prone in an infant with accompanying lung disease, although this position should be avoided as the infant is being prepared for discharge.

Sensory Stimulation

Several modes of sensory stimulation have been proposed for the prevention of apnea of prematurity. Somatic sensory stimulation has been shown to induce spontaneous regular breathing already in utero and was proposed as a prophylactic therapeutic intervention in preterm infants. Systematic review of randomized controlled clinical trials using repeated cutaneous stimulation with an oscillating mattress or other form of kinesthetic stimulation for the prevention or treatment of apnea revealed no evidence of effect on short- or long-term outcomes and could not support this approach (27, 28).

Skin-to-skin contact (SSC) between the preterm infant and his/her parent, or "kangaroo care," has achieved widespread acceptance for stable infants, and provides an opportunity for greater parental involvement and bonding. It may potentially benefit premature infants by providing stimuli that are familiar to the infants from their prenatal experience, thus improving the integrity of their natural sleep. SSC is widely believed to be free of adverse side-effects, although controlled clinical studies have yielded conflicting results. Heart rate, respiratory rate and temperature may increase, decrease or remain unchanged during SSC, while the rate of oxygen desaturation, apnea and bradycardia episodes is unchanged in most studies (29–31). Bohnhorst et al. have presented data suggesting an increase in the rate of bradycardia and desaturation in premature infants during SSC (32). Additional well-designed randomized controlled trials of SSC nursing care are still needed, although this approach seems reasonable, except in the most fragile patients.

Olfactory stimulation also may have an effect on respiration. A promising novel approach suggests that introduction of a pleasant odor to the incubator has a therapeutic value in diminishing apnea and bradycardia unresponsive to pharmacologic therapy (33). Clearly such an approach needs to be reproduced if it has any chance of gaining acceptance in clinical practice.

Modification of Inspired Gas or Oxygen-Carrying Capacity

Oxygen Supplementation

The optimal target oxygen saturation for preterm infants is an issue of considerable interest that is yet to be resolved. One might anticipate that desaturation accompanying apnea will be greater at lower baseline oxygen saturation (SaO_2), but this has not been well documented. Despite a decrease in subclinical apnea, periodic breathing and bradycardia, which was evident in a series of asymptomatic premature babies receiving low-flow supplemental oxygen (34), there is currently insufficient evidence to support oxygen supplementation or increased baseline saturation as a strategy to prevent or treat clinical apnea of prematurity.

CARBON DIOXIDE SUPPLEMENTATION

Supplementation of inspired air with a very low concentration (0.5%) of carbon dioxide (CO_2) has been proposed to increase respiratory drive and decrease apnea (35). The efficacy and safety of this approach require further investigation.

BLOOD TRANSFUSION

It has been assumed that enhanced oxygen-carrying capacity, as with red blood cell transfusions, may decrease the likelihood of hypoxia-induced respiratory depression and resultant apnea. Some studies have suggested a decrease in the frequency of apnea after transfusion of anemic premature infants, while others found little effect. A recent, large, randomized, controlled trial of higher versus lower blood transfusion thresholds did not find infants in the lower hemoglobin concentration transfusion threshold to require significantly more interventions for apnea (36). On the other hand, infants in the restrictive-transfusion group of a different randomized controlled trial had more frequent apneic episodes as well as intraparenchymal brain hemorrhages and periventricular leucomalacia (37). The presence of apnea of prematurity on its own should probably not be an indication for blood transfusion, but rather should be taken into account when forming guidelines for blood transfusion in premature babies.

Control of Hyperbilirubinemia

Yellow staining of various brain regions, including the brainstem, is found in kernicterus, a complication of severe hyperbilirubinemia in newborn infants. Apnea of prematurity is believed to be a manifestation of immaturity of brainstem-mediated respiratory control. Hyperbilirubinemia and transient bilirubin encephalopathy have been linked to an increased incidence of apnea in premature infants (38). Mesner et al. have demonstrated, in a rat pup model, a persistent inhibitory effect of acute hyperbilirubinemia on respiratory drive, as well as blunting of the responses to hypercapnia and hypoxia (39). These abnormalities of respiratory control may underlie the increased incidence of apnea in formerly jaundiced premature babies.

Further research is required to determine whether more stringent control of hyperbilirubinemia can decrease the incidence of apnea in such infants.

Nutritional Modification

L-CARNITINE

L-Carnitine is an important biological cofactor which plays a role in mitochondrial ß-oxidation of fatty acids and the production of adenosine triphosphate. Premature infants on total parenteral nutrition (TPN) are susceptible to L-carnitine deficiency due to insufficient in utero placental transport, immature biosynthesis and lack of exogenous L-carnitine. Carnitine deficiency results in decreased energy production at the muscular level. Despite initial reports of decrease in episodes of apnea and periodic breathing in infants with carnitine deficiency following treatment with oral carnitine, randomized, blinded, placebo-controlled trials have not demonstrated any reduction in apnea of prematurity following its administration. (40)

CREATINE

Supplementation of creatine, a substrate in the non-oxidative phosphorylation of ATP, has been proposed to potentially improve hypoxic ventilatory depression and muscle fatigue. Despite the theoretical benefit, a randomized controlled trial of oral creatine supplementation in premature babies did not demonstrate any beneficial effect on symptoms of apnea of prematurity (41). Larger-scale studies with a higher dose or duration may be needed to demonstrate an effect.

Doxapram

Doxapram is a respiratory stimulant, widely used in some countries for the treatment of methylxanthine-resistant apnea of prematurity. The use of doxapram is controversial, due to short- and long-term side-effects. A reduction of the frequency of apnea, bradycardia and hypoxemia has been demonstrated in premature infants with caffeine-resistant apnea of prematurity (42). Nevertheless, a systematic review of randomized controlled studies has identified only one small study, in which doxapram had a short-term, non-significant beneficial effect (43). Short-term adverse effects include sleeplessness, jitteriness, seizures, feeding intolerance and life-threatening cardiac conduction disorders. Even more concerning are findings of decreased cerebral flow velocity and decreased oxygen delivery, coupled with increased cerebral oxygen consumption in preterm infants receiving doxapram (44). These findings may explain a suggested association between mental developmental delay and prolonged doxapram therapy in very low birth weight infants (45). Careful evaluation of risk and benefit must be used in prescribing this drug.

Anti-Reflux Medication

Gastro-esophageal reflux (GER) has been implicated in causing apnea, but such an attribution should be made cautiously. Although early studies implied a relationship between apnea and GER, more recent studies have failed to support this relationship (46). Both apnea and GER commonly occur in this infant population. However, even when these events coincide, GER does not prolong the concurrent apnea (47). A criticism of these studies is the limitation of the pH probe in detecting non-acid-based reflux. However, new technology utilizing a combined impedance and pH probe for detection of both acid and non-acid GER have confirmed no overall relationship between GER and apnea (48). Although physiological experiments in animal models reveal that reflux of gastric content into the larynx induces reflex apnea, treatment of reflux has been shown to have no effect on the frequency of apnea in premature infants (49). Pharmacologic management of GER with agents that decrease gastric acidity or increase gut motility should be reserved for infants who exhibit signs of emesis or regurgitation of feedings, regardless of whether apnea is present. Future studies might focus on the identification of a possible subgroup of preterm infants in whom such a therapy might decrease apnea.

RESOLUTION AND OUTCOME

Although the use of heart rate, oxygen saturation, or apnea monitoring is almost universal in the hospital setting, there is great discrepancy in the recommendations for monitoring in the home regarding both need and duration. Since studies have failed to show a clear association between both apnea or home monitoring and the incidence of sudden infant death syndrome (SIDS) the American Academy of Pediatrics (AAP) has stated that prevention of SIDS is not an acceptable indication for home monitoring (17). Although the CHIME study (2) revealed an increased incidence of extreme cardiorespiratory events in preterm infants when compared with healthy term infants, there were no differences between infant groups after 43 weeks post-conceptional age. If home monitoring in preterm infants is pursued this would suggest discontinuation after 43 weeks post-conceptional age if there have been no documented events.

Studies performed during hospitalization have shown a link between both the number of days in which apnea occurred (50) and the persistence of such events beyond 35 weeks (51) with impairments in both mental and psychomotor developmental indices. Further evaluation of such events as recorded by home monitoring have shown a relationship between the incidence of five or more cardiorespiratory events and lower mental developmental index (MDI) scores when compared to preterm infants having no cardiorespiratory events (52). There is, therefore, some degree of uncertainty as to how aggressively to treat apnea of prematurity, given that there is no available information whether treatment improves neurodevelopmental outcome.

REFERENCES

1. Johnston BM, Gluckman PD. Lateral lesions affect central chemosensitivity in unanesthetized fetal lamb. J Appl Physiol 1989; 67:1113–1118.
2. Ramanathan R, Corwin M, Hunt CE, et al. Cardiorespiratory events recorded on home monitors: comparison of healthy infants with those at increased risk for SIDS. J Am Med Assoc 2001; 285:2199–2207.
3. Nock ML, Di Fiore JM, Arko MK, Martin RJ. Relationship of the ventilatory response to hypoxia with neonatal apnea in preterm infants. J Pediatr 2004; 144:291–295.
4. Gerhardt T, Bancalari E. Apnea of prematurity. Lung function and regulation of breathing. Pediatrics 1984; 74:58–62.
5. Abu-Shaweesh JM. Maturation of respiratory reflex responses in the fetus and neonate. Sem Neonatol 2004; 9:169–180.
6. Olsson A, Kayhan G, Lagercrantz H, et al. IL-1β depresses respiration and anoxic survival via a prostaglandin-dependent pathway in neonatal rats. Pediatr Res 2003; 54:326–331.
7. Martin RJ, Di Fiore JM, Jana L, et al. Persistence of the biphasic ventilatory response to hypoxia in preterm infants. J Pediatr 1998; 132:960–964.
8. Vento M, Asensi M, Sastre J, et al. Resuscitation with room air instead of 100% oxygen prevents oxidative stress in moderately asphyxiated term neonates. Pediatrics 2001; 107:642–647.
9. Gauda EB, McLemore GL, Tolosa J, et al. Maturation of peripheral arterial chemoreceptors in relation to neonatal apnoea. Sem Neonatol 2004; 9:181–194.
10. Bookatz GB, Mayer CA, Wilson CG, et al. Effect of supplemental oxygen on initiation of breathing after resuscitation of rat pups. Pediatr Res 2007; 61:698–702.
11. Gozal D, Reeves SR, Row BW, et al. Respiratory effects of gestational intermittent hypoxia in the developing rat. Am J Respir Crit Care Med 2003; 167:1540–1547.
12. Darnall RA, Kattwinkel J, Nattie C, et al. Margin of safety for discharge after apnea in preterm infants. Pediatrics 1997; 100:795–801.
13. Farre R, Montserrat JM, Rotger M, et al. Accuracy of thermistors and thermocouples as flow-measuring devices for detecting hypopnoeas. Eur Respir J 1998; 11:179–182.
14. Weese-Mayer DE, Corwin MJ, Peucker M, et al. Comparison of apnea identified by respiratory inductance plethysmography with that detected by end-tidal CO_2 or thermistor. Am J Respir Crit Care Med 2000; 162:471–480.
15. Bohnhorst B, Peter CS, Poets CF. Detection of hyperoxaemia in neonates: data from three new pulse oximeters. Arch Dis Child Fetal Neonatal Ed 2002; 87:F217–F219.
16. Bohnhorst B, Corinna SP, Poets CF. Pulse oximeters' reliability in detecting hypoxemia and bradycardia: Comparison between a conventional and two new generation oximeters. Crit Care Med 2000; 28:1565–1568.
17. Policy Statement. American Academy of Pediatrics: apnea, sudden infant death syndrome, and home monitoring. Pediatrics 2003; 111(4):914–917.
18. Perlman JM, Volpe JJ. Episodes of apnea and bradycardia in the preterm newborn: impact on cerebral circulation. Pediatrics 1985; 76:333–338.
19. Di Fiore JM, Zadell A, Walsh M, et al. Progressive increase in incidence of episodic desaturation in very low birth weight infants during the first month of life. Abstract, submitted to Pediatric Academic Societies Meeting, 2006.
20. Lemyre B, Davis PG, de Paoli AG. Nasal intermittent positive pressure ventilation (NIPPV) versus nasal continuous positive airway pressure (NCPAP) for apnea of prematurity. Cochrane Database Syst Rev 2002.
21. Robertson NJ, McCarthy LS, Hamilton PA, Moss AL. Nasal deformities resulting from flow driver continuous positive airway pressure. Arch Dis Child 1996; 75:F209–F212.
22. Walsh M, Engle W, Laptook A, et al. Oxygen delivery through nasal cannulae to preterm infants: can practice be improved? Pediatrics 2005; 116(4):857–861.
23. Sreenan C, Lemke RP, Hudson-Mason A, et al. High-flow nasal cannulae in the management of apnea of prematurity: a comparison with conventional nasal continuous positive airway pressure. Pediatrics 2001; 107:1081–1083.
24. Heimler R, Langlois J, Hodel DJ. Effect of positioning on the breathing pattern of preterm infants. Arch Dis Child 1992; 67(3):312–314.

25. Kurlak LO, Ruggins NR, Stephenson TJ. Effect of nursing position on incidence, type, and duration of clinically significant apnoea in preterm infants. Arch Dis Child Fetal Neonatal Ed 1994; 71:16–19.

26. Keene DJ, Wimmer JE Jr, Mathew OP. Does supine positioning increase apnea, bradycardia, and desaturation in preterm infants? J Perinatol 2000; 20(1):17–20.

27. Henderson-Smart DJ, Osborn DA. Kinesthetic stimulation for preventing apnea in preterm infants. [Systematic Review] Cochrane Database Syst Rev 2005.

28. Henderson-Smart DJ, Osborn DA. Kinesthetic stimulation for treating apnea in preterm infants. [Systematic Review] Cochrane Database Syst Rev 2005.

29. Conde-Agudelo A, Diaz-Rossello JL, Belizan JM. Kangaroo mother care to reduce morbidity and mortality in low birth weight infants. Cochrane Database Syst Rev 2005.

30. Anderson GC, Moore E, Hepworth J, Bergman N. Early skin-to-skin contact for mothers and their healthy newborn infants. Cochrane Database Syst Rev 2005.

31. Ludington-Hoe SM, Anderson GC, Swinth JY, et al. Randomized controlled trial of kangaroo care: cardiorespiratory and thermal effects on healthy preterm infants. Neonatal Netw 2004; 23(3):39–48.

32. Bohnhorst B, Gill D, Dördelmann M, et al. Bradycardia and desaturation during skin-to-skin care: no relationship to hyperthermia. J Pediatr 2004; 145:499–502.

33. Marlier L, Gaugler C, Messer J. Olfactory stimulation prevents apnea in premature newborns. Pediatrics 2005; 115(1):83–88.

34. Simakajornboon N, Beckerman RC, Mack C, et al. Effect of supplemental oxygen on sleep architecture and cardiorespiratory events in preterm infants. Pediatrics 2002; 110(5):884–888.

35. Al-Aif S, Alvaro R, Manfreda J, et al. Inhalation of low (0.5%-1.5%) CO_2 as a potential treatment for apnea of prematurity. Semin Perinatol 2001; 25(2):100–106.

36. Whyte R, Kirpalani H, Andersen C, et al. A randomized controlled trial of low vs. high hemoglobin thresholds for transfusion in extremely low-birth-weight infants. Pediatric Res 2004; 56(3):510.

37. Bell EF, Strauss RG, Widness JA, et al. Randomized trial of liberal versus restrictive guidelines for red blood cell transfusion in preterm infants. Pediatrics 2005; 115(6):1685–1691.

38. Amin SB, Charafeddine L, Guillet R. Transient bilirubin encephalopathy and apnea of prematurity in 28 to 32 weeks gestational age infants. J Perinatol 2005; 25(6):386–390.

39. Mesner O, Miller MJ, Iben SC, et al. Hyperbilirubinemia diminishes respiratory drive in a rat pup model. Abstract, submitted to the Pediatric Academic Societies' Meeting, 2006.

40. O'Donnell J, Finer NN, Rich W, et al. Role of L-carnitine in apnea of prematurity: a randomized, controlled trial. Pediatrics 2002; 109(4):622–626.

41. Bohnhorst B, Geuting T, Peter CS, et al. Randomized, controlled trial of oral creatine supplementation (not effective) for apnea of prematurity. Pediatrics 2004; 113(4):e303–307.

42. Poets CF, Darraj S, Bohnhorst B. Effect of doxapram on episodes of apnoea, bradycardia and hypoxaemia in preterm infants. Biol Neonate 1999; 76(4):207–213.

43. Henderson-Smart D, Steer P. Doxapram treatment for apnea in preterm infants. Cochrane Database Syst Rev 2004; 18(4):CD000074.

44. Dani C, Bertini G, Pezzati M, et al. Brain hemodynamic effects of doxapram in preterm infants. Biol Neonate 2005; 89(2):69–74.

45. Sreenan C, Etches PC, Demianczuk N, et al. Isolated mental developmental delay in very low birth weight infants: association with prolonged doxapram therapy for apnea. J Pediatr 2001; 139(6):832–837.

46. Molloy EJ, Di Fiore JM, Martin RJ. Does gastroesophageal reflux cause apnea in preterm infants? Biol Neonate 2005; 87(4):254–261.

47. Di Fiore JM, Arko M, Whitehouse M, et al. Apnea is not prolonged by acid gastroesophageal reflux in preterm infants. Pediatrics 2005; 116(5):1059–1063.

48. Peter CS, Sprodowski N, Bohnhorst B, et al. Gastroesophageal reflux and apnea of prematurity: no temporal relationship. Pediatrics 2002; 109:8–11.

49. Kimball AL, Carlton DP. Gastroesophageal reflux medications in the treatment of apnea in premature infants. J Pediatr 2001; 138:355–360.

50. Janvier A, Khairy M, Kokkotis A, et al. Apnea is associated with neurodevelopmental impairment in very low birth weight infants. J Perinatol 2004; 27:763–768.

51. Cheung PY, Barrington KJ, Finer NN, et al. Early childhood neurodevelopment in very low birth weight infants with predischarge apnea. Pediatr Pulmonol 1999; 27:14–20.

52. Hunt CE, Corwin MJ, Baird T, et al. Cardiorespiratory events detected by home memory monitoring and one-year neurodevelopmental outcome. J Pediatr 2004; 145:465–471.

Chapter 21

Strategies for Prevention of Apneic Episodes in Preterm Infants: Are Respiratory Stimulants Worth the Risk?

Dirk Bassler MD MSc • Barbara Schmidt MD MSc

An Introduction to Respiratory Stimulants

History of Respiratory Stimulant Use for Apnea of Prematurity

Current Use of Respiratory Stimulants in Preterm Infants

Possible Adverse Effects of Respiratory Stimulants on the Developing Brain

What is the Evidence?

Summary Points

AN INTRODUCTION TO RESPIRATORY STIMULANTS

Caffeine

Caffeine is an alkaloid that is naturally found in numerous plant varieties, such as coffee, tea, and cocoa. Coffee beans were chewed rather than infused in the highlands of Ethiopia. However, the most popular formulation of caffeine has been, and still is, as a beverage. Tea has been consumed for thousands of years in Asia. The Taoists and Zen Buddhists relied on the caffeine in tea for their meditations. Bodhidharma was a legendary Buddhist monk who founded the school of meditation that evolved into Zen Buddhism. One legend tells that Bodhidharma cut off his own eyelids in anger for having fallen asleep after nine continuous years of meditation. The eyelids fell to the ground and took root, transforming into tea bushes that would sustain meditations forever after (1).

In the 15th century, Sufis may have been the first to use caffeine expressly for its pharmacological effects. Sufism, a branch of Islam, requires of its followers that they perform the *dhikr* through continuous repetition of God's holy name or passages from the Koran. The Sufis of Yemen used coffee to stay awake during such extensive sessions of prayer and meditation (1). During the 16th century coffee houses spread throughout the Arabic world. However, their controversial reputation led to periodic prohibitions. Conservative muslims argued that the consumption of coffee, like the consumption of alcohol, was forbidden by the Koran because of coffee's stimulating effects. At one point Mecca's police chief banned the use of coffee. Soon after, the Sultan of Cairo, a coffee drinker himself, reversed the ban, agreeing with those who were fond of coffee because it helped them to keep alert and awake (1).

Around 1650 the first coffeehouses were opened across Europe. They served as information exchanges for writers, businessmen and scientists. They were also centers of political dissent. This is why Charles II of England declared coffeehouses to be "very evil and dangerous" in 1675.

In 1819, caffeine was isolated for the first time by the German chemist Friedrich Ferdinand Runge. This scientific achievement has been attributed to an encounter between Runge and Johann Wolfgang von Goethe, one of the world's great poets. Goethe was intrigued by the results of Runge's investigations into belladonna extract. The poet subsequently presented the chemist with a small box of rare Arabian mocha beans for a similar analysis. Within a few months, Runge had successfully isolated the world's first relatively pure caffeine sample (1).

Today, caffeine is thought to be the most widely used psychoactive drug (2). Maternal caffeine intake during pregnancy has been blamed as a risk for spontaneous abortions, although the evidence for a causal link remains inconclusive (3). Moderate consumption of caffeine is compatible with breast-feeding.

Aminophylline and Theophylline

Caffeine is one of a group of purine alkaloids called methylxanthines. This group also includes aminophylline, theophylline and theobromine (found in chocolate). All methylxanthines stimulate the central nervous system and the cardiac muscle, and promote diuresis. Methylxanthines have been used to treat asthma (4) and other obstructive lung diseases because they relax smooth muscle. Like caffeine, theophylline is naturally found in plants such as black tea and to a lesser extent in coffee and cocoa. The ability of theophylline to stimulate the respiratory system was first recognized in patients with Cheyne-Stokes respiration (5).

Doxapram

Doxapram was introduced as a new respiratory stimulant in the 1960s (6). It is not chemically related to the methylxanthines. Doxapram hydrochloride stimulates peripheral chemoreceptors and central respiratory centers in the medulla in a dose-dependent fashion (7). Higher doses of this analeptic drug progressively stimulate other parts of the brain as well as the spinal cord.

HISTORY OF RESPIRATORY STIMULANT USE FOR APNEA OF PREMATURITY

In 1973, Kuzemko and Paala published the first report of methylxanthine therapy for apnea in 10 preterm infants (8, 9). They used suppositories containing 5 mg of aminophylline to treat apneic attacks (8). North American investigators soon confirmed these observations, using either rectal aminophylline (10) or oral theophylline (11, 12). In 1975, Lucey concluded: "Out of a simple rediscovered observation may come a series of very important therapeutic advances." However, he also cautioned that the possible risks of therapy should be carefully balanced against the treatment gains (13).

In 1977, Aranda et al. reported the first use of caffeine for apnea of prematurity in the English biomedical literature (14). Dutch pediatricians are said to have used caffeine treatment for apneic spells as early as the 1950s (15).

Doxapram was first used to treat apnea of prematurity in the 1970s (16). Doxapram increases minute ventilation by increasing tidal volumes rather than respiratory rate (7, 17).

CURRENT USE OF RESPIRATORY STIMULANTS IN PRETERM INFANTS

"The Netherlands can be divided into two parts, above and below the Rhine River. Above the river the population is predominantly Protestant, drinking tea and coffee, below the river the population is predominantly Roman Catholic, drinking beer and alcohol. So above the river Rhine, pediatricians ... used small amounts of caffeine to treat apneic spells in premature babies. Below the Rhine, a drop of cognac is given after feeding to prevent apneic spells." (15)

Although it has not been reported what became of the Dutch practice of treating apnea of prematurity with alcohol, a number of recent drug surveys have shown that methylxanthines have become one of the most commonly used classes of drugs in neonatal medicine in Holland (18) and elsewhere (19–23). This is despite the fact that prescriptions of methylxanthines for apnea of prematurity are either unlicensed or off-label in most countries. Conroy et al. reviewed recent studies of unlicensed and off-label medicine use in neonatal intensive care units. A methylxanthine was the most commonly used drug in four of the five studies involving preterm infants (23).

Aminophylline and theophylline are used "off label" as respiratory stimulants for apnea of prematurity, since they are not licensed for this indication. Caffeine citrate is currently licensed only in the USA, and only for the "short-term treatment of apnea of prematurity in infants between 28 and < 33 weeks gestational age" (24). However, despite this narrow label, methylxanthines are frequently used in less mature infants and the duration of use is often prolonged (25). Data from the Neonatal Research Network of the National Institute of Child Health and Human Development in the USA showed that methylxanthines were still used at a postmenstrual age of 36 weeks in 44% of very low birth weight infants who met a stringent physiological definition of BPD, and in 21% of infants without BPD (26).

Doxapram seems to be very popular in France. A questionnaire-based practice survey was recently conducted to determine the use of doxapram in all 236 French neonatal special care and intensive care units. The response rate was 67% (27). Doxapram was used in 64% of the nurseries if methylxanthines failed to reduce the frequency of apneic spells. We have been unable to find data on recent doxapram use in other countries.

POSSIBLE ADVERSE EFFECTS OF RESPIRATORY STIMULANTS ON THE DEVELOPING BRAIN

Methylxanthines

Methylxanthines are non-specific inhibitors of two of the four known adenosine receptors (28). Adenosine is a purine nucleoside that is produced naturally in human tissues, including the brain. Adenosine is involved in the regulation of sleep and arousal, susceptibility to seizures and analgesia (28). Extracellular concentrations of adenosine rise in the brain when energy demand outstrips energy supply and brain cells are at risk of dying. Hypoxia and ischemia are among the situations that cause such an imbalance between ATP synthesis and ATP breakdown (28). Adenosine slows things down in order to preserve precious energy. Numerous animal experiments suggest that this is an important mechanism to protect the brain from permanent injury (28, 29).

Thurston et al. were the first to warn clinicians about the possible risks of methylxanthine therapy for apnea of prematurity. These investigators exposed weanling mice in pairs of littermates to an atmosphere of nitrogen. One member of each pair was pre-treated with aminophylline. Ten of the 16 untreated controls survived this anoxic insult, but all 16 methylxanthine-treated animals died (30). Very preterm infants frequently experience bradycardias and desaturations, both off (31, 32) and on the ventilator (33, 34). Is the blockade of adenosine receptors in the brain with methylxanthines detrimental during these episodes of hypoxia and ischemia? Only a sufficiently large randomized controlled trial with long-term follow-up will be able to answer this question conclusively.

Several small observational follow-up studies have failed to detect adverse effects of methylxanthines on growth or on cognitive, neurologic, and ophthalmologic development (15, 35–38). However, two reports from Australia have raised more concern. Kitchen et al. followed over 400 surviving very low birth weight infants who were born between 1977 and 1982 to the age of 2 years. These authors found that theophylline administration was significantly associated with an increased risk of cerebral palsy (39). Davis et al. reported the status at 14 years for 130 children from Kitchen et al.'s original inception cohort. Again, theophylline was significantly associated with an increased risk of cerebral palsy. However, children who had received theophylline achieved higher psychological test scores (40).

Doxapram

Like methylxanthines, doxapram has the potential to worsen ischemic brain injury. Following bilateral carotid artery occlusion in newborn rats, Uehara et al. observed that doxapram increased white matter damage in these experimental animals (41). A few observational studies in human infants also point to possible harm. Doxapram has been reported to reduce cerebral blood flow velocity in preterm infants (42) and to increase the cerebral consumption of oxygen (43). Sreenan et al. performed a case-control study to examine the variables associated with isolated mental delay in 80 infants with birth weights below 1250 g. Mental delay was defined as a mental developmental index < 70 (Bayley Scales of Infant Development II) at a corrected age of 18 months. Many different neonatal therapies and complications were included in the analyses. Only the degree of exposure to doxapram differed significantly between cases and controls. Cases had received greater cumulative doses and longer duration of treatment (44). Lando et al. provided further evidence to support the hypothesis that doxapram may have adverse effects on the developing brain. These authors administered the Revised Prescreening Developmental Questionnaire during a structured telephone interview to the parents of 88 extremely preterm children when their children had reached a corrected age of 9–15 months. Doxapram treatment was associated with some developmental delay (45).

A statistical association does not necessarily prove causation. The dose and duration of doxapram therapy may simply be a marker for infants who have cerebral dysfunction and especially pernicious apneic spells. A randomized controlled trial with long-term follow-up will be required to determine whether doxapram contributes to neonatal brain injury.

WHAT IS THE EVIDENCE?

Overview of Randomized Controlled Trials (RCTs)

Theophylline and aminophylline have been compared with placebo or no treatment for apnea of prematurity in eight randomized trials (Table 21-1). The largest of these studies was conducted in 1985 and enrolled 43 infants with a gestational age less than 37 weeks (46). In two additional trials, theophylline has been compared with non-pharmacologic interventions, continuous positive airway pressure

Table 21-1   **RCTs of Aminophylline/Theophylline vs. Placebo/No Treatment**

First author/ Year of publication	Patients	Intervention	Control	Outcomes	Notes
Gupta 1981 (65)	29 infants; GA 26–34 weeks; with apnea	Theophylline p.o. loading: none; maintenance: 4 mg/kg 6 hourly, increased to 6 mg/kg 6 hourly if no response	Placebo: same vehicle as for theophylline preparation	Reduction of apnea frequency; death before discharge	As per Cochrane Review on "Methylxanthine treatment for apnea in preterm infants" this study was terminated early
Greenough 1985 (66)	40 infants; GA < 34 weeks; on the ventilator for RDS	Theophylline p.o. loading: 5 mg/kg; maintenance: 1.25 mg/kg 6 hourly	Placebo: same vehicle as for theophylline preparation	Lung compliance; time to extubation; morbidities incl. IVH; pneumothorax	Primary outcome was lung compliance
Sims 1985 (46)	43 infants; GA < 37 weeks; with apnea	Theophylline i.v. loading: 6.8 mg/kg; maintenance: 1.4 mg/kg 8 hourly	No treatment	Reduction of apnea frequency; need for mechanical ventilation; death	
Viscardi 1985 (67)	26 infants; BW < 1250 g; on the ventilator	Theophylline i.v. or p.o. loading: 6 mg/kg; maintenance: 2 mg/kg 12 hourly	Placebo: normal saline	Failed extubation	
Durand 1987 (68)	42 infants; BW < 1250 g; on the ventilator	Aminophylline i.v. loading: 7 mg/kg; maintenance: 1.5 mg/kg 8 hourly	No treatment	Failed extubation; morbidities incl. BPD; NEC; ROP	
Peliowski 1990 (69)	20 infants; GA < 35 weeks; with apnea	Theophylline i.v. loading 8 mg/kg; maintenance: 0.5 mg/kg/h	Placebo: normal saline for loading; 5% glucose for maintenance	Reduction of apnea frequency; need for mechanical ventilation	In a third arm 11 infants were randomized to receive doxapram
Pearlman 1991 Unpublished	26 infants; BW < 2000 g; on the ventilator for RDS	Theophylline i.v. loading: 7 mg/kg; maintenance: 2.5 mg/kg 8 hourly	Placebo: type of solution not specified	Failed extubation; BPD; NEC	Data from this unpublished study are reported in the Cochrane Review on "Prophylactic methylxanthines for extubation in preterm infants"; in a third arm 19 infants were randomized to receive caffeine
Barrington 1993 (70)	20 infants; GA < 35 weeks; BW < 2500 g; on the ventilator	Aminophylline i.v. loading: 4 mg/kg; maintenance: 2.5 mg/kg 6 hourly × 3; then 1.5 mg/kg 6 hourly	Placebo: type of solution not specified	Airway pressure after occlusion; maximal inspiratory force; failed extubation; reduction of post-extubation apnea frequency	Primary outcome was airway pressure after occlusion

Abbreviations: BPD, bronchopulmonary dysplasia; BW, birth weight; CPAP, continuous positive airway pressure; GA, gestational age; i.m., intramuscular; i.v., intravenously; IVH, intraventricular hemorrhage; NEC, necrotizing enterocolitis; p.o., per os; PMA, postmenstrual age; PVL, periventricular leucomalacia; RDS, respiratory distress syndrome; ROP, retinopathy of prematurity.

Table 21-2	RCTs of Theophylline vs. Non-pharmacologic Interventions				
First author/ Year of publication	Patients	Intervention	Control	Outcomes	Notes
Jones 1982 (71)	32 infants; GA < 33 weeks; with apnea	Theophylline i.v. loading: 6.2 mg/kg; maintenance: 4.4 mg/kg/day	Mask CPAP: 2–5 cm water; CPAP level could be increased to 4–5 cmH$_2$O if no response	Reduction of apnea frequency; need for mechanical ventilation; death; NEC	As per Cochrane Review on "Continuous positive airway pressure versus theophylline for apnea in preterm infants," this study was terminated early
Saigal 1986 (72)	20 infants; BW 750– 1750 g; with apnea	Theophylline p.o. loading 6 mg/kg; maintenance: 2 mg/kg 12 hourly	Oscillating water bed 12–14 regular cycles/min	Reduction of apnea frequency; need for mechanical ventilation; sleep states; behavioral and developmental assessments at term, 3, 6 and 12 months corrected age	

For abbreviations see Table 21-1.

(CPAP) in one study, and an oscillating water bed in the other (Table 21-2). Caffeine is the best-studied methylxanthine. However, with the exception of the Caffeine for Apnea of Prematurity (CAP) trial, the number of study infants in each study has been small and the length of follow-up has been very short (Table 21-3). Doxapram has been investigated in 6 small trials, and compared with placebo or no treatment (Table 21-4), and with aminophylline or theophylline (Table 21-5).

Systematic Reviews from the Cochrane Collaboration

The Cochrane Collaboration is an international non-profit and independent organization. It consists mostly of health-care professionals who wish to produce up-to-date, accurate information about the effects of healthcare (47). This information is condensed in systematic reviews that are readily available worldwide through the Cochrane Library. The review groups are the heart of the Cochrane Collaboration (47). The neonatal group is one of the few review groups that deals with a certain population and age group, rather than with specific organ systems. The neonatal review group was registered in 1993, the year of the foundation of the international Cochrane Collaboration. The group is "dedicated to improving outcomes of newborn infants through the collection and synthesis of the highest quality evidence" that derives from randomized controlled trials (48).

The Cochrane neonatal review group has approached the evaluation of respiratory stimulants by conducting multiple narrow reviews, each focusing on a specific indication and treatment comparison. This "splitting" rather than "lumping" of the available evidence is also apparent in the numerous reviews that have been performed for other common neonatal treatments: examples include surfactant therapy and the use of postnatal corticosteroids (48).

Although it may be easier for the reviewer to focus on narrow questions the resulting systematic reviews may be of limited use to the clinician. Narrow reviews often include only a very small number of randomized controlled trials. Moreover, the number of trials that contribute to the pooled results for the individual

Table 21-3 RCTs of Caffeine vs. Placebo/No Treatment

First author/ Year of publication	Patients	Intervention	Control	Outcomes	Notes
Murat 1981 (73)	18 infants; PMA < 36 weeks; with apnea	Caffeine citrate i.m./p.o. loading: 20 mg/kg; maintenance: 5 mg/kg/day	No treatment	Reduction of apnea frequency	
Bucher 1988 (74)	50 infants; GA < 33 weeks; breathing spontaneously	Caffeine citrate i.v. loading: 20 mg/kg; maintenance: 10 mg/kg/day	Placebo: normal saline	Reduction of episodes of hypoxemia and bradycardia	
Levitt 1988 unpublished	54 infants; GA < 31 weeks	Caffeine citrate i.v./p.o? loading: 20 mg/kg; maintenance: 5 mg/kg/day	Placebo: normal saline	Reduction of apnea frequency; need for mechanical ventilation	Data from this unpublished study are reported in the Cochrane Review on ''Prophylactic methylxanthine for preventing apnea in preterm infants''
Welborn 1988 (75)	20 infants; GA < 38 weeks; PMA < 45 weeks; undergoing general anesthesia for inguinal hernia repair	Caffeine i.v. citrate or base? single dose: 5 mg/kg after induction of anesthesia	Placebo: normal saline	Reduction of post-operative apnea frequency	
LeBard 1989 (76)	26 preterm infants undergoing general anesthesia	Caffeine i.v. citrate or base? single dose: 10 mg/kg after induction of anesthesia	Placebo: normal saline	Reduction of post-operative apnea frequency	Study published only as abstract
Welborn 1989 (77)	32 infants; GA < 38 weeks; PMA < 45 weeks;	Caffeine i.v. citrate or base? single dose: 10 mg/kg after induction of anesthesia	Placebo: normal saline	Reduction of post-operative apnea frequency	

Table continued on following page

Table 21-3   RCTs of Caffeine vs. Placebo/No Treatment (Continued)

First author/ Year of publication	Patients	Intervention	Control	Outcomes	Notes
	undergoing general anesthesia for inguinal hernia repair				
Pearlman 1991 unpublished	26 infants; BW < 2000 g; on the ventilator for RDS	Caffeine i.v. citrate or base? loading: 10 mg/kg; maintenance: 2.5 mg/kg/day	Placebo: type of solution not specified	Failed extubation; BPD; NEC	Data from this unpublished study are reported in the Cochrane Review on "Prophylactic methylxanthines for extubation in preterm infants"; In a third arm 12 infants were randomized to receive theophylline
Muro 1992 (78)	18 infants; BW < 1750 g; on the ventilator for RDS	Caffeine citrate i.v./p.o. loading: 20 mg/kg; maintenance: 5 mg/kg/day	Placebo: normal saline	Time to extubation; pulmonary function	Study published only as abstract
Erenberg 2000 (79)	85 infants; PMA 28–32 weeks; with apnea	Caffeine citrate i.v./p.o. loading: 20 mg/kg; maintenance: 5 mg/kg/day	Placebo: citric acid/sodium citrate	Reduction of apnea frequency; Side-effects; NEC	
Schmidt 2006 (63)	2006 infants; BW 500–1250 g; candidate for methylxanthine during first 10 days of life	Caffeine citrate i.v./p.o. loading: 20 mg/kg; maintenance: 5–10 mg/kg/day	Placebo: normal saline	Death or neurosensory impairment; growth; morbidities incl. BPD; brain injury; NEC	Follow up to the corrected ages of 18-21 months and 5 years is in progress

For abbreviations see Table 21-1.

Table 21-4 RCTs of Doxapram vs. Placebo/No Treatment

First author/ Year of publication	Patients	Intervention	Control	Outcomes	Notes
Peliowski 1990 (69)	21 infants; GA < 35 weeks; with apnea	Doxapram i.v. loading: 3 mg/kg; maintenance: 1.5 mg/kg/h	Placebo: normal saline for loading; 5% glucose for maintenance	Reduction of apnea frequency; need for mechanical ventilation	In a third arm 10 infants were randomized to receive theophylline
Barrington 1998 (80)	56 infants; GA < 30 weeks; BW < 1251 g; on the ventilator	Doxapram i.v. loading: 3.5 mg/kg; maintenance: 1 mg/kg/h	Placebo: normal saline	Death before discharge; failed extubation; side-effects; home oxygen	
Huon 1998 (81)	29 infants; GA < 34 weeks; BW ≤ 1251 g; on the ventilator	Doxapram i.v. loading: none; maintenance: 0.5 mg/kg/h; dose could be doubled if no response	Placebo: normal saline	Death before discharge; failed extubation; side-effects; oxygen therapy at 28 days; apnea; IVH or PVL; infection; NEC; ROP	Following randomization, all infants were also treated with caffeine

For abbreviations see Table 21-1.

outcomes may be even smaller than the total number of studies that are included in the review (Tables 21-6 and 21-7). This often leads to imprecise and inconclusive estimates in meta-analyses. On the other hand, broad systematic reviews may produce heterogeneous results that are also of limited use for the clinician. To avoid unacceptable heterogeneity, reviewers should ensure that the study populations, interventions and outcomes in the eligible studies are reasonably similar. Clinical

Table 21-5 RCTs of Doxapram vs. Methylxanthines

First author/ Year of publication	Patients	Intervention	Control	Outcomes	Notes
Eyal 1985 (82)	16 infants; GA? Mean observed GA: 30 +/- 2.2 weeks; with apnea	Doxapram i.v. loading: none; maintenance: 2.5 mg/kg/h	Aminophylline i.v. loading: 6 mg/kg; maintenance: 1.5 mg/kg 8 hourly	100% reduction of apnea frequency; > 50% reduction of apnea frequency	
Peliowski 1990 (69)	21 infants; GA < 35 weeks; with apnea	Doxapram i.v. loading: 3 mg/kg; maintenance: 1.5 mg/kg/h	Theophylline i.v. loading: 8 mg/kg; maintenance: 0.5 mg/kg/h	Reduction of apnea frequency; need for mechanical ventilation	In a third arm 10 infants were randomized to receive placebo
Romeo 1991 (83)	19 infants; GA? mean observed GA 30 +/- 0.4 weeks; with apnea	Doxapram i.v. loading: none; maintenance: 1.5 mg/kg/h	Aminophylline i.v. loading: 5 mg/kg; maintenance: 2.5 mg/kg/day	100% reduction of apnea frequency; > 50% reduction of apnea frequency	

For abbreviations see Table 21-1.

Table 21-6   Ten Systematic Reviews from the Cochrane Collaboration of Respiratory Stimulants in Preterm Infants: Description of Included Trials

Ref. no. Patients	Intervention	Control	Total number of included studies	Median number of studies per outcome	Total number of included patients
(50) Preterm infants with recurrent apnea	Any methylxanthine	Placebo or no treatment	5	4.5	192
(51) Preterm infants treated for apnea of prematurity	Caffeine	Theophylline	3	2	66
(52) Preterm or low birth weight infants being weaned from IPPV	Prophylactic methylxanthines	Placebo or no treatment	6	4	197
(53) Preterm infants at risk for recurrent apnea, bradycardia, and hypoxic episodes	Prophylactic methylxanthines	Placebo or no treatment	2	1	104
(54) Preterm infants with recurrent apnea	Doxapram	Methylxanthine	3	2	56
(55) Preterm infants with recurrent clinical apnea	Kinesthetic stimulation	Methylxanthine	1	1	20
(56) Preterm or low birth weight infants being weaned from IPPV with planned extubation	Doxapram	Placebo or no treatment	2	1.5	85
(57) Preterm infants with clinical recurrent apnea/bradycardia	CPAP	Methylxanthine	1	1	32
(58) Preterm infants undergoing general anesthesia at term	Caffeine	Placebo	3	2.5	78
(59) Preterm infants with recurrent apnea	Doxapram	Placebo	1	1	21

judgment must be used and supplemented by statistical methods to test for heterogeneity (49).

As of January 2006, there were 209 completed neonatal systematic reviews (Cochrane Library issue 1/2006). The efficacy of respiratory stimulants in preterm infants has been the subject of the following 10 reviews (Tables 21-6 and 21-7).

1. Methylxanthine Treatment for Apnea in Preterm Infants (50)

This review includes five trials with a total of 192 infants.

The authors conclude: "Methylxanthines are effective in reducing the number of apneic attacks and the use of mechanical ventilation in the 2 to 7 days after starting treatment. In view of its lower toxicity, caffeine would be the preferred drug. The effects of methylxanthines on long-term outcome are not known and this should be addressed in any new trials."

2. Caffeine versus Theophylline for Apnea in Preterm Infants (51)

This review includes three trials with a total of 66 infants.

The authors conclude: "Caffeine appears to have similar short-term effects on apnea/bradycardia as does theophylline, although caffeine has certain therapeutic advantages over theophylline. The possibility that higher doses of caffeine might be

Table 21-7   **Ten Systematic Reviews from the Cochrane Collaboration of Respiratory Stimulants in Preterm Infants: Results**

Ref no. Outcome	No. of studies	Total no. of participants	Effect size RR WMD	95% Confidence interval
(50) Failed treatment after 2–7 days	5	192	0.43	0.31–0.60
Use of mechanical ventilation	5	192	0.34	0.12–0.97
Side-effects	4	149	4.69	0.24–89.88
Death before discharge	3	154	0.49	0.14–1.78
(51) Continuing apnea at 1–3 days	2	50	1.49	0.56–3.98
Continuing apnea at 5–7 days	1	20	1.5	0.32–7.14
Mean rate of apnea at 1–3 days	3	60	0.40	0.33–0.46
Mean rate of apnea at 5–7 days	2	36	0.01	−0.05–0.07
Side-effects	3	66	0.17	0.04–0.72
(52) Failed extubation	6	197	0.47	0.32–0.70
Side-effects	2	56	5.53	0.28–107.97
(53) Apnea (more than 4/day)	1	54	0.87	0.52–1.45
Apnea (more than 10/day)	1	54	0.86	0.49–1.50
Bradycardia (more than 12/day)	1	50	No estimate	
Bradycardia (more than 24/day)	1	50	1.18	0.84–1.64
Hypoxemic episodes (more than 12/day)	1	50	1.16	0.89–1.51
Withdrawal for definitive caffeine treatment	1	54	0.89	0.40–1.96
Use of IPPV	2	104	0.60	0.15–2.36
Tachycardia	2	104	4.00	0.48–33.51
Hyponatremia	1	54	1.71	0.80–3.68
(54) Failed treatment in the first 48 h	3	63	1.16	0.43–3.13
Failed treatment before 7 days	1	28	1.30	0.72–2.36
(55) Daily rate apnea/bradycardia/cyanosis and stimulation	1	20	3.36	−0.07–6.79
Daily rate apnea/bradycardia/cyanosis or stimulation	1	20	4.48	0.33–9.43
Death	1	20	2.24	0.26–22.80
Use of IPPV or CPAP	1	20	8.40	0.49–144.05
Neurological abnormality in survivors	1	17	4.13	0.19–88.71
Neurological abnormality in survivors or death	1	20	3.67	0.46–29.49
Bayley MDI at 6 months	1	17	6.00	−7.00–19.00
Bayley PDI at 6 months	1	17	15.00	3.10–26.90
Bayley MDI at 12 months	1	17	6.00	−5.90–17.90
Bayley PDI at 12 months	1	17	7.00	−5.17–19.17
(56) Failed extubation	1	29	0.80	0.22–2.97
Death before discharge	2	85	1.43	0.34–6.01
Days of IPPV	2	85	−0.36	−2.85–2.13
Side-effects causing cessation of therapy	2	85	3.21	0.53–19.43
Oxygen at 28 days	1	29	3.20	0.14–72.63
Oxygen at discharge in survivors	1	51	0.88	0.39–1.99
(57) Failed treatment	1	32	2.89	1.12–7.47
Use of IPPV	1	32	3.09	1.42–6.70
Death in the first year	1	32	2.57	0.97–6.82
Necrotizing enterocolitis	1	32	0.64	0.06–6.39
Major disabilities in survivors at 12–24 months	1	20	0.78	0.10–6.05
Death or major disability at 12–24 months	1	32	1.65	0.82–3.32
(58) Postoperative apnea/bradycardia	3	78	0.09	0.02–0.34
Postoperative oxygen desaturations	2	58	0.13	0.03–0.63
(59) Failed treatment in first 48 h	1	21	0.45	0.20–1.05
Use of IPPV in first 48 h	1	21	0.31	0.01–6.74

Abbreviations: CPAP, continuous positive airway pressure; IPPV, intermittent positive pressure ventilation; MDI, mental development index; PDI, psychomotor development index; RR, relative risk; WMD, weighted mean difference.

more effective in extremely preterm infants needs further evaluation in randomized clinical trials."

3. Prophylactic Methylxanthines for Extubation in Preterm Infants (52)

This review includes six trials with a total of 197 infants.

The authors conclude: "Methylxanthines increase the chances of successful extubation of preterm infants within 1 week. One trial suggests that this benefit is principally in infants of extremely low birth weight extubated in the first week. There is insufficient information to assess side-effects or longer-term effects on child development."

4. Prophylactic Methylxanthines for Prevention of Apnea in Preterm Infants (53)

This review includes two trials with a total of 104 infants.

The authors conclude: "The results of this review do not support the use of prophylactic caffeine for preterm infants at risk of apnea, bradycardia or hypoxemic episodes."

5. Doxapram versus Methylxanthine for Apnea in Preterm Infants (54)

This review includes three trials with a total of 56 infants.

The authors conclude: "Intravenous doxapram and intravenous methylxanthine appear to be similar in their short-term effects for treating apnea in preterm infants, although these trials are too small to exclude an important difference between the two treatments or to exclude the possibility of less common adverse effects. Longer-term outcome of infants treated in these trials has not been reported."

6. Kinesthetic Stimulation versus Theophylline for Apnea in Preterm Infants (55)

This review includes one trial with a total of 20 infants.

The authors conclude: "The results of this review should be treated with caution. Theophylline has been shown in one small study to be superior to kinesthetic stimulation at treating clinically important apnea of prematurity."

7. Prophylactic Doxapram for the Prevention of Morbidity and Mortality in Preterm Infants undergoing Endotracheal Extubation (56)

This review includes two trials with a total of 85 infants.

The authors conclude: "The evidence does not support the routine use of doxapram to assist endotracheal extubation in preterm infants who are eligible for methylxanthine and/or CPAP. The results should be interpreted with caution because the small number of infants studied does not allow reliable assessment of the benefits and harms of doxapram."

8. Continuous Positive Airway Pressure versus Theophylline for Apnea in Preterm Infants (57)

This review includes one trial with a total of 32 infants.

The authors conclude: "Theophylline is more effective than mask CPAP for preterm infants with apnea. Since CPAP is no longer administered by mask, the results of this review have limited importance for current clinical practice."

9. Prophylactic Caffeine to Prevent Postoperative Apnea following General Anesthesia in Preterm Infants (58)

This review includes three trials with a total of 78 infants.

The authors conclude: "Caffeine can be used to prevent postoperative apnea/bradycardia and episodes of oxygen desaturation in growing preterm infants if this is deemed clinically necessary. In view of the small numbers of infants studied in these trials and uncertainty concerning the clinical significance of the episodes, caution is warranted in applying these results to routine clinical practice."

10. Doxapram Treatment for Apnea in Preterm Infants (59)

This review includes one trial with a total of 21 infants.

The authors conclude: "Although intravenous Doxapram might reduce apnea within the first 48 hours of treatment, there are insufficient data to evaluate the precision of this result or to assess potential adverse effects. No long-term outcomes have been measured."

Comments

The decision by the Cochrane reviewers to produce separate reviews for the prophylactic and therapeutic use of respiratory stimulants is an example of the "splitting" approach to the topic. Although it makes sense in many medical conditions to distinguish between prophylaxis and treatment, it is questionable whether this holds true for apnea of prematurity. Apnea is very common in preterm babies and presents soon after birth. Henderson-Smart reported that the incidence of recurrent apnea at 30–31 weeks gestation was 54% (60). The first apnea was detected on day 1 or 2 of life in 77% of preterm infants (60). Barrington and Finer studied 20 healthy preterm infants <34 weeks gestation with continuous polygraphic recordings and found that – before 24 hours of age – all had apneic spells of greater than 15 s duration which were accompanied by hypoxia or bradycardia (61). The distinction between methylxanthine therapy for prophylaxis and for the treatment of apnea of prematurity seems to be unnecessary because of the early onset of the condition and the almost certainty of its occurrence. Lumping studies that assess the efficacy of prophylactic and therapeutic methylxanthines for apnea in very preterm infants together in a single systematic review may yield more clinically meaningful and statistically precise estimates of treatment efficacy.

The Caffeine for Apnea of Prematurity (CAP) Trial

The existing Cochrane reviews confirm that methylxanthines reduce the frequency of apnea and the need for mechanical ventilation during the first week of therapy. Beyond these two short-term outcomes, very little has been known about the effects of this common neonatal therapy. Inappropriately small numbers of study infants in past trials and the failure to measure clinically important outcomes are chiefly to blame for the long-standing uncertainty about the benefits and risks of respiratory stimulants for apnea of prematurity (Tables 21-6 and 21-7).

The Caffeine for Apnea of Prematurity (CAP) trial was launched to resolve this uncertainty (29, 62). This international, multicenter, placebo-controlled randomized trial of caffeine was designed to determine whether survival without neurodevelopmental disability at a corrected age of 18 months is improved if apnea of prematurity is managed without methylxanthines in infants at high risk of apneic attacks. The CAP study is a large, simple and pragmatic trial. Infants with birth weights 500–1250 g were enrolled during the first 10 days of life if their clinicians considered them to be candidates for methylxanthine therapy (63).

Two thousand and six infants were randomly assigned to receive either caffeine or placebo. Short-term outcomes before the first discharge home were recently published (63). Follow-up assessments at the corrected ages of 18 months (primary outcome) and at 5 years continue (64). To date, the CAP trial has shown that caffeine reduces the incidence of bronchopulmonary dysplasia: BPD rates (O_2 at 36 weeks) were 36% with caffeine and 47% with placebo; OR 0.63, 95% CI 0.52–0.76, $P < 0.001$. Caffeine also reduces weight gain for the first 3 weeks after the start of therapy. Head circumference is not affected. Importantly, the rates of death, ultrasonographic signs of brain injury and NEC were similar in the caffeine and placebo groups of the CAP trial (63).

SUMMARY POINTS

- Respiratory stimulants have been used routinely for the treatment of apnea of prematurity for the past 30 years.
- Respiratory stimulants reduce the frequency of apneic spells.
- Respiratory stimulants may have adverse effects on the developing brain.
- Published randomized controlled trials of respiratory stimulants have been small and focused on very short-term outcomes. The long-term efficacy and safety of respiratory stimulants remain uncertain.
- Of all the respiratory stimulants, doxapram has been studied the least. Its use should only be considered in selective infants with troublesome apnea who fail to respond to methylxanthines and nasal CPAP.
- The methylxanthines aminophylline, theophylline and caffeine have similar short-term effects on apnea. However, caffeine is the preferred drug because of its pharmacological properties: it has a wide therapeutic range and regular measurements of blood concentrations are not needed.
- The international Caffeine for Apnea of Prematurity (CAP) Trial has enrolled more than 2000 very low birth weight infants and will evaluate rigorously the short- and long-term benefits and risks of methylxanthines.
- To date, the CAP trial has shown that caffeine reduces the incidence of BPD.
- Caffeine also reduces weight gain for the first 3 weeks after the start of therapy.
- Follow-up of infants who participate in the CAP trial is under way to the corrected ages of 18 months and 5 years. Until these follow-up data become available, caffeine should continue to be used with caution.

REFERENCES

1. Weinberg BA, Bealer BK. The world of caffeine: the science and culture of the world's most popular drug. London: Routledge; 2002.
2. Fredholm BB. Astra Award Lecture. Adenosine, adenosine receptors and the actions of caffeine. Pharmacol Toxicol 1995; 76:93–101.
3. Signorello LB, McLaughlin JK. Maternal caffeine consumption and spontaneous abortion: a review of the epidemiologic evidence. Epidemiology 2004; 15:229–239.
4. Mitra A, Bassler D, Goodman K, et al. Intravenous aminophylline for acute severe asthma in children over two years receiving inhaled bronchodilators. Cochrane Database Syst Rev 2005; Ap. 18(2):CD001276.
5. Vogel A. Euphyllin. Wien Klin Wochenschr 1927; 40:105–108.
6. Wasserman AJ, Richardson DW. Human cardiopulmonary effects of doxapram, a respiratory stimulant. Clin Pharmacol Ther 1963; 4:321–325.
7. Bairam A, Faulon M, Monin P, et al. Doxapram for the initial treatment of idiopathic apnea of prematurity. Biol Neonate 1992; 61:209–213.
8. Kuzemko JA, Paala J. Apnoeic attacks in the newborn treated with aminophylline. Arch Dis Child 1973; 48:404–406.
9. Kuzemko JA. Use of methylxanthines in the management of apneic attacks in the newborn. NeoReviews 2003; 4:e62–4.
10. Bednarek FJ, Roloff DW. Treatment of apnea of prematurity with aminophylline. Pediatrics 1976; 58:335–339.
11. Shannon DC, Gotay F, Stein IM, et al. Prevention of apnea and bradycardia in low-birthweight infants. Pediatrics 1975; 55:589–594.
12. Uauy R, Shapiro DL, Smith B, et al. Treatment of severe apnea in prematures with orally administered theophylline. Pediatrics 1975; 55:595–598.
13. Lucey JF. The xanthine treatment of apnea of prematurity. Pediatrics 1975; 55:584–585.
14. Aranda JV, Gorman W, Bergsteinsson H, et al. Efficacy of caffeine in treatment of apnea in the low-birth-weight infant. J Pediatr 1977; 90:467–472.

15. Koppe JG, de Bruijne JI, de Boer P. Apneic spells and transcutaneous PO$_2$: treatment with caffeine, 19-year follow-up. Birth Defects Orig Artic Ser 1979; 15:437–445.

16. Burnard ED, Moore RG, Nichol H. A trial of doxapram in the recurrent apnea of prematurity. In: Stern L, Oh W, Fris-Hansen B, eds. Intensive care in the newborn I. New York: Masson Press; 1978: 143–148.

17. Barrington KJ, Finer NN, Peters KL, et al. Physiologic effects of doxapram in idiopathic apnea of prematurity. J Pediatr 1986; 108:124–129.

18. 't Jong GW, Vulto AG, de Hoog M, et al. A survey of the use of off-label and unlicensed drugs in a Dutch children's hospital. Pediatrics 2001; 108:1089–1093.

19. Conroy S, McIntyre J, Choonara I. Unlicensed and off label drug use in neonates. Arch Dis Child Fetal Neonatal Ed 1999; 80:F142–F145.

20. Avenel S, Bomkratz A, Dassieu G, et al. The incidence of prescriptions without marketing product license in a neonatal intensive care unit. Arch Pediatr 2000; 7:143–147.

21. Barr J, Brenner-Zada G, Heiman E, et al. Unlicensed and off-label medication use in a neonatal intensive care unit: a prospective study. Am J Perinatol 2002; 19:67–72.

22. O'Donnell CP, Stone RJ, Morley CJ. Unlicensed and off-label drug use in an Australian neonatal intensive care unit. Pediatrics 2002; 110:e52.

23. Conroy S, McIntyre J. The use of unlicensed and off-label medicines in the neonate. Semin Fetal Neonatal Med 2005; 10:115–122.

24. New drug application: CAFCIT (NDA) 020793. Washington, DC: Food and Drug Administration; 2000.

25. Eichenwald EC, Aina A, Stark AR. Apnea frequently persists beyond term gestation in infants delivered at 24 to 28 weeks. Pediatrics 1997; 100:354–359.

26. Walsh MC, Yao Q, Gettner P, et al. Impact of a physiologic definition on bronchopulmonary dysplasia rates. Pediatrics 2004; 114:1305–1311.

27. Benard M, Boutroy MJ, Glorieux I, et al. Determinants of doxapram utilization: a survey of practice in the French Neonatal and Intensive Care Units. Arch Pediatr 2005; 12:151–155.

28. Dunwiddie TV, Masino SA. The role and regulation of adenosine in the central nervous system. Annu Rev Neurosci 2001; 24:31–55.

29. Millar D, Schmidt B. Controversies surrounding xanthine therapy. Semin Neonatol 2004; 9:239–244.

30. Thurston JH, Hauhard RE, Dirgo JA. Aminophylline increases cerebral metabolic rate and decreases anoxic survival in young mice. Science 1978; 201:649–651.

31. Poets CF, Stebbens VA, Richard D, et al. Prolonged episodes of hypoxemia in preterm infants undetectable by cardiorespiratory monitors. Pediatrics 1995; 95:860–863.

32. Adams JA, Zabaleta IA, Sackner MA. Hypoxic events in spontaneously breathing premature infants: etiologic basis. Pediatr Res 1997; 42:463–471.

33. Bolivar JM, Gerhardt T, Gonzalez A, et al. Mechanisms for episodes of hypoxemia in preterm infants undergoing mechanical ventilation. J Pediatr 1995; 127:767–773.

34. Dimaguila MA, Di Fiore JM, Martin RJ, et al. Characteristics of hypoxemic episodes in very low birthweight infants on ventilatory support. J Pediatr 1997; 130:577–583.

35. Gunn TR, Metrakos K, Riley P, et al. Sequelae of caffeine treatment in preterm infants with apnea. J Pediatr 1979; 94:106–109.

36. Nelson RM, Resnick MB. Long-term outcome of premature infants treated with theophylline. Semin Perinatol 1981; 5:370–373.

37. Ment LR, Scott DT, Ehrenkranz RA, et al. Early childhood developmental follow-up of infants with GMH/IVH: effect of methylxanthine therapy. Am J Perinatol 1985; 2:223–227.

38. LeGuennec JC, Sitruk F, Breault C, et al. Somatic growth in infants receiving prolonged caffeine therapy. Acta Paediatr Scand 1990; 79:52–56.

39. Kitchen WH, Doyle LW, Ford GW, et al. Cerebral palsy in very low birthweight infants surviving to 2 years with modern perinatal intensive care. Am J Perinatol 1987; 4:29–35.

40. Davis PG, Doyle LW, Rickards AL, et al. Methylxanthines and sensorineural outcome at 14 years in children < 1501 g birthweight. J Paediatr Child Health 2000; 36:47–50.

41. Uehara H, Yoshioka H, Nagai H, et al. Doxapram accentuates white matter injury in neonatal rats following bilateral carotid artery occlusion. Neurosci Lett 2000; 281:191–194.

42. Roll C, Horsch S. Effect of doxapram on cerebral blood flow velocity in preterm infants. Neuropediatrics 2004; 35:126–129.

43. Dani C, Bertini G, Pezzati M, et al. Brain hemodynamic effects of doxapram in preterm infants. Biol Neonate 2006; 89:69–74.

44. Sreenan C, Etches PC, Demianczuk N, et al. Isolated mental developmental delay in very low birth weight infants: association with prolonged doxapram therapy for apnea. J Pediatr 2001; 139:832–837.

45. Lando A, Klamer A, Jonsbo F, et al. Doxapram and developmental delay at 12 months in children born extremely preterm. Acta Paediatr 2005; 94:1680–1681.

46. Sims ME, Yau G, Rambhatla S, et al. Limitations of theophylline in the treatment of apnea of prematurity. Am J Dis Child 1985; 139:567–570.

47. Chalmers I. The Cochrane collaboration: preparing, maintaining, and disseminating systematic reviews of the effects of health care. Ann N Y Acad Sci 1993; 703:156–163.

48. Davis PG. Cochrane reviews in neonatology: past, present and future. Semin Fetal Neonatal Med 2006; 11:111–116.

49. Sterne JA, Juni P, Schulz KF, et al. Statistical methods for assessing the influence of study characteristics on treatment effects in "meta-epidemiological" research. Stat Med 2002; 21:1513–1524.

50. Henderson-Smart DJ, Steer P. Methylxanthine treatment for apnea in preterm infants. Cochrane Database Syst Rev 2001; (3):CD000140.

51. Steer PA, Henderson-Smart DJ. Caffeine versus theophylline for apnea in preterm infants. Cochrane Database Syst Rev 2000; (2):CD000273.

52. Henderson-Smart DJ, Davis PG. Prophylactic methylxanthines for extubation in preterm infants. Cochrane Database Syst Rev 2003; (1):CD000139.

53. Henderson-Smart DJ, Steer PA. Prophylactic methylxanthine for preventing of apnea in preterm infants. Cochrane Database Syst Rev 2000; (2):CD000432.

54. Henderson-Smart DJ, Steer P. Doxapram versus methylxanthine for apnea in preterm infants. Cochrane Database Syst Rev 2000; (4):CD000075.

55. Osborn DA, Henderson-Smart DJ. Kinesthetic stimulation versus theophylline for apnea in preterm infants. Cochrane Database Syst Rev 2000; (2):CD000502.

56. Henderson-Smart DJ, Davis PG. Prophylactic doxapram for the prevention of morbidity and mortality in preterm infants undergoing endotracheal extubation. Cochrane Database Syst Rev 2000; (3):CD001966.

57. Henderson-Smart DJ, Subramaniam P, Davis PG. Continuous positive airway pressure versus theophylline for apnea in preterm infants. Cochrane Database Syst Rev 2001; (4):CD001072.

58. Henderson-Smart DJ, Steer P. Prophylactic caffeine to prevent postoperative apnea following general anesthesia in preterm infants. Cochrane Database Syst Rev 2001; (4):CD000048.

59. Henderson-Smart D, Steer P. Doxapram treatment for apnea in preterm infants. Cochrane Database Syst Rev 2004; (4):CD000074.

60. Henderson-Smart DJ. The effect of gestational age on the incidence and duration of recurrent apnoea in newborn babies. Aust Paediatr J 1981; 17:273–276.

61. Barrington K, Finer NN. The natural history of the appearance of apnea of prematurity. Pediatr Res 1991; 29:372–375.

62. Schmidt B. Methylxanthine therapy in premature infants: sound practice, disaster, or fruitless byway? J Pediatr 1999; 135:526–528.

63. Schmidt B, Roberts RS, Davis P, et al. Caffeine therapy for apnea of prematurity. N Engl J Med 2006; 354:2112–2121.

64. Schmidt B. Methylxanthine therapy for apnea of prematurity: evaluation of treatment benefits and risks at age 5 years in the international Caffeine for Apnea of Prematurity (CAP) trial. Biol Neonate 2005; 88:208–213.

65. Gupta JM, Mercer HP, Koo WW. Theophylline in treatment of apnoea of prematurity. Aust Paediatr J 1981; 17:290–291.

66. Greenough A, Elias-Jones A, Pool J, et al. The therapeutic actions of theophylline in preterm ventilated infants. Early Hum Dev 1985; 12:15–22.

67. Viscardi RM, Faix RG, Nicks JJ, et al. Efficacy of theophylline for prevention of post-extubation respiratory failure in very low birth weight infants. J Pediatr 1985; 107:469–472.

68. Durand DJ, Goodman A, Ray P, et al. Theophylline treatment in the extubation of infants weighing less than 1,250 grams: a controlled trial. Pediatrics 1987; 80:684–688.

69. Peliowski A, Finer NN. A blinded, randomized, placebo-controlled trial to compare theophylline and doxapram for the treatment of apnea of prematurity. J Pediatr 1990; 116:648–653.

70. Barrington KJ, Finer NN. A randomized, controlled trial of aminophylline in ventilatory weaning of premature infants. Crit Care Med 1993; 21:846–850.

71. Jones RA. Apnoea of immaturity. 1. A controlled trial of theophylline and face mask continuous positive airways pressure. Arch Dis Child 1982; 57:761–765.

72. Saigal S, Watts J, Campbell D. Randomized clinical trial of an oscillating air mattress in preterm infants: effect on apnea, growth, and development. J Pediatr 1986; 109:857–864.

73. Murat I, Moriette G, Blin MC, et al. The efficacy of caffeine in the treatment of recurrent idiopathic apnea in premature infants. J Pediatr 1981; 99:984–989.

74. Bucher HU, Duc G. Does caffeine prevent hypoxaemic episodes in premature infants? A randomized controlled trial. Eur J Pediatr 1988; 147:288–291.

75. Welborn LG, de Soto H, Hannallah RS, et al. The use of caffeine in the control of post-anesthetic apnea in former premature infants. Anesthesiology 1988; 68:796–798.

76. LeBard SE, Kurth CD, Spitzer AR, et al. Preventing postoperative apnea by neuromodulator antagonists. Anesthesiology 1989; 71:A1026.

77. Welborn LG, Hannallah RS, Fink R, et al. High-dose caffeine suppresses postoperative apnea in former preterm infants. Anesthesiology 1989; 71:347–349.

78. Muro M, Perez-Rodriguez J, Garcia MJ, et al. Efficacy of caffeine for weaning premature infants from mechanical ventilation. Effects on pulmonary function. J Perinat 1992; 20:315 Suppl.1.

79. Erenberg A, Leff RD, Hack DG, et al. Caffeine citrate for the treatment of apnea of prematurity: a double-blind placebo-controlled study. Pharmacotherapy 2000; 20:644–652.

80. Barrington KJ, Muttitt SC. Randomized, controlled, blinded trial of doxapram for extubation of the very low birthweight infant. Acta Paediatr 1998; 87:191–194.

81. Huon C, Rey E, Mussat P, et al. Low-dose doxapram for treatment of apnoea following early weaning in very low birthweight infants: a randomized, double-blind study. Acta Paediatr 1998; 87:1180–1184.

82. Eyal F, Alpan G, Sagi E, et al. Aminophylline versus doxapram in idiopathic apnea of prematurity: a double-blind controlled study. Pediatrics 1985; 75:709–713.

83. Romeo MG, Proto N, Tina LG, et al. A comparison of the efficacy of aminophylline and doxapram in preventing idiopathic apnea in preterm newborn infants. Pediatr Med Chir 1991; 13:77–81.

Index

Page numbers with boxes have suffix **b,** those with figures have suffix **f,** and those with tables have suffix **t**

A

AAP *see* American Academy of Pediatrics
ABCA3 *see* amino-acid polypeptide
A/C *see* assist/control ventilation
ACTA2 *see* alpha smooth muscle actin
acute respiratory distress syndrome (ARDS), 93, 94, 137
Ahdab-Barmada, M., 343, 344
Ahlstrom, H., 363
alpha smooth muscle actin (ACTA2), 11, 12
alveolar homeostasis in the newborn, 42–49 *see also*
    surfactant as basis for clinical treatment strategies
  clinical perspectives, 48, 49
  inherited disorders of surfactant homeostasis, 45–48
    disorder of lamellar body formation ABCA3, 48
    hereditary SP-B deficiency, 45–47
      mutations in *SFTPB,* 46
    heredity SP-C deficiency, 47, 48
      mutations in *SFTPC,* 47, 48
    views of lung histology, 46**f**
  lung maturation and surfactant homeostasis, 42–44
    components of the surfactant system in the
        alveolus, 43, 44
      view of surfactant homeostasis, 44**f**
    type II epitheal cells, 43
  surfactant proteins (SP), 44, 45
Aly, H., 88, 89
American Academy of Pediatrics (AAP), 216, 266, 267, 453,
    454, 458
amino-acid polypeptide (ABCA3), 48
angiogenesis, defined, 28, 29, 54
angiopoietins (ang), 58, 59
apnea of prematurity (AOP), 362, 403, 450
  adverse effects of stimulants, 463, 464
    doxapram, 464
    methylxanthines, 463, 464
  caffeine for apnea of prematurity trial, 473, 474
    shows that caffeine reduces the incidence of BPD,
      473, 474
  defined, 453, 454
  history of respiratory stimulants, 462
    current use, 463
  management, 454–458
  use of respiratory stimulants, 461–474
    aminophylline and theophylline, 462
    caffeine, 461, 462
      history of use, 461–462
    comments on the reviews, 473
    doxapram, 462
    overview of randomized controlled trials (RCT), 464–474
      aminophylline/theophylline vs placebo/no
        treatment, 465**t**
      caffeine vs placebo/no treatment, 467t–468t
      description of ten trials, 470**t**
      doxapram vs methylxanthines, 469**t**
      doxapram vs placebo/no treatment, 469**t**
      results of ten trials, 471**t**
      theophylline vs non-pharmacologic
        interventions, 466**t**
    reviews, 470–473
      caffeine vs theophylline for apnea, 470–472

apnea of prematurity (AOP) *(Continued)*
      continuous positive airway pressure vs theophylline
        for apnea, 472
      doxapram treatment for apnea, 473
      doxapram vs methylxanthine for apnea, 472
      kinesthetic stimulation vs theophylline for
        apnea, 472
      methylxanthine treatment for apnea, 470
      prophylactic caffeine to prevent apnea, 472, 473
      prophylactic doxapram for extubation, 472
      prophylactic methylxanthines for extubation, 472
      prophylactic methylxanthines for prevention of
        apnea, 472
apoptosis, 276
Aranda, J.V., 462
ARDS *see* acute respiratory distress syndrome
arginine therapy, 270, 271
assist/control ventilation (A/C), 395
atelectasis, 253
Australian National Health and Medical Council
    Fellowship, 373

B

Bajaj, N., 324, 325
Bancalari, E., 234
basic helix-loop-helix transcription factors (bHLH),
    25, 26
Bauer, A.R., 334
Bayley Scale of Infant Development (BSID), 355, 464
Bell, Alexander G., 392
Benefit of Oxygen Saturation Targetting (BOOST) trials of
    oxygenation, 349, 356
Beractant (surfactant), 94, 95
Bhatt, A,J., 66
bHLH *see* basic helix-loop-helix transcription factors
Blayney, M., 303, 304
BMP signalling factors, 11–12, 279, 280
Bohnhorst, B., 456
BOOST trials of oxygenation *see* Benefit of Oxygen
    Saturation Targetting
bosentan, 274, 275
Bradley, S., 350, 351
bradycardia, 454, 455
bronchopulmonary dysplasia (BPD), 187–203, 208–226 *see*
    also inflammation/infection in the fetal/newborn lung;
    injury in the developing lung; pathogenesis of neonatal
    lung disease
  changes in clinical presentation, 187–190
    proportion of infants breathing normally, 189**f**
    X-ray of infant with stage 4 BPD, 188**f**
    X-ray of mild BPD, 189**f**
  clinical definition, 234–237
    initially proposed by Bancalari, 234
    NIH consensus definition, 235, 236, 235**t**
    physiologic definition, 236, 237
      impact on diagnosis, 237**f**
      variation in impact, 237**f**
    table of BPD definitions, 236**t**
    table of outcomes associated with diagnosis of BPD, 234**t**
  defined, 51

bronchopulmonary dysplasia (BPD) *(Continued)*
  diagnosis, 208–211
  epidemiology, 195, 196
    incidence of BPD according to different diagnostic
      criteria, 196**t**
  lung injury, 210
  management, 221–226
    antibiotics for postnatal infection, 224, 225
    bronchodilators, 224
    diuretics, 223, 224
    immunization and monoclonal antibodies, 225
    late inhaled glcocorticoids, 223
    late systemic postnatal glucocorticoids, 222, 223, 222**t**
    mechanical ventilation harmful, 221
    mucolytics, 224
    other anti-inflammatory drugs, 224
    pentoxifylline, 225
    sildenafil, 225
  'new' BPD, 238
    oxygen patterns of neonates, 238**f**
  normal lung development, 209, 210
  oxidative stress and lung inflammation, 210, 211
  pathogenesis, 190–195
    blood transfusions, 194, 195
    early adrenal insufficiency, 194
    fluid administration, pulmonary edema, and PDA,
      192, 193
      perinatal and postnatal risk factors for BPD, 193**f**
      table of risk analysis, 194**t**
    immaturity of lung development, 190
    increased airway resistance, 193, 194
      genetic factors, 194
    inflammation and infection, 191, 192
      hyaline membrane disease, 191, 192
      postnatal infection, 192
    markers of BPD, 195
    nutritional deficencies, 193
  pathogenic possibilities, 191**f**
  pathology, 209
  postnatal intervention, 214–221
    antibiotic treatment, 218
    antioxidant therapy, 218, 219
    bronchodilators, 217
    caffeine, 217, 218
    cytokines and anticytokines, 220, 221
    early inhaled postnatal glucocorticoids, 216, 217
    early systemic postnatal glucocortoids, 215, 216
    inhaled nitric oxide, 219, 220
    inositol, 215, 215**t**
    other anti-flammatory agents, 217
    prostaglandin synthetase inhibitors, 217
    proteinase inhibitors, 219
    surfactant therapy, 214, 215, 214**t**
  predictors of BPD, 238, 239
    scores to predict risk of BPD, 239**t**
  prevention, 196–203, 211–221
    antenatal prevention, 197
      preventing antenatal oxidative stress, 197
      preventing preterm labor/acceleration of lung
        maturity, 197
    neonatal interventions, 197–203
      exogenous antioxidants, 199
        N-acetylcysteine (NAC), 199
      fluid restriction, 200
      inhaled nitric oxide, 199, 200
      inositol, 201
      mechanical ventilation, 197, 198
        'gentle ventilation,' 198
      oxygen therapy, 198
        supplemental therapeutic oxygen for prethreshold
          retinopathy of prematurity (STOP-ROP), 198

bronchopulmonary dysplasia (BPD) *(Continued)*
      surfactant therapy, 197
      vitamin A, 201, 202
    nutritional issues, 200–202
      general undernutrition, 200
      lipid nutrition, 200, 201
      polyunsaturated fatty acids (PUFA), 200, 201
    prenatal intervention, 211–214
      prevention of preterm birth, 211, 212
      prevention of respiratory distress syndrome, 213,
        214
        glucocorticoids, 213
        prenatal thyrotrophin-releasing hormone, 214
      table of interventions, 212**t**
    reduction of lung inflammation, 202, 203
      cortocosteroids, 202
      methylxanthines, 203
      proteinase inhibitor, 202
      recombinant human clara cell, 202, 203
Bry, K., 126–128
BSID *see* Bayley Scale of Infant Development

C

Caddell, J.L., 193
caffeine for apnea of prematurity trial, 473, 474
Calfactant (surfactant), 95, 96
Campbell, K., 356
Campbell, Kate, 334, 335
Canadian Oxygen Trials (COT), 356
CAP *see* congenital alveolar proteinosis
Cassin, S., 340
CDH *see* congenital diaphragmatic hernia
CDP *see* continuous distending pressure
CFTR *see* cystic fibrosis transmembrane regulator
Chang, C., 54, 219
Cheah, F.C., 122–124
Chernick, V., p0280
Chien, Y.H., 306
Choi, C.W., 122–124, 137
chorioamnionitis, 120–122, 128, 129, 134–138
Chow, L., 346–348
chronic lung disease (CLD), 154
chronic pneumonitis of infancy (CPI), 47
CINRGI *see* Clinical Inhaled Nitric Oxide Research Group
citrulline therapy, 271
Clara *see* nonciliated columnar cells
CLD *see* chronic lung disease
Clinical Inhaled Nitric Oxide Research Group (CINRGI),
  260
Coalson, J.J, 192
Cochrane Library, 330, 361, 470
Cochrane Review, 223, 322, 363–365
Cogo, P.E., 92, 93
Colfosceril Palmitate (synthetic surfactant), 94, 95
Collard, K.J., 114
Collins, P., 343, 344
Columbia University, 78, 124, 125, 257, 258
Comroe, Julius, 356
congenital alveolar proteinosis (CAP), 45
congenital diaphragmatic hernia (CDH), 281, 282
Conroy, S., 463
continuous distending pressure (CDP), 367
continuous positive airway pressure (CPAP), 78, 88–90,
  177, 178, 351, 352
corticosteroids, 202
COT *see* Canadian Oxygen Trials
CPAP *see* continuous positive airway pressure
CPI *see* chronic pneumonitis of infancy
Crosse, Mary, 334, 335
CRYO-ROP *see* multicenter trial of cryotherapy of
  prematurity

Cummings, J.J., 215, 216
Cunningham, C.K., 306
cysteine-rich secretory protein (LCCL), 17, 18
cystic fibrosis transmembrane regulator (CFTR), 143

D

Davidson, D., 263, 264
Davis, P.G., 464
Dawes, G.S., 340
DCA *see* dichloracetate
de Felice, C., 190
deMello, D.E., 55
Developmental Test of Visual-Motor Integration, 309
dichloracetate (DCA), 278, 279
Doppler echocardiography, 284
doxapram, 458, 462, 464
Doyle, L.W., 302–306
Drosophila, 10, 11, 15
ductus arteriosus, 339–341

E

ECM *see* extracellular matrix molecules
ECMO *see* extracorporeal membrane oxygenation
E.coli endotoxin, 131
Ehrenkranz, R.A., 236
ELBW *see* extremely low birthweight
endothelial monocyte activating peptide (EMAP), 61
endothelial progenitor cells (EPC), 51, 54, 63, 281
endothelins, 247, 248
Enhorning, Goran, 87, 88
EPC *see* endothelial progenitor cells
epitheal cells, 43
European Association of Perinatal Medicine, 216
extracellular matrix molecules (ECM), 3, 4, 54
extracorporeal membrane oxygenation (ECMO), 254,
    255, 258, 260
extremely low birthweight (ELBW), 300

F

Farel, A.M., 309
Fas (endogenous ligand), 167, 168
FBM *see* fetal breathing movements
FDA *see* Food and Drug Administration
Ferrara, N., 29
fetal breathing movements (FBM), 27, 28
FGF *see* fibroblast growth factor
FGFR *see* tyrosine kinase receptors
fibroblast growth factor (FGF), 4–7, 8, 13
FiO$_2$ *see* fraction of inspired oxygen
Fletcher, B.D., 234
fluid balance in neonatal lung disease, 142–158
    clearance of lung liquid at birth, 147–149
        epithelial sodium absorption in fetal lung, 148f
        Na,K-ATPase activity, 149
        role of epithelial Na channels, 149
    composition and dynamics of fetal lung liquid, 143–145
        concentration of K in fetal lung liquid, 145
        increase of liquid in the lung lumen, 145
        table of composition of lung luminal liquid,
            144t
    decrease of lung liquid before birth, 145, 146
        sections of lungs from lambs, 146f
    hormonal effects on fetal lung liquid, 146, 147
        epithelium becomes Na-absorbing membrane, 147
        inhibition of production, 147
    lung fluid balance during development, 152, 153
        schematic showing forces affecting liquid removal,
            153f
    pathways for removal of fetal lung liquid, 152
    postnatal clearance of fetal lung liquid, 149–151
        mechanisms of liquid removal, 150–151

fluid balance in neonatal lung disease *(Continued)*
        photographs of sections of rabbit lung, 150f
        stages of transepitheleal movement, 151
    pulmonary edema, 153–160
        factors delaying removal of fetal liquid, 153, 154
        features of neonatal respiratory distress
            syndromes (RDS), 154–160
                variables related to fluid balance, 156t
                vulnerability of immature lung to edema, 154t
        increased lung protein permeability, 155, 156, 157f,
            histological section of lungs, 158f, 159f
        strategies for reducing lung edema after premature
            birth, 160t
    secretion of fetal lung liquid, 142, 143
        diagram of fluid compartments of fetal lung, 143f
        drawing showing lung epithelium, 144f
        protein concentration of lung liquid, 142
        transport of Cl ions, 142–143
Food and Drug Administration (FDA), 260
FOX proteins, 22–24
fraction of inspired oxygen (FiO$_2$), 408, 409
fumagillin, 66

G

glucocorticoids, 213
Goldenberg, R.L., 121, 122
Google Scholar, 330
Gray, P.H., 308
Gregory, George, 363, 371, 392
GREM signalling factors, 12
Guthrie, S.O., 263
Gyllensten, L., 343, 344

H

Hall, R.T., 363
Hall, S.M., 55
Halvorsen, T., 301, 302
Hamilton, P.A., 372
Han, V.K., 32
Hannaford, K., 122–124
Harding, G.W., 26, 27
Haynes, R.L., 343, 344
Healy, A.M., 33
hedgehog family of morphogens (HH), 15
HFNC *see* high-flow nasal cannula
HFV *see* high-frequency ventilation
HH *see* hedgehog family of morphogens
HIF *see* hypoxia inducible factor
high-flow nasal cannula (HFNC), 351, 352, 370
high-frequency ventilation (HFV), 377–388
    classification of high-frequency ventilators, 382–383, 382t
        high frequency
            flow interruption, 383
            jet ventilation, 382, 383
            oscillatory ventilation, 383
            positive pressure ventilation, 382
    clinical applications, 383–388
        bronchopleural fistula/pneumothorax, 387
        bronchoscopy and airway and thoracic surgery, 388
        impaired cardiac function, 387, 388
        preterm infants with respiratory distress syndrome,
            383–387
            importance of ventilator settings, 387
            individual results for BPD, 386f
            overall results of trials, 384f
            plot of survival without BPD, 386f
            results of subgroup for BPD, 385f
            results of subgroup for intraventricular haemorrage, 385f
        pulmonary hypertension, 387
    CO$_2$ elimination, 379, 380
        correction of hypercapnia, 380f

high-frequency ventilation (HFV) *(Continued)*
gas exchange, 377–382
mechanisms, 378, 379
augmented diffusion, 378
convective screening, 364**f**, 378
direct alveolar ventilation, 378
entrainment, 378
non-uniformity of exchange, 378
pendelluft, 379
oxygenation during HFV, 380–382
correction of hypoxemia, 381**f**
mechanism of improved oxygenation, 381, 382
Hitti, J., 122–124
HMD *see* hyaline membrane disease
Hoeper, M., 275, 276
Holbert, D., 370
Horbar, J.D., 88
Hospital Virgen del Consuelo, Valencia, 323, 324
Howard, P.J., 334
HOX family of transcription factors, 24, 25
HRE *see* hypoxia response element
Hughes, C.A., 310
human surfactant protein C (SFTPC), 9, 10
hyaline membrane disease (HMD), 154, 191, 192
hypoxia, 252
hypoxia inducible factor (HIF), 30, 31
hypoxia response element (HRE), 30, 31

I

impact of perinatal lung injury in later life, 300, 311
neurological outcomes, 307–310
controversies, 307–310
neurosensory prolems in BPD survivors, 307, 308
specific effects of BPD on psychological
outcomes, 308–310
academic performance, 310
attention, 308
behavioural problems, 310
executive skills, 309, 310
general cognitive functioning, 308
language, 309
memory and learning, 309
visual-spatial perception, 309
summary of controversies, 310
effect of postnatal corticosteroids, 310, 311
methodological issues, 307
respiratory outcomes of BPD, 300–307
controversies, 301–307
change of respiratory function with age,
303, 304
data show no significant effect, 303
effect of smoking, 305, 306
respiratory function worse in smokers, 305, 306
other health issues, 306
BPD survivors require more hospital
readmissions, 306
pulmonary outcomes for oldest survivors
of BPD, 301–303
effect of low birthweight, 302
reductions in airflow, 303
table of respiratory function in early
adulthood, 302**t**
respiratory outcome change with use of surfactant,
304, 305
advent of 'new BPD,' 304
increase in ELBW infants survival rate, 304
no clear effect from surfactant, 305
table of respiratory function pre- and post-
surfactant in Australia, 305**t**
summary of controversies, 306, 307
methodological issues, 300, 301

IMV *see* intermittent mandatory ventilation
Infant Flow Driver, 369
inflammation/infection in the fetal/newborn lung, 119–138,
128, 129 *see also* fluid balance in neonatal lung disease;
injury in the developing lung; pathogenesis of neonatal
lung disease
antenatal corticosteroid treatments, 132–134
effects on fetal outcomes, 133**t**
maternal betamethasone effects on inflammation,
133**f**, 134**f**
chorioamnionitis, 120–122, 128, 129, 134–138
defined, 120
effect of lung maturation, 128, 129
inconsistency in variables, 124
increased risk of BPD, 137, 138
lymphocytes in bronchoalveolar lavage from preterm
lambs, 138**f**
occurrence of BPD not clearly related to
chorioamnionitis, 137, 138
injury to fetal lung, 134–136
adaption to chronic inflammation, 135, 136
effects of intra-amniotic endotoxin, 136**f**, 136**f**
hydrogen peroxide production by cord blood
monocytes, 135**f**
lung gas volume of fetal sheep, 134**f**
occurrence, 121, 122
outcomes with use of CPAP, 125**f**, 126**t**
overview of outcomes, 124**f**
relationship between diagnosis and age, 122**f**
table of PCR for ureaplasma, 121**t**
timeline for involvement of chorioamnionitis in
BPD, 126**f**
variation with severity of BPD, 125**f**
Venn diagram of diagnoses, 121**f**
clinical associations, 122–126
age with tracheal aspirate cultures, 123**t**
preterm premature rupture of membranes, 123**t**
fetal inflammation overview, 119, 120
fetal lung response to inflammation, 130, 131
inflammation mediated lung maturation, 131
blockage of endo-toxin induced lung
inflammation, 132**f**
link between fetal exposure and lung maturation,
126–128
cord plasma cortisol values following injection of
endotoxin, 128**f**
injection of endotoxin in fetal sheep, 127**f**
time course of lung injury in fetal sheep, 127**f**
mediators to induce fetal lung responses, 129, 130
toll-like receptors (TLR), 129
ureaplasma, 129, 130**t**
inhaled nitric oxide (iNO), 260–267
inhaled nitric oxide therapy for PPHN, 260–267
dosing recommendations, 262, 263
starting dose, 262, 263
timing of response and duration of therapy, 263
infants to be treated with iNO therapy, 260–262
age limitations, 260, 261
gestational, 260
postnatal, 261
congenital heart disease, 262
severity of hypoxemia, 261, 262
underlying pulmonary pathology, 262
overall safety profile of iNO, 266, 267
strategies for weaning iNO, 264–266
choice of oxygen or nitric oxide in weaning, 265
dose reduction strategies, 265
recommended strategy, 266
starting weaning, 264, 265
use of echocardiogram, 265
use of adjunctive therapies with iNO, 264

injury in the developing lung, 101–114 *see also*
  bronchopulmonary dysplasia; impact of perinatal lung
  injury in later life; inflammation/infection in the fetal/
  newborn lung
  antioxidants, 106–108
    albumin and sulfhydryl groups, 107
    catalase, 107, 108
    defined, 106
    glutathione, 107
    lung antioxidant levels in the preterm infant, 108
    superoxide dismutase (SOD), 107
    thioredoxins and peroxiredoxins, 108
    transferrin and ceruloplasmin, 107
    urates, 106
    vitamins, 106
  free radicals, 103–105
    arachidonic acid oxidation, 105
    cytochrome P-450 system, 105
    defined, 103
    mechanism of production, 104, 105
    mitochondrial respiratory chain, 104
    myeloperoxidase, 104, 105
    NADPH enzyme, 104
    physiological role of oxidative stress, 105
    table of all relevant species, 103t
    transition metals, 105
    xanthine oxidase, 105
  lung development, 101–103
    airway epithelial barrier, 102, 103
      protects against oxidative stress, 102, 103
    embryology, 101, 102
    five stages of development, 102
  mechanical ventilation induced lung injury (VILI),
    112, 113
    biotrauma, atelectotrauma, volutrauma, 112, 113
    cause of hypercoagulability, 113
  oxidant-antioxidant balance, 111
    blood transfusion, 111
    maternal role, 111
    possible interventions, 111
  oxidative stress injury
    defined, 109
    infection, 110
    lipid peroxidation, 108–111
    matrix metalloproteins, 109, 110
    neutrophils and macrophages, 110
    nitric oxide and peroxynitrite, 110, 111
  susceptibility of premature infant, 114
  susceptibility of the lung to oxidative damage, 101
iNO *see* inhaled nitric oxide
inositol, 201, 215
intermittent mandatory ventilation (IMV), 393
isoprostanes, 247
Ito, T., 12, 13
Ivy, D.D., 269, p1550

J
Jobe, A.H., 166, 167
John Hopkins University, 47

K
Karg, E., 319
Kendig, J.W., 87, 88
keratinocyte growth factor (KGF), 13, 195
Kinsella, J.P., 219, 220
Kinsey, V.E., 334, 335
Kitchen, W.H., 464
Klinger, G., 321
Kopelman, A.E., 370
Korhonen, P., 304
Kotecha, S., 26, 27, 192

Koumbourlis, A.C., 303, 304
Kuzemko, J.A., 462

L
Lando, A., 464
Lavoisier, Anton, 334
LCCL *see* cysteine-rich secretory protein
left-right determination factors (LEFTY), 26
leukotrienes, 246
Liljedahl, M., 192
Listeria monocytogenes, 119, 120
Locke, R.G., 351, 352, 370
Lu, M.M., 12
Lucey, J.F., 462
Lucinactant (synthetic surfactant), 94, 95
lung circulation, 51–68
  anatomy of postnatal pulmonary circulation,
    51–53
    bronchial circulation, 52
    lymphatic system, 52, 53
    pulmonary artery, 51, 52
  clinical implications of disruption of lung vascular
    development in BPD, 53–68
    abnormal vascular growth, 66–68
      effect of NO treatment, 67, 68
      effect of thalidomide and fumagillin, 66
      therapeutic potential for angiogenic growth factor
        modulation, 66–68
      use of anti-PECAM-1 antibody, 66
    pulmonary vascular disease in BPD, 64–66
      'new' BPD, 64
      pulmonary hypertension, 66
      schematic of the abnormalities of the pulmonary
        circulation, 65f
  regulation of vascular growth, 57–61
    epigenetic factors, 61
      hemodynamic forces, 62f, 62, 63
        endothelial progenitor cells (EPC), 63
        intrauterine pulmonary hypertension in fetal
          sheep, 62f
      O$_2$ tension, 61–61
    genetic factors, 57–61
      angiopoietins (ang), 58, 59
      endothelial monocyte activating peptide
        (EMAP), 61
      notch signaling, 60
      role of VEGF signaling, 58f
      VEGF critical regulator, 57
      views of disruption of angiogenesis, 59f
      Wnt proteins, 60
  vascular growth in developing lung, 53–57
    bronchial circulation, 56, 57
    embryonic period, 53, 54
    fetal period, 55, 56
      canalicular stage, 55
      pseudoglandular period, 55
      saccular stage, 55, 56
    five stages of growth, 53
    postnatal period, 56
      alveolarization stage, 56
      intussusceptive growth, 56
      microvascular maturation, 56
      sprouting angiogenesis, 56
    table of stages of vascular growth, 53t
    vascular morphogenesis, 54, 55
      angiogenesis, vasculogenesis and vascular
        fusion, 54–54
      vascular endothelial growth factor (VEGF), 55
  Wnt proteins, 60
lung development *see* molecular basis for lung
  development

M

magnesium sulfate, 259, 260
Manar, M.H., 194
Masimo Radical Oximeters, 355
mask pneumotachograph, 452
Maudlana Azad Medical College, New Delhi, 322, 323
Mazzella, M., 369, 370
McCormick, M.C., 306
MDK *see* midkine growth factor
mechanical ventilation developments, 393–412 *see also*
    high-frequency ventilation; non-invasive respiratory
    support; pulmonary function testing; respiratory
    control
  conventional mechanical ventilation, 393–403
    limitations, 393, 394
    patient-ventilator asynchrony, 393
  experimental modalities of neonatal mechanical
    ventilation, 404–412
    automated adjustment of inspired oxygen, 408–410
      adjustment of basal FiO2, 408–410
      clinical experience, 408–410
      regulation during hypoxemia, 410f
    dead-space reduction techniques, 407, 408
      continuous tracheal gas insufflation (CTGI), 407
      continuous washout of the flow sensor, 408
      intracheal ventilation, aspiration of dead space and
        distal bias flow, 407
    liquid ventilation, 410, 411
      clinical evidence, 411
      partial liquid ventilation (PLV), 411
      total liquid ventilation (TLV), 411
    neurally adjusted ventilatory assist (NAVA), 407
    proportional assist ventilation (PAV), 404, 405
      physiologic effects and clinical evidence, 404, 405
    targeted minute ventilation, 405, 406
      adaptive mechanical backup ventilation, 406
      apnea backup ventilation, 406
      graphical comparison with SIMV, 406f
      mandatory minute ventilation (MMV), 406
  future directions, 412
  new modalities, 394–403
    advantages/limitations of synchronised ventilation,
      396, 397
      avoidance of asynchrony, 396
      disadvantage in delayed triggering, 396
      physiological benefits, 396
    clinical and physiological differences between
      synchronised modalities, 398, 399
      combined use, 400f, 399
      differences between SIMV and A/C modalities,
        398, 399
    clinical evidence with synchronised ventilation, 397–399
      relative effect on respiratory outcome, 398f, 411
      trials showed no clear benefit, 397–397
    synchronised mechanical ventilation, 394, 395
      abdominal wall motion, 394
      air flow, 395
      airway pressure, 395
      esophageal pressure, 394, 395
      synchronised methods, 394, 395
      thoracic impedance, 395
    ventilatory modalities, 395, 396
      assist/control ventilation (A/C), 395
      pressure support ventilation (PSV), 396
      synchronised intermittent mandatory ventilation
        (SIMV), 395, 396
    volume targeted ventilation, 399–403
      physiologic and clinical evidence, 401–403
        possible beneficial effects, 401–403
      pressure-regulated volume-controlled (PRVC), 401
      volume-assured pressure support (VAPS), 400, 401

mechanical ventilation developments *(Continued)*
      volume-controlled (VC), 400
      volume guarantee (VG), 401
    noninvasive ventilation of the newborn, 403, 404
      clinical evidence, 403, 404
      dependent on maintenance of the airway, 404
mechanical ventilation-induced lung injury (VILI), 112, 113
mesenchymal stem cells (MSC), 281
methylxanthines, 203, 455
midkine growth factor (MDK), 31
Miller, L.A., 15
Moa, G., 369
Moens, C.B., 21
Moessinger, A.C., 26, 27
molecular basis for lung development, 4–34 *see also* injury
    in the developing lung; lung circulation; surfactant as
    basis for clinical treatment strategies
  developmental stages, 4–8
    early lung development, 4–7
      murine lung branching, 6f
    late lung development, 8
    mid lung development, 7, 8
    mouse and human pulmonary development, 6f
    table of stages of lung formation, 5t
  diagram of putative molecular interactions across the
    epithelial-mesenchymal border, 34f
  growth factors, 15
    early growth factors, 8–12
      BMP signalling factors, 11, 12
      FGF9, 10
      FGF10, 8–10
    late growth factors, 15
      FGFR, 15
    mid growth factors, 12–14
      FGF1, 12, 13
      FGF7, 13
      SMAD, 14
      TGFB, 13, 14
  importance of molecular oxygen, 3, 4
  lung asymmetry, 26
    view of left and right murine pulmonary
      isomerism, 27f
      left-right determination factors (LEFTY), 26
  morphogens, 15–18
    CRISPLD2, 17, 18
    SHH, 15, 17
  physical determinants, 26–28
    forces on the lung, 26, 27
      fetal breathing movement (FBM), 27, 28
      lung fluid, 26, 27
      peristaltic airway contractions, 27, 28
  receptors, 18, 19
    PTC receptor, 18
    retinoic acid (RA), 18, 19
  transcription factors, 19–26
    early transcription factors, 19–22
      GATA6, 21
      GLI family, 20, 21
      NMYC phenotype, 21
      TITF1, 21
    mid transcription factors, 22–26
      FOX proteins, 22–24
      helix-loop-helix (bHLH), 25, p0480
      HOX proteins, 24, 25
  vascular development, 28–33
    alternative theories, 28, 29
    angiogenesis, 28, 29
    hypoxia inducible factor (HIF), 30, 31
    hypoxia response element (HRE), 30, 31
    midkine growth factor (MDK), 31
    molecular mediators, 29–33

molecular basis for lung development (Continued)
   vascular endpthelial growth factor (VEGFA), 29
   nitric oxide synthase 3 (NOS3), 32
   proximal-distal vessel fusion, 28, 29
   vasculogenesis, 28, 29
monocrotaline, 277
Mortola, J.P., 321
MSC see mesenchymal stem cells
mucolytics, 224
multicenter trial of cryotherapy of prematurity
   (CRYO-ROP), 350
myeloperoxidase, 104, 105

N

N-acetylcysteine (NAC), 199
NADPH see nicotinamide adenosine dinucleotide phosphate
Na,K-ATPase (epithelial cell), 145, 147–149
nasal continuous positive airway pressure (NCPAP), 361
National Institute of Child Health and Human
   Development, 195, 463
National Institute of Health (NIH), 138, 213, 235, 236
National Library of Medicine, 330
NBW see normal birthweight
NCPAP see nasal continuous positive airway pressure
near-infrared spectroscopy (NIRS), 339
Neonatal Inhaled Nitric Oxide Study Group (NINOS), 260
'new' BPD, 166, 167, 175, 179, 208, 238
Newborn Lung Project, 234
NICHD Neonatal Research Network, 192, 193, 201, 202,
   220, 236, 307, 308
nicotinamide adenosine dinucleotide phosphate
   (NADPH), 104, 317
NIH see National Institute of Health
NINOS see Neonatal Inhaled Nitric Oxide Study Group
NIRS see near-infrared spectroscopy
nitric oxide, 248, 249, 260–267
nitric oxide synthase 3 (NOS3), 32
Nogawa, H., 12, 13
non-invasive respiratory support, 362–373
   complications of NCPAP, 372
   CPAP failure, 372
   high flow nasal cannulae, 370, 371
      technique needs further evaluation, 370
   invasive and non-invasive neonatal ventilation, 363
   nasal intermittent positive pressure ventilation
      (NIPPV), 365, 366
      comparison of NIPPV vs NCPAP, 365f, 366f
   NCPAP devices, 369f, 369, 370
      single or double prong NCPAP, 370f
   NCPAP for babies with RDS, 366–368
      continuous distending pressure (CDP) better than no
         CDP, 367f, 368f, 367
      CPAP in the 'surfactant era,' 368
      prophylactic CPAP or no assisted ventilation, 367f, 366
   NCPAP for post-extubation care, 363–365
      NCPAP for extubation, 364f, 364f
   physiological principles, 362–362
      apnea of prematurity, 362
      respiratory distress syndrome (RDS), 362
      role of nasal continuous positive airway pressure
         (NCPAP), 362
   use of supporting pressure, 371, 372
      analysis by pressure used, 371f
   weaning from NCPAP, 372, 373
      best method not certain, 372
nonciliated columnar cells (Clara), 4–8, 172, 202, 203
normal birthweight (NBW), 300, 301
Northway, W.H., 154, 187, 188, 190, 208, 225, 226, 233,
   234, 301, 302, 392, 393
NOS3 see nitric oxide synthase 3
notch signaling, 60

novel and experimental therapies for iNO, 267–275
   antioxidant therapy, 271–273
      mechanisms for ROS-mediated vasoconstriction, 272
      reactive oxygen species (ROS), 271, 272
      superoxide dismutase, 271, 272
   arginine therapy, 270, 271
      'arginine paradox,' 270
      inadequate clinical trials, 271
   citrulline therapy, 271
   COX-prostaglandin pathway, 273, 274
      prostacyclin analogues, 273, 274
         prostacyclin (PGI₂) mainstay of therapy, 273
      thromboxane synthase, 274
   endothelin pathway, 274, 275
      bosentan, 274, 275
      selective endothelin-A receptor antagonists, 275
   NO-cGMP pathway, 267–283
      alternative means of delivering nitric oxide, 268
      phosphodiesterase inhibitors, 268–270
      schematic of three biochemical pathways, 268f
Novogroder, M., 363

O

O'Brodovich, H., 234, 307
oxygenation in preterm infants, 334–356
   clinical outcomes of oxygen therapy, 349–351
      long term outcomes, 350–351
         multicenter trial of cryotherapy of prematurity, 350
      neonatal mortality, 349, 350
   controversies on oxygen therapy, 351–353
      continuous non-invasive monitoring, 352
         functional and fractional saturation, 353b
      continuous positive airway pressure (CPAP) or
         oxygen, 351, 352
      optimum oxygen saturation variation with age, 353
      'restrictive' or 'liberal' approach, 351
   critical threshold of fetal oxygenation, 338, 339
      fetal pulse oximetry, 338
      near-infrared spectroscopy (NIRS), 339
   historical perspectives, 334–336
      graphs of oxygen saturation, 336f
      incidence of ROP (1940-1990), 334f
      monitoring oxygen levels, 335, 336
      'randomized controlled trial' methodology, 336
      use of oxygen for newborn infants, 334
   multicenter randomized controlled trials, 355, 356
      double blind strategy, 355
   normal levels of oxygenation in newborns, 344, 345
   optimal levels of oxygenation in preterm infants, 345–349
      neonatal period, 345–348
         limits within which oxygen saturation varied, 348f
         meta-analysis of three trials of eye disease, 345f
         'restrictive oxygen approach,' 346
         survey of recent studies, 347t
         table of one year survivors, 348t
      post-neonatal period, 348, 349
         American STOP-ROP trial, 348, 349
         Australian BOOST trial, 349
   oxygen toxicity in preterm infants, 341–344
      oxygen and brain, 343, 344
         glutathione as antioxidant, 343, 344
         vulnerability to oxygen neurotoxicity, 342, 343
      oxygen and eye, 341–343
         pathogenesis of ROP, 342f
         retinal neovascularization, 342
         vascular endothelial growth factor (VEGF), 341
      oxygen and lung, 344
         experiment on lambs demonstrated oxygen
            toxicity, 344
         premature babies and oxidative stress, 344
   oxygenation during fetal to neonatal transition, 339–341

oxygenation in preterm infants *(Continued)*
    ductus arteriosus, 339–341
        physiology of premature infants, 339
        pulmonary vascular conductance, 340**f**
    physiological considerations, 336–338
        fetal oxygenation, 337, 338
        graph of age with P_{50}, 338**f**
        hemoglobin 50% figure (P_{50}), 337
        oxyhemoglobin dissociation curve, 337**f**, 336, 337
    resolving uncertainty, 353–355
        graph of oxygen saturation monitoring policy in
            UK, 354**f**
        'ideal' randomized control trial, 354, 355

P

Paala, J., 462
PAF *see* platelet activating factor
Palta, M., 234
PAP *see* pulmonary alveolar proteinosis
Parera, M.C., 54, 55
Parida, S.K., 259
pathogenesis of neonatal lung disease, 167–180 *see also*
        bronchopulmonary dysplasia
    adherence and cellular-endothelial interaction,
        168**f**, 168, 169
    alveolar capillary permeability, 174, 175
        schematic of inflammatory mediators, 175**f**
    chemotactic and chemokinetic factors, 169, 170
        graph of chemotactic activity, 170**f**
    deformability and chemotaxis, 169
    factors inducing pulmonary inflammation, 179**f**, 176–179
        chorioamnionitis, 176, 177
        hyperoxia, 178
        hypoxia, 179
        infection, 177
        mechanical ventilation, 177, 178
    neutrophils and macrophages in pulmonary
        tissue, 167, 168
        neutrophil the predominant cell in inflammation, 167
    'new' BPD, 166, 167, 175, 179
    oxidative damage, 173, 174
        phagocytosis changes cellular oxygen
            metabolsm, 173, 174
        preterm infants can be exposed to hyperoxia, 174
        role of toxic oxygen metabolites, 172, 173
        schematic showing elastolytic and oxidative damage to
            the alveolar capillary unit, 173**f**
    pro- and anti-inflammatory cytokines, 170–172
        Clara cell protein 10, 172
        postnatal factors induce pro-inflammatory
            cytokines, 171**f**
        synthesis of proinflammatory cytokines, 170, 171
        Toll-like receptors (TLR), 171
    proteolytic damage, 172, 173
        neutrophil granules as source of proteolytic
            enzymes, 172
    repair mechanisms and growth factors, 175, 176
Patz, Arnall, 334, 335
PAV *see* proportional assist ventilation
PCR *see* polymerase chain reaction
PDGF *see* platelet-derived growth factor
PEEP *see* positive end expiratory pressure
pentoxifylline, 225
Perni, S.C., 120, 121
persistent pulmonary hypertension of the newborn
        (PPHN), 241–285
    clinical management and therapeutic interventions,
        256–285
        combination therapies, 275, 276
        novel and experimental therapies for iNO (*see* novel
            and experimental therapies for iNO)

persistent pulmonary hypertension of the newborn
        (PPHN) *(Continued)*
    therapies for PPHN, 257–267
        evidence-based, 260–267
            inhaled nitric oxide (*see* inhaled nitric oxide
                therapy for PPHN)
            surfactant therapy, 267
        unproven, 257–260
            hyperventilation and alkaline infusion, 258, 259
            magnesium sulfate, 259, 260
            oxygen therapies, 257, 258
            sedation and paralysis, 259
            tolazoline, 259
    presentation and clinical management of PPHN, 254–256
        epidemiology of neonatal respiratory failure and
            PPHN, 254
        etiologies of PPHN, 255, 256
        presentation and diagnosis of PPHN, 254, 255
            extracorporeal membrane oxygenation
                (ECMO), 254, 255
    targeting vascular remodelling, 276–281
        bone morphogenic protein (BMP) signaling and the
            survivin gene, 279, 280
        dichloracetate (DCA), 278, 279
        endothelial progenitor cell (EPC) and stem cell
            therapy, 281
        hydroxy-methylglutaryl-coenzyme A, 280
            statins, 280
        inhibitors of serine elastase activity, 277
            monocrotaline, 277
        platelet-derived growth factor (PDGF) receptor
            antagonists, 279
        rho/rho associated kinase inhibitors, 280, 281
        voltage-gated potassium channels (K channels),
            277–279
            redox theory, 277, 278
    therapies for abnormalities associated with
        PPHN, 281–283
        bronchopulmonary dysplasia (BPD), 282, 283
            stimulation of lung growth needed, 282, 283
        congenital diapragmatic hernia (CDH), 281, 282
            pulmonary vascular changes, 281, 282
    transitional physiology, 241–254
        biochemical mediators of fetal pulmonary
            vasoconstriction, 246–248
            cyclooxygenase products of arachidonic acid
                metabolism, 246
            cytochrome P450 metabolites of arachidonic
                acid, 246, 247
            endothelins, 247, 248
            isoprostanes, 247
            leukotrienes, 246
            rho/rho kinese, 248
        biochemical mediators of fetal pulmonary vasodilation,
            248, 249
            cyclooxygenase-dependent vasodilators, 248
            nitric oxide, 248, 249
        determinants of fetal pulmonary vascular tone,
            244–246
            importance of physical laws, 244, 245
            role of oxygen, 246
        events critical to postnatal circulatory adaptation,
            244**b**, 243, 244
        factors involved in failed circulatory adaptation,
            252–254
            atelectasis, 253
            hypothermia and polycythemia, 252
            hypoxia, 252
            impact of postnatal age, 253, 254
            pH, 252
            pulmonary hypoplasia and structural changes, 253

persistent pulmonary hypertension of the newborn (PPHN) *(Continued)*
  factors involved in successful circulatory adaptation, 249–252
    biochemical events, 249–252
    mechanical events, 249
    fetal circulatory anatomy, 242**f,** 242, 243
  unmet challenge, 283–285
    development of appropriate therapies, 285
    Doppler echocardiography, 284
platelet activating factor (PAF), 193, 194
platelet-derived growth factor (PDGF), 279
PNEC *see* pulmonary neuroendocrine cell
Polin, R.A., 372
polymerase chain reaction (PCR), 120, 121
polyunsaturated fatty acids (PUFA), 200, 201
Poractant Alpha (surfactant), 94, 95
positive end expiratory pressure (PEEP), 178, 427–429
Post, M., 20, 21
Poulsen, J.P., 319
PPHN *see* persistent pulmonary hypertension of the newborn
Priestley, Joseph, 317, 334
proportional assist ventilation (PAV), 404, 405
prostacyclin (PGI$_2$), 273, 274
PUFA *see* polyunsaturated fatty acids
pulmonary alveolar proteinosis (PAP), 43
pulmonary function testing, 420–442 *see also* mechanical ventilation developments
  measurement of pulmonary mechanics, 420–423
    intrapatient variability of measurements, 421, 422
    lack of correlation between compliance measurement and gas exchange, 422, 423
    lack of normal reference values, 422
    limitations of pulmonary function measurements, 423
    methodological problems, 420, 421
  ventilator graphics in neonatal ventilation, 423–442
    asynchrony between infant and ventilator, 439–441
      asynchrony during IMV, synchrony during SIMV, 439**f**
      automatic termination of inspiration, 440**f**
      poor synchrony during A/C, 440**f**
      variability of inspiratory duration, 441**f**
    automatic termination of inspiration, 433
      effect on duration of inspiration, 433**f**
    changes in compliance, 427
      graphs showing improvement in compliance, 427**f**
    circuit flow, 429–431
    clinical relevance of pulmonary function data, 441, 442
      uses for ventilator graphics, 441, 442
    duration of expiration and gas trapping, 434–436
      effect of shortened expiratory duration, 435**f**
    duration of inspiration, 431, 432
      importance of a proper duration of inspiration, 432
      influence of inspiratory time on waveforms of pressure, 431**f**
    effect of pressure on tidal volume, 425
      graph of airway pressure, 424**f**
      pressure and volume for breath, 425**f**
    effects of PEEP, 428**f,** 429**f,** 429, 427–429
      P/V loops, 430**f**
    future implications, 442
    graphic display of flow, volume and pressure, 423–441
      normal trace of flow, 424**f**
    increased pulmonary resistance, 433, 434
      effect of high airway resistance on flow, 434**f**
      P/V loops with resistance, 435**f**
    leaks around the endotracheal tube, 436–439
      effect of inspiratory leak on flow, 436**f**
      effect of leak on automatic termination, 437**f**

pulmonary function testing *(Continued)*
      leak during expiratory phase, 438**f,** 438**f**
    pulmonary overdistention, 426, 427
      change in airway pressure, 426**f**
      pressure and volume for breath, 426**f**
      shown by loops of previous breaths, 421
pulmonary neuroendocrine cell (PNEC), 4–7
pulse oximetry, 452, 453

R
RA *see* retinoic acid
Ramji, S., 322, 323
Ramsey, P.S., 122–124
randomized controlled trials (RCT), 464–474
Rasanen, J., 340, 341
RCT *see* randomized controlled trials
RDS *see* respiratory distress syndrome
reactive oxygen species, 271, 272
respiratory control, 449–459 *see also* apnea of prematurity
  diagnostic dilemmas, 452, 454
    definition of events, 453, 454
    heart rate, 453
    oxygen saturation, 452, 453
      pulse oximetry, 452, 453
    respiratory monitoring, 452
      mask pneumotachograph, 452
      respiratory inductance plethysmography (RIP), 452
  management options of apnea of prematurity (AOP), 454–458
    table of therapeutic interventions, 454**t**
    therapeutic interventions requiring further study, 456–458
      anti-reflux medication, 458
        gastro-esophageal reflux (GER), 458
      blood transfusion, 457
      body positioning, 456
      carbon dioxide supplementation, 457
      control of hyperbilirubinemia, 457
      doxapram, 458
      nutritional modification, 457, 458
        creatine, 457, 458
        l-carnitine, 457
      oxygen supplementation, 456
      sensory stimulation, 456
        skin-to-skin contact (SSC), 456
    therapeutic interventions with proven benefit, 455–455
      methylxanthines, 455
      positive airway pressure, 455
        benefits and problems, 455
  physiologic considerations, 449–452
    fetal breathing movements, 449, 450
      importance of muscle activity, 449, 450
    postnatal respiratory patterns, 450
      apnea of prematurity, 450
    ventilatory responses to hypercapnia, 450
      decreased response to CO$_2$, 450
    ventilatory responses to hypoxia, 450–452
      apneic episodes, 451, 452
      inhibition at the ventral medulla, 451**f**
  resolution, 458, 459
respiratory distress syndrome (RDS), 30, 31, 42, 43, 45, 76–79, 154, 362
respiratory inductance plethysmography (RIP), 452
resuscitation of newborn infants, 317–330 *see also* oxygenation in preterm infants
  basic science, 317–320
    free radicals, 317, 318
      view of free oxygen radical formation, 320**f**
    hyperoxic states, 318, 319
    human data, 320–325

resuscitation of newborn infants *(Continued)*
  clinical trials exploring resuscitation, 321**b**
  concern about hyperoxia, 321
  multicenter study by Saugstad, 323
  randomized trial by Bajaj, 324, 325
  retrolental fibroplasia damage to newborn, 320, 321
  room air vs oxygen for resuscitation, 322**f**
  study by Ramji, 322, 323
  Vento trials, 323, 324, 324
  potential clinical impact, 327, 328
  table of limited neurodevelopmental outcome
      data, 328**t**
  use of information, 326, 327
  caution needed, 327
  validity of trial data, 325, 326
  way forward, 328, 329
  consider which is the best comparison to
      explore, 328, 329
  practice statements published recently, 330**b**
retinoic acid (RA), 18, 19
retinopathy of prematurity (ROP), 67, 334, 335, 349, 350
retrolental fibroplasia *see* retinopathy of
  prematurity (ROP)
Revised Prescreening Developmental Questionnaire, 464
rho/rho kinese, 248, 280, 281
Rhodes, P.G., 363
RIP *see* respiratory inductance plethysmography
Robertson, Bengt, 87, 88
Robertson, N.J., 372, 372
ROP *see* retinopathy of prematurity
ROS *see* reactive oxygen species
Royal Women's Hospital, Melbourne, 300, 302, 303,
  305, 306
Runge, Friedrich Ferdinand, 462
Rutter, M., 20, 21

S
Saigal, S., 307
Sakai, M., 281, 282
saturated phosphatidylcholine (Sat PC), 92, 93
Saugstad, O.D., 323, 327
Schachtner, S.K., 28, 29
Scheele, Karl, 334
Schmidt, B., 350
Schulze, A., 340, 341
Schwarz, M., 33, 61
SFTPC *see* human surfactant protein C
Shennan, A.T., 234
SHH *see* sonic hedgehog
SIDS *see* sudden infant death syndrome
sildenafil, 225, 269, 269
Silverman, William A., 333
Silvers, K.M., 194, 195
SIMV *see* synchronised intermittent mandatory ventilation
Sjöstrand, U., 382
Smith, J., 19, 20
Solas, A.B., 319
sonic hedgehog (SHH), 4–7, 20, 21
SP *see* surfactant proteins
Speer, C.P., 120, 190, 191
Spry gene, 10, 11
Sreenan, C., 351, 352, 370, 464
Steel, J.H., 120, 121
Stevenson, D.K., 259
STOP-ROP *see* supplemental therapeutic oxygen for
  prethreshold retinopathy of prematurity
Strang, L.B., 142, 333
Subhedar, N.V., 219, 220
sudden infant death syndrome (SIDS), 458
Sun, J., 346–348
Supp, D.M., 26

supplemental therapeutic oxygen for prethreshold
  retinopathy of prematurity (STOP-ROP), 198, 221,
  222, 348, 349
surfactant as basis for clinical treatment strategies, 73–96
  see also alveolar homeostasis in the newborn; lung
      circulation; molecular basis for lung development
  bronchopulmonary dysplasia, 91–93
  increase in surfactant in lungs of baboons, 94**f**
  surfactant proteins increase with age after preterm
      birth, 92**f**
  table of metabolic variables for sat PC, 93**t**
  table of surface tension of airway samples, 93**t**
  controversy about RDS, 76–79
  changes in diagnosis of RDS, 78
  clinical outcomes of CPAP therapy, 78**f**
  pathophysiology of RDS, 77**f**
  surfactant function in infants with RDS, 79–91**f**
  surfactant required for use of CPAP, 79**f**
  use of continuous positive airway pressure
      (CPAP), 78, 79
  factors that influence surfactant in the preterm
      lung, 79–91
  antenatal corticosteroid effects on surfactant, 82–84
      dose-response curves, 84**f**
      graph of effects of treatment, 83**f**
      table of outcome of preterm infants, 84**t**
  factors that modify surfactant function, 80**t**
  inactivation of surfactant, 79, 80
  number of doses of surfactant, 90
      second dose not usually needed, 90
  surfactant activation, 80–82
      improvement of surfactant function, 82**f**
      phased response to surfactant treatment, 82**f**
      relationship between PO_2 and surface tension, 81**f**
  surfactant distribution with treatment, 84–87
      aeration of preterm lungs, 85**f**
      how surfactant treatment should be given, 87
      importance of treatment technique, 85–87
      maldistribution of ventilation, 87
      plots of different surfactant distributions, 86**f**
      table of variables for distribution of surfactant, 85**t**
  table of mechanisms of inactivation, 80**t**
  use of surfactant for other problems, 90, 91
  when surfactant should be given, 87–90
      characteristics of infants at delivery, 90**f**
      outcomes for infants with low birth weight, 89**t**
      table of outcomes of quality improvement
          initiative, 89**t**
      timing of early treatment of infants at risk, 88
  meconium aspiration syndrome, 91
      experimental 'lung lavage,' 91
      surfactant inhibited by meconium, 91
  sepsis/pneumonia syndromes, 93, 94
  surfactant composition and metabolism, 74–76
      catabolism and clearance of surfactant, 76
      composition, 74
      pathways for surfactant metabolism, 75**f**
      timing of surfactant phospholipid labeling, 76**f**, 75, 76
  surfactant during normal fetal lung development, 73, 74
      graph of lung maturity using amniotic fluid, 74**f**
  treatment of lung injuries, 94–96
      comparison of surfactants, 95**t**
surfactant proteins (SP), 44, 45
synchronised intermittent mandatory ventilation
  (SIMV), 395, 396

T
Tadalafil, 270
targeting vascular remodelling, 276–281
Taylor, H.G., 309, 309, 310
Temesvari, P., 319

TGFB *see* transforming growth factor B
thalidomide, 66
Thebaud, H., 281, 282
thromboxane synthase, 274
Thurston, G., 463, 464
Tin, W., 346, 350
TLR *see* toll-like receptors
TNT *see* transient tachypnea
tolazoline, 259
toll-like receptors (TLR), 129, 171
Tooley, WH, 234
transforming growth factor B (TGFB), 11
transient tachypnea (TNT), 153
Turing, Allan, 15
tyrosine kinase receptors (FGFR), 8–10, 15

U

Uehara, H., 464
University of Miami/Jackson Memorial Medical Center, 196
ureaplasma urealyticum, 120–124, 129, 134, 192
Usher, R., 345, 346

V

Van Marter, L.J., 122–124
Van Meurs, K.P., 220
Van Tuyl, M., 29, 30, 33

vascular endothelial growth factor (VEGF), 29, 55, 58, 195, 341
vasculogenesis, defined, 54
VEGF *see* vascular endothelial growth factor
Venn diagram of diagnoses, 121f
Vento, M., 323, 324, 324
Vermont-Oxford Network, 88, 89, 346–348
very low birth weight (VLBW), 122–124, 134, 300, 310
VILI *see* mechanical ventilation-induced lung injury
VLBW *see* very low birth weight

W

Walsh, W.F., 236, 351, 352
Watterberg, K.L., 122–124, 194
Weaver, M., 11, 12
websites
    hopkinsmedicine.org, 47
    nichd.nih.gov/cochrane/default.cfm, 361
Whyte, R.K., 349, 350
Wilson-Mickity syndrome, 134, 238
Wung, Jen, 257–259

X

xanthine oxidase, 105

Z

Zhou, L., 23, 24